CHRONIC HEADACHES: BIOLOGY, PSYCHOLOGY, AND BEHAVIORAL TREATMENT

CHRONIC HEADACHES:
BIOLOGY, PSYCHOLOGY,
AND BEHAVIORAL TREATMENT

Jonathan M. Borkum

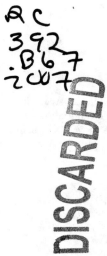 LAWRENCE ERLBAUM ASSOCIATES, PUBLISHERS
2007   Mahwah, New Jersey   London

Senior Acquisitions Editor: Debra Riegert
Editorial Assistant: Rebecca Larsen
Cover Design: Tomai Maridou
Full-Service Compositor: MidAtlantic Books and Journals, Inc.

This book was typeset in 10/12 pt. Times, Italic, Bold, and Bold Italic, with Gill Sans.

Lawrence Erlbaum Associates, Inc., Publishers
10 Industrial Avenue
Mahwah, New Jersey 07430
www.erlbaum.com

CIP information for this volume can be obtained from the Library of Congress.

Library of Congress Cataloging-in-Publication Data

ISBN 978-0-8058-4973-8 — 0-8058-4973-4 (case)
ISBN 978-0-8058-6199-0 — 0-8058-6199-8 (paper)
ISBN 978-1-4106-1583-1 — 1-4106-1583-9 (e book)

Books published by Lawrence Erlbaum Associates are printed on
acid-free paper, and their bindings are chosen for strength and durability.

Printed in the United States of America

10 9 8 7 6 5 4 3 2 1

Dedication

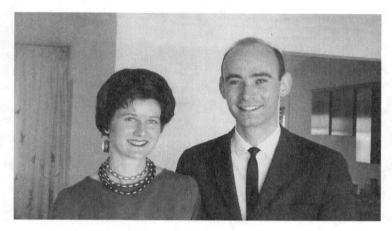

Judith and David B. Borkum, Nov. 1961

If the knowledge in this book goes back to the early days of our chronic pain program, its soul goes back much further, to the small study in our house in Syosset, New York. There, in a white short-sleeve dress shirt, barometer and geode nearby, with slide rule and finely marked graph paper, my father conducted calculations for work, and technical analyses of stocks. Just to his right, on shelves up to the ceiling, his books on electrical engineering, philosophy, and classical studies mingled with my mother's on natural history and the romance languages. At night, when the wooden cover was up on the hi-fi he had built, the vacuum tubes glowed—bright orange filaments below, ghostly blue-violet auras above—and the warm tones of Beethoven filled the room. By day, when the window was open, there were the sounds of the street and of kids on bicycles. All of Long Island was new then, every building fresh and bright, and the belief that human logic, integrity, values and science could create a more perfect world, was as self-evident as sunlight.

Because this book is dedicated to my father, I shall tell one story about him. It is from early in his work in avionics, before the E–2C radar plane at Grumman Aerospace, before the radar on the lunar module. At that time, as a young engineer with an even younger family, he was asked to pass a submarine design in an internal quality review. He refused, he refused again, and ultimately he forced a redesign. The sub's electrical equipment had been located near its only hatchway. If a fire had broken out there would have been no means of escape.

Now from my home by the Stillwater River in Maine, moonlight on the falls and a long-desolate electric plant, more than a generation has passed, and the bright promise of those early days is still waiting. I think of other nights in the unfathomable past, as an undergraduate on the edges of Cornell University. In those archaic times, even my questions were unformed, but the impressions were indelible. On warm Ithaca nights, sublime scholarship seemed to move through the air like wind moving the branches under the street lights by Fall Creek. To me, the first lesson of Talmud was this: The Divine Presence lives in knowledge. You can feel it.

Contents

PART I.   FOUNDATIONS

PART II.   PRINCIPAL TYPES OF HEADACHES: PHYSIOLOGY AND PSYCHOLOGY

PART III.   CLINICAL GUIDE TO HEADACHES

**PART IV.   BEHAVIORAL MEDICINE TREATMENT
OUTCOME LITERATURE**

Foreword

Chronic Headaches is the book I have been hoping would be written. It is comprehensive, scientifically rigorous, skillfully written and, unlike edited books, conceptually integrated. Key contributions from biology and psychology are skillfully interwoven to provide a comprehensive and sophisticated history, overview, and analysis of the field. Concepts and technical findings in biology and psychology are clearly explained, and often accompanied by surprising and entertaining historical or biographical notes. Dr. Borkum accomplishes the most difficult of tasks. He has written both the best available introduction for the student new to the area, and, at the same time, an indispensable reference for the experienced clinician and investigator.

Headaches are almost a universal experience, with clinical headache disorders common. Headache disorders also are an important cause of impaired social and occupational functioning, have a significant impact on the family, as well as create enormous personal suffering. Despite their prevalence and their familiarity, primary headache disorders are frequently untreated, not treated effectively, fail to respond to treatment, or worse, progress and become more disabling. Moreover, paradoxes abound in primary headache disorders. Obvious, but nonetheless intriguing, is the headache itself: repeated episodes of disabling pain, the body's adaptive response to injury, in the absence of injury. Possibly less obvious, but equally intriguing: pain medicines provide initial relief, but then reverse their action increasing the frequency of headaches. Jonathan Borkum argues for psychology's role in solving these puzzles, paradoxes, and treatment problems. Fortunately, it is the 21st century when advances in neuroscience are revealing not only the brain's role in generating and maintaining pain, but simultaneously revealing the biological correlates of psychological variables shown to play a role in the development, persistence and amelioration of pain. Thus, the possibility of success is growing daily.

This is the tale Jonathan Borkum tells in his synthesis of 50 years of research. Basic research from psychology and biology, results from clinical trials in both psychology and medicine, and astute clinical observations are brought together for a psychological view of the current state of the clinical science.

Students in psychology, medicine and in other health sciences can profitably read this book in at least two ways: just for the excellent overview of the psychobiology and psychological management of headaches, or also for the analysis and thoughtful integration of research findings within and across topics. Clinicians will find excellent coverage of psychological treatment and, in the psychological analysis of treatment processes and accompanying clinical observations, fresh ideas. Physicians with an interest in headaches but untutored in psychology, might select just the relevant chapters for an excellent treatment of the psychology of pain and headache. Finally, the investigator working with headache disorders will find a goldmine of stimulating ideas. Pick a topic you are familiar with, or better yet, one which you are less familiar with than you would like to be, and see what you find.

I am already looking forward to the second edition.

Kenneth Holroyd, Ph.D.
August, 2006

Preface

This book is about the theory, research, and treatment of chronic headaches. It is designed to make the tools of assessment and therapy widely accessible, while placing them firmly in the context of fundamental knowledge about how the disorders arise. Clinical experience and laboratory data are brought together, to help in understanding, selecting, and individualizing treatment. Moreover, the physiology and psychology of pain and headache are integrated in a manner accessible to both psychologists and medical care providers, to facilitate comprehensive therapy and collaboration across disciplinary boundaries. Further, chronic headaches are discussed against the background of what is known about chronic pain. It is often the chronic pain aspects of a case that prove most vexing to physicians, and call for psychologists' participation in treatment.

This is the first book on the behavioral treatment of chronic headaches to appear in 14 years, a time that has seen enormous advances in our understanding of headaches, and of pain in general. Moreover, the book is designed to be comprehensive: All the major forms of chronic benign headache are covered—migraine, tension-type, posttraumatic, cervicogenic, temporomandibular dysfunction, trigeminal neuralgia, cluster headache, and the various types of chronic daily headache.

This book will be useful to healthcare providers who want a deeper understanding of headaches, including psychologists, primary care physicians, neurologists, physiatrists, counselors, dentists, and specialists in pain medicine. Academicians and researchers will find a substantive and useful coverage of the neuroscience of pain and headache, and a discussion of unfinished research problems. Further, the book is designed to be accessible to graduate students, interns and residents treating headaches, and in graduate courses on chronic pain, health psychology, and behavioral medicine. Introductions and summaries of key sections make the material more digestible. Each new term is thoroughly defined, and an extensive glossary will help readers in psychology and medicine understand each other's vocabulary. Key chapters were reviewed carefully by graduate students of varying backgrounds and reworked several times over for clarity.

The book has at its core a guide to evaluation and treatment. In various chapters, the headache interview, diagnosis, triggers, medications, nutraceuticals, and psychological assessment and interventions are all covered. Moreover, a range of practical tools are incorporated. Key sections of the 2004 International Headache Society diagnostic criteria are reproduced. Separate tables allow rapid look-up of the various headache disorders and their distinguishing characteristics, referral patterns of myofascial trigger points relevant to headache, and the comparative advantages, disadvantages, and contraindications of triptan medications and migraine preventives. Blank headache diaries appropriate to various stages of treatment are presented as models for patients to use. A relaxation exercise is included. For biofeedback practitioners, surface electromyography (muscle tension) norms for pericranial muscles are collected from the literature and the hand temperature norms of Blanchard et al. are given.

In Part I, the foundations are set. The diagnostic interview introduces the major types of chronic benign headaches, and their clinical presentation. As noted, a table allows for rapid look-up of the various disorders to narrow the diagnostic possibilities, while relevant areas of the 2004 International Headache Society diagnostic criteria provide for more exact diagnosis, to facilitate treatment matching in the clinic and case assignment in research.

Part I also includes a definitive coverage of pain, including the types of neural plasticity that underlie its transition from the acute to chronic state and their interplay with psychological factors. We will draw on this grounding when discussing specific headache types, and the actions of pharmacological and psychological treatments. After each major variable is examined, its clinical implications are developed—how the material arises in patients' descriptions of their experience, and how it can guide treatment. It is from this foundation that psychological treatment first emerges as an applied neuroscience.

In Part II, the major forms of chronic benign headache are covered. For each headache type, the physiological underpinnings, the perturbations and triggering induced by the psyche, and the ramifications for psychological and pharmacological treatment are reviewed. A sense of the disorder, and of the person who has the disorder, is provided, to guide the assessment and the selection of treatments. Brief vignettes illustrate how each disorder presents clinically.

In Chapter 4 the physiology of migraine is covered—our current knowledge and theories, and those theories, still of heuristic value, on which the sun has set (but perhaps to rise again). Migraines have generated psychological theory too, back to the time of Galen, principally of emotional triggers, and we will review these thoughts as well. The impact and economic burden of migraine, on the individual and on society, are discussed.

A key point of intersection between psychology and migraine is the physiological stress response—vascular, neural, and inflammatory—and in Chapter 5 we will summarize the weight of literature in this field. This psychophysiological literature allows us to understand, individualize, and refine biofeedback treatments.

In Chapter 6 we examine tension-type headaches, a process that leads us to consider muscle pain and the psychological variables that affect its intensity. Following this thread brings us into the realm of pain sensitization in the central nervous system, and the earlier, foundational material becomes immediately relevant.

Chronic daily headache, common in the clinic and often intractable, forms our next focus, in Chapter 7. Here, we review what is known about medication overuse headache, hemicrania continua, new daily persistent headache, and the overlapping categories of chronic and transformed migraine. For medication overuse headache, we will discuss both the ways in which analgesics, curiously, can induce pain, and the psychological variables that can bring people into such a maladaptive corner.

Cluster headaches have been little studied psychologically, but cause so much suffering that it is worthwhile for us to gather our paltry knowledge about them, and the few hints of psychological triggers, as we do also in Chapter 7.

Secondary headaches—cervicogenic, temporomandibular, and posttraumatic, as well as trigeminal neuralgia—bring us into the realm of spine, joints, muscle, and nerve—fields as prone to theory and schools of thought as psychology, and with elucidating literatures on which we will draw in Chapter 8. As with the other forms of headache, the physical brings us to the psychological, and vice versa.

While children suffer from the same types of benign headaches as adults, the presentations, triggers and treatments can vary enough to deserve separate consideration, which we will give in Chapter 9.

The third part of this book is a clinical guide to headaches, on which practitioners can draw when seeing patients.

Triggers are discussed in Chapter 10 in terms of their empirical data and implications for therapy.

In Chapter 11, acute and preventive medications, herbals, and nutraceuticals are then reviewed in depth, along with their indications, contraindications, and interactions. The tables mentioned above permit rapid comparison of the various triptan medications for acute migraine treatment and similarly the various migraine preventives. Of course the chapter cannot stand alone—knowledge of the patient, the judgment of the prescriber, and familiarity with the drug and its *Physician's Desk Reference* listing are crucial.

The assessment chapter, 12, extends the coverage of the interview begun in Chapter 1, before progressing to psychometrics and the psychophysiological (biofeedback) evaluation. Standardized questionnaires for disability and common psychological comorbidities are reviewed. The *Migraine Disability Assessment Scale (MIDAS)* and Ken Holroyd's *Headache Specific Locus of Control Scale* are included in their entirety. Normative surface EMG (muscle tension) values are given. Diagrams show the standard electrode placements. As noted, blank headache diaries appropriate to various stages of treatment are given as models.

The treatment chapter, 13, includes both discussion of the traditional interventions for headaches—relaxation training, biofeedback, and cognitive therapy—and chronic pain therapies, for use when, as in chronic daily headache, pain sensitivity may be a more useful target than muscles, blood vessels, or stress. Resources for home-based treatment are reviewed. Case vignettes illustrate the varying paths by which recovery unfolds in practice.

Lest the application of psychological treatments to physiological disorders seem purely an act of faith, the last part of this book returns to empirical underpinnings, but this time of the treatments themselves. Successive chapters cover the outcome literature—how well the treatments work—through the lens of meta-analysis (Chapter 14), process studies of the mechanisms behind the efficacy (Chapter 15), and our preliminary knowledge and practical guidelines for patient selection and treatment matching (Chapter 16), including the relative merits of stepped- and stratified-care.

Lastly, Chapter 17 deals with long-term outcome studies, some 5 to 10 years after therapy. We then conclude with some thoughts about the great unfinished business in this field—a small sampling of research questions poised but still unanswered. A glossary completes the text, to help make psychological and physiological terms accessible to people from varying disciplines. Each term that appears in the glossary is bold-faced when first introduced in the text.

And so we will travel, from the clinical consideration of the diagnostic interview, to the laboratory knowledge of pain and headache, to clinical assessment and treatment, and then back to the empirical process and outcome literature, always seeking the day when chronic benign headaches will be enshrouded, not by ignorance, but by irrelevance, as they join the great diseases of the past.

ACKNOWLEDGMENTS

This book has its roots in the chronic pain program at Mid-Maine Medical Center in Waterville (now MaineGeneral), which I joined as a Ph.D. student two decades ago. This was when the woolen mills and shoe factories and paper plants were in full swing, old smoky brick buildings, some a quarter-mile long, on snowy river banks. Inside, ancient machinery, fantastic contraptions, would gee and yaw and screech and clank and jam. And with stochastic certainty give rise, in ghastly byproduct, to industrial injuries. It is here that I first learned about the complex problems of chronic pain. My first debt, then, is to Bruce Cummings and Ralph Gabarro who founded the program, to Dayton Haigney, MD and Ira Lipsky, M.Ed. who ran it, and to Ken Kindya, Ph.D., who brought me into its fold.

Of course, if Waterville were only an industrial town, this book could not have been born; I am grateful to the many other people who have helped turn rural New England into an oasis of knowledge.

Jeff Matranga, Ph.D., ABPP, became our program leader close to the beginning, and brought a sophisticated knowledge of chronic pain from his year of post doc. He has consistently set a stan-

dard of achievement—in board certification, in a second master's degree in clinical psychopharmacology, in certification for prescription privileges—with which the rest of us struggle to keep pace.
Christine Gray, Psy.D., helped launch this book by suggesting headaches as a topic for a talk we co-
presented in 1998, and then gave helpful suggestions on the manuscript nearly eight years later. Jeri
Wilson, O.T., provided the business acumen to keep us solvent, while Cora Damon, librarian, preserved and extended our scholarly resources, Barbara Jones and her staff at the University of Maine
procured many hundreds of interlibrary loan articles. And Jeff Leonards, Ph.D., Peter Flournoy,
Ph.D., Laura E. Holcomb, Ph.D., Peter Bridgman, MD, Willy White, M.A., Bruce Mehler, M.A., Vee
Burden, R.N., Natalie Morse, Health Educator, Sandy Picurro, PT, Martha Works, PT, Alice Van-
derwerken, O.T., Marsha Hashinsky, O.T., Mary McMorrow-Adams, LCSW, Lydia Parsons, LCSW,
Trish Hildreth, Ann Grout, Eleanor Ellis, Jan Hoffman, and Angela McMahon each enriched our
knowledge and spirit.

Will Taylor, MD, brought surface electromyography alive to us in a magical day of instruction back in 1992, a lesson continued in informative talks by Bruce Mehles, MA and the quiet,
exceptional competence of Altaf Ahmed, MD. Jim Fegan, MD's restless intellect (he has also been
an executive, statistician, engineer, fighter pilot and jazz guitarist) delighted in turning up new
knowledge and in challenging us with simple yet paradoxically unanswerable questions. As he
struggled to find answers to chronic pain, he enlightened all around him. Other physiatrists—John
Ditri, MD, John Hall, MD, and Douglas Pavlak, MD, and his colleagues—likewise shared their
knowledge and clinical discoveries. The chance to interact with anesthesiologists Jonathan Her-
land, D.Sc., MD, Peter Leong, MD, Ben Zolper, MD, Peter Thompson, MD, and David Landry,
MD, added still further to our development.

Still, this book would have been far less thorough, academically and clinically, and much
harder to read, were it not for the incisive recommendations of Ken Holroyd, Ph.D., Paul Duckro,
Ph.D., Steven Baskin, Ph.D., Frank Andrasik, Ph.D., and an anonymous reviewer, as well as
Teresa Edenfield, Barbara Hermann, Diana Higgins, Stephanie Lamattina, and Janell Schartel.
Their questions were much better than my answers, however, and the inadequacies that remain are
purely my responsibility.

Meanwhile, as a Ph.D. student and beyond, my knowledge and life have been wonderfully
enriched by my involvement with Prof. Colin Martindale's laboratory, and his unendingly creative
invisible college. I am grateful to him, and to Professors Larry Smith, Joel Gold, Sandy Sigmon,
Alan Rosenwasser, and Marie Hayes, and to department chair Jeff Hecker, for the opportunity to
continue my connections with the University of Maine, in the Department of Psychology and
the Neurosciences Program.

Debra Riegert, senior editor at Lawrence Erlbaum Associates, was remarkably effective,
sure-handed, and supportive throughout the publication process.

Julie King and Mary Edmonds-Sutton sparked many fascinating discussions. Angie and
coworkers at the Bangor Mall Staples made the manuscript look like a book long before it was one.
Marc Mytar, Ph.D. gave support at a key time.

Further back, at Stony Brook, Jack Riley paid me a great and undeserved honor by treating me
as a peer. In those days of Univac computers, Professor Bernard J. Baars showed us the early con-
nections between clinical psychology and the neurosciences. At the Syracuse NY VA, psychologists Tim Hayes, Robert P. Sprafkin, and their colleagues taught how the consulting room is a
source of knowledge and discovery about human nature.

Finally, as this book ends its long gestation in my word processor and takes its first steps, I
thank my brother Roger and his wife Celeste; my sister Debi and her son Christopher; my aunts
and uncles Sumner and Sandy Borkum; Marjorie and George Schiering, and Edward and Joan
After; my cousins Sandy and Richard Bertman, and their children; and my parents, David and
Judith, to whom this book is dedicated.

Headache roams over the desert, blowing like the wind,
Flashing like lightning, it is loosed above and below . . .
This man it has struck, and
Like one with heart disease he staggers,
Like one bereft of reason, he is broken . . .
Headache whose course like the dread windstorm none knows,
None knows its full time or its bond.

Sumerian text, c. 3000–4000 B.C.
(cited in McHenry, 1969)

PART I

Foundations

CHAPTER 1

Headache Nosology and Warning Signs

"The good man would not hear of migraine, since the often excessive pains were not one-sided as is the case with migraine but consisted in a raging torment in and above both eyes, and moreover were considered by the physician to be a secondary symptom."

—Thomas Mann (1947), Dr. Faustus (cited in G. D. Perkin, 1995a)

When the medical epics of our own era are written, I suppose there will be little mention of headaches. Prions and viruses, cancer and heart disease, ALS and MS, these will be the true antagonists against whom our mortal battles are waged. Yet as those who have had chronic migraines or cluster headaches, or who have struggled with the long-term sequellae of head injury can attest, headaches are no small players in the course of human suffering. Among chronic pain conditions, headaches seem to be a little more intrusive, a little more disabling, a little closer to where "we" are, than pain at more distal locations. As the saying goes, "If it can kill you, it's not a migraine; if it can't kill you but you wish it would, it probably is a migraine."

It is this capacity of headaches to be intense, distressing, and disruptive, as well as their sheer prevalence, that leads us to seek out knowledge, indeed expertise, about them.

And there are other reasons to study headaches as well. They are unique among pain conditions in their degree of responsiveness to combined medical and psychological intervention. As a result, the field of headaches is a terrain on which the bridge between body and mind can be seen with particular clarity. Moreover, to truly understand headaches one must understand pain more generally. Thus, the tools that we learn here can serve us well when dealing with other types of chronic pain.

Headaches are not primarily psychological phenomena, but neither can they be fully understood, prevented, and treated if psychological factors are ignored. In the pages that follow, we will explore their nature on the psychological, the neural, and sometimes even the molecular planes. Traveling between these levels, and finding their interconnections, will be part of the intellectual reward for our efforts.

But before embarking on this project, we must first understand what the principal types of headaches are.

There are, of course, **migraines**:[1] paroxysmal bouts of moderate-to-severe, pulsating head **pain**, joined with nausea, sometimes vomiting, and an intolerance of light, sound, and activity. Their impact on functioning, and even on thinking, can be profound; they can dampen success

---

[1]Terms in bold are defined in the glossary.

in a career, or in life. Yet by their very starkness, migraines leave a trail—in neuroimaging, bio-chemistry, psychophysiology, and the subtle cognitive and perceptual tests of experimental psychology. Very gradually, migraines are yielding their secrets, and as they do so, we can gather clues about how to prevent and treat them.

Tension-type headache—a usually mild-to-moderate, squeezing pain, not accompanied by the flagrant autonomic signs of migraine—would seem to be at a very inconsequential end of the headache spectrum. And inconsequential they are, unless you are among the 2.8 percent of women or 1.4 percent of men who have tension-type headaches more than half the days of the month, for 6 months or more. These chronic tension-type headaches can be disabling, and constitute one subtype of chronic daily, or near daily, headache. And while tension-type headaches are often mild, this is, unfortunately, only an optional feature, not a necessary one, for their diagnosis.

To understand tension-type headaches, and chronic daily headaches, we will first delve into a study of the muscles, and then of the nerve pathways along which pain is transmitted and inhibited. There, deep in the brain and spinal cord, physiology and psychology merge into a picture of the phenomenon itself. And in this picture, too, we will find tools for prevention and treatment.

Cluster headaches, like migraines, are stark and distinctive, and as precise in their clinical features as in their clockwork timing. So far they have kept more of their secrets than migraines, but not all of them, and we will be able to discern recent progress. And we will see that even here, on this harsh physiological terrain, self-management has had victories of its own.

On then to headaches whose physiology is well enough understood that they are called "sec-ondary" (to a physical disorder): myofascial pain, temporomandibular joint dysfunction, dis-orders of the **zygapophyseal joints** of the cervical spine, and occipital and trigeminal neuralgia. Self-management has a role to play in the first two disorders, less so in the last three. As in all types of headaches, we will stop respectfully at the border, and admire the work of neurolo-gists, neurosurgeons, anesthesiologists, orthopedic surgeons, physiatrists, dentists, and the experts in manual medicine.

Posttraumatic headache too—a group of disparate disorders joined only by the fact that they start with an injury to the head or neck—requires, we will see, the diagnostic and treatment acumen of several specialties, including psychology as one facet of the overall effort.

But our success, when we find it, will be in the details. And it is to those details, beginning with a review of the International Headache Society's diagnostic system, that we now turn.

THE IHS DIAGNOSTIC SYSTEM

At first, diagnosing headache seems simple enough. But consider the entry for migraine in what was the standard diagnostic system from 1962 to 1987, that of the Ad Hoc Committee on Clas-sification of Headache:

> "Vascular Headaches of Migraine Type.—Recurrent attacks of headache, widely varied in inten-sity, frequency, and duration. The attacks are commonly unilateral in onset; are usually associ-ated with anorexia and, sometimes, with nausea and vomiting; in some are preceded by, or associated with, conspicuous sensory, motor, and mood disturbances; and are often familial" (Ad Hoc Committee, 1962, p. 717).

The entry is rather vague, even for describing prototypical cases. And the system offers us no guidance—no actual criteria—for assigning those common but ambiguous cases that fall in the borderland between two categories. In contrast, the demarcations are sharper, the assignments clearer, under the system that followed, created by the Headache Classification Committee of the International Headache Society (IHS):

"Migraine without aura.
A) At least 5 attacks fulfilling B–D
B) Headache attacks lasting 4–72 hours (untreated or unsuccessfully treated)
C) Headache has at least two of the following characteristics
 1. Unilateral location
 2. Pulsating quality
 3. Moderate or severe intensity
 4. Aggravation by walking stairs or similar routine physical activity
D) During the headache at least one of the following
 1. Nausea and/or vomiting
 2. Photophobia and phonophobia"
(Headache Classification Committee, 1988)

The IHS diagnostic system was revised in 2004. The criteria for the forms of chronic benign headache most likely to come to the attention of psychologists are excerpted in Table 1–2, later in this chapter. As is apparent, all of the categories are similarly well demarcated.

The criteria were developed through expert consensus rather than any one study or set of studies (Olesen, 1990; Headache Classification Subcommittee, 2004). They were intended to standardize research and clinical work, and to provoke further research into the criteria themselves. That they are a work in progress is suggested, for example, by the criteria for **cervicogenic headache**. Such research scrutiny has not been focused yet on the 2004 criteria, of course, but the second edition seems likely to share the strengths of its predecessor, whose criteria were quite precise and replicable (e.g., Honkoop, Sorbi, Godaert, & Spierings, 1999).

On the other hand, there is much less evidence that anyone is actually using the IHS system, at least in clinical practice. Thus, Marcus and coworkers mailed four vignettes to members of the American Headache Society (AHS). Each vignette contained enough information to make an unambiguous diagnosis under IHS criteria, along with extra, "decoy" information. The 405 people who responded were typical of the AHS membership, and represented 60 percent of the sample. Of course, they would be expected to have greater familiarity than the average practitioner with the IHS criteria.

Now, of the 405 respondents, the number who correctly diagnosed at least three of the four vignettes was exactly 2, or 0.50 percent. Actually, the respondents showed good agreement with each other, but they did not agree at all with the IHS criteria. How can this be? The decoy information included headache features that would not be expected with the actual headache type. For example, the tension-type headaches were influenced by hormonal factors or were relieved by ergotamine, while the migraines included neck muscle spasms, did not improve with propranolol, and/or were not found in the patient's relatives. Moreover, in a separate part of the same survey, respondents indicated that in their clinical practice, non-IHS criteria were important in their diagnostic work (Marcus, Nash, & D. C. Turk, 1994). Thus, we might speculate that the practitioners were not using exact criteria, but rather were matching the patient's characteristics to cognitive prototypes representing the different diagnoses. The prototype with the closest match became the assigned diagnosis. This interpretation is uncertain, but it seems to fit with the way people in general make category assignments (Rosch & Mervis, 1975).

The results of Marcus et al. should be qualified by the fact that the survey was conducted in approximately 1992, not long after the 1988 introduction of the IHS framework. Presumably the respondents were familiar with the criteria, but perhaps it takes longer than 4 years to change one's diagnostic practice. Also, the thorny issue of validity is not addressed in this study. It may be that in clinical practice, knowing which medications a patient has responded to, for example, is more important than knowing the official diagnosis. Still, use of the IHS system allows one's clinical work to share in its precision, and to link to the large body of research data in which the criteria are used.

Limitations. A weakness of the 1988 criteria was that in them, only one type of chronic daily headache was recognized: chronic tension-type headache. To rectify this problem, Hemicrania Continua and New Daily Persistent Headache were added to the 2004 revisions, the section on Medication Overuse Headache was markedly expanded, and Chronic Migraine was developed by analogy to Chronic Tension-Type Headache. For comparison, a supplementary nosology proposed by N. T. Mathew (1997a), is given in Table 1–3. The main difference from the IHS revisions is the category, "Migraine chronic tension-type headache complex." We will discuss this category, and the other types of chronic daily headache, in Chapter 7.

The second main area of weakness in the IHS system had been in applying the criteria to migraine and episodic tension-type headache in children. We will discuss this area further in Chapter 9, which focuses on pediatric headache.

A note on migraine diagnosis. Rapoport and Edmeads (2000) note that the Sumerian text with which we started this book may be referring to a migraine. The description seems to capture poetically the randomness ("like the wind"), head pain and nausea ("loosed above and below") and cognitive impairment ("Like one bereft of reason") often found in migraines. On the other hand, the symptoms could be signs of a greater problem, such as meningitis (Rapoport & Edmeads, 2000). We cannot be certain of the diagnosis in the poem, of course, but we need to be absolutely sure when it comes to our patients. For while the vast majority of headaches are benign, the ones that are not can be ominous indeed.

WARNING SIGNS

Recently at our clinic we received a referral from a primary care physician, of a man in his early 40s. The referral was for treatment of migraines and for assessment of adult attention deficit disorder. The patient had brought up the second concern to his physician after seeing a television show on it. A few days before the evaluation, it was canceled. The message from the patient said simply that he had been diagnosed with lung cancer. Presumably, both the "migraines" and the difficulty attending were due to brain metastases.

Suppose this referral had slipped through. How much behavioral treatment would the patient have received? How much **biofeedback** would have been directed toward the "migraines?" Hopefully, the answer would have been "none." Attention difficulties are a neurological symptom, and presumably it would have emerged at the evaluation that the problem had arisen only recently. New onset neurological symptoms should *always* be reported to the patient's health care provider,[2] and this is even truer in the context of new onset headaches.

---

[2]By phone. Do not assume that the evaluation report will be read anytime soon.

Throughout the rest of this work we will assume that the disorder is one or more of the benign primary headache types noted above. Thus, we assume that referral to the psychologist has been made by the patient's physician, physician's assistant, or nurse practitioner, and that ominous causes of the headaches have been ruled out medically, including those requiring immediate medical attention. But of course, physicians make mistakes too. And while it is neither within a psychologist's competence nor within their responsibility to rule out a disease process giving rise to the headaches, there are warning signs that, if followed, can help prevent the occasional inappropriate referral from becoming a tragically misdirected course of treatment.

A *partial* list of these warning signs—indications that a headache requires further medical work-up on an emergency basis—include the following (adapted from Rapoport & Silberstein, 1992; Silberstein, Lipton, & Goadsby, 1998):

First or worst headache of one's life

Severe, rapid-onset, recurrent headache

Accelerating pattern of headaches; headache worsens over days or weeks

Progressive or new daily persistent headache

Change in the frequency, severity or clinical features of the headache

Headache begins after age 50

New onset headache in a patient with cancer or HIV

Headache with fever, stiff neck, rash, or other sign of systemic illness

Papilledema (swelling of the optic disk, on the retina)[3]

Neurological symptoms that do not meet the criteria of migraine with typical aura, or which themselves warrant investigation

Persistent neurological defects

Alteration or loss of consciousness; change in cognition

Headache has no obvious identifiable etiology

Papilledema is a warning sign because it indicates elevated pressure of cerebrospinal fluid, due, for example, to a tumor, a blood clot blocking the venous outflow from the brain (cerebral venous thrombosis; Quattrone, Bono, R. Oliveri, Gambardella, Pirritano, Labate, et al., 2001), or arising without known cause (idiopathic intracranial hypertension; pseudotumor cerebri). Even when there is no abnormality except the elevated CSF pressure, treatments not often used for headaches, such as the diuretics furosemide (Lasix) and acetazolamide (Diamox) may be effective (N. Mathew, Ravishankar, & Sanin, 1996). This is important not only for the headache, but for preventing damage to the visual system (D. I. Friedman, 1999). When papilledema is absent, we should nonetheless note carefully any reports of **tinnitus**, a ringing or buzzing in the ears, in synchrony with the pulse. Although by no means a sure sign, it is sometimes the only indication of intracranial hypertension (S.-J. Wang, Silberstein, S. Patterson, & W. B. Young, 1998).

As a general rule, the rarer the headache disorder, the more likely imaging studies are to be useful. Thus, in migraine, lesions are found with no greated frequency than in the general population, but in migraine with motor aura, which is much less common, abnormalities are

---

[3]Admittedly, not something a psychologist will usually know, but included here for completeness.

occasionally present. Trigeminal neuralgia, which is relatively rare, found almost exclusively above age 40, and whose symptoms suggest nerve compression or damage, is particularly appropriate for diagnostic work-up (Zakrzewska, 2002). At tertiary care centers, which tend to accumulate worst-case scenarios, trigeminal neuralgia is secondary to a tumor or other lesion in 8–10 percent of cases (Cheng, Cascino, & Onofrio, 1993; Scrivani, Keith, Mathews, & Kaban, 1999).

Also, a headache that follows a recent head trauma is appropriate for further workup. There can be intracranial hemorrhages or hematomas even if there was no loss of consciousness and no impairment on the Glasgow Coma Scale at the time of injury (Shah, 1991).

Moreover, in the IHS criteria it is noted that "occipital headache in children, whether unilateral or bilateral, is rare and calls for diagnostic caution; many cases are attributable to structural lesions" (Headache Classification Subcommittee, 2004, p. 25).

For migraines specifically, there is evidence to support the use of imaging studies when there is an unexplained abnormality on neurological examination (Frishberg et al., 2000).

THE HEADACHE INTERVIEW

Once it is clear that we are dealing with a benign headache, we must rely on the clinical interview, perhaps supplemented by daily headache records. At this point, diagnosis rests on careful inquiry about the headache's characteristics, that is, its:

- *Location*, including whether it spreads from an initial focal point, whether it is unilateral and, if unilateral, whether it is always on the same side ("side-locked")
- *Quality*, whether it is pulsatile (throbbing in time to the pulse), a dull ache, sharp and stabbing, boring/piercing, or a pulling pain;
- *Duration*, which, among chronic headaches, can vary from seconds to pain that is continuous over years;
- *Intensity*, which similarly can span the full range;
- *Associated Features*, including autonomic (e.g., nausea, lacrimation, rhinorrhea, bloodshot eyes), anatomic (chronically restricted neck movements), and behavioral (resting quietly vs. pacing with agitation);
- *History*, especially changes in the frequency, intensity, or characteristics of the headaches, whether these changes were rapid over days and weeks or gradual over months and years, whether they followed a clear trauma, and whether they were recent;
- *Triggering Factors*, including lifestyle (e.g., **stress**, diet), environmental (e.g., weather, glare), time of day, and mechanical (neck movements, pressure to tender areas).

For the main forms of chronic benign headache, the clinical features are summarized in Table 1–1. Table 1–1 is intended for rapid look-up, to enable practitioners to narrow their search to a few diagnostic possibilities. For exact diagnosis, the International Headache Society Criteria, given in Table 1–2, should then be consulted.

As we have seen, *Migraines*, untreated or unsuccessfully treated, last for 4 to 72 hours in adults. The pain has at least two of: unilateral location (but often not the same side every headache), pulsating quality, moderate or severe intensity, and aggravation by (or causing avoidance of) routine physical activity. Moreover, migraines are accompanied by painful aversion to both light and conversational sound levels (**photophobia** and **phonophobia**, respectively) and/or by nausea or vomiting. Informally, it is this intolerance of stimulation, even faint smells

(*text continued on page 19*)

TABLE 1–1
Principal Features of Benign Headache Disorders

Type	Location	Intensity	Quality	Duration	Features	Prevalence[1]	Onset	Triggers	Other
Migraine	Supraorbital, temporal; often initially unilateral	Moderate-to-severe	Pulsing	4–72 hours untreated	Nausea, photophobia, phonophobia, osmophobia, intolerance of routine activity	~10% 3:1 female (without aura); 1–2% 1:1 female (with aura)	Childhood, teens, or early adult	Menses (esp. without aura), stress, sensory stimulation	
Tension-Type	Forehead, temples; or neck, occiput	Mild-to-moderate	Pressing, tightening	Widely varying	*Episodic* May have one of photophobia, phonophobia, may have anorexia; *Chronic* May have one of: photophobia, phonophobia, mild nausea	~80% 1.3:1 female (episodic); ~2% 2:1 female (chronic)	Often after major life events stress	Stress, muscle tension	
Medication-Overuse	Usually diffuse, bilateral	Varies	Usually pressing, tightening	Often continuous	For triptan overuse, may be same as migraine; otherwise none	~1% (population); 7–15% (clinic) more female	Intake of symptomatic medications ≥10 days per month for ≥3 months		Patient may fear headache recurrence
Temporomandibular Dysfunction	Temple, ear, in front of ear	Varies	Dull soreness; may be sharp when chewing	Varies	Jaw may be tender; joint sounds may be present with chewing	~5% (Adol. population) ~8% (Adult population). 1.7:1 female (population). 4:1 female (clinic)	Childhood, teens, or early adult	Worse with jaw movements, chewing hard food	
Cervicogenic	Spreads from neck or occiput to eye, temple, forehead on same side; usually unilateral & side-locked	Usually moderate, can be severe	Dull, aching, boring, pulling (not pulsatile or lancinating)	Usually hours to days; may become continuous	Reduced neck range of motion; mild autonomic signs may be present	14–18% (clinic); 0.25–4% (population); 3:1 female (clinic)	May follow neck trauma	Neck movements, posture, pressure to tender areas in neck or occiput	Relief with diagnostic nerve block; no response to triptans; not abolished by indomethacin

(continued)

9

TABLE 1–1 (*Continued*)
Principal Features of Benign Headache Disorders

Type	Location	Intensity	Quality	Duration	Features	Prevalence[1]	Onset	Triggers	Other
Cluster	At, behind, or above eye; temple; unilateral	Very severe	Piercing, boring	15–180 minutes, untreated	Agitation; nasal congestion, lacrimation, rhinorrhea, on the affected side, or other local parasympath. symptoms	~0.1% 4:1 male	Any age, but typically late 20's, early 30's	Heat, alcohol, ?hypoxia	Frequency: once every other day–8 per day; 92% are current or former smokers
Paroxysmal Hemicrania	At, behind, or above eye; temple; jaw; forehead; unilateral	Moderate to very severe	Varies	2–30 minutes	Same as Cluster Headache	Unknown. 2–3:1 female (chronic) 1:1 female (episodic)	Any age	In some, neck movements	Frequency usually >5/day; completely prevented by indomethacin
Hemicrania Continua	Unilateral	Moderate, with severe episodes	May have superimposed jabs and jolts	Continuous	Nasal congestion, rhinorrhea; conjunctival injection, lacrimation; ptosis, miosis	Considered rare		None known	Completely prevented by indomethacin
New Daily Persistent Headache	Location varies; usually bilateral	Mild or moderate	Pressing, tightening	Usually continuous; daily and unremitting from within 3 days of onset	May have one of: photophobia, phonophobia, mild nausea; sometimes tinnitus, dizziness or paresthesias	Unknown. ?1.4–2.5:1 female	?20's–40's Possibly after cold- or flu-like illness	None known	Usually not aggravated by routine physical activity; Rule Out CSF leak

	Location	Severity	Quality	Duration	Associated symptoms	Incidence/Prevalence[1]	Age/Onset	Triggers	Other considerations
Posttraumatic Headache	Varies; often at temples and across forehead	Varies	Varies, but usually resembles migraine or tension-type headache	Usually continuous	Varies; often with impaired concentration & memory, irritability, fatigue, dizziness & blurred vision	Incidence 0.03%/year. ? more male	Within 7 days of head trauma	Often, mental and physical exertion	Look for myofascial problems, other neck disorders, and medication overuse
Trigeminal Neuralgia	Often cheeks, jaw, lower face. Unilateral 98% of time	Severe	Sharp, stabbing	<1 second to 2 minutes		Incidence ~.004%/year. 1.5:1 female	Usually ages 40–70	Chewing, talking, brushing against trigger zones on cheek	Rule out tumor, demyelinating disorder
Occipital Neuralgia	Back of head; unilateral; sometimes radiates to forehead, eyes	Severe	Quick stabbing, sometimes on a burning or aching background	Seconds	Responds to nerve block		May follow trauma to neck or head	Neck movements; pressure to Occ. nerve, C2 spinous process, or top of head	

Note. Sources of information: Anthony (2000); J. N. Campbell & Sciubba (2005); D. W. Dodick & J. K. Campbell (2001); Drangsholt & LeResche (1999); Dubuisson (1999); S. F. Dworkin, Huggins, et al. (1990); Evers, Suhr, Bauer, Grotemeyer, & Husstedt (1999); Haldeman & Dagenais (2001); Headache Classification Subcommittee (2004); D. Li & Rozen (2002); Martelletti & van Suijlekom (2004); L. C. Newman & Goadsby (2001); Ramadan & Keidel (2000); B. K. Rasmussen (2001); B. K. Rasmussen, R. Jensen, Schroll, & J. Olesen (1991); Rozen, Capobianco, & Dalessio (2001); B. S. Schwartz, Stewart, Simon, & Lipton (1998); Silberstein & Lipton (2001); S. Solomon (1997); S. Solomon & Färkkilä (2000); Vanast (1986)

[1]Prevalence is with respect to the general population unless otherwise specified.

TABLE 1–2
Diagnostic Criteria for Headaches (International Headache Society, 2nd Edition, Excerpts)

1.1 Migraine without aura
   A) At least 5 attacks fulfilling criteria B–D
   B) Headache attacks lasting 4–72 hours (untreated or unsuccessfully treated)
   C) Headache has at least 2 of the following characteristics:
      1. Unilateral location
      2. Pulsating quality
      3. Moderate or severe pain intensity
      4. Aggravation by or causing avoidance of routine physical activity (e.g., walking or climbing stairs)
   D) During the headache at least one of the following:
      1. Nausea and/or vomiting
      2. Photophobia and phonophobia
   E) Not attributed to another disorder
1.2 Migraine with aura
   A) At least 2 attacks fulfilling criterion B
   B) Migraine aura fulfilling criteria B and C for one of the subforms 1.2.1–1.2.6
   C) Not attributed to another disorder
      1.2.1 Typical aura with migraine headache
         A) At least 2 attacks fulfilling criteria B–D
         B) Aura consisting of at least one of the following, but no motor weakness:
            1. Fully reversible visual symptoms including positive features (e.g., flickering lights, spots or lines) and/or negative features (i.e., loss of vision)
            2. Fully reversible sensory symptoms including positive features (i.e., pins and needles) and/or negative features (i.e., numbness)
            3. Fully reversible dysphasic speech disturbance
         C) At least two of the following:
            1. Homonymous visual symptoms and/or unilateral sensory symptoms
            2. At least one aura symptom develops gradually over ≥5 minutes, and/or different aura symptoms occur in succession over ≥5 minutes
            3. Each symptom lasts ≥5 minutes and ≤60 minutes
         D) Headache fulfilling criteria B–D for 1.1 *Migraine without aura* begins during the aura or follows aura within 60 minutes
         E) Not attributed to another disorder
      1.2.2 Typical aura with non-migraine headache
      1.2.3 Typical aura without headache
      1.2.4 Familial Hemiplegic Migraine (FHM)
         A) At least two attacks fulfilling criteria B and C
         B) Aura consisting of fully reversible motor weakness and at least one of the following:
            1. Fully reversible visual symptoms including positive features (e.g., flickering lights, spots or lines) and/or negative features (i.e., loss of vision)
            2. Fully reversible sensory symptoms including positive features (i.e., pins and needles) and/or negative features (i.e., numbness)
            3. Fully reversible dysphasic speech disturbance
         C) At least two of the following:
            1. At least one aura symptom develops gradually over ≥5 minutes and/or different aura symptoms occur in succession over ≥5 minutes
            2. Each aura symptom lasts ≥5 minutes and <24 hours
            3. Headache fulfilling criteria B–D for 1.1 *Migraine without aura* begins during the aura or follows onset of aura within 60 minutes
         D) At least one first- or second-degree relative has had attacks fulfilling these criteria A–E
         E) Not attributed to another disorder
      1.2.5 Sporadic Hemiplegic Migraine [same criteria as Familial Hemiplegic Migraine, except:
         D) No first- or second-degree relative has attacks fulfilling these criteria A–E]
      1.2.6 Basilar-Type Migraine
         A) At least two attacks fulfilling criteria B–D

(continued)

TABLE 1–2 (*Continued*)

B) Aura consisting of at least two of the following fully reversible symptoms, but no motor weakness:
   1. Dysarthria
   2. Vertigo
   3. Tinnitus
   4. Hypacusia
   5. Diplopia
   6. Visual symptoms simultaneously in both temporal and nasal fields of both eyes
   7. Ataxia
   8. Decreased level of consciousness
   9. Simultaneously bilateral paresthesias

C) At least one of the following:
   1. At least one aura symptom develops gradually over ≥5 minutes and/or different aura symptoms occur in succession over ≥5 minutes
   2. Each aura symptom lasts ≥5 minutes and ≤60 minutes

D) Headache fulfilling criteria B–D for 1.1 *Migraine without aura* begins during the aura or follows aura within 60 minutes

E) Not attributed to another disorder

1.3 Childhood periodic syndromes that are commonly precursors of migraine

    1.3.1 Cyclical vomiting

      A) At least 5 attacks fulfilling criteria B and C

      B) Episodic attacks, stereotypical in the individual patient, of intense nausea and vomiting lasting from 1 hour to 5 days

      C) Vomiting during attacks occurs at least 4 times/hour for at least 1 hour

      D) Symptom-free between attacks

      E) Not attributed to another disorder

    1.3.2 Abdominal migraine

      A) At least 5 attacks fulfilling criteria B–D

      B) Attacks of abdominal pain lasting 1–72 hours (untreated or unsuccessfully treated)

      C) Abdominal pain has all of the following characteristics:
        1. Midline location, periumbilical or poorly localized
        2. Dull or "just sore" quality
        3. Moderate or severe intensity

      D) During abdominal pain at least 2 of the following:
        1. Anorexia
        2. Nausea
        3. Vomiting
        4. Pallor

      E) Not attributed to another disorder

    1.3.3 Benign paroxysmal vertigo of childhood

      A) At least 5 attacks fulfilling criterion B

      B) Multiple episodes of severe vertigo, occurring without warning and resolving spontaneously after minutes to hours

      C) Normal neurological examination and audiometric and vestibular functions between attacks

      D) Normal electroencephalogram

1.4 Retinal migraine

  A) At least 2 attacks fulfilling criteria B and C

  B) Fully reversible monocular positive and/or negative visual phenomena (e.g., scintillations, scotomata or blindness) confirmed by examination during an attack or (after proper instruction) by the patient's drawing of a monocular field defect during an attack

  C) Headache fulfilling criteria B–D for 1.1 *Migraine without aura* begins during the visual symptoms or follows them within 60 minutes

  D) Normal ophthalmological examination between attacks

  E) Not attributed to another disorder

(*continued*)

TABLE 1–2 (*Continued*)

1.5 Complications of migraine
    Comment: Code separately for both the antecedent migraine subtype and for the complication
       1.5.1 Chronic migraine
          A) Headache fulfilling criteria C and D for 1.1 *Migraine without aura* on ≥15 days/month for >3 months
          B) Not attributed to another disorder
    "When medication overuse is present and fulfills criterion B for any of the subforms of 8.2 *Medication overuse headache,* it is uncertain whether criterion B for 1.5.1 *Chronic migraine* is fulfilled until 2 months after medication has been withdrawn without improvement." (p. 32)
       1.5.2 Status migrainosus
          A) The present attack in a patient with 1.1 *Migraine without aura* is typical of previous attacks except for its duration
          B) Headache has both of the following features:
             1. Unremitting for >72 hours
             2. Severe intensity
          C) Not attributed to another disorder
       1.5.3 Persistent aura without infarction
          A) The present attack in a patient with 1.2 *Migraine with aura* is typical of previous attacks except that one or more aura symptoms persists for >1 week
          B) Not attributed to another disorder
       1.5.4 Migrainous infarction
       1.5.5 Migraine-triggered seizure
1.6 Probable migraine
       1.6.1 Probable migraine without aura
          A) Attacks fulfilling all but one of criteria A–D for 1.1 *Migraine without aura*
          B) Not attributed to another disorder
       1.6.2 Probable migraine with aura
          A) Attacks fulfilling all but one of criteria A–D of 1.2 *Migraine with aura* or any of its subforms
          B) Not attributed to another disorder
       1.6.5 Probable chronic migraine
          A) Headache fulfilling criteria C and D for 1.1 *Migraine without aura* on ≥15 days/month for >3 months
          B) Not attributed to another disorder but there is, or has been within the last 2 months, medication overuse fulfilling criterion B for any of the subforms of 8.2 *Medication-overuse headache*
2.1 Infrequent episodic tension-type headache
    A) At least 10 episodes occurring on <1 day per month on average (<12 days per year) and fulfilling criteria B–D
    B) Headache lasting from 30 minutes to 7 days
    C) Headache has at least two of the following characteristics:
       1. Bilateral location
       2. Pressing/tightening (non-pulsating) quality
       3. Mild or moderate intensity
       4. Not aggravated by routine physical activity such as walking or climbing stairs
    D) Both of the following:
       1. No nausea or vomiting (anorexia may occur)
       2. No more than one of photophobia or phonophobia
    E) Not attributed to another disorder
       2.1.1 Infrequent episodic tension-type headache associated with pericranial tenderness
          A) Episodes fulfilling criteria A–E for 2.1 *Infrequent episodic tension-type headache*
          B) Increased pericranial tenderness on manual palpation
       2.1.2 Infrequent episodic tension-type headache not associated with pericranial tenderness
          A) Episodes fulfilling criteria A–E for 2.1 *Infrequent episodic tension-type headache*
          B) No increased pericranial tenderness
2.2 Frequent episodic tension-type headache
    [Same as 2.1 *Infrequent episodic tension-type headache* except
    A) At least 10 episodes occurring on ≥1 but <15 days per month for at least 3 months (≥12 and <180 days per year) and fulfilling criteria B–D]

TABLE 1–2 (*Continued*)

2.2.1   Frequent episodic tension-type headache associated with pericranial tenderness
2.2.2   Frequent episodic tension-type headache not associated with pericranial tenderness
2.3 Chronic tension-type headache
A) Headache occurring on ≥15 days per month on average for >3 months (≥180 days per year) and fulfilling criteria B–D
B) Headache lasts hours or may be continuous
C) Headache has at least two of the following characteristics:
   1. Bilateral location
   2. Pressing/tightening (non-pulsating) quality
   3. Mild or moderate intensity
   4. Not aggravated by routine physical activity such as walking or climbing stairs
D) Both of the following:
   1. No more than one of photophobia, phonophobia or mild nausea
   2. Neither moderate or severe nausea nor vomiting
E) Not attributed to another disorder
   ". . .2.3 *Chronic tension-type headache* evolves over time from episodic tension-type headache; when these criteria A–E are fulfilled by a headache that, unambiguously, is daily and unremitting within 3 days of its first onset, code as 4.8 *New daily-persistent headache.* When the manner of onset is not remembered or is otherwise uncertain, code as 2.3 *Chronic tension-type headache.* . . When medication overuse is present and fulfills criterion B for any of the subforms of 8.2 *Medication-overuse headache*, it is uncertain whether this criterion E is fulfilled until 2 months after medication has been withdrawn without improvement." (pp. 39–40)
   2.3.1   Chronic tension-type headache associated with pericranial tenderness
   2.3.2   Chronic tension-type headache not associated with pericranial tenderness
2.4 Probable chronic tension-type headache
[Same as for 2.3, *Chronic tension-type headache*, except:
E) Not attributed to another disorder but there is, or has been within the last 2 months, medication overuse fulfilling criterion B for any of the subforms of 8.2 *Medication overuse headache*.]
3.1 Cluster headache
A) At least 5 attacks fulfilling criteria B–D
B) Severe or very severe unilateral orbital, supraorbital and/or temporal pain lasting 15–180 minutes if untreated
C) Headache is accompanied by at least one of the following:
   1. Ipsilateral conjunctival injection and/or lacrimation
   2. Ipsilateral nasal congestion and/or rhinorrhea
   3. Ipsilateral eyelid edema
   4. Ipsilateral forehead and facial sweating
   5. Ipsilateral miosis and/or ptosis
   6. A sense of restlessness or agitation
D) Attacks have a frequency from one every other day to 8 per day
E) Not attributed to another disorder
   3.1.1   Episodic cluster headache
       A) Attacks fulfilling criteria A–E for 3.1 *Cluster headache*
       B) At least two cluster periods lasting 7–365 days and separated by pain-free remission periods of ≥1 month
   3.1.2   Chronic cluster headache
       A) Attacks fulfilling criteria A–E for 3.1 *Cluster headache*
       B) Attacks recur over >1 year without remission periods or with remission periods lasting <1 month
3.2 Paroxysmal hemicrania
A) At least 20 attacks fulfilling criteria B–D
B) Attacks of severe unilateral orbital, supraorbital or temporal pain lasting 2–30 minutes
C) Headache is accompanied by at least one of the following:
   1. Ipsilateral conjunctival injection and/or lacrimation
   2. Ipsilateral nasal congestion and/or rhinorrhea
   3. Ipsilateral eyelid edema

(continued)

TABLE 1–2 (*Continued*)

4. Ipsilateral forehead and facial sweating
5. Ipsilateral miosis and/or ptosis
6. A sense of restlessness or agitation

D) Attacks have a frequency above 5 per day for more than half of the time, although periods with lower frequency may occur
E) Attacks are prevented completely by therapeutic doses of indomethacin
F) Not attributed to another disorder

". . . In order to rule out incomplete response, indomethacin should be used in a dose of ≥150 mg daily orally or rectally, or ≥100 mg by injection, but for maintenance smaller doses are often sufficient" (p. 46)

3.2.1 Episodic paroxysmal hemicrania
    A) Attacks fulfilling criteria A–F for 3.2 *Paroxysmal hemicrania*
    B) At least two attack periods lasting 7–365 days and separated by pain-free remission periods of ≥1 month

3.2.2 Chronic paroxysmal hemicrania
    A) Attacks fulfilling criteria A–F for 3.2 *Paroxysmal hemicrania*
    B) Attacks recur over >1 year without remission periods or with remission periods lasting <1 month

3.4 Probable trigeminal autonomic cephalalgia
  A) Attacks fulfilling all but one of the specific criteria for one of the subtypes of trigeminal autonomic cephalalgia [e.g., cluster headache or paroxysmal hemicrania]
  B) Not attributed to another disorder
    3.4.1 Probable cluster headache
    3.4.2 Probable paroxysmal hemicrania

4.7 Hemicrania continua
  A) Headache for >3 months fulfilling criteria B–D
  B) All of the following characteristics:
    1. Unilateral pain without side-shift
    2. Daily and continuous, without pain-free periods
    3. Moderate intensity, but with exacerbations of severe pain
  C) At least one of the following autonomic features occurs during exacerbations and ipsilateral to the side of pain:
    1. Conjunctival injection and/or lacrimation
    2. Nasal congestion and/or rhinorrhea
    3. Ptosis and/or miosis
  D) Complete response to therapeutic doses of indomethacin
  E) Not attributed to another disorder

4.8 New daily persistent headache
  A) Headache for >3 months fulfilling criteria B–D
  B) Headache is daily and unremitting from onset or from <3 days from onset
  C) At least two of the following pain characteristics:
    1. Bilateral location
    2. Pressing/tightening (non-pulsating) quality
    3. Mild or moderate intensity
    4. Not aggravated by routine physical activity such as walking or climbing stairs
  D) Both of the following:
    1. No more than one of photophobia, phonophobia, or mild nausea
    2. Neither moderate or severe nausea nor vomiting
  E) Not attributed to another disorder

[Sections 5–12 of the IHS system are for headaches secondary to other disorders, such as arteritis, low cerebrospinal fluid pressure, viral infection, intracranial hematoma or neoplasm. Several of these, including headaches secondary to head trauma, to medication overuse, to temporomandibular joint disease, or to disorders of the neck, may come to the attention of psychologists.]

5.1 Acute post-traumatic headache
    5.1.1 Acute post-traumatic headache attributed to moderate or severe head injury
      A) Headache, no typical characteristics known, fulfilling criteria C and D

(*continued*)

TABLE 1–2 (*Continued*)

    B) Head trauma with at least one of the following:
        1. Loss of consciousness for >30 minutes
        2. Glasgow coma scale (GCS) <13
        3. Post-traumatic amnesia for >48 hours
        4. Imaging demonstration of a traumatic brain lesion (cerebral hematoma, intracerebral and/or subarachnoid hemorrhage, brain contusion and/or skull fracture)
    C) Headache develops within 7 days after head trauma or after regaining consciousness following head trauma
    D) One or other of the following:
        1. Headache resolves within 3 months after head trauma
        2. Headache persists but 3 months have not yet passed since head trauma

5.1.2 Acute post-traumatic headache attributed to mild head injury
[Same as for 5.1.1 *Acute post-traumatic headache attributed to moderate or severe head injury* except:
    B) Head trauma with all the following:
        1. Either no loss of consciousness, or loss of consciousness of <30 minutes' duration
        2. Glasgow Coma Scale (GCS) ≥13
        3. Symptoms and/or signs diagnostic of a concussion
    C) Headache develops within 7 days after head trauma]

5.2.1 Chronic post-traumatic headache attributed to moderate or severe head injury
5.2.2 Chronic post-traumatic headache attributed to mild head injury
[Same as for acute post-traumatic headache, but persisting for >3 months after injury]

5.3 Acute headache attributed to whiplash injury
  A) Headache, no typical characteristics known, fulfilling criteria C and D
  B) History of whiplash (sudden and significant acceleration/deceleration movement of the neck) associated at the time with neck pain
  C) Headache develops within 7 days after whiplash injury
  D) One or other of the following:
      1. Headache resolves within 3 months after whiplash injury
      2. Headache persists but 3 months have not yet passed since whiplash injury

5.4 Chronic headache attributed to whiplash injury
[Same as 5.3 *Acute headache attributed to whiplash injury* except
  D) Headache persists for >3 months after whiplash injury]

8.2 Medication-overuse headache (MOH) [Includes revisions from Silberstein, J. Olesen, et al. (2005)]
  A) Headache present on ≥15 days/month fulfilling criteria C and D:
  B) Regular overuse for >3 months of one or more drugs that can be taken for acute and/or symptomatic treatment of headache.
  C) Headache has developed or markedly worsened during medication overuse.
  D) Headache resolves or reverts to its previous pattern within 2 months after discontinuation of overused medication.

    8.2.1 Ergotamine-overuse headache
      A) Headache fulfilling criteria A, C and D for 8.2 *Medication-overuse headache*
      B) Ergotamine intake on ≥10 days/month on a regular basis for >3 months
    8.2.2 Triptan-overuse headache
      A) Headache fulfilling criteria A, C and D for 8.2 *Medication-overuse headache*.
      B) Triptan intake (any formulation) on ≥10 days/month on a regular basis for >3 months
    8.2.3 Analgesic-overuse headache
      A) Headache fulfilling criteria A, C and D for 8.2 *Medication-overuse headache*.
      B) Intake of simple analgesics on ≥15 days/month on a regular basis for >3 months
    8.2.4 Opioid-overuse headache
      A) Headache fulfilling criteria A, C and D for 8.2 *Medication-overuse headache*.
      B) Opioid intake on ≥10 days/month on a regular basis for >3 months
    8.2.5 Combination analgesic-overuse headache
      A) Headache fulfilling criteria A, C and D for 8.2 *Medication-overuse headache*.

(continued)

TABLE 1–2 (*Continued*)

B) Intake of combination medications on ≥10 days/month on a regular basis for >3 months
"Combination medications typically implicated are those containing simple analgesics combined with opioids, butalbital and/or caffeine" (p. 95)

8.2.6 Medication-overuse headache attributed to combination of acute medications
- A) Headache fulfilling criteria A, C and D for 8.2 *Medication-overuse headache*.
- B) Intake of any combination of ergotamine, triptans, analgesics and/or opioids on ≥10 days/month on a regular basis for >3 months without overuse of any single class alone.

8.2.7 Headache attributed to other medication overuse
- A) Headache fulfilling criteria A, C and D for 8.2 *Medication-overuse headache*.
- B) Regular overuse for >3 months of a medication other than those described above.

8.2.8 Probable medication-overuse headache
- A) Headache fulfilling criteria A and C for 8.2 *Medication-overuse headache*.
- B) Medication overuse fulfilling criterion B for any one of the subforms 8.2.1–8.2.7
- C) One or other of the following:
  1. Overused medication has not yet been withdrawn
  2. Medication overuse has ceased within the last 2 months but headache has not so far resolved or reverted to its previous pattern

  ". . .Many patients fulfilling the criteria for 8.2.8 *Probable medication-overuse headache al*so fulfill criteria for either 1.6.5 *Probable chronic migraine* or 2.4.3 *Probable chronic tension-type headache*. They should be coded for both until causation is established after withdrawal of the overused medication. Patients with 1.6.5 *Probable chronic migraine* should additionally be coded for the antecedent migraine subtype (usually 1.1 *Migraine without aura*)." (Silberstein, J. Olesen, et al., 2005, p. 462)

11.2 Headache attributed to disorder of neck

11.2.1 Cervicogenic Headache
- A) Pain, referred from a source in the neck and perceived in one or more regions of the head and/or face, fulfilling criteria C and D
- B) Clinical, laboratory and/or imaging evidence of a disorder or lesion within the cervical spine or soft tissues of the neck known to be, or generally accepted as, a valid cause of headache
- C) Evidence that the pain can be attributed to the neck disorder or lesion based on at least one of the following:
  1. Demonstration of clinical signs that implicate a source of pain in the neck
  2. Abolition of headache following diagnostic blockade of a cervical structure or its nerve supply using placebo- or other adequate controls
- D) Pain resolves within 3 months after successful treatment of the causative disorder or lesion

  ". . .cervical spondylosis and osteochondritis are NOT accepted as valid causes fulfilling criterion B. When myofascial tender spots are the cause, the headache should be coded under 2. *Tension-type headache*" (p. 115)

11.7 Headache or facial pain attributed to temporomandibular joint (TMJ) disorder
- A) Recurrent pain in one or more regions of the head and/or face fulfilling criteria C and D
- B) X-ray, MRI and/or bone scintigraphy demonstrate TMJ disorder
- C) Evidence that pain can be attributed to the TMJ disorder, based on at least one of the following:
  1. Pain is precipitated by jaw movements and/or chewing of hard or tough food
  2. Reduced range of or irregular jaw opening
  3. Noise from one or both TMJs during jaw movements
  4. Tenderness of the joint capsule(s) of one or both TMJs
- D) Headache resolves within 3 months, and does not recur, after successful treatment of the TMJ disorder

12.1 Headache attributed to somatization disorder

12.2 Headache attributed to psychotic disorder

13.1 Trigeminal neuralgia

13.1.1 Classical trigeminal neuralgia
- A) Paroxysmal attacks of pain lasting from a fraction of a second to 2 minutes, affecting one or more divisions of the trigeminal nerve and fulfilling criteria B and C
- B) Pain has at least one of the following characteristics
  1. Intense, sharp, superficial or stabbing
  2. Precipitated from trigger areas or by trigger factors

(continued)

TABLE 1–2 (*Continued*)

	C)	Attacks are stereotyped in the individual patient
	D)	There is no clinically evident neurological deficit
	E)	Not attributed to another disorder
13.8		Occipital neuralgia

13.8 Occipital neuralgia

    A) Paroxysmal stabbing pain, with or without persistent aching between paroxysms, in the distribution(s) of the greater, lesser and/or third occipital nerves

    B) Tenderness over the affected nerve

    C) Pain is eased temporarily by local anesthetic block of the neck

       "Occipital neuralgia must be distinguished from occipital referral of pain from the atlantoaxial or upper zygapophyseal joints or from tender trigger points in neck muscles or their insertions" (p. 128)

Note. Excerpted from "International Classification of Headache Disorders (2nd ed.)," by the Headache Classification Subcommittee of the International Headache Society, 2004, *Cephalalgia, 24* (Supplement 1). Copyright 2004 by the International Headache Society. Reprinted with permission.

TABLE 1–3
Supplemental Nosology for Chronic Daily Headache (N. T. Mathew, 1997a)

  I. Chronic tension-type

  II. Migraine chronic tension-type headache complex

    A. Transformed migraine

      1. With analgesic overuse

      2. Without analgesic overuse

    B. Evolved from tension-type headache

      1. With analgesic overuse

      2. Without analgesic overuse

  III. New persistent daily headache

  IV. Cervicogenic headache

    A. Idiopathic

    B. Post-neck trauma

  V. Post-head trauma headache

    A. With migrainous features

    B. Without migrainous features

Note. From "Transformed Migraine, Analgesic Rebound, and Other Chronic Daily Headaches," by N. T. Mathew, 1997, *Neurologic Clinics, 15*(1), p. 168. Copyright 1997 W. B. Saunders Co. Reprinted with permission.

or room lighting, that seems particularly characteristic. The person looks and feels ill during a migraine episode.

At least five migraine attacks are required before the person is considered to have the disorder, unless the attacks are preceded by an aura—fully reversible neurological symptoms that develop gradually or successively over at least five minutes, or that are unilateral on the body or in the visual field. In case of aura, only two attacks are needed for diagnosis. The usual symptoms are visual—scintillating lines or patches, and/or blind spots. But the same types of symptoms may be translated into the somatosensory realm: a region of tingling, or of diminished sensation. Auras often "march" across the field of vision, or down an arm or leg. Temporary dysphasic speech disturbance (e.g., difficulty finding words) may also be an aura symptom. (Retinal Migraine is very similar to other migraines with visual aura, except that the aura symptoms are in one eye rather than one visual field.)

Motor aura symptoms (e.g., Hemiplegic Migraine) such as reversible weakness are especially important to note because they point to possible medication options that are ineffective (acetazolamide) or only moderately effective (verapamil) in the more common types of migraine. We will discuss medications in detail in Chapter 11.

Similarly, basilar-type aura symptoms such as dysarthria, **vertigo**, **tinnitus**, diminished hearing, double vision, aura occurring in both visual fields or on both sides of the body, ataxia, or decreased consciousness are important to note, as they may indicate that vasoconstrictive acute migraine medications are not warranted (Silberstein, Saper, & Freitag, 2001). Most important of all, of course, are aura symptoms that do not fully reverse; these require prompt medical work-up.

Besides current frequency, duration, and intensity, which are best gathered from a headache diary, described in Chapter 12, we should ask about changes in occurrence over time. A pattern of increasing headache frequency should motivate intensive treatment, even if a lesion has been excluded and even if most of the headaches are tension-type. For here we may have the opportunity to prevent evolution to **transformed migraine**, chronic daily headache. Overuse of acute medications, recent major life stresses, and certain other factors, discussed below, also carry risk for chronic daily headache. Significant disability and, possibly, major depression, suggest a more refractory disorder, for which a higher intensity of treatment may be indicated.

We may inquire, too, of the extent to which the patient is aware of triggers, circumstances of onset, and early signs of impending headache. Is there a clear prodrome, with changes in mood (e.g., elation, irritability, dysphoria), appetite, or bodily functions (e.g., diarrhea, diuresis, water retention, feeling unwell, a progressive coolness at the hands)? Do the migraines reliably follow stress by a given period of time, possibly as long as 3 or 4 days? Do the migraines occur preferentially in certain high pressure or overly stimulating environments, or after predictable changes in routine? In Chapter 10, we will look at triggers much more closely, and in Chapter 12 we will discuss a format by which a person with headaches can become more aware of the patterns. Here, our interest is on the degree to which the migraines are experienced as being predictable and controllable.

The history of pharmacological and other interventions can be helpful, for understanding the patient's story, and often for identifying surprising gaps in treatment. Remember, too, that "when nothing has worked, everything can still work"—that is, treatments that have failed as single modalities may be effective as parts of a multidisciplinary approach (Duckro, W. Richardson, J. E. Marshall, Cassabaum, & G. Marshall, 1999).

Tension-type Headaches are much of what migraines are not. The pain has at least two of: bilateral location, pressing or tightening (not pulsating) quality, mild or moderate intensity, without aggravation by routine physical activity. The person may lose their appetite, and in chronic forms may have mild nausea, but moderate or severe nausea, or vomiting, exclude the diagnosis. So, too, would an aversion to both light and conversational sound levels.

The duration can vary widely—from 30 minutes to 7 days in the criteria—as can frequency. When the headaches average less than 1 day a month (infrequent episodic tension-type headache) they are unlikely to come to professional attention. When they occur at least one day a month but less than half the month they may be more troublesome, but still fall within the rubric of (frequent) episodic tension-type headache. Chronic tension-type headache occurs at least 15 days a month, on average, for at least three months, and is thus a subset of chronic daily headache.

With tension-type headache, we enter the murky borderland between muscle problems, pain sensitization, and uncommon but important emotional comorbidities. Thus, in part we want to be alert to signs of myofascial pain—restricted neck range of motion, a clenched jaw, a chronically tense, corrugated forehead, or continuously hunched shoulders, perhaps with signs of ergonomic problems at home or in the workplace. Secondly, we want to note whether the person's pericranial region is sensitive to pressure—they may report a tender, bruised feeling, or pressure from their pillow or hand may bring on a headache, or even combing their hair may be painful. From still a third perspective, we want to gauge how the person handles the pain. Do they think about it constantly? Does it make them fearful, depressed, ruminative, or downtrodden? Are clinical depression and/or an anxiety disorder present? All of these may need to be addressed if treatment is to be successful. If the headache is worsened by stress or concentration, it may make outside stressors feel more negative, impactful, and uncontrollable, potentially leading to a vicious cycle of stress exacerbation (Ehde & Holm, 1992; Holm, K. A. Holroyd, Hursey, & Penzien, 1986). Thus, the person's main stressors and characteristic ways of handling them should also be assessed.

As with migraines, the degree to which a person is aware of their headache patterns—the conditions that trigger or exacerbate, the earliest symptoms or warning signs—and any skills they have developed for preventing them, are important to note as is, of course, the treatment history.

Chronic Tension-type Headaches can be intermittent but frequent, or continuous and unremitting. In the latter case they should be distinguished from New Daily Persistent Headache (NDPH), which is identical to a chronic tension-type headache except that NDPH is continuous from within three days of onset. In contrast, chronic tension-type headache evolves from episodic tension-type headache over weeks, months, or years.

Chronic daily headaches are, in large majority, chronic tension-type headaches in their clinical appearance, with or without migrainous exacerbations, and will often have evolved from episodic tension-type headache or migraine. Chronic Migraine can also occur, however, in which prototypical migraine attacks occur on at least half the days of the month, on average, for at least three months.

We want to be alert, too, for the symptoms of *Hemicrania Continua*: pain that is continuous, always on the same side, moderate with severe exacerbations, and accompanied by at least one autonomic sign on the same side as the pain. Autonomic signs may include nasal congestion or runny nose, tearing or conjunctival injection, pupillary constriction or a drooping of the upper eyelid. Detecting possible hemicrania continua is important because of an additional diagnostic criterion: For unknown reasons, the disorder *always* responds to therapeutic doses of indomethacin.

When we encounter chronic daily headache, or a history of increasing frequency of migraine or tension-type headache suggesting transformation to a chronic state, then we should also look carefully for known and suspected risk factors. These include high use of symptomatic (vasoconstrictive and analgesic) medications (S.-R. Lu, Fuh, W. T. Chen, Juang, & S. J. Wang, 2001; S. J. Wang, Fuh, C. Y. Liu, Hsu, P. N. Wang, & H. C. Liu, 2000; Zwart, Dyb, K. Hagen, Svebak, & J. Holmen, 2003), low socioeconomic status (K. Hagen, Vatten, Stovner, Zwart, Krokstad, & Bovim, 2002), being divorced, widowed, or separated (Scher, Stewart, Ricci, & Lipton, 2003), or (other) recent history of major **life events**-type stress (Stewart, Scher, & Lipton, 2001). Also predictive are physical variables such as obesity, diabetes, and, independently, frequent snoring or sleep problems (Scher, Lipton, & Stewart, 2002; Scher, Stewart, & Lipton, 2002; Scher, Stewart, Ricci, & Lipton, 2003). Addressing these factors is a logical part of treatment, even though their causal role has not been definitely established.

Here, too, the person's awareness of triggers and patterns of exacerbation is important to assess, for a part of treatment is making the headaches more predictable and, ultimately, preventable.

The pain in *Cluster Headaches* is unilateral, severe or very severe, relatively brief (15–180 minutes untreated) and located in or above the eye, or at the temple. The attacks occur from once every two days to eight per day, and are accompanied by a sense of restlessness or agitation, and/or at least one autonomic sign on the same side as the pain: swelling or drooping of the eyelid, constriction of the pupil, forehead and facial sweating, nasal congestion or runny nose, tearing or conjunctival injection. The patient must have had at least five such attacks to be diagnosed with certainty.

The relatively short duration, quick onset and offset, frequent, often clock-like occurrence, and agitation seem to distinguish cluster headaches. The unilateral tearing, runny nose, congestion, or eyelid drooping, although striking, can occur with migraines too (where they may suggest the efficacy of intranasal lidocaine), and even with myofascial pain or a neck injury. Thus, the autonomic symptoms should not necessarily generate a diagnosis of cluster headache, and even less a diagnosis of "cluster-migraine," commonly used in some communities. Moreover, when the attacks are quite frequent (above five per day for more than half the time), brief (2–30 minutes), and there have been more than 20 of them, then we must consider *Paroxysmal Hemicrania*—a disorder in which headaches are completely preventable by therapeutic doses of indomethacin.

The treatment of cluster headaches has largely been the domain of medications, but there is circumstantial evidence for smoking and alcohol as risk factors, and for vasodilation (e.g., hot baths) and possibly the letdown following strong emotions as trigger factors (L. Kudrow, 1993). The role of behavioral treatment has not been well defined for cluster headaches, but locating gaps in treatment, identifying and changing triggers and risk factors, and cognitive-behavioral work in pain tolerance are all logical elements.

Post-traumatic Headaches have no known characteristic symptoms, except that they develop within 7 days after a head trauma. The trauma may be mild, and indicated only by "symptoms and/or signs diagnostic of concussion." (Headache Classification Subcommittee, 2004, p. 60). Thus, for treatment we need supplementary information. Did the accident give rise to **Posttraumatic Stress Disorder**? Is the course complicated by overuse of analgesic or acute migraine medications? Are other post-concussive symptoms generating stress, life disruption, or emotional upset? Are cognitive symptoms, such as difficulty concentrating, compounded by avoidance, out of fear of betraying deficits, or of having to face that basic skills have been lost? Some patients, healthy except for the headaches, seem to see themselves as profoundly disabled after attending rehabilitation alongside severely brain-injured people. Very high levels of pericranial muscle tension, especially in the frontalis region, can be missed without specific assessment such as surface **electromyography** (discussed in Chapter 12).

For all headaches, it is helpful to know the amount, pattern, and changes over time in medication use, from which overuse, misuse, and gaps in treatment can often be identified. Preventive medication trials should have been for a minimum of 4 weeks, and are not valid when symptomatic medications are being overused at the same time. The refractoriness of the headaches to appropriate medication is useful in gauging the degree to which intervention may need to be multidisciplinary, and/or include chronic pain **coping**.

Headache-related disability is also important, as a reflection of the impact of headaches, as an outcome measure, and as an indication of natural history. For disability, once acquired, does not appear to resolve on its own. In a prospective population study, 92 percent of people with moderate or high disability from headaches were still disabled 3 years later. Only 12 percent of non-disabled headache subjects became disabled over the same time period (Von Korff, Ormel, Keefe, & Dworkin, 1992). Thus, it is useful to know the number of days of absenteeism from work, school, and household activities, especially in migraine and chronic daily headache. Absenteeism is less likely in episodic tension-type headache, but should be checked all the same. Perceived impairment and reduced effectiveness is also relevant, but its estimation may be influenced by mood. For their validation and standardization, psychometrics are useful for quantifying disability, and are covered in Chapter 12.

We should also note signs of pain sensitization: reported tenderness to reasonably light pressure, whether this is localized to the head or present throughout the body, and specific to the headache state (most common in migraines) or continuous (most common in chronic tension-type headaches).

And although the vast majority of persons with chronic headaches do not have a psychiatric condition, the interview should include a screening for the more common comorbidities, including clinical depression, generalized anxiety, and panic disorder. Here, too, psychometrics are useful, and are discussed in Chapter 12.

Certain constructs from the chronic pain field are useful for headaches as well. How confidently does the patient cope with pain, how versatile and resourceful are they in reducing it, and how involved are they with non-pain activities? Catastrophic thinking and fear of pain may be particularly important in medication overuse. They can be gauged psychometrically, and may need to be reassessed periodically as treatment proceeds. At the interview, frequent and intrusive **pain behaviors** may suggest pain-related anxiety, or that the person has fallen into an illness role.

Thus, it is helpful to use the interview to establish the type of chronic benign headache we are dealing with, and then to get a fuller sense of its context. This information will allow us to draw from the basic and applied literature in developing a treatment plan. In the pages that follow, we will explore this literature, on headaches, and on pain in general, deeply. Then, better grounded, we will return to a more detailed discussion of clinical assessment and treatment.

CHAPTER 2

Pain Neurophysiology and Perception

> *Nerve injuries maintain an evolutionary potential . . . Clinical calm does not mean that all is done. Time does not exist for our tissues.*
> —Leriche, 1951, p. 1281 (cited in Schott, 2001)

Amber's husband is incarcerated now, but for 10 years, at random times, he would beat her until she was nearly unconscious. She slept poorly, hated to be at home, and assumed that one day he would accidentally kill her. In an odd way she felt sorry for him. When he went to jail she could first glimpse a life without fear, but over the next few months she grew progressively more fatigued, weak, and painful. Within a year she had been diagnosed with fibromyalgia and lupus, an autoimmune disorder.

By what process does a keen, vigorous person, poised before life's pleasures and goals, develop chronic pain? How does one back strain, one sinus infection, one migraine too many, lead in one stroke, or with imperceptible subtlety, to a course of futile x-rays, desperate surgeries, and medications that at best merely palliate? What happened to this person's path through life? Through what trapdoor did they fall?

In this chapter and the next, we will explore this topic systematically, first on the biological plane, and then on the psychological. We will seek out the processes that underlie conversion from the acute to chronic state, and find clues at every level, from receptors in the skin to the highest levels of cortex. We will find that the potential for chronic pain is inherent in the **nociceptive** system. The knowledge we gain will have bearing on preventing chronic pain, and on reversing it insofar as possible.

DETECTING HARM

In introductory courses we learn that noxious stimuli are transduced by "free nerve endings" in the skin (e.g., R. J. Sternberg, 1998). But how can a simple nerve ending, with no specialized sensory apparatus, transduce anything at all? The answer, at least for the skin and at least for certain stimuli, is the vanilloid receptor, VR1 (Julius & Basbaum, 2001). On its most primitive level, VR1 is an ion channel—a pore—found on sensory nerves (Caterina & Julius, 2001). Warming the cell membrane above 45 °C, the heat pain threshold, causes the pore to open. This allows positively charged ions such as sodium, potassium, magnesium, and especially calcium to rush inside, bringing the neuron closer to firing (Caterina, Schumacher, Tominaga, T. A. Rosen, J. Levine, & Julius, 1997). Thus, VR1 channels enable the neuron to detect noxious levels of heat.

But VR1 is also complicated: In the presence of acid (injured tissue is acidic) VR1 opens at lower temperatures, down to 35 °C, making even body temperature feel painfully hot (Caterina &

Julius, 2001). A chemical, **prostaglandin** E_2, produced by injured tissue as part of the inflammatory response, has the same effect. No wonder inflammatory pain is a burning sensation, and can be relieved by ice. The channel is opened, too, by capsaicin, a chemical that resembles vanilla structurally, and that gives chili peppers their ability to produce pain (Julius & Basbaum, 2001). Naturally, pharmaceutical companies have taken a keen interest in blocking VR1 (Cortright & Szallasi, 2004; Szallasi & Appendino, 2004).

In contrast, little is known about the receptor for pressure pain, except that it is thought to be a nonselective ion channel like VR1 (J. Hu, Milenkovic, & Lewin, 2006). Presumably, the channels are structured in such as way as to open when the axonal membrane is deformed by outside forces.

Here in the skin, far from the synapses of the central nervous system, we can begin to see the transition from acute to chronic pain. For in certain chronic pain conditions, the DNA for VR1 may be over-transcribed, causing a greater concentration of vanilloid receptors in the cell membrane (Cortright & Szallasi, 2004). This implies that chronic pain is not simply a psychological condition. We will see below, however, how psychology interweaves the process at many points.

Now, only a few structures in the head are pain-sensitive that they could be a source of headaches. There is the skin, of course, and the pericranial muscles. Inside the cranium there is the dura mater, especially around its arteries and the venous sinuses. The extracranial blood vessels and the large arteries within the brain are similarly sufficiently innervated to play a role in headache pain (G. Solomon, 1999). All of these structures are potential entrance points for toxins or mechanical insult. It is not surprising that a warning system such as pain receptors would be stationed mostly at the gates (Moskowitz, 1991).

The pain signal is then conveyed to the central nervous system by two types of sensory nerve fibers: myelinated fibers, called **Aδ**, that transmit the pain signal relatively quickly, and unmyelinated **C fibers** that transmit the pain relatively slowly. Now one may ask, what is the biological use of a nerve that transmits pain information *slowly*? In fact, C fibers have two rather unique properties that make them quite useful indeed.

The first is found at the distal end, where the nerve endings pick up information on noxious levels of pressure (**mechanoreceptors**), or noxious levels of pressure, heat, or chemicals (polymodal nociceptors). Although the primary role of the nerve endings is to transduce the noxious stimulation, they also contain **neuropeptides** such as **substance P** and **calcitonin gene-related peptide** (Davidoff, 1998). When the nerve endings are sufficiently activated they release these chemicals, causing inflammation, sensitizing nearby pain receptors, and causing the leakage (**extravasation**) of proteins out of the plasma and into blood vessel walls, which then swell. After injury other chemicals can sensitize pain receptors (Davidoff, 1998), including **bradykinin** (from the plasma), **serotonin** (from the platelets), and certain **prostaglandins** (locally acting hormones produced by tissue in response to an injury). The area shifts to a hyperalgesic, pain-sensitive state. But the neuropeptides released by the nerve endings of C fibers are particularly important because they set up a positive feedback loop: The receptors, when stimulated, sensitize other, nearby receptors. And as we shall see in Chapter 4, this process seems to play a key role in migraines. (See Figure 2–1).

The second unusual property of C fibers is found at their proximal end, where they synapse with the spinal cord. We will discuss this property shortly.

Thus, injury does not merely stimulate nociceptors, it also sensitizes them. This hints at a key difference between acute and chronic pain: With chronicity, the pain system itself has been altered. But sensitization of nerve endings takes place and subsides quickly. To appreciate the full scope of plasticity, we must follow the sensory pathways along their course.

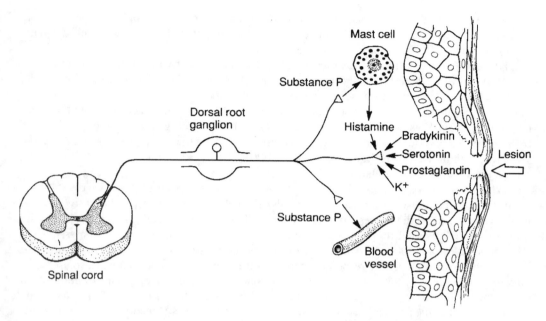

FIGURE 2–1.   Pain pathways from peripheral C-fiber to the dorsal horn. Notice that some sensory nerve endings not only transduce noxious stimuli, they also secrete chemicals such as substance P and calcitonin gene-related peptide. These chemicals dilate blood vessels, stimulate mast cells to release histamine, and sensitize nearby nerve endings. From "Pain and Analgesia," by T. M. Jessell and D. D. Kelly, 1991, in E. R. Kandel, J. H. Schwartz, and T. M. Jessell (Eds.), *Principles of Neural Science* (3rd edition, page 387), Norwalk, CT: Appleton and Lange. Copyright 1991 by Appleton and Lange. Reprinted with permission.

SENSORY NERVES

Recall that sensory nerves have projections in one direction, to the structures they innervate, and projections in the other direction, to the central nervous system. In between these two projections are the cell bodies, which for the head are found in the trigeminal ganglion (also called the Gasserian ganglion), inside the skull at around the level of the ear. For sensory nerves in the rest of the body, the equivalent structures are the dorsal root ganglia, which run alongside the length of the spine (see Figure 2–1).

Now there are few synapses within the trigeminal ganglion. However, it seems that the cell bodies themselves, when stimulated, secrete a neurotransmitter, calcitonin gene-related peptide (Ulrich-Lai, Flores, Harding-Rose, Goodis, & Hargreaves, 2001). We do not know yet what the target of this neurotransmitter is. It might be the blood vessels, so that the blood supply to the ganglion is increased when its nerves are more active. Alternatively however, it might be neighboring nerve cell bodies, lowering their threshold for firing (Ulrich-Lai et al.).

But there is more: Recall that nerve cells communicate with each other by firing: Action potentials travel down the axon, releasing neurotransmitter into the synapse. The action potential is a chain reaction, kindling down the nerve cell on a bed of voltage-gated sodium channels in the cell membrane. If part of the nerve cell is slightly depolarized (say, its interior is raised from $-65\,\text{mV}$ to $-40\,\text{mV}$ by stimulation from neighboring cells) its sodium channels open. The inrush of positively charged sodium ions further depolarizes that part of the neuron, thus opening more sodium channels. In this way, the leading edge of the action potential propagates itself down the axon (M. F. Bear, B. W. Connors, & Paradiso, 2001).

However, human beings have at least eight different types of voltage-gated sodium channels, and not all of them produce action potentials (Waxman, 1999). There are, for example, SNS–2 channels, found only in sensory nerves ("SNS" stands for "sensory nerve specific").[1] These channels have a window of activation between -70 and -45 mV. This upper end of depolarization, -45 mV, is below the threshold, -40 mV, for triggering action potentials. Instead, SNS–2 channels produce waves of slight depolarization along the cell bodies (Waxman, 1999; Waxman, Cummins, Dib-Hajj, & J. A. Black, 2000). The neuron, although nominally at rest, reverberates with subtle oscillations.

What is the purpose of these silent oscillations? Note that the crests of these waves, -45 mV, are just below the threshold for action potentials. The cell would thus respond best to pulses of input that coincide with the crests of its own waves. In this way, the cell's subthreshold oscillations tune it to respond to a particular input frequency, and to fire at this same frequency (Hutcheon & Yarom, 2000; Waxman, 1999). This property is useful in the auditory system, of course, where we want cells to respond to particular frequencies of sound. But it is also useful for information processing more generally, by coordinating the behavior of groups of cells, all of them tuned to the same firing frequency (Hutcheon & Yarom, 2000; Llinás, 2001). This tuning may even underlie the particular coordination we call consciousness (Meador, P. G. Ray, Echauz, Loring, & Vachtsevanos, 2002).

Now, inflammation does more than sensitize nerve endings. The inflamed tissue—especially the Schwann cells surrounding neurons and the **macrophages** drawn to the site of injury—also produces higher amounts of nerve growth factors. These chemicals facilitate healing, but they also increase the number of SNS–2 channels in the cell bodies of pain nerves (Kawamoto & Matsuda, 2004; Waxman, 1999; Waxman, Cummins, et al., 2000).[2] Moreover, injured tissue produces prostaglandin E_2, a locally acting hormone. Prostaglandin E_2 starts a chain of events ending in a structural change—phosphorylation—in the SNS–2 channels, strengthening them (Julius & Basbaum, 2001). As a result, the cell bodies oscillate more readily. And because the voltages crest just below the threshold for action potentials, the cells also fire more readily. And unlike the sensitization of nerve endings, this sensitization of the trigeminal ganglion lasts on the order of months, or longer (Waxman, Cummins, et al.).

Thus, inflammation increases the number and strength of SNS–2 sodium channels in **nociceptive** neurons. In contrast, direct nerve injury cuts a neuron off from nerve growth factors, and the number of SNS–2 channels drops. But in their place, another type of voltage-gated sodium channel, α-III, appears (also termed the $Na_v 1.3$ channel; Waxman, 1999; Waxman, Cummins, et al., 2000). The presence of these channels is abnormal; they are usually found only in embryos (Waxman, Kocsis, & J. A. Black, 1994; J. N. Wood, Boorman, Okuse, & M. D. Baker, 2004). It is as if the neuron, trying to regenerate itself, returns to an earlier stage of development. In the process, enough α-III channels are produced that the injured cell fires more easily. And α-III channels are unusual in that they can sustain very high rates of firing.

Thus, **nociceptive** pain (from tissue damage, inflammation) and neuropathic pain (from nerve damage) involve sensitization, but of different types. And they feel different: In the quick,

---

[1]In recent, standardized nomenclature, SNS-2 channels have been renamed $Na_v 1.9$ channels (A. Goldin et al., 2000).

[2]In some species, nerve growth factors are also secreted in the saliva, which is probably one reason animals lick their wounds (A. K. Li et al., 1980).

sharp stabbing of **neuralgia** (literally, "nerve pain"), one can feel intuitively the spontaneous discharge of an injured nerve. In contrast, the steady burn of inflammation feels like a heightened sensitivity to heat.

It is no surprise at this point, that drugs such as lidocaine or amitriptyline, which inactivate vanilloid receptors and voltage-gated sodium channels, also tend to block neuropathic pain (Catterall & Mackie, 2001; Hirota, Smart, & D. G. Lambert, 2003; G. K. Wang, C. Russell, & S.-Y. Wang, 2004).

Notice that the pain system has changed its threshold—in a sense, it has stored information about past injury—and we have not yet even reached the first synapse! There will be more information storage, of course, when we enter the central nervous system.

At the level of peripheral nerves, we might expect little influence from psychological variables. But, for poorly understood reasons, **norepinephrine**, important in the stress response, increases the oscillations of damaged nerves (Xing, S.-J. Hu, Jian, Duan, 2003). And because these nerves are already sensitized by the α-III channels, each crest of oscillation can in theory become an action potential, causing the damaged cell to fire spontaneously (Xing et al.).

This is one explanation for "sympathetic-sensory coupling"—the **stress** sensitivity seen in neuropathic pain. Patients with **post-herpetic neuralgia** or **reflex sympathetic dystrophy** sometimes report that a few seconds after being startled, they feel an "echo" of pain. In session, they may wince when discussing a stressful topic. Noticing this pattern, and gaining control over it with relaxation skills, can be the beginning of **self-efficacy**—a sense of confidence in one's handling of the pain that is itself therapeutic.

Although we have just begun our journey in understanding pain, the knowledge so far can help us understand our patients' conditions. "Pain," we have seen, is not an undifferentiated construct, but is comprised of at least two subtypes, nociceptive and neuropathic, with different symptoms. We have seen, too, at least here in the periphery, that chronic pain is not an illusion of the psyche, but a shift in threshold of the sensory apparatus. Yet, neither is the psyche absent, for the changes that give rise to neuropathic pain can also make the pain sensitive to the level of stress, fear, or anxiety.

Not all pain, however, is nociceptive or neuropathic. The story is not complete. We must continue down the sensory nerves, to their connections with spine and brain.

TRIGEMINAL NUCLEUS, DORSAL HORN, AND PAIN SENSITIVITY

Now the fibers of the trigeminal nerve go on to enter the brain at the level of the pons, and then head downward to the medulla, where they synapse in the trigeminal nucleus. More specifically, it is in the **caudal** portion of the trigeminal nucleus, and in the adjacent **dorsal horn** of the spinal column at C1 and C2,[3] that pain signals from the head are first truly processed (Goadsby, 1995). (See Figure 2–2). The dorsal horn is part of the gray matter that runs down the center of the spinal cord (see Figure 2–3). The **trigeminal nucleus caudalis** is an extention of the dorsal horn into the lower **brain stem**. It resembles the dorsal horn structurally, and is sometimes called the "medullary dorsal horn" as a result (Craig & Dostrovsky, 1999). At the C1-C2 level, the dorsal horn processes pain signals from the neck, while the trigeminal nucleus processes signals from the head. However, the trigeminal nucleus and the C1-C2 dorsal horns appear to be functionally

---

[3]That is, the dorsal horn at the first and second cervical vertebrae. There is a dorsal horn at each vertebral level, processing signals from the incoming somatosensory nerves.

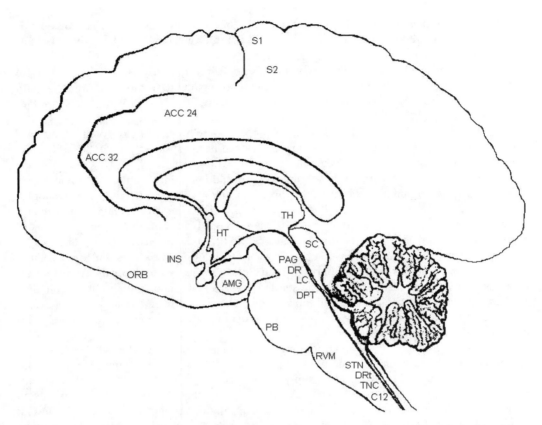

FIGURE 2–2.   Brain (mid-sagittal view), with the main pain processing structures. [a]structure is located in mid-brain; [b]structure is in pons; [c]in medulla; [d]in upper spinal cord. [e]The insula, an inner gyrus of cortex, is a large area beneath the fissure separating the frontal and temporal lobes.

   S1: Primary Somatosensory Cortex; S2: Secondary Somatosensory Cortex; ACC 24: Anterior Cingulate Cortex (Caudal Portion, Brodmann Area 24); ACC 32: Anterior Cingulate Cortex (Rostral Portion, Brodmann Area 32); TH: Lateral and Medial Thalamus; HT: Hypothalmus; SC: Superior Colliculus[a]; PAG: Periaqueductal Gray[a]; INS: Insular Cortex[e]; DR: Dorsal Raphe Nucleus[a]; AMG: Amygdala; LC: Locus Coeruleus[b]; DPT: Dorsal Pontine Tegmentum[b]; ORB: Orbital Frontal Cortex; PB: Parabrachial Nucleus[b]; RVM: Rostral Ventromedial Medulla[c]; STN: Solitary Tract Nucleus[c]; DRt: Dorsal Reticular Nucleus[c]; TNC: Trigeminal Nucleus Caudalis[c]; C12: C1-C2 Dorsal Horn[d].

integrated (Angus-Leppan, G. A. Lambert, & Michalicek, 1997; Edmeads, 1988; Goadsby, 1995). Thus, neck pain can spread into the head, and headaches can involve soreness in the neck.

   Because of their close similarity, we will refer interchangeably to the dorsal horn and the trigeminal nucleus caudalis. What is true of one structure should, in general, be true of the other.

   The primary excitatory neurotransmitter in theses structures appears to be **glutamate** (Storer & Goadsby, 1999). In one theory, chronic pain is due to an excess of glutamate, perhaps a failure of its reuptake from the synapse, which allows ongoing stimulation of the pain pathways. In fact, the glutamate concentration in cerebrospinal fluid *is* elevated in two chronic pain conditions, **fibromyalgia** and chronic migraine, and correlates with average pain intensity in the latter ($r \approx$ 0.55; Peres, Zukerman, Senne Soares, Alonso, Santos, & Faulhaber, 2004; Sarchielli, Alberti, A. L. Floridi, Mazzotta, & A. R. Floridi, 2004).

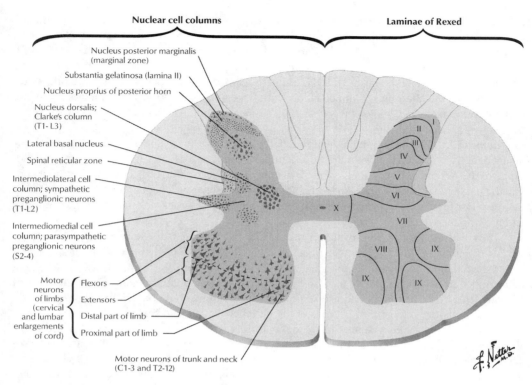

FIGURE 2–3.   Cross section of the spinal cord, showing the gray matter. The dorsal horn corresponds to lamina I through VI. The two most superficial layers, laminae I and II, process nociceptive signals. From *The Ciba Collection of Medical Illustrations. Vol. 1. Nervous System, Part I. Anatomy and Physiology*, A. Brass and R. V. Dingles (Eds.), illustrated by F. H. Netter. West Caldwell, NJ: Ciba Pharmaceutical Company. Copyright by Netter Images/Elsevier. Reprinted with permission.

A key inhibitory transmitter in the trigeminal nucleus caudalis is **serotonin** (Storer & Goadsby, 1999). If we draw analogy to other levels of the dorsal horn, inhibitory neurotransmitters would also include gamma-amino butyric acid (GABA), whose effects last long enough to cumulate over time (temporal summation), and briefer-acting **glycine** (Furue, Katafuchi, & Yoshimura, 2004; Woolf & Salter, 2000). Also involved in inhibition would be the **enkephalins** and **endorphins**, adenosine,[4] and adrenaline, acting via α_2 **adrenoreceptors** in the spinal cord (Pertovaara, 2000).

All of these neurotransmitters are potential targets for drug treatments of chronic pain. So far, medications have mostly potentiated the inhibitory neurotransmitters: narcotics to mimic endorphins, tricyclics and combined **norepinephrine**/serotonin reuptake inhibitors to increase

---

[4]Thus, we might expect that caffeine, an adenosine receptor blocker that readily crosses the blood-brain barrier (Fredholm, 1995) would increase pain sensitivity. In fact, caffeine seems instead to *reduce* pain, at least the type of pain that arises from **ischemia** (Sawynok, 1998). It seems that adenosine receptors are found on sensory nerve terminals in the periphery, and on **mast cells**, where they facilitate pain transduction (Sawynok, 1998). This pain enhancing effect of adenosine usually outweighs any analgesia that might come from its inhibitory role in the spine. Thus, caffeine can have some analgesic properties which, along with its vasoconstrictive effects, may explain its presence in headache medications (S. Diamond & Freitag, 2001).

activity along descending serotonergic and adrenergic pathways. But glutamate and substance P antagonists are logical candidates too, if safe and effective molecules can be developed (Bonney, Foran, Marchand, Lipkowski, & D. B. Carr, 2004; Tambeli, Parada, J. D. Levine, & Gear, 2002). And perhaps we could address neuropathic pain by supplying the injured neurons with nerve growth factors (Boucher, Okuse, D. L. H. Bennett, J. Munson, J. Wood, & S. McMahon, 2000), or by blocking the aberrant sodium channels with lidocaine (Vu, 2004). These methods, too, are under development. In Chapter 11, we shall discuss pain medications in greater depth.

Lamina I.   The trigeminal nucleus caudalis, and likewise the dorsal horn, is comprised of layers of cells, of which the two outermost, laminae I and II, are devoted to pain (see Figure 2–3). Some of the **Aδ** and **C fibers**, then, synapse in lamina I. Here we find projection neurons that convey the pain signal to the brain. And here, at the first synapse, we encounter new types of sensitization. For input to this synapse sets in motion an array of processes that, together, amplify and prolong the signal.

The key excitatory neurotransmitters released by incoming sensory neurons are glutamate for Aδ fibers and, for C fibers, glutamate plus substance P. Now, when glutamate stimulates a nerve cell, the excitatory post-synaptic potential lasts for perhaps 20 milliseconds. However, when the neurotransmitter is substance P, the excitatory post-synaptic potential can last for 20 *seconds* (Woolf, 1996). This is the second useful property of C fibers alluded to above. The C fibers do more than sensitize other nerve endings at the periphery. They also sensitize the receiving neuron in the central nervous system, that is, in the dorsal horn.

Moreover, some of the glutamate receptors are of the **NMDA** variety (named after a chemical that, in the laboratory, stimulates them more strongly than glutamate itself: *N*-methyl-D-aspartate; Curtis & Watkins, 1961). Initially when they are stimulated, these receptors do nothing, because the ion channels they control are blocked by magnesium ions. However, as the excitation increases and the postsynaptic membrane depolarizes, the magnesium ions are jettisoned, and the calcium channels they blocked remain open for *hundreds* of milliseconds (Doubell, Mannion, and Woolf, 1999).

Meanwhile, a different type of receptor, the metabotropic glutamate receptor, produces excitatory changes in the functioning of the postsynaptic cell (including release of calcium from internal stores) that can last for tens of seconds (Doubell, et al.). Thus, through the prolonged action of substance P, metabotropic- and NMDA-type glutamate receptors, the receiving cell can maintain activation on its own long after it is stimulated.

And there are other mechanisms that tend to prolong activation at the synapse. For example, in the postsynaptic neuron, glutamate leads to the production of **nitric oxide**. Nitric oxide is a gas, and can diffuse back to the presynaptic cell and stimulate further glutamate release. Such "retrograde signals" may help to coordinate activity on the two sides of the synapse (Malenka & Nicoll, 1999), but here they prolong the signaling from the pain nerve into the trigeminal nucleus. Moreover, not only the post-synaptic neuron, but also the presynaptic axon terminal can have glutamate receptors ("**autoreceptors**"). Such autoreceptors are usually part of a negative feedback loop (Nestler, Hyman, & Malenka, 2001), allowing the presynaptic cell to "read" how much neurotransmitter is already in the synapse, to avoid overstimulating the receiving cell. However, in the dorsal horn the autoreceptor may be part of a *positive* feedback loop, with the release of glutamate stimulating further glutamate release (Doubell et al., 1999). (See Figure 2–4).

As a result of all of these mechanisms, brief stimulation of the receiving neuron can produce an enduring output, and lower the threshold for future firing. This is one of the reasons that an injured part of the body can become tender to even low-level stimulation.

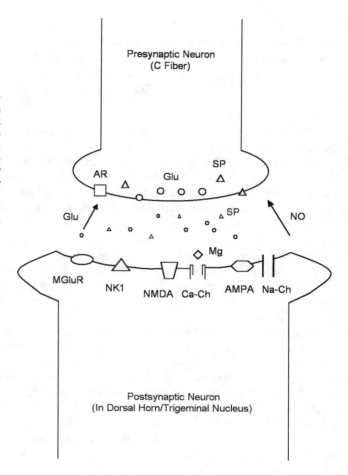

FIGURE 2–4. Processes that facilitate nociceptive transmission across the synapse between the afferent C-fiber and the dorsal horn. These include the long-term effects of substance P and metabotropic glutamate receptors, the phosphorylation of AMPA-type and the unblocking of NMDA-type glutamate receptors, and the back-diffusion of nitric oxide and glutamate, which stimulate further release of neurotransmitter.

AR: Autoreceptors for Glutamate (including metabotropic- and NMDA-type receptors); Glu: Glutamate-containing vesicles (in presynaptic cell); Glutamate (in the synapse); SP: Substance P-containing vesicles (in presynaptic cell); Substance P (in the synapse); NO: Nitric Oxide; Mg: Magnesium ion (blocking calcium channel); MGluR: Metabotropic glutamate receptor; NK1: Substance P receptor (Neurokinin 1); NMDA: NMDA-type glutamate receptor; Ca-Ch: Calcium channel controlled by NMDA receptor; AMPA: AMPA-type glutamate receptor; Na-Ch: Sodium channel controlled by AMPA receptor.

Thus, pain lasting for even a few minutes can produce signs of central sensitization. Physiologically, in the dorsal horn of the spinal cord there is (Coderre, J. Katz, Vaccarino, & Melzack, 1993):

- a decrease in firing threshold
- an increase in spontaneous firing
- a higher firing rate to the same stimulus
- a continuing discharge after the noxious stimulus has ended, and
- a widening of the **receptive fields** of nearby neurons to include the painful site.

These changes seem to have clinical equivalents (Coderre, J. Katz, Vaccarino, & Melzack, 1993):

- **allodynia**: a decrease in pain threshold, so that previously neutral stimuli are perceived as painful,[5]

---

[5]Some researchers also include under "allodynia" a marked distress response to non-noxious stimuli. That is, the light touch or gentle pressure that elicits pain in allodynia also tends to elicit a strong emotional reaction in people and, to all appearances, in animals (Watkins & Maier, 2000).

- ambient pain in the absence of tissue damage,
- primary **hyperalgesia**: an increased sensitivity to painful stimuli at the site of injury,
- persistent pain continuing after a painful stimulus has ended, and
- secondary hyperalgesia: increased sensitivity to pain at undamaged regions near the injury (T. Lewis, 1935; Raja, R. A. Meyer, Ringkamp, & J. N. Campbell, 1999).

Notice, then, that listening to our patients' descriptions of their pain can do much more than build rapport: It can provide clues to the functional state of the pain system.

Other, more qualitative changes occur in the dorsal horn. Palpating a muscle with mild pressure activates low threshold mechanosensitive (LTM) neurons in the dorsal horn, which presumably mediate the feeling of pressure. High levels of pressure activate another population of spinal neurons, which are described as high threshold mechanosensitive (HTM), and which probably convey pressure pain sensations (Mense, 1993). In chronic muscle pain, previously ineffective synapses can become strengthened, new synapses can form, and the low threshold neurons in the dorsal horn can begin sending signals through the same nociceptive pathways as the high threshold neurons (Torebjörk, Lundberg, & LaMotte, 1992). In a sense, the dorsal horn "rewires" itself to become more pain sensitive. This process may underlie the tender, bruised feeling of the scalp in tension-type headache (Bendtsen, Jensen, & Olesen, 1996b) and of the body in **fibromyalgia**.

It is likely that the pathways for various pain sensitive structures converge to a degree, allowing for some cross-sensitization. Thus, Burstein and coworkers report on the results of a careful sensory examination of a migraine patient (who was also a physician) who agreed to forego treatment for the duration of an attack. Now, presumably the migraine pain was originating in the dura mater covering the brain. However, one hour into the migraine, the patient/physician showed drastically reduced pain thresholds to pressure and cold applied to the skin in the region of the migraine pain, above the right eye. After two hours, this allodynia (pain from non-noxious stimulation) was apparent also above the other eye, even though the migraine itself remained unilateral. After four hours, the allodynia included sensitivity to heat, and had extended to the *forearm*, although only on the side ipsilateral to the migraine (Burstein, Cutrer, & Yarnitsky, 2000). The authors suggest that in this sequence, one is witnessing the spread of sensitization to neurons with progressively more convergent input. Where are these neurons found? Presumably in the layers of the first major pain processing structure for the head, the trigeminal nucleus.

This convergence is part of the rationale for various nonspecific treatments of pain. For even if migraines are not caused by muscle tension in the neck, for example, or eye strain, or a sinus infection, or irritation of the facet joints in the spine, input from these structures can presumably lower the pain threshold, and make a migraine more likely. Moreover, the emergence of allodynia in the course of a migraine is highly predictive of whether a **triptan**—a key type of acute antimigraine medication—will work. Once sensitization has occurred, the migraine tends to be out of reach of triptans, which seem to act mostly on blood vessels and C fibers (Burstein, Jakubowski, & D. Levy, 2005).

In lamina I, the synapse is presumably between the incoming sensory nerves and the projection neurons. Thus, sensitization seems to imply a rather direct access of the pain signal to higher brain centers. In fact, however, the signal must traverse a welter of checkpoints. Thus, while the projection neurons in lamina I do send the pain signal further into the brain, it is usually not, as we might expect, to the thalamus and cortex. Rather, the signal's primary destination is a part of the **brain stem**, the *parabrachial nucleus*, responsible for arousal (see Figure 2–2). There, the signal influences a *descending* pain facilitory pathway that terminates back in deeper laminae of the trigeminal nucleus and dorsal horn (Suzuki, Morcuende, Webber, Hunt, & Dickenson, 2002). Here is not transmission, but a loop of activation reverberating between spine and brain stem.

Lamina II.   Meanwhile, some of the incoming sensory nerves bypass lamina I and first synapse in lamina II. Lamina II, also called the **substantia gelatinosa**, looks gelatinous and is dense with mostly inhibitory interneurons (Coggeshall, Lekan, F. A. White, & Woolf, 2001). These inhibitory neurons cause receiving neurons to hyperpolarize, so that they are less likely to fire in response to an incoming stimulus. Now, the computational architecture of lamina II is complex and obscure. Based on the pain system's input-output characteristics, however, Wall and Melzack (1965) proposed a schematic that is of historical, intellectual, and ongoing clinical importance, the **gate control model**. In this model, the "gate" is lamina II.

Gate control.   Imagine stubbing your toe. As painful as this is, the pain will nearly vanish if you rub your foot vigorously near the ankle. Yet, we have done nothing to treat the toe—how can this be?

The classic answer to this question is provided by the gate control model. In this model, no sensory nerves are dedicated to pain. There are simply large diameter fibers (called **Aβ fibers**) and the Aδ and C fibers, which are of small diameter. Now, activation along any of these fibers would tend to transmit signals through the dorsal horn, and up to the brain. But in the theory, impulses along the large fibers also trigger inhibitory processes in the dorsal horn, and thus constrain the ultimate intensity of the signal. In contrast, the small fibers are thought to connect to excitatory feedback loops in the dorsal horn, causing ever increasing activation (Melzack & Wall, 1965). (See Figure 2–5.)[6]

At mild intensities, pressure to the skin causes impulses along both the large and the small fibers, and activation and inhibition are balanced. The total signal transmitted by the dorsal horn is therefore moderate, and interpreted as pressure. The "pain gate" is mostly closed. However, as the stimulus becomes more intense and noxious, activity in the small fibers begins to predominate. This activates the excitatory feedback loops (the gate opens) and the amount of signal transmitted up to the brain increases markedly. At these more intense levels, the signal tends to be interpreted as pain.

Notice, however, that we can close the gate by increasing activation in the large diameter fibers. Rubbing accomplishes this and, as a variable stimulus, tends to keep the large fibers from habituating. Informally, the pressure sensations block the pain.[7]

This is the gate control model in its most circumscribed sense. However, Melzack and Wall also suggest that the dorsal horn receives descending inhibitory input from the brain. This allows such psychological variables as emotion and memories to influence whether the pain gate is open.

---

[6]Why would large fibers inhibit the very mechanism that is designed to transmit their signal to the brain? Actually, this is an oversimplification. The large fibers' **receptive fields**—the territory of the skin or deep tissues that the fibers "read" from, is organized into an "**on-center, off-surround**" format. Signals from the center of the receptive field stimulate the dorsal horn while signals from the immediately surrounding areas inhibit the dorsal horn. This arrangement tells stimulus location more precisely. But because the inhibitory area is larger than the center of the receptive field, the net effect is inhibition of the dorsal horn (Melzack & Wall, 1996).

[7]Notice that in the gate control model we assume that the large fiber and small fiber afferents converge onto the same dorsal horn neurons, which can then be either inhibited or facilitated. In fact, this convergence is true only of some dorsal horn neurons, which are therefore called "wide dynamic range" neurons. Other neurons read only from the small fibers (and are called "nociceptive specific") while still others read from only the large fibers. An open question is whether these different types of dorsal horn cells are hard-wired into their roles, or comprise a distribution of responsiveness that can be shifted with changes in descending signals from the brain (Melzack & Wall, 1996).

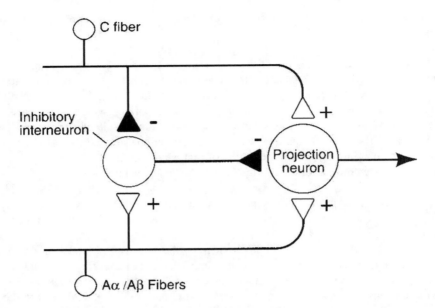

FIGURE 2–5.   Melzack and Wall's Gate Control Model. In the model, both large diameter (Aα and Aβ fibers) and small diameter (Aδ and C fibers) stimulate projection neurons, which send information on stimulus intensity to the brain. But the large diameter fibers also stimulate inhibitory interneurons, and thus constrain the ultimate rate of firing of the projection neurons (i.e., they "close the pain gate"). The small diameter fibers undo this constraint ("open the gate") by inhibiting the inhibitory interneurons. From "Pain and Analgesia," by T. M. Jessell and D. D. Kelly, 1991, in E. R. Kandel, J. H. Schwartz, and T. M. Jessell (Eds.), *Principles of Neural Science* (3rd edition, page 392), Norwalk, CT: Appleton and Lange. Copyright 1991 by Appleton and Lange. Reprinted with permission.

In fact, Melzack and Wall suggested that there might be several such gates, operating at different levels of pain processing.

Clinically, the gate control model has been invoked to explain certain types of neuropathic pain (i.e., when there has been selective death of large diameter fibers), and the effects of counterstimulation such as rubbing. Physicians make use of it, for example tickling a child's arm near the elbow while removing a splinter from the fingertip. And historically, the gate control model served as the impetus for the modern use of electricity as a pain control modality.

Moreover, the model has fared remarkably well in the light of subsequent research (Melzack & Wall, 1996). But even more importantly, the model was a watershed in pain theory for it was the first modern statement that pain is computed by the nervous system, and not simply transmitted.[8] The model set the stage for a research agenda that continues to this day. Indeed, this chap-

---

[8]Indeed, in its simplest form, the gate control theory is a circuit diagram for computing output intensity as a function of large diameter and small diameter input. Thus, the gate control theory fits within the framework of early neural network models. This is not surprising. In the mid 1950s, Patrick Wall, a neurophysiologist, was part of an MIT group headed by Warren McCulloch, which also included Walter Pitts and Jerry Lettvin (M. Devor, 2001). At the time, the McCulloch-Pitts model was the accepted formalism for neural networks, and even helped inspire John von Neuman in the development of digital computers (Anderson & Rosenfeld, 1998, p. 102). Meanwhile Ronald Melzack, a psychologist, was earning his Ph.D. under Donald O. Hebb (Wilentz, 1996). Hebb's ideas about how neural networks can learn through experience are still used in artificial intelligence. In fact, we will encounter a modern version of Hebbian learning below, when we consider how the spinal cord "remembers" pain.

ter and the one that follows are really about the fruits of that research, set in motion by the gate control theory.

PAIN AT THE SPINAL LEVEL

At the dorsal horn and, by extension, the trigeminal nucleus caudalis, we have encountered the first synapse of the pain pathways. There, the intensification, prolongation, and spread of activation lower the threshold for pressure pain, giving rise to a tender, bruised feeling. Not surprisingly, this central sensitization has been proposed as a model of chronic tension-type headache and **transformed migraine**, in which the scalp is sensitive to pressure and pain episodes become increasingly frequent. It has also been proposed as a model for **fibromyalgia**, especially when the pain sensitivity spreads gradually from an initial point of injury to encompass much of the body.

Thus, to the burning pain of inflammation, and the brief lancinating pains of **neuralgia**, we can add a chronic pressure pain mediated by the dorsal horn. The pain from C fibers tends to be dull, aching, and poorly localized (Torebjork, 1985), much like clinical descriptions of chronic pain, again suggesting sensitization at the dorsal horn. Moreover, because various types of input can presumably give rise to sensitization, inflammatory, neuropathic, and other pains can begin to resemble one another experientially as they become chronic.

We have seen hints of new tools as well. With the first synapse comes the potential to block excitatory neurotransmitters, and to up-regulate those that are inhibitory. Meanwhile, the gate control model suggests that self-management can benefit from counterstimulation—electrical stimulation is an example—changing the output of the pain system by changing the input.

And we have seen signs of the system's complexity, in the resonant loop of activation, reverberating between spine and brain stem, and in the descending pain inhibitory pathways assumed in the gate control model. Of course, these descending pathways would flow from higher regions of the nervous system. For a fuller measure of understanding, then, we must proceed further, to examine how the pain signal is processed in the brain.

IN THE BRAIN

So far, we have focused only on the pain processing that occurs in the dorsal horn—the point at which the nociceptive signal first enters the spinal cord. Not surprisingly, given its extreme relevance to survival, the pain signal then goes on to receive extensive subsequent processing in a wide range of brain structures (D. Price, 1999). Together, these structures are sometimes called the "pain neuromatrix," the widespread **neural network** whose activation patterns generate the experience of pain (Melzack, 1990).

The pain system seems "wired" to permit rapid responding. This is implied in Table 2–1, below, in the number of **brain stem** structures—involved in alertness, orienting, arousal, and autonomic responding—that receive pain information (D. Price, 1999, 2000; see also Figure 2–2). It is as if the pain signal, traveling upward through the brain stem, switches on nuclei that prepare for threat. Moreover, at least two pathways from the dorsal horn (the spinohypothalamic and the spinopontoamygdaloid pathway) allow relatively direct access to the pain signal by the hypothalamus and the **amygdala** (D. Price, 2000). As both structures are involved in fight-or-flight responding, the adaptive significance is clear.

The primary pain pathway, however, is the spinothalamic tract (D. Price, 1999): Neurons from the trigeminal nucleus and dorsal horn do ultimately project to the thalamus, which in turn projects to the cortex (Goadsby, 1995). In general, pain signals seem to take two paths through the thalamus. One path is through lateral nuclei, and on to primary and secondary somatosensory

TABLE 2–1
Brain Structures Involved in Afferent Pain Processing

Location	Structure	Functions In Which It May Participate
Medulla	Nucleus Gigantocellularis (in the Rostral Ventromedial Medulla)	Arousal, Escape Behavior (Part of Reticular Formation)
Pons	Parabrachial Nucleus	Autonomic Responding
Midbrain	Superior Colliculus (Deep Layers)	Alerting, Orienting Towards Stimulus
Midbrain	Periaqueductal Gray Region (Central Gray)	Aversiveness, Fear
Diencephalon	Hypothalamus	Sympathetic Activation
Diencephalon	Thalamus: Ventrocaudal Nucleus and Ventroposterior Medial Nucleus	Processing Sensory Pain Information (Location, Quality, Intensity) from Body (Ventrocaudal Nucleus) or Head and Face (Ventroposterior Medial Nucleus); Relay to Primary Somatosensory Cortex
Diencephalon	Thalamus: Central Lateral Nucleus, Medial Dorsal Nucleus, Posterior Nuclear Complex (Ventromedial Part)	Processing Affective/Motivational Pain Information; Relay to Anterior Cingulate Cortex and Other Limbic Structures
Limbic System	Central Nucleus of Amygdala	Fear Conditioning, Fear and Rage Behaviors, Autonomic Responding
Basal Ganglia	Striatum, Globus Pallidus, Substantia Nigra	Various Possible Roles in Pain Perception and Processing
Limbic Cortex	Caudal Portion of Anterior Cingulate Cortex (Brodmann Area 24)	Affective (Unpleasant, Aversive) Aspects of Pain
Limbic Cortex	Insula	? Integration of Sensory Pain Information with Memory and Emotion
Neocortex	Brodmann Area 3a of Primary Somatosensory Cortex	Sensory Aspects of Pain (Location, Quality, Intensity)
Neocortex	Secondary Somatosensory Cortex	Elaboration of Sensory Aspects of Pain
Neocortex	Infraparietal Area (Brodmann Area 7b)	Integration of Sensory Aspects of Pain with Information About Stimulus from Other Sensory Modalities; Computation of Pain as Threat
Neocortex	Frontal Lobe	Cognitive Evaluation of Pain

Note: Information from "*Psychological Mechanisms of Pain and Analgesia*," by D. D. Price, 1999, Seattle: IASP Press; "Psychological and Neural Mechanisms of the Affective Dimension of Pain," by D. D. Price, 2000, *Science*, *288*, 1769–1772; "The Role of the Basal Ganglia in Nociception and Pain" by E. H. Chudler and W. K. Dong, 1995, *Pain*, *60*, 3–38; and "Imaging Cognitive Modulation of Pain Processing," by P. Petrovic and M. Ingvar, 2002, *Pain*, *95*, 1–5.

cortex. This lateral pathway seems to convey the sensory aspects of the pain: its location, intensity, and quality (Treede, Kenshalo, Gracely, & Jones, 1999). The other path is through medial thalamic nuclei, and on to the **insula** and the **caudal** portion (**Brodmann Area** 24) of **anterior cingulate cortex**.[9] This medial pathway, with its connections to the limbic system, may encode the affective and motivational (unpleasant) qualities of pain (Treede, Kenshalo, et al.). Thus, the idea that pain contains separate sensory and emotional components (Melzack & Casey, 1968; Merskey & Spear, 1967; D. Price, Harkins, & Baker, 1987) seems reflected in neurophysiology (Derbyshire, Jones, Gyulai, Clark, Townsend, & Firestone, 1997).

---

[9]The lateral thalamic nuclei are, for pain from the body, the ventrocaudal nucleus, and for pain from the head and face, the ventral posteromedial thalamus (Goadsby, 1995; D. Price, 1999). The relevant medial thalamic nuclei are the central lateral nucleus, the medial dorsal nucleus, and the posterior nuclear complex, ventromedial part (D. Price, 1999).

We can see this division in daily life. Rejection and loss also activate the back (caudal) portion of anterior cingulate cortex (Eisenberger & M. D. Lieberman, 2004; Eisenberger, M. D. Lieberman, & K. D. Williams, 2003). The activation rarely spills into the sensory system, so we usually cannot locate the pain of rejection in a particular region of the body. Rather, it suffuses us, ghostly and inchoate—pain without location, an ache without form. In the clinic an especially anxious patient may relate that when their physical pain is severe they can no longer identify its location, suggesting a shift from sensory to emotional processing.

Conversely, pleasant emotions, and interpreting the pain sensation as less unpleasant, deactivate area 24, and soften or remove the distressing quality of the pain, while leaving its sensory aspects unchanged (Rainville, Duncan, D. D. Price, Carrier, & Bushnell, 1997). This is one reason for the widespread use of relaxation training in pain treatment programs.

Of course we would expect primary somatosensory cortex (S1), where the sensory homunculus resides, to be involved in pain perception. But it is more complicated: There are actually four homunculi, or complete maps of the body, in S1, corresponding to **Brodmann Areas** 3a, 3b, 1, and 2 (Kaas, R. J. Nelson, Sur, Lin, & Merzenich, 1979). And it is only in area 3a, far down on the back wall of the central sulcus, that pain is represented (Tommerdahl, Delemos, Favorov, Metz, Vierck, & Whitsel, 1998). It turns out, however, that as pain intensity increases, the activated area in primary somatosensory cortex also increases. Moreover, activation in the pain area 3a seems to inhibit the nearby region, Brodmann Area 1 (and possibly 3b) that is involved in the perception of vibratory stimuli (Rosso et al., 2003; Tommerdahl et al.). This suggests that there is competition at the level of the cortex among different types of somatosensory stimulation, and that a high pain level tends to block perception of vibration. This is supported as well by psychophysical studies (Apkarian, Stea, & Bolanowski, 1994; Bolanowski, Maxfield, Gescheider, & Apkarian, 2000).

Physical therapists seem to make use of this competition all the time. Hot packs, ice, electrical stimulation and massage may address themselves to the cortex as much as to the muscles.

In theory, this intracortical inhibition could be another reason that a pressure sensation (e.g., rubbing one's ankle) can inhibit a nearby pain source (e.g., a stubbed toe). In fact, Tommerdahl et al. found no inhibition of pain by vibration, only an inhibition of vibration by pain, in studies of brain physiology (Tommerdahl, Delemos, Favorov, Metz, Vierck, & Whitsel, 1998). This is surprising because we know from perceptual studies that vibration can indeed reduce pain intensity. Perhaps the locus of action is subcortical (Yarnitsky, Kunin, Brik, & Sprecher, 1997). Alternatively, the effectiveness of vibration may depend on the degree to which we attend to it in place of the pain (Longe et al., 2001). That is, counterstimulation and control of attention may be mutually reinforcing tools in pain self-management.

Moreover, there seems to be a subset of patients with unexplained pain who describe being unable to perceive warmth in the affected area. They sometimes scald themselves, in the shower or with a heating pad, in an effort to override the pain. It would be useful to know whether this selective hypesthesia means that the pain has become embedded in the strength of intracortical inhibition.

Regardless, this pattern, in which the activation of pain-encoding regions tends to spread while non-pain regions become inhibited, is mirrored elsewhere in cortex. Under high intensity pain, much of the "pain matrix" is firing, while regions devoted to vision and audition show decreased activation (D. Price, 1999). It seems that for an individual in severe pain, much of the nervous system is involved. Conversely, processing information from other sensory modalities seems to go along with decreased activity in pain-encoding regions (Villemure & Bushnell, 2002).

Patients often resonate to this image on an intuitive level. They feel as if the pain is taking over more and more of their lives, more and more of their central nervous system. But by engaging in and attending to non-pain stimuli, they can begin taking back that control.

Now, all of this seems to suggest that pain affect and pain sensation are processed in parallel: Pain affect through relatively direct paths to the hypothalamus and **amygdala**, and by way of the thalamus to the anterior cingulate cortex; pain sensation through the thalamus to primary somatosensory cortex. Price, however, suggests that after the immediate stimulation of emotion and arousal centers, things become more complex (D. Price, 2000). He traces a path from primary somatosensory cortex, to secondary somatosensory cortex, to the infraparietal region, and on to the insula. Along this path, the sensory information is presumably integrated with information about the stimulus from other sensory modalities, and with the internal representation of the body ("**body schema**"), to develop a cognitive sense of the threat. This information is then "fed forward" to the posterior portion of the anterior cingulate cortex, which seems to encode the emotional valence of pain (unpleasantness) and to participate in setting response priorities (D. Price, 1999). Presumably, the anterior cingulate cortex also receives considerable input from the adjacent frontal lobes. In this pathway, pain affect appears to follow in series the extraction of sensory information. Price suggests that immediately following the stimulus, pain affect is triggered directly and processed in parallel with pain sensation. If the pain persists and ultimately becomes chronic, pain affect comes to depend to a greater extent on cognitive factors (D. Price, 1999). (See Figure 2–6).

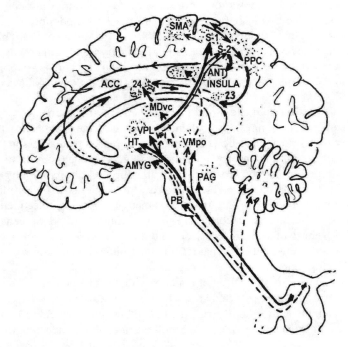

FIGURE 2–6.   Primary projection areas for pain. Notice the primary pathway (solid line), up from the dorsal horn, through the spine and brain stem, to the periaqueductal gray (PAG), hypothalamus (HT), and lateral thalamic nuclei (VPL and VPI). In turn, the lateral thalamic nuclei project to primary and secondary somatosensory cortex (S–1 and S–2). From there, the signal travels to the supplementary motor area (SMA), posterior parietal cortex (PPC), anterior insula (ANT INSULA), and ultimately to Brodmann area 24 of anterior cingulate cortex (ACC). Meanwhile, a medial thalamic nucleus (MDvc) projects directly to Brodmann area 24. Also seen on the diagram are secondary pathways from the dorsal horn to the parabrachial nucleus (PB), amygdala (AMYG) and hypothalamus (HT), and the close ties between anterior cingulate cortex and the prefrontal cortex to its left. From *Psychological Mechanisms of Pain and Analgesia* (p. 126) by D. D. Price, 1999, Seattle: IASP Press. Copyright 1999 by IASP Press. Reprinted with permission.

Thus, in the cortex our understanding of counterstimulation has broadened to include other sensory modalities and the role of selective attention towards or away from pain. Indeed, non-pain activities of all types can be thought of as counterstimulation, broadly conceived, if they reduce the relative activation in the pain matrix.

Particularly noteworthy is the role of the medial (emotional) pain system, especially the back portion of anterior cingulate cortex. Activated by both emotional and noxious sensory stimuli, it is a potential point of intersection between depression and pain. We will examine the effects of attention, activity and emotions on pain processing later in this chapter, and in the next.

HOW PAIN BECOMES CHRONIC

Dorsal horn and trigeminal nucleus.   We have seen, then, that following an injury the dorsal horn can become sensitized, and the injured part of the body tender. Of course, this is ordinarily temporary. The person recovers, and their pain sensitivity returns to normal. A question of enormous clinical importance is this: Is the sensitization process always fully reversible, or can the dorsal horn become permanently hyperresponsive? At this point, we do not know. There are at least two theories, however, that suggest how sensitization can become permanent.

The first theory focuses on the excitatory changes that take place in the dorsal horn: the unblocking of NMDA receptors as magnesium ions are jettisoned, the opening of voltage-dependent calcium channels, and the activation of metabotropic glutamate receptors. Now, the NMDA receptors cause calcium channels to open, voltage-dependent calcium channels are of course conduits for calcium, and the metabotropic glutamate receptors cause release of calcium from intracellular stores. So, one effect of the excitatory processes is to cause a sharp rise in the calcium concentration in the postsynaptic neuron.

Now, in the hippocampus, this process seems to underlie the formation of memories (T. H. Brown, Ganong, Kairiss, Keenan, & Kelso, 1989). The increased calcium levels activate certain enzymes that attach phosphate groups to a subunit of a different type of glutamate receptor, **AMPA**, increasing the receptor's activity, and strengthening the synapse ("long-term potentiation;" Lee, Barbarosie, Kameyama, Bear, & Huganir, 2000). There also seems to be an increase in the total number of functioning AMPA receptors, which are moved into place at the synapse from nearby locations on the cell membrane (Malenka & Nicoll, 1999; Tocco, Maren, Shors, Baudry, & Thompson, 1992), or from within the cell (Bear, W. F. Connors, & Paradiso, 2001), making the synapse more sensitive still. Ultimately, the active surface of the synapse may get larger through the growth of axonal boutons (presynaptically) and dendritic spines (postsynaptically), strengthening the synapse in a fairly permanent, structural way, at least in young animals (Huntley, Benson, & Colman, 2002; Magee & Johnston, 1997). Thus, short-term memory, encoded in a pattern of strengthened synapses, consolidates into a long-term store.

It is a relatively small leap to say that the types of changes that give rise to memory formation in the hippocampus are taking place as well in the dorsal horn and trigeminal nucleus (H. Ikeda, Heinke, Ruscheweyh, & Sandkühler, 2003; Woolf & Salter, 2000). That is, glutamate and substance P may bring about a long-term activation of their synapses, leading in turn to changes in gene transcription, activity and number of AMPA receptors, and dendritic spine formation, which increase the excitability of the post-synaptic membrane at that synapse (Sandkühler, 2000; Wilcox, 1991; Woolf, 1991). This could be called a "memory model" of pain. Of course it is not memory in any ordinary sense, as it is taking place in the spinal cord and medulla rather than in higher brain centers. A more neutral term might be "information storage model" (Sandkühler, 2000).

The second theory focuses not on the excitatory processes, but on the network of inhibitory connections that tend to block the pain signal. We have seen that synapses can become stronger, when AMPA-type receptors are phosphorylated and moved into position. But AMPA-type receptors can also be *de*-phosphorylated and moved *out* of position, weakening a synapse ("long-term depression" of synaptic strength; Malenka & Nicoll, 1999). If the inhibitory synapses are weakened the net effect would be equivalent to pain sensitization (Woolf & Salter, 2000).

There is also a second version of this "disinhibition theory" in which an even more permanent change is posited. Recall that the excitatory neurotransmitter in the dorsal horn is glutamate. High concentrations of glutamate are thought to be toxic to neurons, for example contributing to the damage in **ischemic** stroke (Berg-Johnsen, Haugstad, & Langmoen, 1998; Dirnagl, Iadecola, & Moskowitz, 1999). In the second theory, overstimulation of the nociceptive pathways leads to the death of small inhibitory neurons through glutamate toxicity (Dubner, 1991).

"Permanent" is a relative term, and we do not know whether synaptic strengthening and weakening in the dorsal horn, if they truly do take place, will eventually decay back to baseline. In the hippocampus, long-term potentiation can last for the lifetime of an animal; some memories are forever. However, studies of this type have not yet been conducted on nociceptive pathways.

Many of the details of these models remain theoretical. For example, although there is indeed evidence for a loss of GABA-mediated inhibition in the dorsal horn (Coggeshall, Lekan, F. A. White, & Woolf, 2001; Whiteside & Munglani, 2001), technical difficulties abound and there have been noteworthy failures to replicate (Polgár, Hughes, Riddell, Maxwell, Puskár, & A. J. Todd, 2003). And although dendritic spines are found on a subset of neurons in laminae I (Cheunsuang & R. Morris, 2000; J. Schoenen, 1982) and II (Y. Q. Li, H. Li, Kaneko, & Mizuno, 1999; J. Schoenen, 1982) of the dorsal horn, we do not know whether their density changes with experience. Perhaps pain sensitivity does not consolidate, the way long-term memory in the brain does. Persistent changes in pain threshold might be maintained by malleable, "reverberant loops" of activation—firing that echoes from the dorsal horn to the brain stem and back again. We have already encountered one example, between the dorsal horn and the parabrachial nucleus. Reverberant loops imply that descending signals are important in pain. Later in the chapter, we will see evidence that they are.

In general, the same types of injuries that send a volley of pain signals to the central nervous system also sensitize the peripheral nerves. We have seen that inflammation and nerve damage lower the firing thresholds of sensory neurons. As a result, the peripheral nerves may fire spontaneously, in what is called "ectopic discharge." Some researchers suggest that this extra stimulation from the peripheral nerves is enough to maintain central sensitization (Pertovaara, 2000; Treede, Handwerker, Baumgärtner, R. Meyer, & Magerl, 2004) or to contribute to the death of inhibitory interneurons (Woolf & Salter, 2000).

Before leaving the dorsal horn, let us reflect for a moment on the concept of long-term depression of synaptic strength as an opposing process to long-term potentiation (Linden, 1999; Sandkühler, 2000). If we accept an analogy to classical conditioning, old learning might not decay so much as be written over by new learning. But whether the dorsal horn can be "re-taught" normal pain processing is entirely unknown. In Chapter 3 we will encounter a psychological theory that people can habituate to pain provided fear and avoidance do not get in the way. We will also encounter seminal studies by Pavlov suggesting that animals can selectively learn to not experience certain types of pain. And in Chapter 15 we will encounter a little bit of data, of unknown reliability, that chronic pain can sometimes be permanently reversed with a psychological intervention, **hypnosis**.

Thalamus.   Higher-level structures may also play a direct role in central sensitization. For example, in some cases of chronic pain, electrical stimulation of the thalamus reproduces the clinical pain, suggesting that this structure, too, becomes sensitized (Gorecki, Hirayama, Dostrovsky,

Tasker, & Lenz, 1989; Nathan, 1985). The activity of inhibitory interneurons may perhaps diminish (A. K. P. Jones, Kulkarni, & Derbyshire, 2003), and portions of the thalamus may atrophy (Apkarian, Sosa, Sonty, et al., 2004).

CHRONIC PAIN AND THE CORTEX

Sensitization at lower levels seems to have consequences at the cortex. In fact, one of the types of evidence that a cortical neuron encodes pain is that it shows sensitization and an enlarged **receptive field** after peripheral injury (Treede, Kenshalo, Gracely, & Jones, 1999).

Cortical reorganization.   Moreover, the cortex itself may undergo changes in chronic pain. Flor and coworkers studied the magnetic field response evoked from primary somatosensory cortex by a painful electrical stimulus.[10] The early component of the evoked magnetic field had greater power in patients with chronic low back pain than in healthy matched controls, and in fact the power increased linearly with chronicity (Flor, Braun, Elbert, & Birbaumer, 1997). That a stronger cortical response was being elicited at ten years post-injury than at five years suggests that pain sensitization continues to develop over many years. Moreover—and this is key—in patients with the greatest chronicity, the location of maximum magnetic activity shifted, raising the possibility of a functional reorganization of the cortex in cases of very chronic low back pain.

Amputation, too, should cause a functional reorganization of primary somatosensory cortex and this indeed has been demonstrated, using evoked magnetic potentials (T. Yang, Gallen, B. Schwartz, F. E. Bloom, Ramachandran, & Cobb, 1994): In somatosensory cortex, contralateral to an arm amputation, the evoked response to light pressure at the lower face shifts in location. The evoked response for the face "invades" the region that had encoded the now missing hand. The extent of the shift can be large, several centimeters over the cortex, and has been used as a measure of the amount of reorganization.

Now, Flor and coworkers found that this degree of reorganization was unrelated to the subject's age, age when the amputation occurred, time since amputation, amount of stump pain, nonpainful sensations of the stump, and nonpainful phantom limb sensations. However, there was a remarkably strong correlation across the 13 subjects ($r = 0.93$, $p < .0001$) between the amount of reorganization and the subjects' ratings, on a 0 to 5 scale, of the amount of **phantom pain** they experienced (Flor, Elbert, et al., 1995). As this is a correlational study, we do not know whether the cortical reorganization is a cause or an effect of the phantom pain, or if they are both manifestations of some other process. Certainly, however, we must entertain the possibility that changes in primary somatosensory cortex play a role in the development of chronic pain.

Now, when **phantom limb pain** is due, say, to a neuroma, a tangle of nerves and connective tissue in the stump, the therapy is generally to remove the neuroma surgically. But what treatment is appropriate if the pain has become embedded in the cortex? Surely not brain surgery. But what is inaccessible to surgery may be amenable to psychology, for everyday training and education are, most likely, subtle, guided changes in central nervous system connectivity.

---

[10]This "magnetoencephalography," or MEG, is analogous to ordinary electroencephalography, the EEG, except that magnetic fields are read in place of electrical fields. Because magnetic fields are not distorted as they pass through the skull, the source of the evoked activity can be better localized than with the EEG (Wheless, et al., 2004). An illustration of evoked potential EEG is shown in Figure 2–7.

Ramachandran and Rogers-Ramachandran[11] may have found such an effect in a study of people who had lost one of their arms to illness or accident. In the study, each subject sat with a box before them. The front and top of the box had been cut away, and a mirror had been placed down the middle, so that when the subject inserted their intact arm, it looked as if the other arm were in the box too. The investigators asked people to mentally place their phantom arm in the box, and to position their intact arm so that the image was superimposed on the phantom arm. Looking into the box, the subjects "saw" a left and right arm. Of five subjects who had felt that their phantom hands were locked in a painful spasm, four obtained temporary relief by making a fist with their intact hand, and then mentally unclenching both hands simultaneously. It seems that the intention to unclench (signals from the motor cortex) plus the visual feedback, were enough to change the somatosensory experience. Particularly noteworthy were the results from a sixth patient, who practiced the procedure at home for 15 minutes a day for three weeks. After this period, most of his phantom limb was gone, and along with it, the phantom pain. The pain had still not returned when he was contacted six months later (Ramachandran & Rogers-Ramachandran, 1996).

In a second study, Flor and coworkers randomly assigned 10 upper extremity amputees to receive either intensive assessment plus standard treatment (the control group), or sensory discrimination training (the experimental group). In the training, participants practiced identifying the frequency and place of non-painful electric pulses delivered to closely spaced locations on the stump. This was designed to expand the cortical representation of the stump, pushing back the representation of the face, and partially reversing the cortical reorganization. The phantom limb pain (but not pain in the stump) improved in the group that received the training, and it remained improved at three month follow-up. Patients in the control group did not improve. Moreover, for the experimental group, the degree of improvement correlated with the degree to which cortical reorganization, measured from **evoked potential** EEG, was reversed (Flor, Denke, Schaefer, Grüsser, 2001). To my knowledge, this is the first form of psychological therapy to be developed out of functional neuroimaging results.

With phantom limbs, we have encountered a new type of pain: It is neither nociceptive (from tissue damage) nor neuropathic (from nerve damage), but generated de novo by the central nervous system because of the loss of sensory input ("deafferentation"). Here is the clearest possible illustration, for ourselves and our patients, that pain is not the inevitable consequence of tissue damage, but an experience constructed by the nervous system. For in the phantom limb, it is the quietude, the loss of sensory input, which is interpreted as pain.

Thus, phantom limb pain seems to be responsive to a behavioral intervention. But if psychological processes are important in reversing cortical reorganization, do they play a role in generating it in the first place? The answer, at least for short-term changes, seems to be "yes." Specifically, Buchner and coworkers used a local anesthetic to block sensation from the middle three fingers in medical student volunteers (Buchner, Reinartz, Waberski, Gobbele, Noppeney, & Scherg, 1999). When the volunteers were distracted, the representations of digits 1 and 5 moved closer together, suggesting that the cortical area devoted to the anesthetized fingers had decreased. When the volunteers were not distracted (and hence were presumably attending to the "feeling" of anesthesia) the area devoted to the anesthetized fingers seemed to increase. Thus, attention may play a role in cortical reorganization, at least in its very earliest stages.

And it may not take an amputation for the cortex to generate a phantom-like pain. The origins of complex regional pain syndrome (CRPS), with its intense pain, sensitivity to light moving

---

[11]I am indebted to a member of our lab, Audrey Dailey, Ph.D. (1943–1998), for telling me about the existence of this research.

stimuli such as the brush of clothing against the skin, localized swelling, changes in blood flow, sweating, and skin temperature, pronounced guarding of the affected limb, and associated changes in motor cortex (Eisenberg, Chistyakov, Yudashkin, B. Kaplan, Hafner, & Feinsod, 2005), have long been mysterious. But in its early stages, CRPS responds readily to Ramachandran's mirror therapy (McCabe, Haigh, Ring, Halligan, P. D. Wall, & Blake, 2003). If the condition becomes chronic, the pain can be reduced by stimulating motor cortex, whether through implanted electrodes (Son, M. C. Kim, Moon, & Kang, 2003) or magnetic pulses from a coil outside the head (**transcranial magnetic stimulation**; Pleger, Janssen, Schwenkreis, Völker, C. Maier, & Tegenthoff, 2004).

But we do not always need invasive technology. Visualizing movements of the affected limb also activates motor cortex, and can lead to a long-term reduction in pain (Moseley, 2004). Thus, when extreme, prolonged guarding of a limb is medically unnecessary, it might be aggravating the pain through a loss of inhibitory feedback from motor cortex. In those cases, a psychological treatment—**imaginal desensitization** to movement, followed by in vivo desensitization—can be part of the recovery. Of course, such combined psychological-physical intervention calls for close coordination in the treatment team.

How does the disorganization of somatosensory cortex, or of the closely connected motor cortex (T. Weiss, Miltner, Liepert, Meissner, & E. Taub, 2004), lead to pain? Possibly, it is by inducing a mismatch between motor intention and the absent or altered proprioceptive feedback. Perhaps such a discrepancy produces phantom pain, the way a discrepancy between visual and vestibular input produces nausea (A. J. Harris, 1999; McCabe, Haigh, Halligan, & Blake, 2003a, 2003b). This might explain why mirror therapy—a restoration of congruent sensory feedback— seems to work. Our scalp does not provide much proprioceptive feedback, and we cannot see it, so perhaps sustained muscle tension there generates tension-type headaches through this same cortical mechanism (Harris, 1999).

The discovery of functional reorganization in phantom limb pain was not surprising. Well before the brain imaging results there were the psychophysical—unusual patterns of referred sensation, in which stroking the cheek, for example, was felt in the phantom limb (J. P. Hunter, J. Katz, & K. D. Davis, 2003). Patients sometimes describe other phenomena that seem to hint at cortical reorganization. For example, a person with a 10-year history of low back pain, for whom heat has never been useful at their lumbar region, may discover accidentally that applying warmth to their feet eliminates the back pain. In my experience, it is when counterstimulation shows such unusual referral patterns that it is most likely to have cumulative benefit in reducing pain over weeks and months of conscientious application.

Atrophy.   Other changes in cortex may be involved as well in chronic pain. Grachev, et al., used **magnetic resonance spectroscopy** to look at the concentration of various chemicals in selected brain regions, for people with vs. without chronic back pain (Grachev, Fredrickson, & Apkarian, 2000). The people with chronic back pain showed lower concentrations of glucose and **N-acetylaspartate** in the dorsolateral prefrontal cortex.[12] This area of cortex has been implicated in chronic pain by brain imaging studies (Grachev, et al.), and may play a role in the top-down control of pain (Lorenz, Minoshima, & Casey, 2003). Moreover, this region has been associated with several executive functions, including selective attention, sustained monitoring of

---

[12]The dorsolateral region is, broadly, the outer surface of the frontal lobes, the part you would see if you looked at the brain from the side. Other major divisions include cingulate cortex on the inner surface of the frontal lobes, and orbital cortex at the bottom of the lobes (Fuster, 1997). Of course this division is rather coarse, and undoubtedly conceals a within-region diversity of function (Fuster, 1997).

an aspect of sensation, and the use of knowledge of a stimulus for planning a response to it (Dubois, Levy, Verin, Teixeira, Agid, & Pillon, 1995). Meanwhile, N-acetylaspartate, an amino acid found almost exclusively in nerve cells, seems to be a marker for neuronal integrity and functioning (Tsai & Coyle, 1995). Reductions in N-acetylaspartate correlate with cognitive decline in Alzheimer's dementia (Jessen et al., 2001), severity of head injury (Signoretti, Marmarou, Tavazzi, Lazzarino, Beaumont, & Vagnozzi, 2001), and demyelination in multiple sclerosis (Tsai & Coyle, 1995).

In chronic pain, the correlate may be loss of brain tissue. Apkarian et al. found that the volume of gray matter in dorsolateral cortex was lower by 14 percent in subjects with musculoskeletal chronic low back pain, and by 27 percent in those with chronic neuropathic back pain, as compared with matched controls (Apkarian, Sosa, Sonty, et al., 2004). Pain duration, intensity and, especially in neuropathic pain, the distressing affective quality of the pain, correlated with the decline. In contrast, use of pain medications, and more general measures of anxiety and depression, were not related to cortical volume.

Now, chronic pain is certainly not thought of as a cause of neurological trauma. But, on the other hand, neuropsychological deficits seem to be common in chronic pain (Iezzi, Archibald, Barnett, Klinck, & M. Duckworth, 1999), including deficits in controlled attention (Grisart & Van der Linden, 2001) and in judgment under risk (Apkarian, Sosa, Krauss, et al., 2004). In Chapter 3 we will see evidence that this is accounted for by the distracting effects of the pain's emotional characteristics. However, Apkarian's results suggest an alternative possibility, that a portion of the deficit is in fact a physiological impairment. Such an impairment might have important consequences for behavioral pain **coping**. Some patients, particularly those who use effortful pain suppression, describe a sense of "coping fatigue." One wonders whether some type of depletion at the dorsolateral frontal lobe may play a role. Moreover, Fuster notes that damage to the dorsolateral frontal lobe sometimes produces a syndrome clinically indistinguishable from endogenous depression (Fuster, 1997).

The fact that cortical reorganization and perhaps atrophy can emerge well after the pain has crossed the threshold of "chronic" suggests that our treatment is always preventive, if not of the injury, or of the pain, or of chronicity, then of its further embedding in the cortex.

Certainly, additional research in this area is critically important, and will hopefully shed light, not only on chronic pain, but on ways of preventing or reversing it. Especially intriguing is the question of whether cortical atrophy is driven by the stimulus characteristics of the pain, or is the product of a particular type of effort to control it. Similarly, is the influence of unpleasantness in neuropathic pain a measure of some bottom-up aspect of neural firing that is especially toxic, or is the unpleasantness best understood as a modifiable deficit in pain coping? We will touch on the prevention of chronic pain in Chapter 3.

Grachev et al. also found that the pattern of correlations among the concentrations of different chemicals, between and within brain regions, was different in the chronic back pain patients than in the healthy volunteers (Grachev, Fredrickson, & Apkarian, 2000). This might suggest differences in information processing induced by (or inducing) the chronic pain.

CHRONIC PAIN AND COGNITIVE PROCESSING

Now, the use of magnetic resonance spectroscopy to study information processing is very new, and it is not clear how the results should be interpreted. However, differences in information processing have been suggested using other methods as well. For example, Lutzenberger et al. note that the EEG at the left parietal and frontal regions is more complex when individuals with vs. without chronic pain recall a painful experience (Lutzenberger, Flor, & Birbaumer,

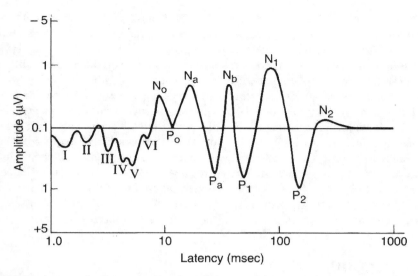

FIGURE 2–7.   An example of an event-related potential, here recorded following an auditory stimulus (from
J. H. Martin, 1991). Here, the negative (N) and positive (P) components have been labeled with roman numerals,
letters, and ordinal numbers. An alternative scheme is to label them by their approximate latency. Then, N1 would
be called N100, as it occurs approximately 100 msec after the stimulus. From "The Collective Electrical Behavior
of Cortical Neurons: The Electroencephalogram and the Mechanisms of Epilepsy," by J. H. Martin, 1991, in E. R.
Kandel, J. H. Schwartz, and T. M. Jessell (Eds.), *Principles of Neural Science* (3rd edition, page 780), Norwalk, CT:
Appleton and Lange. Copyright 1991 by Appleton and Lange. And from "Human Auditory Evoked Potentials.
I: Evaluation of Components," by T. W. Picton, S. A. Hillyard, H. I. Krausz, and R. Galambos, *Electrophysiology and
Clinical Neurophysiology* (vol. 36, page 181). Copyright 1974 by Elsevier. Reprinted with permission.

1997).[13] Presumably this greater complexity, recorded at the brain's working memory regions,
shows that the associative network involving the pain is more elaborate, and involves the activation of a greater number of cell assemblies (Lutzenberger, Preißl, & Pulvermüller, 1995). A
possible result is that a wider range of stimuli might serve as reminders of the pain (Lutzenberger, Flor, & Birbaumer, 1997). Note, however, that primary somatosensory cortex did not
show the increased signal complexity, and that exposure to acute thermal pain did not elicit the
complexity, even in individuals with chronic pain. Hence, the EEG finding appears to relate
specifically to cognitive processing of personally relevant pain.

Other information processing differences have been suggested. Flor, Knost, and Birbaumer
compared the EEG **event-related potentials** of people with chronic upper back pain and healthy
control subjects to very briefly (tachistoscopically) presented words. Event-related potentials
are subtle changes in an EEG signal following presentation of a stimulus. These perturbations
show up as a series of peaks and troughs in voltage measured at the scalp (see Figure 2–7). The
authors report that for the patients, but not the healthy control subjects, the amplitude of the N100
and N200 components of the visual **evoked potential** (the negative voltage peaks around 100 and
200 msec post-stimulus) was greater for pain-related words than for neutral words. Also, the
research participants who had pain, but not the healthy controls, showed a greater electrodermal
response to the pain words than to the neutral words. Now, for visual presentation, N100 is the
earliest component of the event-related potential to be significantly strengthened by selective

---

[13]That is, the autocorrelation matrix had a greater number of non-noise eigenvectors, or principal components, implying a greater number of dimensions of information in the EEG signal.

attention to the stimulus (Fabiani, Gratton, & M. G. H. Coles, 2000). Thus, the authors suggest that in pain patients there may be a greater preconscious allocation of attention to stimuli related to pain (Flor, Knost, & Birbaumer, 1997).

In the Flor et al. study, later components of the evoked potential, and the ability to recognize the pain-related words, were not enhanced in the patients. Other studies, however, have found more explicit information processing differences in people who have chronic pain. For example, Edwards and S. A. Pearce (1994), in what was ostensibly an "experiment on language" asked individuals with chronic pain, healthy volunteers from the general population, and health professionals to complete word stems (e.g., to write down words that begin with "ten__" or "sha__"). Both health professionals and patients generated more words that had to do with illness. However, the patients generated more words dealing with pain sensation than either the health professionals or the volunteers. The cognitive **schema** for pain seems to have remained active, even during a theoretically neutral task (Edwards & S. A. Pearce, 1994).

Does a cognitive schema emphasizing pain perception have clinical consequences? In Chapter 3 we will see indirect evidence that it does.

PAIN MODULATION

Thus, as we traced the pain system along stimulus-driven, bottom-up pathways, we encountered pain sensitization at every stage—the release of **neuropeptides** at sensory nerve endings, the change in sodium channel density at the dorsal root ganglion, long-term synaptic potentiation in the dorsal horn and presumably the brain, possibly the death of inhibitory interneurons, and a reverberant loop of activation between the dorsal horn and the brain stem's parabrachial nucleus. Like other sensory modalities, the pain system adapts to stimulation. But unlike other modalities, the adaptation seems to occur only in the direction of increased sensitivity. In its stimulus-driven mechanisms, the pain system does not seem to habituate.

Why, then, does not all pain become chronic? Part of the reason may be the inertia caused by inhibitory processes, for example in lamina II (Doubell, Mannion, and Woolf, 1999). By blunting the response of the dorsal horn, and constraining the amount of pain signal sent on to higher structures, the local inhibition may keep the pain system below a threshold for sensitization. Additional explanation, however, is provided by descending pain modulatory circuits.

The endorphin system. So far, we have discussed pain sensitization as if it were a purely bottom-up process, the inevitable result of a noxious stimulus of sufficient intensity and duration. But in fact, as surmised in the Gate Control Model, there are projections down from the brain that set the tonic level of activity in the dorsal horn (Fields, 2000; Gjerstad, Tjølsen, & Hole, 2001). Indeed, descending inhibitory pathways can synapse directly on the central axon terminals of peripheral sensory neurons, reducing the amount of signal transmitted into the dorsal horn. Thus, neurons from the brain can inhibit the pain signal even from entering the central nervous system in the first place.

The best understood of the descending circuits involves a pathway from the **periaqueductal gray** area of the midbrain to the rostral ventromedial medulla area[14] and on to the dorsal horn and the trigeminal nucleus caudalis (Fields, 2000). Also involved is the dorsolateral pontine tegmentum, which sends efferent signals to the rostral ventromedial medulla (see Figure 2–2). These pathways use **endorphins** as neurotransmitters, and are sometimes called the "lower opioid system" (Petrovic & Ingvar, 2002, p. 2). This system has a slow rise time, several minutes, during which the pain gradually declines (Fields, 2000; D. Price & Barrell, 2000).

---

[14]Important components of the rostral ventromedial medulla include the nucleus raphe magnus (Millan, 2002) and the nucleus reticularis gigantocellularis (Calejesan, S. J. Kim, & Zhuo, 2000).

Now the term "lower opioid system" implies that there is an "upper opioid system," and indeed there is. More exactly, there are a number of higher brain regions that seem connected to, and capable of activating, the endorphinergic system in the periaqueductal gray. These regions, and the possibly relevant processes they subserve, are (Fanselow, 1994; Fields, 2000; Petrovic & Ingvar, 2002): the medial and lateral frontal cortex (cognitive evaluation of the situation in which the pain stimulus is embedded), the amygdala (fear conditioning), hypothalamus (fight or flight response), and the **rostral** part of the anterior cingulate cortex (Brodmann Area 32; prioritizing emotionally meaningful stimuli for response).[15]

In particular, the portion of the anterior cingulate cortex that seems responsible for hypnotic analgesia (Faymonville et al., 2000) is rich in endorphin receptors (Petrovic & Ingvar, 2002) and there seems to be a path linking it to the deeper endorphinergic structures such as the periaqueductal gray (Fanselow, 1994). Moreover, Petrovic, et al. found in an imaging study that activation in the rostral part of the anterior cingulate cortex covaried with activation in the periaqueductal gray area (Petrovic, Kalso, Petersson, & Ingvar, 2001), suggesting that the two are functioning as part of the same pain control process (Petrovic & Ingvar, 2002).

The pathways from the medial frontal cortex and the anterior cingulate cortex may provide a mechanism by which selective attention can inhibit pain. Because selective attention would thus ultimately involve activation of endorphinergic synapses, and because opioid medications mimic the endorphins, we might expect distraction and narcotics to have qualitatively similar effects on pain. We will see evidence below that they do. In essence, we can measure the analgesic effects of distraction in milligrams of morphine.

Diffuse noxious inhibitory controls.   The process by which pain in one part of the body inhibits pain in another part appears to involve a reflex through the dorsal reticular nucleus of the medulla, rather than the full endorphin system (see Figure 2–2; Bouhassira, Bing, & Le Bars, 1990; Millan, 2002; Roby-Brami, Bussel, Willer, & Le Bars, 1987). Intuitively, we might assume that pain in one part of the body simply distracts us from pain in another part. Then, the pain-on-pain inhibitory pathways (which are called "**diffuse noxious inhibitory controls**" or DNIC) are simply those that mediate attention. In psychophysical studies, however, remote pain and distraction have distinct effects. Distraction, like morphine, inhibits all pain by a discrete amount. Remote pain decreases only those target pains of moderate intensity; low-intensity and high-intensity target pains are not affected (Plaghki, Delisle, & Godfraind, 1994).[16] Speculatively, the efficacy of TENS units,[17] acupuncture, and other "counter-irritant" procedures has been ascribed to diffuse noxious inhibitory controls (Dar, Ariely, & Frenk, 1995; Sandkühler, 2000).

---

[15]Note that this is a different part of anterior cingulate cortex than that encoding the emotional qualities of pain.

[16]Note that the selectivity of pain-on-pain inhibition also tends to rule out adaptation-level theory (Dar, Ariely, & Frenk, 1995; Helson, 1964) as an explanation. Adaptation-level is a cognitive theory, in which the experience of an intense stimulus changes one's internal reference points, so that lesser pains are regarded as milder than they had been.

[17]"TENS" stands for "transcutaneous [across the skin] electrical nerve stimulation." TENS units are the size of walkmans and affix to one's belt. Small wires from the unit attach via adhesive pads to the surface of the skin near the painful area. The electrical stimulation from the unit produces a tingling or vibrating sensation that masks the pain. TENS units were invented by Patrick Wall (M. Devor, 2001) based on the gate control model: The electrical stimulation of large sensory nerves should balance out the noxious input from small sensory nerves and make the dorsal horn less responsive. However, the analgesia from a TENS unit can last for hours after the unit is switched off. This is hard to explain with the gate control model, and suggests instead that the unit activates the descending pain control system, perhaps by functioning as a mild irritant. We should add, too, that "electrical anesthesia" was used as a research tool in the early days of experimental psychology (Goldscheider, 1889; Pillsbury, 1901; J. E. Winter, 1912), and seems to have been tried in surgery as early as 1847 (Wright, 1996), more than a century before the gate control model. In fact, the technique is mentioned in an ancient Roman text, where an electric fish is recommended for producing numbness and pain relief (Kane & A. Taub, 1975).

Pain Facilitation.   Within the endorphin system, not all of the descending signals from the rostral ventromedial medulla are certain to be inhibitory. Neurons that facilitate pain transmission ("**On cells**") also project to the dorsal horn, possibly increasing its sensitivity (Fields, 2000; Zhuo & Gebhart, 1997). As we will see in Chapter 7, on cells play an important role in opioid analgesia and possibly in the rebound pain of medication overuse headaches (Fields, 2001). Many other structures involved in descending pain inhibition seem to play a role in descending facilitation as well, including the **solitary tract nucleus**, the dorsal reticular nucleus (of the medulla), the periaqueductal gray, and the hypothalamus (Millan, 2002). Indeed, in animals, pain facilitatory pathways have been traced rostrally as far as the anterior cingulate cortex and the frontal lobes (Calejesan, S. J. Kim, & M. Zhuo, 2000), suggesting that in people, cognitive and emotional factors might be able to up-regulate activity in the dorsal horn.

Non-opioid analgesia.   There seem to be other mechanisms, not nearly as well understood as the endorphinergic pathways, by which the central nervous system modulates pain (Field, 2000). For example, fight-or-flight responding seems to activate a second analgesic pathway in the periaqueductal gray that does not use endorphins (Bandler, J. L. Price, & Keay, 2000). And there are direct, monosynaptic projections from the somatosensory, frontal, and motor areas of the cortex, back down to the nociceptive parts of the dorsal horn (Field, 2000; Millan, 2002). We should add, too, that the endorphins, while important, are not the only, or even the primary, neurotransmitter involved in descending pain control. Others include norepinephrine, dopamine, **acetylcholine**, and serotonin. These same four transmitters are involved in descending facilitation, along with **cholecystokinin**, substance P, **histamine**, and melanocortin (Millan, 2002).

So far, we have focused on pain modulatory systems that extend down to the brain stem and the dorsal horn. It is possible, however, for the brain to modulate pain at the highest levels of the central nervous system. For example, the frontal lobes appear able to inhibit thalamocortical pathways (Gracely, 1995; Vuilleumier, Chicherio, Assal, Schwartz, Slosman, & Landis, 2001), the **basal ganglia** (Vuilleumier et al.), and the amygdala (Petrovic & Ingvar, 2002), suggesting that pain intensity and emotional consequences can be modified by the frontal lobes.

Pain modulation and central sensitization.   Thus, through the endorphinergic pathways, the brain may be thought of as operating a "gain" or "volume" control at the earliest processing station for pain in the spinal column. Top down endorphinergic processes influence the firing rates of nociceptive neurons in the dorsal horn. Not surprisingly, then, there is evidence that the level of descending inhibition affects proneness to developing central sensitization (Sandkühler, 2000). Moreover, the level of descending inhibition is regulated in part by psychological variables such as distraction. This raises the possibility that psychological variables may help determine whether dorsal horn synapses become physiologically sensitized, and hence whether chronic pain develops (Sandkühler, 2000). A connection of this type would help explain, for example, why psychometric tests such as the **MMPI** are reasonably good predictors of pain-related outcomes from back surgery (e.g., Sørensen, 1992; Sørensen, Mors, & Skovlund, 1987; Wiltse & Rocchio, 1975), or why emotional reactions to injury predict the persistence of pain in whiplash (e.g., Drottning, Staff, L. Levin, & U. F. Malt, 1995). So far, however, there is no direct evidence linking psychology with central sensitization. There is a study that comes close, however. Harris and coworkers found that classically conditioned **hypoalgesia**, which we will study further below, suppressed the expression of genes in dorsal horn neurons associated with neuronal excitation (Harris, Westbrook, Duffield, & Bentivoglio, 1995).

If it turns out that inhibition at the dorsal horn can prevent central sensitization, what could we say about pain coping that occurred purely at the forebrain, for example by inhibition of thalamocortical pathways? Such a coping mechanism might allow us to persist at a painful task, all the while exposing our dorsal horns to noxious stimulation. That is, a pain coping strategy that functioned entirely at the forebrain could inadvertently be a psychological risk factor for chronic pain. Now, at this point we do not know if there truly are mechanisms with such isolated effects—perhaps all pain inhibitory processes involve efferent paths to the dorsal horn. But the caution is worth thinking about, and we will return to it again in Chapters 3 and 15.

A similar question pertains to the long-term use of opiates. Vanderah and associates provide evidence that chronic morphine administration leads to tonic facilitation from on cells in the rostral ventromedial medulla to the dorsal horn, causing **hyperalgesia** and **allodynia**. This facilitation seems to occur even during continuous administration, in the absence of withdrawal (Vanderah, Ossipov, J. Lai, Malan, & Porreca, 2001; Vanderah, Suenaga, Ossipov, Malan, J. Lai, & Porreca, 2001). Meanwhile, the morphine continues to function as an analgesic at higher brain centers (Roerig, O'Brien, Fujimoto, & Wilcox, 1984). At this point we know very little about the long-term effects of the specific treatments for chronic pain, behavioral or pharmacological.

Pain modulation and chronic pain.   Deficits in pain inhibition may play a role in chronic pain. For example, if the right upper trapezius and deltoid muscles are contracted to the point of fatigue, the threshold for pressure pain increases. This resistance to pressure pain is not likely to be a local effect of fatigue because there is also an increase in threshold at the *left* upper trapezius and deltoid, even if there was no coactivation of these muscles (Persson, Hansson, Kalliomäki, Moritz, & Sjölund, 2000). Rather, it appears that the sustained contraction induces central antinociceptive activity. In people with fibromyalgia, however, isometric contraction does not increase pressure pain thresholds, suggesting a deficit in central pain inhibition (Kosek, Ekholm, & Hansson, 1996).

Descending pain facilitation may also be important, at least for certain types of pain. In animal studies, descending facilitation has not had significant long-term effects on local inflammatory pain following injury (Re & Dubner, 2002). However, the facilitation does seem to have considerable impact on the long-term sensitivity of the region *surrounding* the injured tissue (secondary hyperalgesia; Re & Dubner, 2002).

Moreover, descending facilitation may be crucial to the long-term maintenance of neuropathic pain, at least in animals (Burgess et al., 2002). In the Burgess, et al. study, neuropathic pain faded after four days when pain facilitatory pathways were blocked. In control animals, the pain persisted for at least twelve (Burgess et al.). Similarly, destruction of on cells in the medulla seems to prevent the development of neuropathic pain in animals, while leaving ordinary nociception unchanged (Porreca, Burgess, et al., 2001).

It appears that synapses in the pain modulatory circuits can undergo the same types of synaptic strengthening that we saw in the dorsal horn, and with the same general mechanisms: an increase in the number of AMPA- and NMDA-type glutamate receptors, and phosphorylation of the AMPA types (Re & Dubner, 2002). This suggests that one's ability to inhibit or facilitate pain can be gradually, and perhaps inadvertently, strengthened over time.

Top-down processes can also cause clinically important *hypo*algesia. There is abundant evidence that individuals with high blood pressure, indeed even those who are merely at risk for high blood pressure, have significantly dampened pain perception (C. R. France, 1999). This can be good, for example, if one is recovering from surgery, or bad, if one is having a heart attack. Hypertension-associated hypoalgesia has been offered as an explanation for silent **myocardial infarctions** (C. R. France, 1999). It appears that blood pressure receptors ("**baroreceptors**") in the carotids and the aorta send projections to the hypothalamus, which in turn projects to the periaqueductal gray region, activating the endorphin system. In fact, one theory of high blood pressure holds that it is a (presumably unconscious) learned response that is reinforced by reductions in pain and stress (C. R. France, 1999).

Of course not all brain-mediated hypoalgesia is bad. We will encounter a rather beneficial example, the placebo response, in Chapter 3. Indeed, with descending pain modulation we enter upon the full symphony of pain processing. For pain is not simply a signal written on the brain's tablet, but an experience which many regions of the central nervous system help create. Here, then, is the field on which psychological variables can exert a great deal of influence. But before we begin examining this influence, before we look at the pain system's "inherent psychology," let us consider what we have learned from the standpoint of patient assessment.

THE EXAM AS CLINICAL LABORATORY

We have encountered three broad types of pain—nociceptive, neuropathic, and deafferentative— each springing from a separate source. But perhaps these three types are not discrete categories so much as dimensions or ingredients that can be present in varying degrees. Perhaps any given pain condition might receive contributions from

- An ongoing peripheral source
- Central sensitization at the dorsal horn and/or thalamus
- Decreased descending pain inhibition
- Increased descending pain facilitation
- Cortical changes, such as a disorganization of the somatosensory homunculus
- And possibly cumulative damage to pain control structures.

This may be one reason that chronic pain is so difficult to assess and treat. Because we cannot easily or precisely image central nervous system processes, we are left with one equation and six unknowns. Yet we have also seen that sensory information itself is informative. Primary and secondary hyperalgesia are defined as a reduction in pain threshold. The degree to which exercise of an unrelated body part or induced pain at a distant location can raise this threshold tells us about the effectiveness of endorphinergic processes. The organization of somatosensory cortex can be inferred from the ability to localize and discriminate tactile stimuli (Hodzic, Veit, Karim, Erb, & Godde, 2004; Pleger, Dinse, Ragert, Schwenkreis, Malin, & Tegenthoff, 2001), and from referred sensations to light touch (McCabe, Haigh, Shenker, J. Lewis, & Blake, 2004). Referral of pain from painful stimuli seems to be a particular marker for distortion of the homunculus (Grusser et al., 2001). Responsiveness to drugs may also be instructive. For example, extradural motor cortex stimulation seems to benefit patients whose **central pain** responds to barbiturates, but not those whose pain responds only to morphine (Canavero & Bonicalzi, 2002). In the future, functional neuroimaging of pain pathways may become a tool for clinical diagnosis (Borsook, Burstein, & Becerra, 2004). But so, too, can the clinical exam, and especially its recasting in quantitative terms via psychophysics, provide a noninvasive means of characterizing the functional state of the pain system in a given patient.

Psychophysics of chronic pain.   Just as a patient's intuitive description of their pain can convey the state of the nociceptive system, so too can precise sensory testing be informative. Thus, one approach to studying chronic pain is through **psychophysics**: Determining the quantitative relationship between the amplitude of the painful stimulus and the intensity of the resulting pain. This relationship is often depicted as a graph, termed the stimulus-response, or SR, curve, of pain rating as a function of stimulus intensity.

Several changes in the SR curve are informative. The simplest is a drop in the y-intercept, with no change in slope. All pain intensities are reduced by a constant amount. This type of change reflects an increase in descending pain inhibition, whether from opioid medication or distraction (Bendtsen, Jensen, & Olesen, 1996b; Plaghki, Delisle, & Godfraind, 1994).

Alternatively, the curve's shape may change, for example when pain intensity is reduced at moderate levels of stimulation, while pain at high and low levels of stimulation is unchanged. This type of change, which appears as a plateau in the SR curve, is produced by diffuse noxious inhibitory controls (Plaghki, Delisle, & Godfraind, 1994).

A third change, also of shape, may be seen at the low end of the curve, when the stimulation is from pressure. In healthy subjects, there is little pain below a certain threshold. Above the threshold, pain increases rapidly. The SR curve can be described as a step function, or else as a **power function** with a very strong positive acceleration. In people with tension-type headache, however, even low levels of pressure are painful, and the SR curve is linear (Bendtsen, Jensen, & Olesen, 1996b). As it turns out, these two types of curve—step function vs. linear—characterize two types of **mechanoreceptors** in muscle (at least in rats; You & Mense, 1990). Ordinarily, low threshold mechanoreceptors convey pressure as a linear function of stimulation. High threshold mechanoreceptors signal pain as a step function. Thus, the change in stimulus-response curve suggests that, in tension-type headache, input from low threshold mechanoreceptors has been re-routed in the dorsal horn through pain pathways usually reserved for the high threshold mechanoreceptor input. This is part of the evidence that the dorsal horn rewires itself in chronic pain.

Additional information is conveyed by "windup"—a response to noxious stimulation repeated at long intervals. Over trials, the pain response increases, not merely linearly, which would indicate temporal summation of the stimuli, but in an accelerating manner. This acceleration was one of the earliest demonstrations of a form of central sensitization (Woolf, 1996). And even when we do not test for it, patients may report it anyway. For some, the first sign of a flare-up may be that one's daughter's insistent tapping on the arm during a car ride cumulates into pain. Or in physical therapy, pulses of electrical stimulation, well below the pain threshold at first, may quickly become intolerable for some people with chronic pain.

At this point, the use of pain psychophysics for studying diagnostic groups is still in its infancy. Certainly it is too soon to know if it will have the necessary sensitivity and specificity for use in assessing individual patients. However, this is an important area of clinical research, to which experimental psychologists are well positioned to contribute.

THE PAIN SYSTEM'S INHERENT PSYCHOLOGY

Our knowledge of the pain system hints at treatment. Stimulus-driven sensitization of the dorsal horn suggests that **pacing** one's activities may be important, not only to prevent short-term flare-ups but also to prevent a long-term erosion of pain thresholds. When pain more likely arises from cortex, sensorimotor reeducation, exemplified in mirror therapy, guided motor imagery, and discrimination training, is suggested. But it is in the descending pathways, inhibitory and facilitory, that the full power of the central nervous system to control pain is realized. It is from this substrate that most of our behavioral tools derive. To understand these tools it will help to explore the inherent purpose of descending pain control—the adaptive value of shifts in pain sensitivity.

Conditioned Hyperalgesia

We have seen that central sensitization can develop as the result of exposure to acute pain. But, as the brain is involved, we would not be surprised to find that learning is involved as well. Thus, Duncan et al. demonstrated that when monkeys are trained to respond to a painful stimulus, over trials some nociceptive neurons in the trigeminal nucleus begin to fire at the warning signal, before the painful stimulus actually begins (Duncan, Bushnell, R. Bates, & Dubner, 1987). Thus, it seems that with repeated exposure to pain, a **priming** of neurons encoding pain can be conditioned. Certainly it seems reasonable that the central nervous system use its past experience with a situation to fine-tune its perceptual focus.

Pain conditioning, however, does not require actual exposure to pain. For example, Wiertelak and coworkers produced nausea (by injecting lithium chloride) or malaise (by injecting bacteria-derived lipopolysaccharides, which stimulate an immune response) in rats. Within a few minutes of the injections, the rats showed an increased sensitivity to heat pain and inflammatory pain, but not to innocuous pressure stimuli (Wiertelak et al., 1994). Other researchers have found lower thresholds for pressure pain after injecting immune system chemicals such as interleukin–1β (Ferreira, Lorenzetti, Bristow, & Poole, 1988). In the trigeminal nucleus caudalis specifically, lipopolysaccharides have been shown to cause hyperalgesia to noxious chemical stimulation (Kemper, Spoelstra, Meijler, & Ter Horst, 1998). Presumably, a systemic illness that does not involve pain will nonetheless produce a sensitization to pain.

The mechanism behind this effect is gradually becoming clearer (Watkins & Maier, 2000). For example, during an infection, certain white blood cells produce **cytokines**, chemicals that help coordinate the immune response. One of these cytokines is the above-noted interleukin–1, and remarkably, there appear to be sensory nerves in the abdomen with receptors for it. Thus, the nerves can detect an immune response. Signals from these sensory nerves are transmitted in turn to the vagus nerve, the **solitary tract nucleus** in the medulla, the nucleus raphe magnus which is also in the medulla, and ultimately the dorsal horn, where it triggers hyperalgesia (Watkins & Maier, 2000).[18] Thus, an increase in pain sensitivity, alongside fever and a need to rest, can be elicited by infection. This adds to the impression that hyperalgesia is an adaptive response by the body (Wiertelak et al., 1994), at times implemented through descending pain facilitatory pathways (Porreca, Ossipov, & Gebhart, 2002).

Now, behaviorists will note that nausea and malaise, induced by lithium and/or lipopolysaccharides, are key ingredients in **conditioned taste aversion**. If an animal experiences nausea or malaise after ingesting a somewhat novel food, the animal will avoid that food for a long time to come. Conditioned taste aversion is an unusually rapid form of classical (Pavlovian) conditioning. This leads us to a question: When an animal acquires a conditioned taste aversion is it also acquiring a conditioned hyperalgesia? In the study by Wiertelak et al., the lithium chloride or lipopolysaccharide injections followed a taste of saccharine water. Later, the conditioned animals were exposed to a small amount of saccharine water, without the injection. In the conditioned animals, but not in control animals, the hyperalgesia was elicited all over again, and with the same time course as occurred after the injection (Wiertelak et al., 1994).

Note that pain itself does not appear to have been conditioned. The animals displayed no **pain behaviors** in the absence of noxious heat or inflammation. But a sensitivity to pain was learned, apparently automatically.

---

[18]In addition to signaling through the vagus nerve, cytokines gain entrance to the brain through active transport and by diffusion in places where the blood-brain barrier is weak. Also, cytokines can cause blood vessels to produce prostaglandins and nitric oxide, which enter the brain as "second messengers" (Licinio & M.-L. Wong, 1997).

Perhaps then, with signs of illness, when the danger is inside, the brain shifts focus, and lowers the pain threshold so that relevant information is getting through. We have barely begun to explore whether this phenomenon has clinical effects in people. But who among us is aware of our pain thresholds? All we know is that we feel pain, or that we do not feel pain. If our pain thresholds are lower, we simply hurt more. For a person who has been housebound with chronic pain for weeks, months, or years, the home environment can surely become saturated with reminders of feeling unwell.

In the study by Wiertelak and coworkers, the pain sensation itself was not conditioned. We can ask, however, whether pain *can* be elicited purely through classical conditioning. I have come across only one apparent example, and it may be the exception that proves the rule. Ramachandran and Rogers-Ramachandran describe the case of a woman with phantom pain in her fingers following an arm amputation. She had had arthritis in the hand before the amputation, and the phantom pain, like the arthritic pain before it, would flare up in damp weather (Ramachandran & Rogers-Ramachandran, 1996). Note, however, that in phantom limb pain the brain does not receive corrective, somatosensory feedback from the limb. Perhaps it is only when the brain's representation of pain is cut off from true sensory information that the pain can become a purely conditioned response (Ramachandran & Rogers-Ramachandran, 1996).

Now, our brains can do much more than form simple associations. What if we conclude based on rational grounds that a given stimulus might be dangerous. Would that be enough to lower the pain threshold? Logically, of course, the answer is yes. And there is some evidence that this is true empirically as well.

Expectancy Effects

Can the expectation of pain produce pain? There is some evidence that it can, in what is called "**nocebo** responding." The term seems to have been coined by Kennedy (1961), and derives from the Latin, "I will harm" (Wall, 1999). It has been examined by Kissel and Barrucand (1964), Schweiger and Parducci (1981), and Hahn (1997). Nocebos are like placebos, except that they elicit pain or other symptoms instead of reducing them.

In a particularly striking demonstration, Bayer and coworkers attached sham electrodes to the foreheads of subjects during what was nominally a reaction time study. The electrodes were attached to a machine with a clearly visible intensity dial and a just-audible hum. When the dial setting was increased the hum's volume stayed the same but its frequency incremented by 10 Hz. The subjects were told that they would receive an "undetectable electrical current to measure its effect on reaction time and that the current was 'safe but often painful'" (Bayer, Baer, & Early, 1991, p. 46). In all, 55 percent of subjects in the experimental group reported a headache, and average pain ratings were a monotonic increasing function of the stimulator's fake intensity setting (Bayer et al., 1991).

Now, the headaches were probably not due to stress because heart rate was not different, and the number of **skin conductance responses** was lower, in the subjects who reported pain vs. those who did not. And the headaches were probably not false reports designed to satisfy the experimenters' expectations, because subjects who believed that their pain levels were being monitored electronically ("**bogus pipeline**") did not report pain less often. Rather, the combination of drawing attention to the topic of headaches and building an expectation that a headache would occur was enough to actually induce a headache (Bayer et al., 1991).

This seems adaptive. The volunteers in Bayer et al.'s experiment were recruited from an unemployment line; most were uneducated. We would not expect them to entirely trust the experimenters or the strange machine. Under the circumstances, it would make sense for the subjects to lower pain thresholds for the head, so as to detect harm and react to it as quickly as possible, before any physical damage could occur. Presumably, the subjects unconsciously lowered their pain thresholds to the point that background neural activity was experienced as pain.

Or neural activity may have increased, for the anticipation of pain is enough to increase firing in the same corical regions as are involved in pain perception. Ordinarily, expectation is only about one-third as potent as an actual pain stimulus (Porro et al., 2002),[19] but perhaps this depends on how strong the expectation is.

Whether nocebo responding is clinically relevant is not yet certain. To the participants in Bayer, et al.'s study the pain felt very real; they were surprised when debriefed afterwards about the experimental setup. However, the pain was also mild and abated quickly after the "current" was switched off. If Bayer et al.'s results do transfer to a clinical setting, they raise the question of whether frequent tension-type headaches might produce the expectation of having more headaches, and hence become a self-sustaining cycle. If so, then **cognitive therapy** to reduce the expectation might have efficacy for tension-type headache.

Stress-Induced Analgesia

Psychological factors can reduce pain as well as increase it. In the next chapter we will discuss perhaps the most salient example of this, the placebo effect. Here, let us consider a case in which the adaptive significance is even greater: **Stress-induced analgesia**.

When a person is exposed to a severe stressor, such as when a veteran is exposed to reminders of battle, pain sensitivity is markedly reduced. When the feared stimulus is inescapable, the analgesia seems to be due primarily to the endorphin system (Pitman, van der Kolk, Orr, & Greenberg, 1990; Willer & Ernst, 1986) and distraction (S. A. Janssen & Arntz, 1996). When the stimulus is escapable, activating a fight-or-flight response, the analgesia does not seem to work through an endorphinergic mechanism (S. A. Janssen & Arntz, 1999). Possibly, too, there may be a linkage with the immune system: Stress seems to reduce the production of pro-inflammatory cytokines such as interleukin–1β (Kiecolt-Glaser, Marucha, Atkinson, & Glaser, 2001). This in turn seems to delay wound healing (Marucha, Kiecolt-Glaser & Favagehi, 1998), but it could also prevent cytokine-mediated hyperalgesia.

By whatever mechanism, however, the result seems adaptive: When the danger is external and controllable, survival is enhanced by attending to the situation and preparing a fight-or-flight response (Amit & Galina, 1986). For a danger that is external and uncontrollable, being cornered by an attacker, there is a response that sometimes works: playing dead (Amit & Galina, 1986). Preoccupation with pain, of course, would only interfere. This may explain why, after a car accident or other unexpected incident, a person may not feel their injuries for several hours (Beecher, 1946; Wall, 2000).

We might expect that one's adaptation would be even greater if the pain thresholds could be modified in anticipation of the stress. Not surprisingly, then, several investigators have found that stress-induced analgesia, at least of the type mediated by endorphins, can be classically conditioned in animals (Chance, Krynock, & Rosecrans, 1978; Harris, Westbrook, Duffield, & Bentivoglio, 1995; Oliverio & Castellano, 1982), and elicited by the expectation of pain in humans (Willer, Dehen, & Cambier, 1981).

---

[19]"The peculiar theoretic interest of these experiments lies in their showing expectant attention and sensation to be continuous or identical processes" (W. James, 1890/1901, p. 429). James was referring to 19th century reaction time studies, but anticipated Porro's results. See Ploghaus, et al., 1999, note 15.

Of note, however, stress-induced analgesia and its reproduction by classical conditioning seems to be stronger in male than in female animals (Stock, Caldarone, Abrahamsen, Mongeluzi, M. A. Wilson, & Rosellini, 2001). It is not known yet whether this qualification applies to humans as well. In future chapters we will encounter several other examples of sex and gender differences in pain perception (see also the review by Berkley & Holdcroft, 1999).

Clinically, then, does all this mean that relaxation training and **stress management** are misguided? Perhaps pain patients would do better if they were chronically on edge. We cannot, however, attest to the healthful effects of extreme stress. After the analgesic period has ended, it may be replaced by a long-lasting increase in pain sensitivity (Quintero, Moreno, Avila, Arcaya, Maixner, & Suarez-Roca, 2000). In Chapter 7, we will see similar evidence of rebound hyperalgesia when analgesia is induced chemically, that is, with opiate medications.

Exploratory Behavior

We have seen evidence that the brain exerts efferent control over the dorsal horn. In fact, the brain may "reach down" even further than that, as suggested by a study conducted at the Roslin Institute. Gentle and Tilston (1999) produced a temporary joint inflammation in chickens by injecting sodium urate into their left ankles. Chickens returned to their cages showed a number of pain behaviors over the next three hours that to me seem best described as suffering. However, if the chickens were placed in a large, novel pen with another chicken (the birds had been kept in relative isolation until then), pain behaviors were nearly absent. Moreover, inflammation, measured as the temperature difference between the injected and non-injected ankles, was lower in the chickens who had been distracted from their pain. These results are consistent with the view that inflammation is only partly a local reaction of the tissues. A second component of inflammation may be neurogenic and *mediated by the experience of pain*. When the chickens' pain was blocked cognitively by a distracting environment, the neurogenic component of inflammation was reduced (Gentle & Tilston, 1999). The finding that seemingly automatic physiological processes can be influenced by conscious, cognitive variables is one of the bases for biofeedback treatment, about which we will hear much in subsequent chapters.

Now, why would being in a distracting environment reduce pain, let alone inflammation? Actually, as we will see in the next chapter, the term "distracting" is controversial. Momentary distraction (Dowman, 2001) and mere information processing demands do not seem to reduce pain or improve pain coping (McCaul, Monson, & Maki, 1992). Rather, the key seems to be **absorption** in a motivational state that in some ways is the opposite of pain (Lang, Bradley, & Cuthbert, 1997). In the wild, exploration, foraging, and other "appetitive" pursuits often entail some pain. If an animal or a person gives up too easily when they encounter pain, they are less likely to survive (Amit & Galina, 1986). Thus, it is quite helpful if the motivation itself is enough to reduce pain sensitivity.[20]

This, too, is of considerable clinical import. Wilbert Fordyce, who helped develop behavioral chronic pain treatment, regarded as fundamental the reduction in suffering brought about by involvement in important activities (Fordyce, 1988).

---

[20]Of course answering the question of "why" still leaves the difficult question of *how* pain could mediate inflammation. At this point the mechanism, if any, is quite unknown. However, the main components of the immune system are innervated by the peripheral and autonomic nervous systems, with which they sometimes "appear to make synapse-like connections" (E. M. Sternberg, 1997, p. 2,644). Immune cell activity is modulated by a variety of neurotransmitters and neuropeptides, and by the hormone cortisol (E. M. Sternberg, 1997).

Note that this effect of motivation is consistent with what we know of the endorphin system. Recall that pain affect ("unpleasantness") covaries with activation of the back end of the anterior cingulate cortex (D. Price, 2000). Right next to this caudal area, a little more **rostral**, is a second part of the anterior cingulate cortex that seems to play a role in selective attention to emotionally neutral stimuli. And next to that is a third part, the most anterior of the three, that seems to be involved in attention to emotionally meaningful stimuli (Petrovic & Ingvar, 2002). The endorphin system that presumably originates from this region would then adjust pain sensitivity in line with emotional priorities. Successful pain reduction through **hypnosis** (Faymonville et al., 2000), distraction (Frankenstein, Richter, McIntyre, & Remy, 2001), or placebo (Petrovic, Kalso, Petersson, & Ingvar, 2001) involves activation of this third, emotionally relevant, area (Petrovic & Ingvar, 2002). Not surprisingly, activation of the rostral anterior cingulate cortex has been found also in the "non-anatomical" anesthesia of **conversion disorder** (Mailis-Gagnon et al., 2003).

Now, all of the factors we have reviewed so far—conditioning, expectation, fear, and exploration—are psychological. However, none of them necessarily implies that pain sensitivity is a form of psychopathology. Rather, they are adaptive responses, in which pain threshold is adjusted in light of our knowledge of the situation and of the type of danger it is likely to contain.

Presumably, all pain results from the interplay of top-down and bottom-up processes. The division into purely "organic" and purely "psychogenic" pain can refer only to the most unusual and extreme cases, and thus will not generally be useful (D. C. Turk & Okifuji, 2004). In the clinic, "the unprejudiced physician will find some physical defect in every 'functional' case, and some psychical factor in every case of 'organic disease'" (Crookshank, 1926, p. 6). Indeed, even Sigmund Freud, in his case study of Elizabeth R., opined that very rarely, if at all, did pain have a purely psychological origin. Thus, "the circumstances indicate that this somatic pain was not *created* by the neurosis but merely used, increased and maintained by it" (Breuer & Freud, 1893–1895/1957, p. 174). We should inquire instead, then, about which factors are influencing pain sensitivity, in which direction, and whether this is truly adaptive for the individual. We will return to this topic, exploring psychological factors in greater detail, in the next chapter.

CHAPTER 3

Psychological Variables in Chronic Pain

If a slight injury to a joint is gradually followed by a severe arthralgia, no doubt the process involves a psychical element, viz. a concentration of attention on the injured part, which intensifies the excitability of the nerve tracts concerned. But this can hardly be expressed by saying that the hyperalgesia has been caused by ideas.
—Josef Breuer & Sigmund Freud (1893–1895/1957, p. 190)

Medical doctors do and should make every attempt to locate a correctable, physical source for the pain. The progressively more abstruse diagnostic tests and imaging studies in which patients participate are thoroughly justified by this principle. Yet there often seems to be another purpose for pursuing these tests: to be able to frame the pain in concrete and specific terms—to give the patient, as has been eloquently stated, "the dignity of diagnosis" (Bogduk, 1994, cited in Derby, 1996). But **chronic pain syndrome**, viewed from a psychological perspective, is also a diagnosis. It is specific and concrete, and it is often much more treatable than an ambiguous, uncorrectable lesion at the limen of radiographic detection. To make use of this specificity in developing an appropriate behavioral treatment plan, it is first necessary to understand the psychological variables that play a role in chronic pain syndrome.

For chronic headaches will sometimes shade into chronic pain syndrome, in which cognitive, emotional, and behavioral factors complicate pain coping and potentially add to the pain itself. For people with this syndrome, viewing the pain unidimensionally, that is, purely in terms of the physical disorder, can deprive them of additional tools for recovery.

Moreover, the presence of a clear physical diagnosis should not blind us to psychological variables, for the physical and the behavioral are, conceptually, orthogonal dimensions. That is, a thorough understanding of the patient will often require a multiaxial approach, in which physical, psychological, and social factors, and their interactions, are considered (Engle, 1978). We will return to this in the chapter on assessment; first, however, we must consider more deeply the role of psychology in pain.

In the chapter on behavioral treatment, we will have much to say about pain coping tools. However, no programmatic review of treatment can fully prepare us for the myriad constellations of symptoms we will encounter in patients. Thus, it will be very helpful for us to have grounding first in the laboratory data on which psychological therapies are based. It is to this data that we now turn.

COGNITION

Attention and the Control of Pain

Presumably, factors that increase attention to one's pain, increase the pain itself. Thus, Dillmann, et al. asked volunteers to focus on neutral words, or words that expressed sensory or emotional aspects of pain. When thinking of the sensory or emotional words, the EEG somatosensory potential evoked by a painful laser pulse (at 300–370 msec post-stimulus) was higher (Dillmann, Miltner, & T. Weiss, 2000; T. Weiss, Miltner, & Dillmann, 2003). It appears that the nociceptive system responds to cognitive **priming**.

Conversely, various distractions, such as imagining a pleasant scene or focusing on a demanding task, decrease acute pain by (in a **meta-analysis**) approximately 0.5 standard deviations compared with control conditions (Fernandez & D. C. Turk, 1989). This is generally considered a moderate **effect size** (J. Cohen, 1988). In fact, distraction probably exerts a greater effect than this, as some people in the control conditions probably used their own distraction techniques informally. These results may apply to chronic pain as well, as individuals with chronic pain often report spontaneous use of distraction-like techniques (Fernandez & D. C. Turk, 1989).

These results fit well with the idea that activity in higher brain centers can feed back upon and inhibit pain signals in lower centers (Achterberg, 1984). In fact, Petrovic, et al., appear to have captured this effect on film with a positron emission tomography study of regional cerebral blood flow. People whose left (nondominant) hands were immersed in painfully cold ice water (**cold pressor task**[1]) showed brain activation at the expected places: primary somatosensory cortex on the contralateral side, secondary somatosensory cortex on both sides, and certain limbic areas, after correcting for the effects of cold by itself. However, when people solved a maze during the cold pressor task, the pain-related activation virtually disappears, and is replaced by frontal lobe activity presumably related to selective attention (Petrovic, Petersson, Ghatan, Stone-Elander, & Ingvar, 2000). In particular, a region at the lateral orbital area of the frontal lobes seems to project to the **periaqueductal gray** region of the midbrain, where it presumably triggers descending inhibitory controls.

Thus, it appears that a degree of pain control can be achieved through distraction by a competing task. This intuition is widely held. An injured worker, unable to do their usual job, may be brought back to the workplace to sort nuts and bolts, so they are not at home dwelling on their pain. In a deposition, an attorney may ask whether the plaintiff's pain would not improve if they simply dropped their unrealistic expectations and found a menial job. In the clinic, techniques for diverting attention may be taught for pain control. But is distraction really this useful? There are two important caveats.

First, many interventions that nominally sequester attention also arouse interest, motivation, and positive mood, and may produce relaxation and an expectancy for pain control. Thus, the extent to which attention itself is the key variable is not entirely certain. That attention per se might not be important is suggested by an intensive series of studies by McCaul and associates, involving a total of 213 subjects. In a typical study, the subject was shown numbers on a computer screen.

---

[1]The cold pressor task has long been used in psychology to measure pain sensation and tolerance (e.g., Edes & Dallenbach, 1936). In it, a subject is asked to immerse their hand, or their arm up to the elbow, in ice water. In its various implementations, immersion time generally ranges from 60 to 300 seconds, or until the limit of pain tolerance is reached. Dependent variables include pain ratings during and after the immersion, total tolerance time, or both. The task derives its name from its origins in physiology as a technique for eliciting a rise in blood pressure, that is, a "pressor response" (E. Hines & G. E. Brown, 1932, 1933).

The person's task was to indicate when a number was present (easy task), to classify the numbers as even or odd, or as high or low (moderate task), or to classify the numbers as high-odd/low-even or as high-even/low-odd (difficult task). The authors used reaction time and error rate data to verify that the three tasks differed as expected in their amount of attentional load. Simultaneously, the subject was involved in a cold pressor task, periodically rating their degree of distress (McCaul, Monson, & Maki, 1992). Surprisingly, not only did the authors fail to find a dose-response relationship between degree of distraction and distress ratings, they failed to find *any* effect of distraction. Thus, we must entertain the possibility that attention, in the sense of competing information processing demands, is not the relevant variable in bringing about pain reduction.

There are at least four explanations for McCaul, et al.'s, negative results. First, we might hypothesize that the key ingredient is the interest, **absorption**, and challenge brought about by a distractor, and not the cognitive demands. In the last chapter, we saw the role of involvement in a motivated state.

Alternatively, cognitive demands may be important only when the competing stimulus involves similar perceptual or response modalities as the pain. In Chapter 2 we saw how the inhibition of pain by pressure (rubbing) or electricity (**TENS** units) can be explained by the gate control theory, intracortical inhibition, or in certain cases by pain-on-pain inhibition (diffuse noxious inhibitory controls). However, there is also data that the pain modulation is mediated by attention. That is, Longe and associates found that pain ratings and pain-related cerebral activation were reduced by a vibratory stimulus, provided that subjects are attending to the vibration and not the pain (Longe et al., 2001). In theory, pain and vibration may be similar enough that they compete for the same "channel capacity," that is, the same central processing resources.[2]

Third, it may be that sensory stimulation in general is more effective than higher cognitive processes in reducing pain. Strong odors seem to capture attention and reduce pain intensity. If the odors are pleasant, they can also induce a calm, pleasant mood, reducing pain-distress (Villemure, Slotnick, & Bushnell, 2003). In part, pain and smell seem to be processed in **entorhinal cortex**, which perhaps may be a physical basis for a sensory competition (Villemure et al.).

And there is a fourth possible reason as well behind McCaul et al.'s negative results. The experimental task of periodically giving distress ratings may have counteracted the effects of distraction. Consistent with this hypothesis, Christenfeld found that distraction did in fact reduce pain ratings, if the ratings were given after the task was over (Christenfeld, 1997). However, Christenfeld's results may pertain more to memory for pain than to its initial intensity.

In the clinic, each of these theories proves instructive. Thus, from the results so far, we might refrain from asking patients to rate their pain level during a coping activity. We might encourage their attention to the competing, non-pain sensation in a counterstimulation treatment such as TENS. And the case for menial work as a pain coping tool seems weak—sorting nuts and bolts by size is awfully close to sorting numbers into high and low.

Now, competition for central processing resources can be useful in pain management, such as with a TENS unit, but there is at least one scenario in which it is deleterious. It appears that one of the sensations that can compete with pain is the sensation of muscle tension (Knost, Flor, Birbaumer, & Schugens, 1999). Thus, a person who has chronic pain may be subtly reinforced

---

[2]Johnson and coworkers found that trying to detect near-threshold changes in a visual (brightness) or somatic (warmth) stimulus were equally effective in raising pain thresholds—there was no specific advantage for the somatosensory stimulus (M. H. Johnson, Breakwell, Douglas, & Humphries, 1998). Possibly a competing stimulus has to be well above detection threshold to be effective for pain management. Also, we do not know the extent to which the detection tasks induced a motivational state in subjects that may have been the true source of pain reduction.

with pain reduction for increasing tension. This, in turn, may be a risk factor for muscle pain, thus potentially leading to a vicious cycle (Knost et al.). In fact, this process does not seem at all rare clinically. Patients with chronic muscle tension will often experience relaxation as a "pulling" or "tightness." The "stretches" and postural adjustments they adopt on their own to relax the muscle may involve contracting it instead, sometimes quite forcefully. Other patients are aware that they are temporarily overriding an uncomfortable sensation through vigorous tensing.

So far, odors have not been used clinically for pain control, but taste has been: Sugar-water is an analgesic for newborns who need, e.g., to have blood drawn (pacifiers are even better, and may be more effective if sweet; Carbajal, Chauvet, Couderc, & Olivier-Martin, 1999). Similar applications for adults have not been reported, but patients occasionally describe a wonderful endorphinergic-seeming effect of chocolate, with the analgesia dissipating over 90 minutes. In adults, the distraction by pleasant odors may be stronger in women (Marchand & Arsenault, 2002), while the benefits of a sweet taste may be specific to people with low blood pressure (Lewkowski, Ditto, Roussos, & S. N. Young, 2003).

Meanwhile, such tasks as imagery, hypnosis, and absorption in non-pain activities appear quite beneficial, even if the exact mechanism may be more affective than cognitive.

Nonetheless, a second caveat as well pertains to distraction techniques, and this caveat may be of particular clinical importance.

Maladaptive Pain Coping

In the study by Petrovic et al. it appeared that involvement in solving a maze led to activation of descending pain inhibitory circuits, from the lateral orbital frontal lobes, to the periaqueductal gray region, and presumably from there to the medulla and the dorsal horn. This can be quite favorable, for as we have seen a portion of central sensitization takes place at the dorsal horn. But suppose we could reduce pain at higher brain regions without involving descending pain inhibitory circuits? Such a coping strategy would presumably put us at risk for developing or maintaining chronic pain, because we would be able to persist at tasks that were sensitizing the dorsal horn. In fact there is precedence for this effect in medicine: As a rule, general anesthesia markedly reduces brain responsivity to pain without significant effect on spinal nociceptive processing. For this reason, it has become routine practice to administer narcotic analgesics as part of the anesthetic mix, to prevent pain sensitization during surgery (Aida, 2005; Wilder-Smith, 2000; whether preemptive analgesia does in fact prevent central sensitization has not been entirely settled yet; Eisenach, 2000; Guignard et al., 2000).

Are there forms of distraction that are analogous to general anesthesia? We do not know enough about the neurobiology of pain coping to be sure, but there are two plausible candidates: **dissociation**, and pain suppression or blocking.

There are several reasons for suspecting that dissociation does not activate descending pain inhibitory pathways. First, laboratory instructions to use dissociative coping seem to reduce pain-distress and increase pain tolerance, without lowering the sensory intensity of the pain (Giolas & Sanders, 1992). Second, regional cerebral blood flow studies of sensorimotor **conversion disorder** (hysterical paralysis with superficial numbness) suggest that it involves inhibition by the orbitofrontal cortex and the amygdala, of pathways between the thalamus and the cortex, and the **basal ganglia** and the cortex (Vuilleumier, Chicherio, Assal, S. Schwartz, Slosman, & Landis, 2001). There is no evidence so far of more distal involvement. Indeed, the fact that early components of somatosensory evoked potentials do not seem to be affected in conversion disorder (Lorenz, Kunze, & Bromm, 1998) suggests that distal structures may not be involved. This assumes, of course, that conversion disorder involves a type of dissociation. Another condition that is perhaps analogous to dissociation, hypnosis, is similarly thought to involve inhibition of thalamocortical pathways (Crawford, Knebel, Kaplan, & Vendemia, 1998). However, the effects of hypnosis may depend on the type of suggestions given, and we will see evidence in Chapter 15 that some types of suggestion may indeed have effects at the spinal level.

Although attempts to suppress or block out pain bear a superficial resemblance to distraction, they are potential candidates for a maladaptive response. Cioffi and Holloway asked subjects to eliminate awareness of their hand during a cold pressor task (suppression), to focus on detailed imagery of their room at home (distraction), or to examine the location, quality and intensity of their hand sensations (monitoring; Cioffi & Holloway, 1993). Subjects in the three conditions did not differ in their tolerance for the procedure. However, for people in the suppression group, pain abated more slowly after the procedure. The suppressors also had more anticipatory anxiety and a significant reduction in **self-efficacy** for a possible future cold pressor trial. Moreover, suppressors experienced a subsequent vibratory stimulus as less pleasant than did people in the other two groups (Cioffi & Holloway, 1993). And there is some evidence that suppressing thoughts about a procedure beforehand will increase pain subsequently, when the procedure takes place (Sullivan, Rouse, Bishop, & Johnston, 1997).

The reason for this paradoxical effect is not known with certainty. Cioffi and Holloway point out that the only way a person can know whether they have eliminated thoughts of pain is to mentally scan for such thoughts. Not surprisingly, then, suppression leads to intrusive thoughts of the would-be object of suppression. Thus, **thought suppression** may function as an inadvertent thought monitoring condition, but in a sporadic, off-and-on way. Presumably, this lack of focus prevents habituation to the pain, as might have occurred in the intentional pain-monitoring group. Consistent with this hypothesis, the effect of thought suppression prior to a procedure in raising pain during the procedure seems to be mediated by the number of intrusive thoughts (Sullivan, Rouse, Bishop, & Johnston, 1997). Note, too, the decrement in self-efficacy found among suppressors in the Cioffi and Holloway study. Cioffi and Holloway point out that thought suppression, as a very difficult task, may lead to diminished feelings of control, that then spill over into the pain experience. Self-efficacy seems to work in part through endorphin-ergic, that is, descending pain inhibitory, pathways (Bandura, O'Leary, C. B. Taylor, Gauthier, & Gossard, 1987).

A neuropsychological finding may be relevant here as well. Donald Price (1999) discusses a clinical series, first described by Head and Holmes, of individuals who had sustained damage to the thalamus (Head & G. Holmes, 1911). The damage was in the area of the lateral nuclei thought to relay sensory pain information. Thus, we are not surprised to learn that some of these individuals showed diminished responding to mildly painful stimuli. What is unexpected, however, is that people with these lesions also tended to show an exaggerated emotional response to those stimuli that were perceived as painful. It is as if the thalamic nuclei underlying sensory pain processing somehow inhibit the nuclei involved in emotional pain processing (Head & G. Holmes, 1911; D. Price, 1999). If so, then this strange result would imply that dispassionate pain monitoring may indeed turn out to have a clinically useful role.[3]

---

[3]An inhibition of medial thalamic by lateral thalamic nuclei has also been invoked to explain a tragic side effect of treatment. Patients with advanced cancer pain that is no longer responding to medication are occasionally treated with a cordotomy, in which the pain pathways in the spinal cord are lesioned. Touch sensation and motor performance are not affected, but pain and temperature sensation are drastically reduced (Rosso, et al., 2003). However, in a small subset of patients, the brain itself eventually begins to generate a pain signal (**central pain syndrome**), possibly because, in the absence of sensory signals from the periphery, the medial thalamic nuclei become unmasked (Craig, 1998; Rosso, et al.). This phenomenon alone justifies all expenses in researching cancer, and pain.

From all this, we might assume that a dispassionate focus on the sensory qualities of one's pain is a good coping strategy. This indeed appears to be the case for acute, laboratory pain, although the effect may be specific to men (Keogh, Hatton, & Ellery, 2000). For chronic pain, however, the situation is less clear. For example, Keefe et al. found that ignoring pain sensations, as measured on the Coping Strategies Questionnaire, correlated positively with self-efficacy for managing pain, even after controlling for usual pain intensity (Keefe, Kashikar-Zuck, et al., 1997). And Harvey and McGuire found that among chronic pain patients it was instructions to focus on pain, rather than instructions to distract oneself, that led to persistent increases in pain-related thoughts (A. G. Harvey & McGuire, 2000).

How are we to make sense of this? Laboratory pain stimuli tend to intensify over a period of seconds to minutes, making suppression of the sensation quite impractical. In contrast, pain that has been present for months or years may be somewhat easier to disregard. Also, neither the distraction instructions used by Harvey and McGuire, nor the construct of ignoring pain measured by the Coping Strategies Questionnaire seems to capture the rigidity and the intensity of thought suppression.

Despite these differences, I suspect that there are situations in which the laboratory data are relevant to chronic pain coping. Some individuals, especially those who have not accepted their pain or whose **pacing** skills are poor, seem to try to override the pain, and to maintain their activities for as long as possible by brute force. Intuitively, it seems likely that for these individuals the combination of behavioral tolerance, high pain intensity, and the paradoxical effects of thought suppression, would be a risk factor for ongoing chronicity. That is, while laboratory pain may not be a good model of one's usual pain intensity, it may be a good model of pain flare-ups. However, all of this requires empirical examination.

For clinical work, the bottom line seems to be minimizing the degree of vigilance to pain. People who are engaged in unsuccessful attempts to avoid the pain, with frequent intrusions of pain-related experiences, may perhaps benefit from breaking this cycle with focused, dispassionate attention to the pain's sensory qualities.[4] On the other hand, people who are already successful at redirecting their attention should simply be encouraged in their efforts.

Note, too, that distraction does not need to actually reduce pain to be clinically helpful. Distraction might simply prevent a patient from accessing negative expectations that could otherwise impede them from engaging in treatment. For example, M. H. Johnson et al. found that patients with low back pain were able to persist longer at a step-up test, with no deleterious effect on pain level immediately afterwards,[5] if they simultaneously were involved in a cognitive task. This was despite the fact that the task "had little meaning or importance to the subjects, was not particularly interesting, and no incentive was available" (M. H. Johnson & Petrie, 1997, p. 48).

The Intrusiveness of Pain

We have seen, then, that scattered, intrusive thoughts about pain may represent the worst of both worlds. Unlike absorption in a non-pain activity, there is frequent **priming** for awareness of pain. But unlike consistently focused attention to the pain, there is little opportunity to habituate to the

---

[4]One thinks of Freud's definition of psychoanalysis, "complete remembrance in the service of complete forgetting."

[5]The delayed effects of the increased exercise were inconclusive due to low sample size. However, this is really a separate issue. For each patient and condition there is, conceptually, an optimal type and amount of therapy. If negative expectations are interfering with this level of therapy then distraction should be helpful.

sensation, to develop a feeling of mastery, or to make the sensory qualities affectively neutral. Yet in naturalistic circumstances, intrusive thoughts about the pain may not be unusual. Kewman et al. report that 32 percent of patients in their acute and chronic musculoskeletal pain sample showed a clinically significant disruption of attention on neuropsychological testing, even after correcting for depression (Kewman, Vaishampayan, Zald, & Han, 1991). In a series of studies using performance on an attention-demanding task, Eccleston and coworkers have provided more direct evidence that attentional disturbance is due to a redirection of attention by the pain.

What accounts for this effect? Eccleston and Crombez discuss several factors that have been supported empirically. One conclusion is simply that pain by its nature demands attention (Eccleston & Crombez, 1999). The authors suggest that the purpose of pain is to interrupt ongoing activities and substitute escape behavior. The more intense the pain, the more disruptive it tends to be (Eccleston, 1994). Moreover, the authors note that across repeated experimental trials the attention-sequestering effects of pain tend to resist habituation (Crombez, Eccleston, Baeyens, & Eelen, 1997). Thus, Eccleston and Crombez suggest that for some individuals, chronic pain means, cognitively, chronic interruption.

A second explanation focuses on personality characteristics of the person experiencing pain. At least two such characteristics have been explored: a somatic focus, and **catastrophization**. Somatic focus is attention to bodily sensations. It is usually measured as the tendency to report numerous, generalized, non-pain physical experiences. Eccleston et al. note that cognitive disruption tends to occur when individuals with high somatic focus have a disorder with high pain intensity. Neither somatic focus nor high pain level, but rather the catalytic interaction between the two, seems to be crucial in causing attentional interference (Eccleston, Crombez, Aldrich, & Stannard, 1997). Catastrophization is the belief that one will be overwhelmed or unable to cope with pain. In this case, too, a catalytic interaction is seen, in which the anticipation of high pain, when experienced by someone who catastrophizes about pain, disrupts attention (Crombez, Eccleston, Baeyens, & Eelen, 1998a). Not surprisingly, we will have more to say about catastrophizing in the next section. In an analogous result, when an individual is expecting a very painful shock, even mild, non-painful shocks tend to disrupt attention (Crombez, Eccleston, Baeyens, & Eelen, 1998b). It is as if the individual were scanning the environment for signs of the anticipated and dreaded stimulus.

This last result suggests a third explanation. The attention-sequestering effects of pain may depend on its meaning, or more exactly, on how threatening it is. After a physical therapy session, cancer patients' pain and suffering are more intense when seen as a result of their disease rather than the exercise (W. B. Smith, Gracely, & Safer, 1998). We will encounter this result below, in a section on labeling.

Of course this lays the groundwork for a vicious cycle. Fear of the pain can lead to greater attention to the pain, lowered pain thresholds, and consequently more intense pain and more fear of it. Furthermore, fear of pain can be more limiting than the pain itself, and in conditions such as chronic low back pain, can lead to deconditioning and physical vulnerability. Of course Eccleston et al.'s results have important implications for the treatment of chronic pain.

Catastrophizing and Risk of Chronicity

The term "catastrophizing" is due to Meichenbaum (1977). When individuals catastrophize, they see themselves as overwhelmed and as unable to cope with or to withstand the pain (Rosenstiel & Keefe, 1983). Rumination, feelings of helplessness, and an exaggerated appraisal of the negative consequences of the pain seem to be the main components (Sullivan, Bishop, & Pivik, 1995). Catastrophizing seems to exert a particularly malignant effect on pain coping. For example, Keefe et al. studied patients with rheumatoid arthritis (Keefe, G. K. Brown, K. A. Wallston, & Caldwell, 1989). They found that a measure of catastrophizing, from the Coping Strategies Questionnaire, had a test-retest coefficient of 0.81, suggesting that catastrophizing is a stable part of one's outlook and not simply a reaction to a pain flare-up. Moreover, Keefe et al. found that catastrophizing at one point in time predicted level of physical disability six months later, even after controlling for initial physical disability and a variety of potential confounds: duration of the disease (a rough measure of disease severity), disability compensation status, age, socioeconomic status, and gender. Analogous results were found for pain severity and depression: In each case catastrophizing predicted the level of distress six months later, after correcting for baseline distress and the same set of potential confounds. The study does not prove that catastrophizing caused the decline in functioning and well-being, because the correlational design does not exclude a "third variable" explanation. That is, there could be some other process that manifests itself first as catastrophizing, and later as increased pain, depression and a decline in physical functioning. Certainly, however, Keefe et al.'s results raise our suspicion that catastrophizing itself undermines successful pain coping.

Further evidence is provided by Picavet et al. In a population-based study, a measure of catastrophizing predicted low back pain that was severe (**odds ratio** = 2.2, highest vs. lowest tertile), chronic (odds ratio = 2.1) and disabling (odds ratio = 3.1) six months later. Even more striking is that these subjects did not have back pain at the start of the study. Catastrophizing predicted the later development of back pain (Picavet, Vlaeyen, & Schouten, 2002). More specific evidence for a causal association is suggested by treatment studies in which chronicity is prevented in part by addressing catastrophic beliefs (Linton & Andersson, 2000).

How does catastrophizing exert such an effect? It appears that in fibromyalgia (Gracely, et al., 2004), and in healthy individuals (Seminowicz & K. D. Davis, 2006) catastrophization is associated with greater activation in cortical areas subserving the anticipation of and emotional response to pain. Through these cortical regions, catastrophization could intensify the experience of pain. A similar result, an increase in pain-related activation at anterior cingulate cortex, has been found in individuals who tend to be fearful of pain (Ochsner et al., 2006). Moreover, catastrophization may involve decreased activation of dorsolateral prefrontal cortex, implying a lesser degree of top-down inattention to pain (Seminowicz & K. D. Davis, 2006).

In theory, catastrophizing could also raise the level of descending pain facilitation, or lower the amount of descending inhibition, to the dorsal horn. So far, however, evidence for this hypothesis is lacking. C. R. France and colleagues found that scores on the catastrophizing subscale of the Coping Strategies Questionnaire predicted pain thresholds and ratings of pain intensity for electric shock, but not the threshold for the R-III **nociceptive flexion reflex**[6] (C. R. France, J. L. France, al' Absi, Ring, & McIntyre, 2002). The **R-III reflex**, an automatic withdrawal from a painful stimulus, is a measure of pain sensitivity at the spinal level. Thus, in this study, catastrophizing seems to have exerted its effects at supraspinal sites. It may be relevant, however, that the subjects were all pain-free at the start of the study. Descending modulation intensifies in the hours and days after an injury, with long-term changes in synaptic strength along the pain modulatory pathways (Re & Dubner, 2002). It may be in these long-term processes that the effects of catastrophization emerge.

We will examine another hypothesis about catastrophization shortly, in the section on fear-avoidance.

---

[6]The reflex is named after the Type III muscle afferents that help mediate it. Type III nerves are small diameter, myelinated fibers, roughly the equivalent in muscle of Aδ fibers in the skin (Pomeranz, 2001).

Diagnosis and Threat

Catastrophization is generally viewed as a trait—individuals enter a painful situation already high or low on the variable. But situations can also influence how the pain is regarded. For example, Hirsch and Liebert (1998) have provided a demonstration of the effects of how pain is labeled.

Undergraduate volunteers immersed their nondominant arms in cold water of one of three temperatures: 3 °C, 13 °C, or 23 °C. They were also told that the experiment was a study of either "discomfort," "pain," or "vasoconstriction pain." The three labels were crossed with the three water temperatures for a total of nine conditions. Hirsch and Liebert found that behavioral tolerance for the cold-pain (total time the subject was willing to keep her arm immersed) was affected by both label and temperature. The two factors had additive effects and did not interact. For ratings of the unpleasantness of the stimulus, temperature had an effect and there was a trend for label to have an effect. For ratings of the sensory intensity of the stimulus, temperature was important and label did not have an effect. Thus, label helped determine the behavioral response to the pain, and possibly the unpleasantness, but not the sensory intensity of the pain.

Sawamoto et al. have provided another view of this phenomenon using functional magnetic resonance imaging (Sawamoto et al., 2000). Volunteers in their study participated in two conditions on two different days. On one of the days, they were exposed to 20 trials of warm pulses from a laser, delivered to the back of the hand. On the other day, the 20 warm trials were randomly intermixed with 20 trials of painfully hot pulses. The warm pulses themselves were the same on the two days. However, the anterior cingulate cortex was more intensely activated, and a larger area in the neighborhood of secondary somatosensory cortex was activated, when the warm pulses were intermixed with painful ones. This suggests that the expectation of pain was enough to give the warmth a degree of unpleasantness, as the anterior cingulate cortex seems to encode the affective dimension of pain. And, in fact, the volunteers rated the warmth as more unpleasant when it was interleaved with the painful stimulus (Sawamoto et al.). This may be clinically relevant for, as the authors point out, the randomly presented pain from the laser is reminiscent of the random paroxysms of pain in a **neuralgia**, while the acquired unpleasantness of the neutral stimuli reminds one of how pain patients may report a variety of generalized symptoms.

Thus, while labeling seems to have been studied exclusively in laboratory investigations of acute pain, it is presumably relevant to chronic clinical pain as well. For diagnosis, of course, is a label, and how patients understand their diagnoses can affect their expectations for recovery and self-management, and even their long-term outcome (A. K. Burton, Waddell, Tillotson, & Summerton, 1999).

Priming

Thus, pain tends to be increased by attention, and a variety of cognitive, emotional, situational, and personality variables influence the amount of attention that pain receives. But the situation may be subtler than this. Suppose that in the studies above, distraction had been provided not by a maze, a demanding task, or pleasant imagery, but by horrific pictures, say of mutilated accident victims. Would the pain be less, because of the distraction caused by disturbing (and therefore absorbing) scenes, or would the pain be greater because of the strong priming for a pain response implicit in the pictures? Put another way, does a person need to be distracted from his or her own pain only, or from pain in general, for an analgesic effect to occur?

In fact, de Wied and Verbaten (2001) found that unpleasant pictures had as little effect on pain perception as did neutral pictures, provided that the unpleasant pictures were not pain-related. When the pictures suggested bodily injury, the pain on a **cold pressor task** was indeed augmented. The authors note that these findings are consistent with the idea that pain is a response that is constructed to noxious stimuli (Chapman, Nakamura, & Flores, 1999), and that it can be primed on a cognitive level.

In the clinic, such effects do not seem at all rare. A patient whose spouse has dramatic **pain behaviors** of their own, or whose sibling is in failing health, or whose relative passed away in pain (hospice fails sometimes) may have a harder time coping with pain. In the rush of events, even very insightful patients are unlikely to have noticed these connections.

Now, if unpleasant pictures have no more effect than neutral pictures, provided they do not connote pain, then it seems unlikely that negative affect by itself will increase pain. But before we draw this conclusion too firmly we need to look more closely at the interrelationships between pain and affect. We will do so shortly, but first we will consider a clinical area in which learning factors are crucial: the placebo effect.

In the Clinic

Cognitive manipulations in the lab can only hint at what happens when pain becomes an all-consuming focus. When assessing patients, we will want to look closely at the factors that govern attention to pain, or that may otherwise contribute to the development of chronicity:

Situational:

Frightening diagnosis or beliefs about the source of the pain;

Absence of absorbing, enjoyable activities;

Reminders of pain, injury, or poor health, from spouse, friends, lawyer, disability system or even news media

Personality:

Catastrophic thoughts about pain, especially when combined with the threat of a high pain level

Belief that the pain will be uncontrollable

A somatic focus combined with high pain intensity

Pain Quality:

Intermittent high intensity

Coping Strategies:

Forceful thought suppression

Dissociation

Also important are factors that can help ameliorate the pain: coping strategies such as absorption in activities that elicit an appetitive motivational state, dispassionate and sustained monitoring of the pain's sensory qualities, and forms of counterstimulation such as vibration (when attended to), pleasant odors (especially in women), and a sweet taste (especially in people with low blood pressure).

PLACEBO RESPONSE

Having encountered psychological variables that influence pain perception, let us consider a rather dramatic example of their effects: the placebo[7] response. Needless to say, placebo responding is the process by which a theoretically inert medication or other treatment produces a therapeutic response, in this case, analgesia. From our discussion of conditioned hyperalgesia in Chapter 2 we can intuit a possible mechanism for the placebo response: By reassuring the patient that their condition is under (medical) control, we encourage them to decrease their vigilance to the pain, and thus to decrease their pain sensitivity.

More formally, researchers have proposed four mechanisms behind the effectiveness of placebos (Pollo, Amanzio, Arslanian, Casadio, Maggi, & Benedetti, 2001):

1. The placebo may reduce pain, especially its affective dimension (D. Price & Fields, 1997), by reducing anxiety (Evans, 1977).

2. The key process may be classical conditioning. That is, the specific physiological changes induced by a drug may be partially re-created, after repeated exposure, by the stimuli that were associated with the drug (Ader, 1997).

3. Alternatively, the mechanism may be cognitive. That is, the placebo may activate an expectation of relief, perhaps in the form of imagery, based on past experience with pills and injections. The expectation may be stronger, or the image more vivid, when desire for relief is greater (D. Price & Fields, 1997).

4. The fourth explanation is a bit more complicated. Wall suggests that pain is a drive state, analogous to hunger and thirst, and thus may be designed more to motivate a response than to represent a stimulus (Wall, 1999). If a person has presented to a health care provider and received treatment that they trust, pain has at least in part served its purpose, and would decline.[8]

Let us focus on processes (2) and (3). Amanzio and Benedetti (1999) were able to tease apart classical conditioning and cognitive expectation, by repeatedly administering a drug in either a blinded or non-blinded way. (In the blinded trials, the drug was administered from behind a screen, through a continuously running IV.) Of course, the non-blinded trials should generate an additional expectation of pain relief. Now, Amanzio and Benedetti found that expectation-induced relief is mediated through endorphin pathways. Classically conditioned relief, in contrast, depends on which drug was used in the conditioning. If morphine was used, then the conditioning will utilize the endorphin system. If a **nonsteroidal anti-inflammatory drug** (NSAID) was

---

[7]In English, this strange word goes back to at least the 14th century, for it is found in the works of Chaucer (Wall, 1999). In its earliest meaning it is akin to flattery, appealing but vacuous. Not surprisingly, then, in Latin "placebo" means "I will please," (and conversely, "nocebo" means "I will harm" [Wall, 1999]). Wall argues, however, that the term in medicine more likely traces to the book of Psalms, more exactly Psalm 116, verse 9: "Placebo Domino in regione vivorum," "I will walk before the Lord in the land of the living." In light of recent works on the relationship of spirituality to healing, this allusion to the Bible seems precious, but it was probably intended as sarcastic from the beginning. For the verse in question is also the first line of the medieval vespers—prayer—for the dead (Wall, 1999).

[8]Wall's explanation might solve a mystery in our clinic. Here, patients are often referred to psychology by their physicians because of excessive pain behavior. However, in the psychologist's office some of them show no pain behavior whatsoever. Our physicians sometimes suspect that the motive is disability, and the psychologists suspect that the physicians are discriminative stimuli for pain behavior. If Wall is correct, however, the patients might be experiencing a situationally bound increase in pain due to the expectation that medical treatment might be elicited.

used, then the conditioning will partially re-create the NSAID response, rather than activate endorphin pathways.

Notice that expectation and classical conditioning are forms of learning (Fields, 2001). Thus, instead of the "placebo response" we could speak of "learned analgesia."

Learned Inhibition of Pain

We have seen that placebos seem to acquire their pain-reducing qualities through learning. In fact, evidence that analgesia can be learned is found in one of the earliest works of behavioral psychology, Ivan Pavlov's *Conditioned Reflexes*. Pavlov, of course, had demonstrated that a previously neutral stimulus, such as an electric bell, or buzzer, or a ticking metronome, could elicit salivation in dogs if the sound had been repeatedly paired with food. But what if the stimulus was not "previously neutral" like a bell, but highly meaningful, like an electric shock? Can an electric shock bring about salivation, if it is repeatedly paired with food? The answer to this question about the outer limits of classical conditioning is "yes," but there is more: The salivation replaced the usual reaction to pain. "Subjected to the very closest scrutiny, not even the tiniest and most subtle objective phenomenon usually exhibited by animals under the influence of strong injurious stimuli can be observed in these dogs. No appreciable changes in the pulse or in the respiration occur in these animals, whereas such changes are always most prominent when the nocuous stimulus has not been converted into an alimentary conditioned stimulus" (Pavlov, 1927/1960, p. 30).

Pavlov did not imagine that pain perception was infinitely malleable. He noted that the experiment was successful because the unconditioned stimulus (food for the hungry dog) was stronger than the stimulus to become conditioned (the electric shock). If the electric shock were applied to a place near the bone, the defensive reaction it elicited would be too strong to replace with salivation. But at least under some conditions, the pain was inhibited completely.

Until now, we have looked mostly at how pain pathways become sensitized, leading to chronic pain. But synaptic strength can also be decreased, and old learning replaced by new. Pavlov's studies, now almost a century old, hint at the development of behavioral treatment to reverse pain sensitization. The development and testing of such a protocol is one of the great unfinished projects of pain psychology.

AFFECT

In psychotherapy, of course, we are not usually interested in changing cognition alone, but in reducing emotional distress. Can interventions for depression, anxiety, or anger reduce pain? Or is pain, like vision, relatively insulated from the effects of emotions? In the next few pages, we will consider findings from basic research that bear on this question.

Anxiety

Here, we are referring to the effects of anxiety on pain in general. In migraines and tension-type headaches especially there appear to be specific psychophysiological effects of stress that contribute to the disorder, as we will see in the chapters that follow.

The effects of anxiety have been studied in laboratory pain, **phantom limb pain**, and rheumatoid arthritis. The effects seem to depend on the magnitude of the anxiety, the circumstances surrounding it, and characteristics of the person experiencing it.

As we saw in the last chapter, severe anxiety, for example when people with **Posttraumatic Stress Disorder** or simple phobias are exposed to relevant, feared stimuli, seems to produce analgesia, at least in acute pain ("**stress-induced analgesia;**" Amit & Galina, 1986). As noted, the analgesia can be mediated by endorphinergic or non-endorphinergic pathways, depending on whether or not the danger is escapable (S. A. Janssen & Arntz, 1996, 1999; Pitman, van der Kolk, Orr, & Greenberg, 1990; Willer & Ernst, 1986).

Daily **hassles** have also been studied for their ability to predict the next day's pain level (lagged correlation). The hassles seem to play a role for some but not all patients (Affleck, Tennen, Urrows, & Higgins, 1994; Arena, R. A. Sherman, Bruno, & J. D. Smith, 1990). In particular, hassles predict later pain in those rheumatoid arthritis patients who have greater disease severity (joint inflammation and erythrocyte sedimentation rate) and in those who had experienced major life stresses (e.g., death of a spouse) at the start of the study. In fact, daily hassles seemed to have a protective effect for those who had not encountered recent major life stresses, and a deleterious effect for those who had (Affleck et al.). Overall, the results seem to fit with a vulnerability-stress model. The effects were not mediated by mood, which had been partialed out statistically. In fact, the effects of stress on mood were mediated by two different variables: neuroticism (proneness to negative affect) and level of social support (Affleck et al.).

It seems possible that in chronic pain, the stressors (worry about the cause and prognosis of the pain, financial distress, hassles associated with litigation or the workers' compensation system) may redirect attention back to the pain. These stressors, which are most likely more common than the stress modeled by exposure in phobias, would tend to promote attention to the pain, and therefore to increase the pain (Al-Absi & Rokke, 1991; Weisenberg, Aviram, Wolf, & Raphaeli, 1984). Moreover, the hassles associated with one's own pain surely have the potential to prime, and therefore augment, the pain.

In theory, stress that is related to pain could also make the pain more aversive, by adding additional meaning to the physical sensation. The tension from anxiety could add to that from the pain, and hence make the pain harder to tolerate. And in one theory of emotion, the tension might be mislabeled as pain (Nisbett & Schachter, 1966).

Moreover, Ploghaus and associates have noted a direct effect of pain-related anxiety on pain intensity ratings and on cerebral blood flow in the pain neuromatrix. Specifically, anxiety about the pain increased activation initially in **entorhinal cortex** of the hippocampus, followed by the perigenual cingulate and the mid-insula (Ploghaus et al., 2001). In the study's high anxiety condition, subjects did not know whether the next stimulus would be moderately painful or intensely painful. The authors suggest, after Gray and McNaughton (2000) that entorhinal cortex responds to the uncertainty by triggering anxiety (reflected in the cingulate cortex activation) and by increasing the valence of the pain signal (at the mid-insula) so as to prepare for the worst-case scenario.

Again, we are leaving aside effects that are thought to be disorder-specific, such as the painful effects of **epinephrine** or norepinephrine in post-amputation neuromas (S. N. Raja, Abatzis, & Frank, 1998), **reflex sympathetic dystrophy** (Ali, S. N. Raja, Wesselmann, Fuchs, R. A. Meyer, & J. N. Campbell, 2000), and **post-herpetic neuralgia** (Choi & Rowbotham, 1997). As we will see in chapters 4 and 5, cerebral vasoconstriction in migraine may be another example of a disorder-specific stress response.

Anxiety sensitivity.   The role of pain-relevant anxiety is supported by studies showing that people who are high in "anxiety sensitivity" are also more pain sensitive. Anxiety sensitivity is the degree to which sympathetic arousal is interpreted as dangerous or harmful. Individuals with this tendency report more anxiety during painful laboratory procedures (for example, the cold pressor test) and this anxiety in turn appears to mediate increased pain report during the procedures (N. B. Schmidt & Cook, 1999). This has been offered as an explanation for the comorbidity between chronic pain and panic disorder (N. B. Schmidt & Cook, 1999). Note that anxiety-sensitive individuals do not show a stronger psychophysiological response to pain, only a stronger subjective response.

In theory, anxiety sensitivity could play an important role in the transition from episodic to chronic daily headache. Presumably, an individual who found pain-related arousal to be particularly aversive would be more likely to overuse sedating medications and hence to develop rebound headache. Moreover, the anxiety would presumably cause an attentional focus on headaches, perhaps contributing to sensitization and negative expectancies. Pain-related anxiety could foster disability as well, as the individual attempts to prevent exacerbations by avoiding activities (Asmundson, Norton, & Veloso, 1999).

As it turns out, this model so far has worked far better for musculoskeletal pain than for headaches. Asmundson and coworkers found that, contrary to expectations, anxiety sensitivity did *not* predict lifestyle change due to headaches (pain intensity did), nor was there any effect on medication intake (Asmundson, Norton, & Veloso, 1999). Now, it may have mattered that 91 percent of the sample was taking medications, thus losing statistical power to truncated range, and that lifestyle disruption was measured with a single self-report question. Certainly, we would not want to foreclose further research on anxiety sensitivity in headaches. So far, however, in the scant research available, the predictor's promise has not borne fruit.

Now, in anxiety sensitivity we have delved into a personality variable to explain an anxious response to pain. But the situations in which people find themselves can contribute strongly to somatic concerns. Note that when people feel they are in danger, they are biased towards believing information that confirms the danger, and disbelieving indications of safety (Smeets, de Jong, & Mayer, 2000). This is an adaptive bias, erring on the side of safety. As a result, however, once a person has come to believe that they are in danger, the belief becomes relatively insulated from disconfirming data (Smeets, et al.). Moreover, the individual can adopt "ex-consequentia" reasoning: "I wouldn't be this afraid if there weren't a real danger" (Arntz, Rauner, & van den Hout, 1995). Add to this the general human tendency towards a **confirmatory bias**, and a somatic fear can perpetuate indefinitely.

And it seems likely that for some patients with chronic pain, there was much to induce such a fear. There may have been medical tests that were almost other-worldly in their austereness, an emergency surgery, a wait to find out if one is terminally ill, or diagnostic errors and uncertainties. If the headache began with an injury there may have been time out of work, with no income and a nebulous disability status, making the pain highly consequential. From one perspective, it seems surprising that an iatrogenic somatic focus does not occur more often.

The fear-avoidance model of pain.   It seems natural that people will avoid activities that make their pain worse, and that through avoiding they will achieve a measure of control over their pain level. But in one theory of chronic pain, avoidance can be a treacherous strategy. For example, H. C. Philips (1987) notes that, in a cross-sectional study, people whose headaches were more chronic avoided activities to a greater extent, and felt less control over their pain, but they did not report higher pain levels. Philips argues that if avoidance were an effective strategy then people who used it should feel more control over their pain. Moreover, the lack of correlation between pain level and chronicity suggests that over time, avoidance takes on a life of its own.

Now, we can certainly make a case that fear and avoidance predict the amount of disability from pain. This is important in its own right, as it is often disability and lifestyle disruption, more than pain itself, that people find distressing. If some amount of this disability is unnecessary then suffering can be reduced. But do fear and avoidance contribute to the pain itself? In theory they could, through psychophysiological mechanisms such as muscle tension (Vlaeyen, Seelen, et al., 1999), through expectations of pain, through distress contributing to the affective dimension of pain, or through diminished opportunities to habituate to the pain (H. C. Philips, 1987).

So far, however, the expectation model does not seem to have garnered laboratory support. That is, when patients with low back pain overpredict the painfulness of a task, the task does not become more painful, the patients just reduce their predictions the next time (Crombez, Vervaet, Baeyens, Lysens, & Eelen, 1996; McCracken, Gross, Sorg, & Edmands, 1993). The habituation model fares a bit better. Recall from Chapter 2 that synaptic strength can be reduced through learning. In some studies, individuals with more severe chronic pain show increased threshold and tolerance for laboratory pain stimuli (e.g., Dar, Ariely, & Frenk, 1995). However, we do not know if this is a change in pain or in behavioral tolerance, or if it is due to habituation or **diffuse noxious inhibitory controls**. The psychophysiological path seems to be supported by a single study by Vlaeyen and coworkers, in which greater reactivity was found in the back muscles of patients with a higher fear of reinjury (Vlaeyen, Seelen, et al., 1999).

Thus, the fear-avoidance model has some support as a model of disability, but as an explanation for the pain itself the evidence is still very tentative.

Moreover, it is not at all clear that pain patients in general overpredict the amount of pain that an activity will entail. To my knowledge, three studies have examined the question, asking patients to predict the level of pain from an activity, and then to rate their actual pain after performing the activity. Results are shown in Table 3–1, below. As can be seen, patients are not terribly accurate in their predictions, but overall there seems to be no systematic bias towards over- vs. under-predicting.

Thus, if the fear-avoidance model is to be useful, we need some way of knowing which patients may be avoiding activities unnecessarily. In fact, there is some evidence that people who score high in catastrophizing are prone to develop an avoidant response to pain (Vlaeyen, Kole-Snijders, Boeren, & van Eek, 1995).

Of course pain avoidance is likely to have important treatment implications. In one example, patients with chronic benign low back pain participated in a reconditioning program involving an exercise bicycle. The bicycle's resistance was changed frequently by a computer program. Patients who had no cognitive clues to tell them when to expect pain (no clocks, watches, or odometer) showed the same gains in conditioning as non-pain control participants. Patients whose exercise environments contained the usual cues showed essentially no gains (Fordyce, 1979). In Chapter 13 we will return to the fear-avoidance model when we discuss behavioral treatment for chronic pain.

Depression

Patients sometimes report that lapses into depression are followed by a flare-up in pain. For some, mood seems to be the primary determinant of pain intensity. The overwhelmed feeling, inactivity,

TABLE 3–1
Accuracy of Patients with Chronic Pain in Predicting the Painfulness of a Task

Study/Population	% Under-Predicting	% Correctly Predicting	% Over-Predicting
Rachman & Lopatka, 1988 (arthritis)	18%	57%	25%
Rachman & Eyrl, 1989 (headaches)	33%	24%	43%
McCracken, et al., 1993 (low back)	38%	42%	20%
Average	30%	41%	29%

loss of motivation, and inward, somatic focus can all wreak havoc with pain coping. Not surprisingly, then, research on clinical samples suggests a rather high comorbidity between pain and depression (Romano & J. A. Turner, 1985). Logically, the pain may produce depression through a loss of roles and activities, or the depression may produce pain through a lowering of thresholds or tolerance, or pain and depression may be manifestations of a larger process, say, a coping skills deficit or a serotonin deficiency (G. K. Brown, 1990). Surely, the more we understand the links, the more precise our treatments can be.

Yet, surprisingly, the connection between pain and depression seems more tenuous the closer we look. Certainly this is true in the laboratory. Levine and coworkers found that when undergraduates were told they had performed poorly on a reading comprehension test, their pain ratings during a cold pressor task increased. A reasonable explanation is that the perception of failure induced a negative mood, which in turn increased pain report (Levine, Krass, & Padawer, 1993). However, when negative mood was induced in a similar study, by having volunteers read and think about depressing statements, no change in pain level resulted (Zelman, Howland, Nichols, & Cleeland, 1991). Negative mood did lower the average tolerance time for the cold pressor task, but this seems better accounted for as a decrease in persistence than as an increase in pain.

The evidence is no stronger for clinical pain. In presurgical screenings, depression does not usually emerge as a predictor of outcome; when it does, it may be a predictor only over the short-term, say, 6 months post surgery (Sørensen, 1992; Sørensen, Mors, & Skovlund, 1987), unlike somatic preoccupation, which may still be relevant 1–4 years later (Uomoto, J. A. Turner, & Herron, 1988). Nor do fine-grained prospective analyses appear as informative here as they are in pain and daily hassles. In a short-term study, in which depression and rheumatoid arthritis pain were tracked three times a day for 14 days, no relationship was found between changes in pain and in depression (Carter, Feuerstein, & Love, 1986; Feuerstein, Carter, & Papciak, 1987). In a longer-term study, in which the two constructs were tracked every 6 months for 3 years in (after attrition) 243 rheumatoid arthritis patients, pain predicted depression (G. K. Brown, 1990). However, the relationship was modest in degree and held only for the second half of the study. The reverse direction was not supported: Depression did not predict pain. Similarly, von Korff et al. has reported prospective results suggesting that for certain types of pain (chest pain, severe headaches, and possibly temporomandibular dysfunction) depression may be a risk factor, while for others (abdominal pain, back pain) it is not. Moreover, the severity of depression was not predictive (there was no dose-response relationship) although longer duration of depression, prospectively measured, did add to the severe headache risk (Von Korff, Le Resche, & S. F. Dworkin, 1993).

In another approach, Dohrenwend and colleagues interviewed patients with myofascial facial pain, acquaintances of the patients (as controls), and first degree relatives of participants in the two groups. Compared to the control group, there was no increased risk of depression in the patients' first degree relatives, suggesting that the **myofascial pain** and depression were not expressions of the same inherited central nervous system diathesis (Dohrenwend, Raphael, Marbach, & Gallagher, 1999).

Possibly, then, depression does *not* worsen pain. Maybe the comorbidity is an artifact of using clinical samples. Perhaps the combination of pain and depression causes people to present for treatment. If so, then the two conditions might need to be treated separately, consecutively. But before we completely exclude a link from depression to pain, let us examine four possible alternatives.

Subtypes of pain.   In depression, the awareness is turned inwards. Not surprisingly, then, when patients who are clinically depressed are studied in the laboratory, their sensitivity in detecting pain, indeed their attentiveness to any stimulation, is lower than that of healthy control subjects (Dickens, McGowan, & Dale, 2003). However, this relative insensitivity may be specific to electricity, heat, and other stimuli applied to the surface of the body. Internal pain, such as the muscle tenderness of tension-type headache (Janke, K. A. Holroyd, & Romanek, 2004), and the aching of muscular **ischemia**, may be enhanced by depression (Bär, Brehm, M. K. Boettger, S. Boettger, G. Wagner, & Sauer, 2005).

Trait negative affect.   Depression is generally operationalized as a state variable—how the person is feeling at that moment, or perhaps over the past week or month. In contrast, we may consider, as an enduring feature of personality, one's susceptibility to experiencing negative emotions such as depression, anxiety, and anger. In fact, this susceptibility typically emerges as a primary factor in personality studies. It generally clusters with the closely related traits of self-consciousness, low self-esteem, and vulnerability to stress, and is termed "neuroticism" (Costa & McCrae, 1985; Eysenck, 1967), "trait anxiety" (J. A. Gray, 1982), or "trait negative affect" (Watson & Clark, 1984).

Negative affect as a trait disposition and as a temporary mood state may have different consequences for how one experiences one's health status. For example, S. Cohen and colleagues studied objective signs and subjective ratings of upper respiratory illness after exposing volunteers to cold or flu virus. (The psychological measures had been piggybacked onto a drug study.) The authors found that state and trait negative affect each predicted subjective symptoms, but did not interact with each other. Moreover, the state variable seemed to exert its effects on subjective reports by way of increased objective disease severity. People who were more anxious, depressed, and/or hostile when exposed to the virus in fact became physically sicker. In contrast, trait negative affect seemed to exert a direct effect on symptom reporting, independent of disease severity (S. Cohen, Doyle, Skoner, Fireman, Gwaltney, & Newsom, 1995). People with higher trait negative affect reported more symptoms, perhaps because an illness cognitive **schema** was more strongly activated.

Plausibly, then, negative affect as a feature of personality may lead to greater attention to bodily sensations, and a greater tendency to interpret the sensations as signs of disease (Watson & Pennebaker, 1989). Conceptually, trait negative affect should affect pain levels and risk for chronicity. In fact, Price and coworkers present evidence that people high in neuroticism do report higher pain levels (Harkins, D. Price, & Braith, 1989; J. B. Wade, Dougherty, Hart, Rafii, & D. Price, 1992). Not surprisingly, it is specifically the affective/motivational dimension of pain, rather than its sensory/discriminative dimension, that is related to neuroticism. Neuroticism was an even better predictor of one's emotional reaction to the pain. People high in trait negative affect tend not to cope well with stresses, including the stress of chronic pain. However, the pain itself, and specifically the affective/motivational dimension, is higher in high-neurotic individuals.

Thus, it may turn out that the failure to distinguish trait and state aspects of mood helps account for the mixed results found in studies of depression and pain.

A drawback of these studies is their cross-sectional nature. Price et al. note that the trait measures tend not to be affected much by contracting a physical disease. Still, we cannot be sure that longitudinal studies will verify the cross-sectional results. For example, Radanov et al. followed 117 patients beginning one week after whiplash injury. Level of neuroticism, at least as measured by the Freiburg Personality Inventory, did not discriminate those patients whose symptoms went on to persist for the two year study period. On the other hand, chronicity was predicted by a scale on the inventory measuring tendency to somaticize (Radanov, Begré, Sturzenegger, & Augustiny, 1996).

Interaction with stress.   Another possible explanation for the uncertain relationship between depression and pain is that this relationship may change over time. In a study by Potter and coworkers, 41 women with rheumatoid arthritis gave weekly telephone ratings of levels of negative affect, positive affect, and pain. They also completed an instrument measuring the occurrence of stressful **life events** over the preceding week. The authors found that negative affect and pain were mildly correlated on nonstressful weeks ($r = .26, p < .001$), but much more strongly correlated on stressful weeks ($r = .63, p < .001$). Positive affect and pain were not correlated at all when stress was low ($r = .01, ns$), but they were strongly negatively correlated on stressful weeks ($r = -.60, p < .001$). Potter et al. suggest that under stress, information processing becomes simplified and coarser in the interests of rapid decision-making. Pain, negative affect, and the inverse of positive affect, which are relatively independent under nonstressful conditions, are partially conflated into a single dimension when a person is under stress. Hence, one purpose of behavioral treatment may be to improve stress coping, so that emotions and pain have less impact on each other (Potter, Zautra, & Reich, 2000).

Stress hardiness.   "Trait negative affect" implies that people differ in their vulnerability to stress. A second personality variable has been suggested to mediate the effects of stress: There is some evidence that individuals high in "stress **hardiness**," while not actually experiencing fewer hassles, find the hassles to be less intense (Callahan, 2000). What is stress hardiness? The two key features seem to be an internal **locus of control**, or belief that desirable outcomes are under one's own control, and a deep sense of commitment to or involvement in one's activities (Hull, Van Treuren, & Virnelli, 1987; Kobasa, Maddi, & Kahn, 1982). The relevance of this construct to pain is suggested by Callahan's (2000) finding: In his study, patients with temporomandibular dysfunction scored lower in commitment than matched orthodontic-periodontic patients.

These results need to be interpreted cautiously, however. Only 60% of the patients who were recruited actually followed through with the study, so there is plenty of room for sampling bias. And of course the cross-sectional design leaves the direction of causality obscure. It seems quite likely that experiencing chronic pain disrupts one's involvement in outside activities. At this point, all we can say is that stress hardiness is an intriguing concept, particularly for disorders such as tension-type headache in which stress responsiveness seems to play such an important role. Much more research is needed before we will know for certain that hardiness is as relevant as it appears to be.

Positive affect.   We can also ask the question in reverse: Can positive affect reduce pain? The answer seems to be yes. Recall the study by de Wied and Verbaten (2001), in which unpleasant pictures had as little effect on pain as did neutral pictures, provided that the pictures were not pain-related. Suppose that instead of unpleasant pictures we showed pictures that were enjoyable, and that would lead to an approach rather than an avoidance response. That is, suppose the pictures primed, on an affective level, the opposite type of motivation as pain (Lang, Bradley, & Cuthbert, 1997). De Wied and Verbaten included this condition and, in fact, it did reduce pain on a cold pressor task. Moreover, the positive stimuli seemed to have a greater effect on pain than did the negative stimuli. We know from studies of pain coping that tasks such as pleasant imagery are more useful than distractions such as counting. It seems likely that the differential effectiveness is not simply because imagery is more absorbing, but because the positive emotional state itself attenuates pain.

Thus, in addition to treating pain and depression separately, individuals with the two disorders combined may benefit from stress coping skills (e.g., **problem solving therapy**) and induction of positive, motivating affect. When proneness to negative affect is actually a feature of personality, of course, then slower, smaller gains may be likely.

Note, however, that this refers to the relationship between depression and pain in general. We will see that for migraines, tension-type headaches, and possibly temporomandibular dysfunction, depression is more strongly related, and predictive of functioning. Later, we will encounter evidence that depression has differential effects on treatments for tension-type headache, and hence is one factor to consider in treatment matching.

In the Clinic

Certain factors to emerge in formal studies seem directly applicable in patient assessment. Anxiety about pain should be carefully noted and its source clarified: anxiety at the perceived diagnosis, the unpredictability of paroxysms or flare-ups, a fear that the pain will be uncontrollable, anxiety about the experience of sympathetic arousal, and fearful avoidance of activity, can all cause the pain to dominate one's life.

Stresses, too, can be consequential. Major life events stress followed by multiple daily hassles can increase pain by overwhelming one's coping resources. In the context of either life events or daily hassles, distress from pain and stress may blend, even in a typically insightful person, into global negative affect attributed to, and sometimes confused with, pain.

In clinical settings, depression seems to play a larger role than in the laboratory. Perhaps the connection between distress and pain depends on whether they are embedded in the same schema (Clemmey & Nicassio, 1997; Pennebaker, 1982; Pincus & Morley, 2001). The relative insensitivity of depressed patients to electric shock, for example, may reflect the external and somewhat arbitrary nature of the stimulus. In contrast, attention to pain that is internal and part of a negative view of oneself or the world may indeed be enhanced by depression (Rainville, Bao, & Chrétien, 2005). A patient whose chronic pain began unexpectedly with a medical procedure may have flare-ups triggered, not by stress per se, but by other situations in which they feel deceived and betrayed. In practice, then, we will want to understand the degree of depression, its content, and its associations with the pain. The same principle, to understand the schema, applies as well to other forms of distress, such as anger, associated with the pain. Trait negative affect, in which negative schemas are activated with particular ease, may especially need to be taken into account in treatment.

Conversely, we have seen that enjoyable activities, inducing an "approach" or "appetitive" motivational state, tend to reduce pain. So, too, may absorbing activities decrease pain through attentional mechanisms, and commitment to an important cause provides a cushion against stress. Thus, a person can accomplish much in pain coping simply by recognizing enjoyable, absorbing activities that are more important than the pain. If there is any silver lining to an experience as horrible as pain, it is this: Pain impels us to live authentically.

Anger

Little research has been devoted to anger, but studies so far suggest considerable impact on pain sensitivity. Acutely, anger, like other forms of stress, may reduce pain (Janssen, Spinhoven, & Brosschot, 2001), while habitual anger, as a trait, predicts greater sensitivity to laboratory pain (Bruehl, Burns, Chung, Ward, & B. Johnson, 2002).

Anger management style also appears relevant. The tendency to express anger outwardly is correlated with greater pain sensitivity in both healthy individuals and those with chronic pain (Bruehl et al., 2002). The effect has been traced in part to poor endorphinergic tone in those who express anger, but beyond this, the direction of causality is uncertain. Chronic anger might overtax and impair the endorphin system or, alternatively, a limited supply of endorphins might impede control of both anger and pain (Bruehl et al.). People who use narcotic analgesics, even less than daily, tend to express anger and to have poor endorphinergic tone, although whether the narcotics are cause or effect is unknown (Bruehl et al.). Anger expression may also increase pain directly, through chronic muscle tension, at least in men (Burns, 1997), behaviors such as jaw clenching (Gramling, Grayson, T. N. Sullivan, & S. Schwartz, 1997), and perhaps in migraine by intensifying blood flow to the forehead and face (A. Adler, 1931; Drummond & Quah, 2001; Lange, 1885/1922; Stemmler, Heldmann, Pauls, & Scherer, 2001).

The tendency to suppress anger, meanwhile, may increase disability and the unpleasantness of pain, effects that seem to be mediated by depression (Bruehl, Chung, & Burns, 2003; Duckro, Chibnall, & Tomazic, 1995; Tschannen, Duckro, Margolis, & Tomazic, 1992) and anxiety (Gelkopf, 1997).

Of course, anger expression, and especially hostility (cynical mistrust and tendency to impute malicious intent to others; Greenwood, Thurston, Rumble, S. J. Waters, & Keefe, 2003) can disrupt relationships with one's workplace (Vahtera, Kivimaki, Koskenvuo, & Pentti, 1997), spouse (Burns, B. J. Johnson, Mahoney, J. Devine, & Pawl, 1996), and therapist (Burns, Higdon, Mullen, Lansky, & Mei Wei, 1999), causing stress, and furthering disability through the additional burden on coping resources. And as people with chronic pain often feel angry with themselves, their healthcare providers, and, if injured, the person who caused the injury (Okifuji, D. C. Turk, & Curran, 1999), the anger may be part of a cognitive schema that keeps attention focused on the pain (Rainville, Bao, & Chrétien, 2005).

In the clinic, patients may not volunteer anger as a headache trigger or source of stress. It is helpful to ask, and to explore the underlying reasoning and associations closely enough to provide clues for constructive problem solving, or a basis for letting go of the anger as no longer useful. Both cognitive therapy and intensive training in social skills have proved useful in reducing anger (Deffenbacher, Dahlen, R. S. Lynch, C. D. Morris, & Gowensmith, 2000; Deffenbacher, Oetting, Huff, Cornell, & Dallager, 1996).

PSYCHODYNAMIC CONSTRUCTS

Repression

Several investigators have attempted to study the hypothesis that, for some individuals, pain may be a distraction from and an indirect expression of an otherwise unacceptable emotion. The investigations derive broadly from psychodynamic concepts of repression and conversion.

In psychoanalytic thought, repression is an unconscious defensive process, in which an unacceptable thought, image or memory is kep out of consciousness (LaPlanche & Pontalis, 1973/1967). An unconscious, purposeful forgetting of an anxiety-provoking event would be a cardinal example (O. Fenichel, 1945). Repression does not alter perception as profoundly as does denial—the repressed material is stil present, in dreams, in symptoms, and as a half-awareness that something is missing. Among the symptoms that repression can produce is conversion into a physical problem—pain, for example, as a consequence of guilt and self-anger.

The formal research is limited. Burns (2000), for example, operationalized repression as a low score on a psychometric measure of anxiety (the Taylor MAS), combined with a high score on a scale of social desirability (the **MMPI** L scale). He found that individuals with this profile tended not to benefit either subjectively (in depression and pain severity) or objectively (in performance on a lifting task) from multidisciplinary treatment for chronic pain. (In most cases, this was chronic low back pain. Patients with migraines or tension-type headaches were specifically excluded from the protocol.)

Now, the finding that individuals with a particular score configuration are unlikely to benefit from multidisciplinary treatment for certain types of pain is of considerable practical significance. However, we are on less certain ground when we consider the operationalization of "repression." Certainly this is not the psychoanalytic concept, for we have no reason to believe that the process is unconscious. The test results might indicate conscious suppression rather than repression. Alternatively, they might reflect impression management (Weinberger & Davidson, 1994). Possibly, individuals with a high L and low MAS scale were simply, for whatever reason, less cooperative with the assessment. We would not be surprised, then, to find that they went on to benefit less from treatment.

Similarly, the operationalization by Burns et al. does not imply the psychoanalytic concept of conversion, for there is no suggestion that there has been an unconscious symbolic representation of an emotional conflict through a physical symptom (O. Fenichel, 1945, p. 216). On the other hand, repression, defined similarly as in Burns (2000), has been associated with greater physiological reactivity to stress (Pauls & Stemmler, 2003). And for chronic low back pain patients who suppress anger, hostility may raise muscle tension. This effect was specific to the lumbar paraspinals; tension at the trapezius did not change (Burns, 1997). Moreover, the effect was specific to anger suppression; for patients who do not suppress anger, hostility lowers muscle tension. There is also some data, mostly case study or correlational in nature, associating chronic pain with a difficulty in expressing intense emotions (Beutler, D. Engle, Oro'-Beutler, Daldrup, & Meredith, 1986). Thus, there is some possibility that the exclusion of certain emotions (and we do not know if this is conscious, unconscious or somewhere in between) is a risk factor for pain through a symptom-specific psychophysiological mechanism (Burns, 1997).

Analogously, Passchier and coworkers measured repression with a structured projective test, the Defense Mechanisms Inventory. Non-headache subjects who scored high in repression had a greater number of **skin conductance responses** and larger temporal pulse amplitudes at baseline than subjects scoring low in repression. Migraineurs who were high in repression showed lower temporal pulse amplitudes that low-repression migraineurs (Passchier, Goudswaard, Orlebeke, & Verhage, 1988). Thus, there was some evidence that repression facilitated autonomic responding, and that the nature of the response may have been different in migraineurs. However, the study is limited by a rather small sample size relative to the number of variables.

In skin conductance, muscle tension and pulse amplitude at the temples, we have encountered one possible effect of repression: By preventing emotions from being processed and discharged it may intensify the stress response. But what can we say about effects of repression that occur solely in the central nervous system? This question brings us into the realm of conversion disorder.

Conversion

The idea that pain can be purely psychogenic—truly "in one's head"—is by far the most controversial and off-putting in day-to-day clinical work. Clients hate the idea, and clinicians seem to either use it freely or shun it altogether. But before judging it too harshly, let us look at the origins of this unpopular idea.

Freud and Breuer, following other late 19th century thinkers, suggested that a symptom such as pain could come about as an unconsciously generated response to an emotional trauma (Breuer & Freud, 1893/1957, pp. 3–17). Now, Breuer and Freud felt that for most traumas, the strong emotions were dissipated through verbal and physical expression, or by fitting the emotions into one's overall experience. For example, the horrors of an accident might be expressed verbally, or dissipated by thinking about one's subsequent return to safety. But sometimes, it was felt, this dissipation is inhibited, because the trauma is so painful we avoid processing it, or because we encounter the trauma while in a suggestible state, in which the wider context is unavailable. (For example, Freud felt that constricted attention, during the simple repetitive acts of factory work, induced a hypnotic-like mindset.) Then the affect is left undiminished in a separate, wordless consciousness (Breuer & Freud, 1893/1957). When circumstances trigger the unconscious memory, it is expressed in the symbolic, nonverbal language of symptoms.

The symptoms may be idiosyncratic, or a kind of abbreviated reenactment of the original trauma, or the symptoms may be a natural symbolism, for example a physical pain representing a mental pain (Breuer & Freud, 1893/1957).

Not surprisingly, the cure involves restoring the dissipation of trauma related affect, by bringing three processes to bear simultaneously: The eliciting trauma must be recalled. The emotional reaction at the time needs to be accessed. And the emotions must be released or connected with the rest of a person's experience by putting the feelings into words (Breuer & Freud, 1893/1957).

In practice, the concept of conversion disorder has been very difficult to apply responsibly. It is not clear what constitutes a sufficient trauma (Ron, 2001). Indeed, Breuer and Freud noted that people differ in susceptibility, both as a matter of personality, and moment-to-moment. Moreover, often a tragic story comprised of many traumas, each small in itself, is sufficient (Breuer & Freud, 1893/1957). Thus, we cannot definitively infer conversion disorder based on exposure to a trauma. Also, there are no definite physiological markers for pain due to conversion. Thus, in practice conversion becomes a diagnosis of exclusion. Not surprisingly, some disorders that were once thought to be psychogenic (such as cervical dystonia; Dauer, R. E. Burke, P. Greene, & Fahn, 1998; Stacy, 2000) have been reclassified as neurological as knowledge accumulates (Ron, 2001).

Still, despite its difficulties, conversion disorder may truly exist in some cases. Neurological deficits that are medically unexplained will often persist stably for many years (Binzer & Kullgren, 1998; Crimlisk, Bhatia, Cope, David, Marsden, & Ron, 1998). Presumably if there were an undetected neurological disorder, some progression in symptoms would be seen (Ron, 2001). Secondly, there is preliminary evidence on functional neuroimaging that one type of symptom, "hysterical paralysis" (paralysis due to psychological factors) might be mediated by inhibition of the thalamus and basal ganglia by the frontal lobes (Vuilleumier, Chicherio, Assal, S. Schwartz, Slosman, & Landis, 2001).

I generally do not recommend that psychologists diagnose conversion disorder, because we are not able to exclude physical causes for the symptoms. Also, as we have seen, there are many other, and presumably much more common, points of overlap between the psychology and the physiology of pain.

There are exceptions, however, for in psychotherapy practice, symptoms sometimes develop in a manner that implies conversion. For example, a client may feel overwhelmed by affect during a session, and in the process of calming themselves develop dramatic and intrusive medical symptoms that make further focus on the emotions impossible. If vital signs and subsequent medical workup are completely benign, and if conscious intention seems unlikely, then one is left with the definite impression of conversion. In my very limited experience, conversion symptoms seem to call public attention to themselves, often via an obvious loss of functioning. The symptoms seem to go well beyond pain, which is usually endured mostly in private.

Somatization

In its simplest sense, somatization is a failure of insight: The patient experiences the physical signs of an emotion without awareness of its cognitive or affective aspects. Thus, an anxious person might request treatment for an uncomfortable feeling in their stomach, without realizing that the discomfort is because they are nervous.[9]

---

[9]William Matuzas, MD, pointed this out to me during a consult on our inpatient psychiatry unit.

More broadly, "somatization" (or "somatoform disorder" in the parlance of DSM-IV) has meant that psychological factors are thought to be important in generating the physical symptoms, or in the patient presenting with them for treatment (Holder-Perkins & T. N. Wise, 2001). In medical thinking, it is the phrase that precedes the decision to "get a psych consult." Note that as a blanket term, it is not meant to imply a particular psychological mechanism. A person with conversion disorder, a person with frequent stress-related tension-type headaches, and a person who has had a shoulder injury and presents unusually often for treatment because they are experiencing their pain in catastrophic terms, would all be subsumed under the heading of somatization (Mai, 2004). The current chapter is, in a sense, an attempt to shed light on somatization processes as they apply to pain.

Still a third use of the term appears in DSM-IV (American Psychiatric Association, 1994). There, somatization disorder refers to a full-blown syndrome in which, beginning before age 30, a person presents with multiple medically unexplained somatic complaints. Over the course of the disorder, at least four symptoms must involve pain, at least two must be gastrointestinal, at least one must be sexual, and at least one must be pseudoneurological. The diagnosis is not made, of course, if the symptoms are intentionally produced (factitious disorder) or feigned (malingering). Throughout this book, however, we will use "somatization" in the older, broader sense, rather than as the DSM-IV diagnosis.

The origins of somatization are obscure, but risk factors include depression, anxiety, traumatic experiences in childhood, and a personality trait, alexithymia (Heinrich, 2004).

Alexithymia

Alexithymia literally means "no words for feelings" (Sifneos, 1973). The term refers to a difficulty in identifying, differentiating and describing feelings, to a paucity of emotion-related fantasy, and to a tendency to focus on external stimuli and events, rather than on one's internal life (Lesser, 1985; G. J. Taylor, Bagby, & J. D. A. Parker, 1991). In a number of cross-sectional, self-report studies, patients with chronic pain have been found to have higher levels of alexithymia than the members of various control groups, even after correcting for obvious confounds such as depression. This finding requires explanation. Unfortunately, the frequently correlational nature of the research designs leaves open the direction of causality and the possibilities of third variables.

Now, the construct of alexithymia derives from the psychoanalytic literature, and as a starting point, a natural psychodynamic explanation of the association with chronic pain presents itself. People who have difficulty in identifying their feelings might misinterpret the physical sensations of emotion as signs of a medical condition (Lesser, 1985). This does not seem unreasonable. Recognizing a physical sensation as part of an emotion requires integrating knowledge of one's affective and physical states. It would not be surprising for people to differ in their capacity for such a higher level, integrative process.

Note that the somatization process in alexithymia would be somewhat different from that hypothesized to occur in conversion disorder. In psychodynamic theory, conversion is a complex symbolic representation and expression of an unacceptable drive. In alexithymia, a physical symptom may indeed substitute for a feeling, but no complex symbolism is implied (Nemiah, 1996).

Still, there are other plausible hypotheses for the observed relationship between alexithymia and pain (Lumley, Stettner, & Wehmer, 1996). For example, it may be that chronic pain causes alexithymia. Perhaps refocusing attention away from internal experiences is a natural mechanism for coping with pain. Certainly, an external focus may be encouraged by such behavioral strategies as time-contingent rest and medication, and goal-contingent reinforcement. Moreover, the sleep deprivation and use of narcotics often associated with pain, may possibly blunt awareness and expression of affect.

A second possibility is that alexithymia is simply a marker for low socioeconomic status (Lumley, Stettner, & Wehmer, 1996), a disrupted childhood (Berenbaum, 1996), or some other third variable that is the true risk factor for chronic pain. Thus, a life rich in inner experience may be a luxury for those unburdened by a daily struggle to get by. Moreover, people of higher socioeconomic status are likely to have white-collar jobs with lower risk of injury. The association between childhood abuse and chronic pain, and possible explanations, will be discussed below.

A third possibility is that alexithymia is indeed causal, but not because of how physical sensations are labeled. Rather, individuals high in alexithymia may be more likely to drink to excess or otherwise engage in sensation-seeking, perhaps because they are already prone to action rather than fantasy in dealing with problems, or because they lack some of the self-regulation that affect provides. Sensation seeking and/or alcohol use would be risk factors for injury, and hence indirectly for chronic pain. In support of this, Kauhanen and coworkers measured levels of alexithymia in 2297 men, ages 42–60, from in and around the town of Kuopio, Finland. The researchers then followed the men for 5 years, during which 132 deaths took place. Alexithymia predicted all-cause mortality in a dose-dependent manner—the more alexithymic an individual was, the greater his risk of death. Moreover, the association remained after correcting for age, perceived health and known diagnoses at the start of the study, smoking, alcohol use, exercise, obesity, education, income, social support, blood pressure, and HDL and LDL cholesterol fractions (Kauhanen, Kaplan, R. D. Cohen, Julkunen, & Salonen). The risk appears to have been strongest for "external" causes of death (injury, accidental poisoning, suicide, and homicide) although this is uncertain because the small number of such deaths drastically reduced the statistical power.

In a fourth possibility, alexithymia leads to chronically higher sympathetic arousal, because the individual has fewer ways of processing and dealing with negative affect. Although there is a little evidence for this, conflicting results have been reported, and the magnitude of arousal differences may be too low to account for clinical effects (Lumley, Stettner, & Wehmer, 1996; Linden, Lenz, & Stossel, 1996).

Overall, the empirical literature is just beginning to progress beyond the simple finding of an association between alexithymia and chronic pain. An example of the surprises that can emerge is provided in a recent experimental study by Nyklíček and Vingerhoets (2000). As expected, they found that among undergraduates, those scoring higher in alexithymia reported lower pain thresholds and tolerances for electric shock. However, these individuals also had lower thresholds for *detecting* electric shock, long before it became painful. Thus, alexithymia seemed to be associated with greater stimulus sensitivity in general. Not surprisingly, the key component was externally oriented thinking. It seems that individuals oriented to the outside world were more able to detect faint external stimuli.

Clearly, more research is needed to clarify the meaning of the alexithymia-chronic pain correlation, and to shed light on whether the association has implications for assessment and treatment.

BEHAVIORAL FACTORS

Pain Behaviors

The idea that pain intensity is increased by a person's behavioral and verbal expressions of pain is counter-intuitive. We expect the link between behavior and experience to be one-directional: experience causes behavior. However, there is evidence that the link works in the reverse direction as well. In one study, volunteers were administered electric shocks, and were asked to purposefully either exaggerate or conceal the facial expression of pain. Skin conductance responses and pain ratings of the shocks changed in the same direction as facial expression: Reduction in pain expression apparently led to a reduction in stress and subjective pain level (Lanzetta, Cartwright-Smith, & Kleck, 1976).

This result seems extraordinary. In hypnotic analgesia, skin conductance responses to pain are preserved. By this criterion, the deliberate suppression of pain behaviors is more effective than hypnosis. Moreover, we have seen that attempts to suppress awareness of pain often have paradoxical effects—why would suppressing the expression of pain be any different? At this point, we do not know. Lanzetta et al. interpret their results as evidence that facial expression serves a self-regulatory as well as an expressive function (Lanzetta, Cartwright-Smith, & Kleck, 1976). Note too that brain structures involved in selecting or performing motor behaviors (basal ganglia, anterior cingulate cortex) also seem to play a role in pain perception (Chudler & Dong, 1995; D. Price, 2000). Thus, there is perhaps some anatomical basis for thinking of pain as a behavior (Fordyce, 1976).

And clinically, Lanzetta's results are sometimes useful. For when a patient has lost control over much of their life, they can still control their behavior, and this, at least, is a start.

Operant Conditioning

If pain is affected by focus of attention and by overt behaviors, then learning principles that govern attention and behavior should influence level of pain. This is one basis for the operant model of chronic pain, for which a degree of evidence has accrued.

Recall from Chapter 2 a study by Duncan and coworkers, in which monkeys were taught to press a bar when they felt a brief painful stimulus on their upper lip (Duncan, Bushnell, R. Bates, & Dubner, 1987). The pain was preceded by a warning signal (a light) and after awhile, some nociceptive neurons in the trigeminal nucleus caudalis began firing at the light, in advance of the actual pain stimulus. In Chapter 2 we discussed this as evidence that the pain pathways can be primed by expectation. Note, too, however, that when the monkeys detected the pain stimulus and pressed the bar, they were rewarded. This, of course, was necessary for keeping their attention on the experiment. But because there was a reward, the light was not simply a warning signal, it was a **discriminative stimulus**, an indication that pain detection and bar pressing would be reinforced. Thus, Duncan, et al.'s experiment suggests that, on a neurophysiological level, the pain pathways can be trained to fire via behavior modification.

Most likely, this occurs in people as well. In Chapter 2 we encounterd windup—the rapid acceleration of pain with repeated stimulation, reflecting sensitization in lamina I of the dorsal horn. The sensitization process is usually described as the result of stimulus-driven exposure to pain, but it may be more complicated. In the laboratory, the amount of windup can be gradually altered by selectively rewarding increases or decreases in pain perception. This occurs even when the rewards are so infrequent and subtle that people are unaware of the contingency (Hölzl, Kleinböhl, & Huse, 2005). Presumably, such conditioned alterations in windup occur in daily life, too, where interactions with doctors and family, and the subtle pattern of activities accomplished or avoided, give occasional, intermittent reward for changing receptiveness to pain. For, if I persist long enough to experience the joy of achievement, a decrease in my pain sensitivity has been rewarded. If I give up, rest lowers my pain, but could also reinforce an increased sensitivity. But we can also go too far: Extreme persistence, leading to flare-ups, might punish activity and teach further avoidance (Arntz & Peters, 1995). Progressing slowly through a graded hierarchy of pain-inducing tasks may be the most therapeutic approach.

Reinforcing pain behavior (adjusting the intensity of a painful stimulus) may also change pain intensity ratings (Hölzl, Kleinböhl, & Huse, 2005). Similarly, reinforcing higher or lower pain ratings may affect not only the ratings themselves, but also sensory **event-related potentials** as early as 160 msec after the painful stimulus (Lousberg, Vuurman, et al., 2005; however, see Flor, Knost, & Birbaumer, 2002 for conflicting data). Underlying these signs of response generalization is the possibility that in people, operant procedures directed at pain behaviors change not just the expression but the experience of pain.

Perhaps not surprisingly, then, several studies suggest a role for operant factors in clinical populations. For example, Block and coworkers found that patients with solicitous spouses gave higher pain ratings when they thought their spouse was observing them, vs. believing that they were being observed by ward clerks. In contrast, patients whose spouses were not solicitous gave lower pain reports when they thought their spouse was observing (A. Block, Kremer, & Gaylor, 1980). Lousberg and coworkers found that patients had poorer tolerance on a treadmill test in the presence of a solicitous spouse (Lousberg, A. J. Schmidt, & Groenman, 1992). And Flor, et al. found that chronic back pain patients had lower pain thresholds and lower pain tolerances (as assessed in a cold pressor task with the nondominant arm) in the presence of solicitous spouses. Moreover, the patients recalled less use of coping self-statements when a solicitous spouse was present (Flor, Breitenstein, Birbaumer, & Fürst, 1995).

Outside of the laboratory, the interaction between pain behaviors and marital communication is only beginning to be explored. Lauren Schwartz and colleagues, using a modified form of the Response to Conflict Scale, found that in their sample, pain patients were more likely to respond to an argument with pain behaviors (e.g., complaining of pain, rubbing the painful area) than with such conventional responses as yelling or sulking (L. Schwartz, Slater, & Birchler, 1996). Romano et al. found that in 22 to 34 percent of their admittedly nonrandom pain clinic sample, verbal and nonverbal pain behaviors both followed and preceded spouse solicitousness to a greater extent than would be expected by chance. Pain behaviors and more general expressions of spouse support did not show a sequential dependency in patients, nor did solicitous responding seem to affect the probability of pain behaviors in healthy control subjects. In this study, solicitous responding appears to be both a reinforcer and a discriminative stimulus for pain behaviors (Romano, et al., 1992).

Now, why would family members reinforce pain behaviors? The simple explanation, of course, is that the respondents were worried about their spouse's pain and were trying to be helpful. Undoubtedly this is a common source of unintended reinforcement of pain. Family therapists, however, based largely on clinical observations, note that a somatic focus can also arise from a systems pathology. In particular, Minuchin and colleagues felt that a constellation of four processes characterize "psychosomatic families": **enmeshment**, in which family members think and speak for each other, with little sense of individuality; overprotectiveness, in which family members try to prevent each other from experiencing even normal levels of discomfort; rigidity, in which change is strictly resisted; and lack of conflict resolution, in which disagreements are suppressed rather than discussed and resolved (Haggerty, 1983; Minuchin, Rosman, & L. Baker, 1978). We can see how protectiveness, and overprotectiveness, could lead to a focus on physical symptoms. But Minuchin, et al. point out that the four traits together tend to make disagreement anxiety-provoking, and motivate family members to distract themselves from it. Physical symptoms can be a safe, alternative focus that shifts attention from potential areas of conflict.

Kopp et al. found that in families in which the mother had chronic headaches (mothers were selected because there were relatively few men with headaches in the clinic population from which subjects were drawn) members described less openness and communication about feelings than in families in which the mother had chronic back pain, or in which no member had a chronic illness ($p < .00005$; Kopp, Richter, Rainer, Kopp-Wilfling, Rumpold, & Walter, 1995). This could hint that alexithymia plays a role in headaches, or that inhibited communication in families impedes problem solving and creates stress (Kopp, et al.). And improvement in headaches has been reported with couple's therapy (R. Roy, 1989).

In general, however, there is a paucity of evidence for Minuchin's theory, other than the field notes of therapists who feel they have seen the phenomenon in-session. And Kopp et al.'s results could simply reflect that strong emotions can trigger headaches. At this point, the ties between **psychophysiology** and family functioning are in need of further research.

And as Flor, et al. point out, we must hesitate before recommending that a spouse simply be taught to respond less solicitously to pain behaviors. For one thing, pain-contingent solicitousness is positively related to marital satisfaction (Gil, Keefe, Crisson, & Van-Dalfsen, 1987). Clearly we do not want to improve pain coping at the expense of marital adjustment. Moreover, solicitous attention overlaps with the broader construct of social support (Newton-John, 2002). Thus, the predicted increase in pain behaviors from solicitous attention seems to pertain mostly to couples whose marital satisfaction is high (Newton-John, 2002). When the marriage is faltering, or the patient is depressed, or the spouse does not believe the patient is ill, punishing responses may simply add to the patient's stress and burden rather than selectively discouraging pain behaviors. And when the marriage is strong, patients may show less pain tolerance in the presence of a solicitous spouse in part because their blood pressure is lower (Flor, Breitenstein, Birbaumer, & Fürst, 1995). Elevations in blood pressure stimulate **baroreceptors** in the aorta which in turn may lower cortical arousal and pain (Rau, Pauli, Brody, Elbert, & Birbaumer, 1993; see Ghione, 1996 for a review). Self-regulation of pain by means of increased blood pressure is not necessarily advantageous. Thus, pain-contingent solicitous attention calls for a fine-grained idiographic assessment and not blanket assertions (Newton-John, 2002).

Moreover, there is little direct evidence for the role of operant factors in headaches. P. R. Martin et al. report that the most frequent spouse responses to headaches are sympathizing, encouraging the patient to stop what they are doing, and encouraging the patient to sit or lie down (P. R. Martin, Milech, & Nathan, 1993). Certainly this is consistent with an operant model. However, solicitous responding by spouses was positively correlated with treatment outcome, perhaps because it indicated a supportive home environment. In a true conditioning model, solicitous responding would maintain pain behaviors and hence would correlate negatively with outcome. Moreover, Blanchard and coworkers found that patients with daily, intense headaches did not report more avoidance behaviors or family reinforcement than matched patients with less frequent headaches (Blanchard, Appelbaum, Radnitz, Jaccard, & Dentinger, 1989).

Compensation and Litigation

Of course, spouses are not the only source of reinforcement. In the operant model, attention is paid also to compensation and litigation, in which weekly benefits or the prospect of a large settlement can presumably function as disability- and/or pain-contingent reinforcement (T. Hadjistavropoulos, 1999). In the culture at large, this idea is sometimes conflated with malingering. Thus, in 1946 Foster Kennedy cynically opined that chronic symptoms can derive from "a state of mind, born out of fear, kept alive by avarice, stimulated by lawyers, and cured by a verdict" (F. Kennedy, 1946, cited in G. Mendelson, 1992, p. 121). But a reinforcer can exert control over us without our wanting it to—the control exerted by nicotine is an unusually striking example.

Theory, analogy, and rhetoric aside, however, is there any evidence that compensation and litigation are relevant to chronic pain? The dramatic example of a person's functioning miraculously improving a few days after they settle their case seems to be a matter of myth and of a few well-publicized occurrences. In controlled research, there appears to be rather consistent evidence that settling one's case does not lead to an improvement in symptoms or functioning (e.g., R. H. Dworkin, Handlin, Richlin, Brand, & Vannucci, 1985; Guest & Drummond, 1992; Greenough & Fraser, 1989; Kelly & B. N. Smith, 1981). This is not entirely to the detriment of the operant model, however, for it could simply mean that behavior, once changed, is not easily changed back. Moreover, litigation and compensation systems may call upon individuals to repeatedly assert or prove their disability. This type of set-up would be expected to produce a strong conviction in one's disability and pain, through the social psychological mechanisms of cognitive dissonance and self-attribution (Bellamy, 1997; Rohling, Binder, & Langhinrichsen-Rohling, 1995).

Again, however, leaving theory aside: The empirical evidence in favor of litigation and compensation playing a role comes simply from a number of studies showing that these factors are associated with greater pain, prolonged recovery times and poorer response to treatment compared with control subjects (e.g., Connally & Sanders, 1991; Groth-Marnat & Fletcher, 2000; Rohling, Binder, & Langhinrichsen-Rohling, 1995). In particular, Rohling, et al. found in a **meta-analysis** that receiving compensation had an **effect size** somewhere between 0.48 and 0.60, depending on how data was extracted from the individual studies.

Is the influence of litigation and compensation important? This effect size is statistically significant, but whether it is small or large depends on how it is viewed. Classically, an effect size around 0.60 would be considered "moderate" (J. Cohen, 1988). However, if we convert it into a correlation coefficient, $r = 0.24$, compensation accounts for only 6 percent of the variance in pain, disability, and treatment responsiveness. On the other hand, Rohling, et al. note that using Rosenthal's binomial effect size display, eliminating compensation would be statistically equivalent to a drug that cures 24 percent of its patients. (Rohling et al.). In a later meta-analysis the authors reached a similar conclusion, with a similar percent of explained variance, for chronic symptoms following closed head injury (Binder & Rohling, 1996). From this evidence, then, it appears that disability-related payments do indeed exert significant control over pain and functioning.

"Appears," however, may be the operative word. Because patients are not assigned randomly to either receive or not receive compensation,[10] we cannot draw causal inferences with certainty. Rohling et al. note that several studies have matched patients on pretreatment injury or pain severity and still found a significant effect of compensation. However, to my knowledge matching has not been conducted on coping skills, depression, or other psychological variables. Moreover, patients receiving compensation tend to be less educated than those not receiving compensation (Rohling, Binder, & Langhinrichsen-Rohling, 1995), and to have more physically demanding jobs (Teasell, 2001). It is easy to imagine that recovery is affected by these other variables, for which compensation may be functioning as a proxy.

And there are other reasons for doubt. Note that cognitive dissonance and self-attribution processes would play a significant role only for those individuals whose pain was mild before their claim was challenged. In fact, Burns et al. found that compensation predicted poor treatment outcome only for those patients with a history of *high* pain and surgery (Burns, M. L. Sherman, Devine, Mahoney, & Pawl, 1995)—precisely the opposite of what cognitive dissonance theory would predict. The other mediating variable to emerge in the Burns et al. study was pessimism about returning to one's former occupation. All of this points more to a model in which compensation plays a significant role only for individuals whose usual ways of coping are blocked or overwhelmed by the pain.

A similar possibility is raised by the data of Feinstein et al., who found that early seeking of legal counsel was associated with higher levels of self-reported anxiety, depression, and social

---

[10]I suspect that some of my patients would disagree with this statement.

dysfunction (Feinstein, Ouchterlony, Somerville, & Jardine, 2001). And Leavitt has found, not surprisingly, that emotional distress tends to prolong disability in injured workers (F. Leavitt, 1990). Thus, a person's decision to involve a lawyer might serve as a marker for a deficit in coping skills, with the deficit comprising the true risk factor for chronicity.

Of course still another possibility is that the legal system itself is deleterious to recovery (Lishman, 1988). For reinforcement need not be positive. Patients often feel alarmed, mistrustful and angry when they (or their spouses or children) are followed by private investigators. The patients may not want to take any chances with their compensation, and may become very inactive. For conditions such as chronic low back pain, the resulting deconditioning and weight gain can be significant exacerbating factors (Hadjistavropoulos, 1999).

Moreover, the effects of litigation need not be behavioral. Recall the evidence, reviewed above, that positive affect tends to reduce pain and that reminders of pain tend to prime or increase it. Now, the litigation process may include hearings, depositions, independent medical exams, meetings with one's attorney, and seemingly endless correspondence, all of which can be reminders of the accident. Depending on the person's circumstances and perspective, they might also be time away from more enjoyable activities.

So far, we have been assuming that compensation and litigation exert their effects primarily upon the claimant. This assumption may not be justified. Hendler and Kozikowski (1993) found that when patients in the litigation system were referred to their pain clinic, the diagnosis was usually nonspecific, for example "chronic pain". More precise and treatable diagnoses, including myofascial pain, peripheral nerve entrapment, and facet arthropathy, had apparently been overlooked. Hence, it may be the expectations and behavior of the treatment providers, more than those of the patients, that are shaped by the presence of litigation and compensation. Moreover, litigation and the bureaucracy of compensation systems can significantly delay medical interventions, for example postponing back surgery by several months. During the delay, both the physiological aspects (central sensitization) and psychological aspects of chronic pain can intensify, making the condition less responsive to treatment (Gallagher & Myers, 1996).

And yet there remains evidence that the time to return to work can be predicted from the ratio of compensation to post-injury wages: The better the compensation scheme, the more people file for disability, and the more time they spend out of work (Teasell, 2001). In all, then, it seems that the role of compensation and litigation is complex, and probably affects different patients in different ways (Hadjistavropoulos, 1999).

DEVELOPMENTAL FACTORS

It seems logical to presume that genetic factors are important determinants of pain threshold and tolerance, yet the evidence for this is quite mixed. In a large-scale cross-sectional study, Mac-Gregor, et al., found that twins raised in the same household had somewhat similar thresholds for pressure pain. However, the intraclass correlation coefficient (amount of shared variance) was the virtually the same for monozygotic and dizygotic twins. The resulting heritability coefficient was only about 10%, and not statistically significant (A. J. MacGregor, Griffiths, Baker, & Spector, 1997). On the other hand, pain expression in children seems to be strongly related to temperament, that is, general emotionality (Grunau, Whitfield, & Petrie, 1994; Schechter, B. A. Bernstein, A. Beck, Hart, & Scherzer, 1991). To my knowledge, there are no prospective studies examining whether this carries over into adulthood. However, the literature on trait negative affectivity or neuroticism may perhaps be capturing the same phenomenon in adults.

Grunau et al. report a short-term prospective study of preschoolers who had been extremely low birthweight neonates. Mother and child dyads were observed during two structured tasks when the child was three years old, and when the child was four somatization was measured using the Personality Inventory for Children. Maternal involvement with the child correlated positively, and sensitivity to the child's emotional cues correlated negatively, with later reported somatization. This fits with the idea that parents can help children interpret certain physical sensations as being part of an emotional state. These are intriguing results, but quite limited, in that they did not generalize to a sample of full-term children (Grunau, Whitfield, Petrie, & Fryer, 1994). In fact, the most robust predictor of somatic complaints in children appears to be concurrent family stress (Grunau, Whitfield, Petrie, & Fryer, 1994).

Other aspects of the family may also be relevant. For example, Hotopf et al. hypothesized that illness as a child would lead to a tendency to present with medically unexplained symptoms as an adult. To test this, they looked at Great Britain's Medical Research Council National Survey of Health, in which 5362 individuals were followed prospectively from their births in 1946. By age 36, 3322 individuals remained in the study, of whom a small fraction (c. 5 percent) had multiple self-reported symptoms. Excluded from the analysis were those who went on, at age 43, to have a physical disease, in case this could explain the symptoms at age 36. Now, as it turns out, illness in childhood did *not* predict later tendency to report symptoms—in fact the associated **odds ratio** was 1.0. However, illness in the parents during the participants' childhoods did predict later symptom reporting by participants. Survey members whose father's health had been "not very good" were 6.2 times more likely to give multiple somatic complaints compared with those whose fathers' health had been "excellent." For mothers' health, the corresponding odds ratio was 2.5 (Hotopf, Mayou, Wadsworth, & Wessely, 1999). Thus, family **modeling** of illness may be a factor in one's own later perceived poor health.

Abuse and Chronic Stress

A number of researchers have noted high rates of childhood trauma in individuals with chronic abdominal (Drossman, 1994), pelvic (Walker, Katon, Harrop-Griffiths, L. Holm, J. Russo, & Hickock, 1988) or low back pain (Linton, 1997), or headaches (Domino & Haber, 1987). Presumably, the correlation is true of chronic pain conditions in general. Firm conclusions, however, have been limited by the design of the studies, which have invariably been correlational, retrospective, and based on self-report. Thus, we have not been able to rule out reporting bias, or the possibility that the association is due to some unknown factor, say in family structure, that correlates with trauma. Moreover, many of the studies have used clinical samples, and hence it might be health care utilization and not pain itself, that is predicted by childhood trauma.

Nonetheless, the evidence has been consistent and significant. J. Morrison (1989), for example, compared women in treatment for somatization disorder with an age-, education-, and race-matched sample of women with unipolar or bipolar depression. Now, depression should produce a strong recall bias in favor of negative events ("mood congruent recall"; Bower, 1981; Josephson, Singer, & Salovey, 1996; Parrott & Spackman, 2000). Morrison found, however, that while 55 percent of the patients with somatization disorder reported having been sexually molested as children, only 16 percent of the depressed patients did. Moreover, the two groups of patients did not differ in reports of other sexual events.

Linton (1997) conducted a large-scale, population-based study in Sweden, of the relationship between back pain and physical or sexual abuse in childhood or adulthood. Women who reported pronounced pain were 5.1 times more likely to report a history of physical abuse and 4.2 times more likely to report of history of sexual abuse. Noteworthy in this study is that the probability of abuse was the same in the pronounced pain group drawn from the general population as in a clinical sample. Thus, it appears to be the pain itself, and not being a patient, that is predicted by the abuse. Linton did not find significant effects of abuse on pain in men, although the question of interaction with gender is not yet resolved (Fillingim, C. S. Wilkinson, & Powell, 1999). Also, we should add that the 55 percent figure found by Morrison (1989) was not replicated in Linton's study, where 8.1 percent of women with pronounced pain reported an abuse history.

The challenges of studying child abuse prospectively would seem insurmountable. However, Raphael and colleagues were able to circumvent the problems by using court records to identify 676 children below the age of 11 who had experienced severe abuse or neglect (Raphael, Widom, & G. Lange, 2001). These children were matched with 520 others who had not been abused or neglected, on age, sex, race, and neighborhood (as a proxy for socioeconomic status). Twenty years later the children, now around age 29, were contacted and interviewed by assistants blind to the purposes of the study. Now, the subjects' self-reports of abuse and neglect did not match the court records from their childhoods very well. Of those with documented abuse, only 73 percent recalled the abuse at the interview. Among the control subjects, 49 percent reported that some abuse or neglect had in fact occurred, which apparently had not come to the attention of the courts. When the researchers used these retrospective reports, abuse and neglect were associated with physical pain in adulthood, consistent with previous studies. However, when the prospective court data was used, the relationship between abuse and pain evaporated (Raphael et al.). The implication seems to be that it is the recollection of abuse, and not the fact of its having occurred, that is the risk factor for pain.

Perhaps the results of Raphael, et al. should not surprise us. Among Vietnam veterans, it appears to be the presence of Posttraumatic Stress Disorder, and not trauma exposure by itself, that predicts pain reports (Beckham et al., 1997; McFarlane, Atchison, Rafalowicz, & Papay, 1987). In the general population, PTSD seems to be associated with a four-fold increased risk of musculoskeletal pain (B. J. Cox & L. A. McWilliams, 2002), and may mediate the relationship between trauma and fibromyalgia (D. S. Ciccone, D. K. Elliott, Chandler, Nayak, & Raphael, 2005). Moreover, pain intensity seems to correlate specifically with PTSD symptoms that involve reexperiencing the trauma (e.g., intrusive recollections or distressing dreams), rather than symptoms of hyperarousal, avoidance or emotional numbing (Beckham, et al.; McFarlane, et al.). Perhaps the pain is a reminder of the trauma (Asmundson, Coons, S. Taylor, J. Katz, 2002; Beckham et al.), or perhaps cognitive priming from thinking about trauma increases pain sensitivity. Indeed, most of the theoretical mechanisms connecting trauma and pain imply that it is from the sustained emotional effects of the trauma that the vulnerability to pain develops.

What are these theories that would explain the link between trauma and pain? The first is biochemical. Note that severe inescapable stress tends to cause analgesia, at least in part through release of endorphins. Repeated stress could in theory cause an overexposure to endorphins, leading to a compensatory decline in receptor sensitivity, and hence decreased ability to regulate pain. There is some evidence from animal studies that chronic stress does in fact lead to reduced effectiveness of morphine (Gescuk, Lang, & Kornetsky, 1995; Hawranko & D. J. Smith, 1999).

The second theory, also biochemical, draws on parallels between endocrine function in a wide range of pain disorders, and in Posttraumatic Stress Disorder. Specifically, individuals with fibromyalgia (Crofford, et al., 1994), rheumatoid arthritis (Chikanza, Petrou, Kingsley, et al, 1992), chronic pelvic pain (Heim, Ehlert, Hanker, & Hellhammer, 1998), chronic abdominal pain in children (Alfvén, de la Torre, & Uvnäs-Moberg, 1994), chronic whiplash (Gaab, S. Baumann, Budnoik, Gmünder, Hottinger, & Ehlert, 2005) and headaches (Elwan, Abdella, El Bayad, & Hamdy, 1991), tend to show either reduced baseline levels of **cortisol**, or greater suppression of cortisol in response to low-dose dexamethasone. We will see in Chapter 8 that the same may be true for a subset of patients with temporomandibular dysfunction. Generally similar findings have been reported for individuals with Posttraumatic Stress Disorder (Boscarino, 1996; Heim,

Ehlert, Hanker, et al.), suggesting an endocrinological bridge between PTSD and pain. Similarly, al' Absi et al. have found that lower baseline cortisol levels correlate with higher pain ratings during a cold pressor test, although the effect was specific to men ($r = -.44, p < .01$; al' Absi, Petersen, & Wittmers, 2002). Still, a causal connection has not been established, and it is not obvious how reduced cortisol levels or reactivity would lead to pain. In one theory, focus is placed on the fact that cortisol suppresses **prostaglandin** synthesis, and hence presumably inflammation and pain (Heim, Ehlert, Hanker, et al.). Certainly, more research is warranted.

The third theory is psychological. Possibly, childhood trauma might promote negative affectivity, a tendency to experience emotions such as depression and anxiety (R. B. Fillingim, C. S. Wilkinson, & Powell, 1999). This, in turn, could lead to both greater attention to internal sensations, and a stronger tendency to interpret sensations in pessimistic terms (Watson & Pennebaker, 1989). In fact, Fillingim and coworkers found in a college student sample that the relationship between abuse and pain disappeared if they controlled for depression and non-pain somatization (Fillingim et al.).[11]

In the fourth theory, abuse is thought to be a risk factor for catastrophizing, that is, for seeing oneself as unable to cope with stressors (Linton, Lardén, & Gillow, 1996). The diminished cognitive coping resources would then in turn be a risk factor for chronicity if a pain problem develops. In fact, Fillingim and coworkers found greater catastrophizing, but no difference in the use of other coping strategies, in patients with an abuse history (R. B. Fillingim, C. S. Wilkinson, & Powell, 1999).

Clinically, my sense is that when fibromyalgia develops in the weeks following the offset of severe, prolonged stress, the pain is generally accompanied by prominent fatigue and, often, an autoimmune disorder (see Boscarino, 2004; and M. L. Taylor, Trotter, & Csuka, 1995, for preliminary, consistent data). Unfortunately, attempting to boost cortisol by giving oral prednisone appears to be ineffective for fibromyalgia and of little benefit in chronic fatigue (Blockmans, Persoons, Van Houdenhove, Lejeune, & Bobbaers, 2003; S. Clark, Tindall, & R. M. Bennett, 1985; McKenzie et al., 1998). The combination of graded exercise, tricyclics, and cognitive-behavioral therapy remains the treatment of choice (Blockmans et al.), and may (perhaps) help correct underlying neuroendocrine dysfunctions (Geenen, J. Jacobs, & Bijlsma, 2002).

PAIN AND MEANING

We have seen, then, that expectations and attention can change the emotional qualities and even the sensory intensity of pain. This suggests that the meaning given to the pain is an important part of the pain experience (Eimer & A. Freeman, 1998), and leaves much room for depth-oriented psychotherapy that might change this meaning (Grzesiak, Ury, & R. H. Dworkin, 1996). When a person is freed from frequent attention to pain or expectations of having pain, the condition is likely to improve. Which type of therapy brings about this change may vary from patient to patient.

Note, too, that psychological factors do not seem to cause pain *de novo*. Rather, by increasing attention to pain and hence firing rates in the dorsal horn, they may be a contributing factor to central sensitization and hence chronicity. Even someone as committed to psychological fac-

---

[11]Intuitively, negative feelings about one's self might seem relevant as well. However, in structural equation modeling, Harter and Vanecek (2000) found that depression, somatization, and other forms of psychopathology significantly predicted low self-worth, while prediction in the reverse direction was non-significant. That is, low self-worth did not seem to lead to psychological distress so much as psychological distress led to low self-worth. Of course if this result holds up, it has important treatment implications.

tors as Sigmund Freud, recognized this in his first case study, as indicated in the quote at the start of this chapter.

Steps Toward a Unified Model

We have now reviewed physiological and psychological factors relevant to chronic pain. Later in this book we will put these factors to use in the behavioral assessment and treatment of benign headaches. Before taking this step, however, let us pause to consider the intellectual majesty of the model that has emerged. Cognitive, cultural and personal factors influence the meanings given to pain, and therefore the degree to which the pain becomes a focus of attention. The amount of attention influences firing rates in the dorsal horn, and therefore the speed and amount by which calcium ion concentrations rise in the postsynaptic cells. This in turn leads to several changes in enzyme activity in the cell that phosphorylate a specific subunit of AMPA-type glutamate receptors. The phosphorylation increases receptor activity, strengthening the synapse, sensitizing the dorsal horn, and hence leading to chronic pain, with its profound effects on the person's psychological and social world. In a single glance, then, we are able to apprehend a smooth chain of influence, from the historical to the molecular and back again. Our own small corner of the mind-body problem has been solved.[12]

Clinical Implications

We have seen, then, that the intensity of a nociceptive stimulus, and the activity of pain inhibitory and facilitory descending pathways, converge on the dorsal horn, and probably in more proximal structures as well, to determine the degree of central sensitization. This sensitization has as its hallmarks allodynia (the experience of non-noxious stimuli as painful), hyperalgesia and persistent pain (pain that is more intense and that lasts longer than would be expected from the stimulus). Central sensitization, as altered nociception, may be the nucleus around which the affective, behavioral, and social elements of **chronic pain syndrome** coalesce (Loeser, 1982). Ultimately, of course, these concentric spheres and the sensitization at their core, are the targets of chronic pain treatment. Later in this book we will consider in detail strategies for assessment and therapy. For the moment, however, let us mention some broad directions based on the material we have encountered so far. For the physiological and psychological literature on pain processing gives us a foundation for speculating about approaches to enhance pain coping. And although the suggestions that follow are mostly hypotheses in need of testing, or hints of a literature we will explore more deeply in chapters 14–19, they illustrate the intensely practical nature of knowledge about pain.

Chronic pain treatment often includes an emphasis on moderating activity ("pacing") and taking planned, preemptive rest breaks, to reduce the intrusiveness and meaningfulness of the pain. Yet here we see an addition reason: Poor pacing, by maximizing total pain exposure over time, could reasonably lead to a long-term increase in pain sensitivity.

---

[12]The growing evidence of continuity between mind and body, in pain and other parts of the neurosciences, has naturally led to criticism of Descartes. Still, by bringing the study of the body out of the realm of the subjective, and by explicitly comparing the body to a machine, Descartes laid the foundation of scientific medicine. And this was among his goals, for in his *Discourse on Method* he writes that ". . . we might rid ourselves of an infinity of maladies of body as well as of mind, and perhaps also of the enfeeblement of old age, if we had sufficient understanding of the causes from which these ills arise and of all the remedies which nature has provided. It was my intention to devote my whole life to the pursuit of this . . ." (Descartes, 1960/1637, p. 46). If in fact Cartesian dualism is approaching obsolescence, the Cartesian project for a scientific medicine is just beginning to reach its prime.

Conversely, firing rates in the dorsal horn are inhibited by endorphinergic pathways. These pathways are activated in part by activities that have a higher emotional priority than the pain. Thus, absorption in meaningful non-pain activities, especially those that arouse positive affect ("appetitive motivational states") may be helpful not simply for moment-to-moment pain coping, but for long-term reeducation of the afferent pain pathways. Moreover, by limiting attention to the site of pain, such absorption may help prevent the types of cortical changes seen in chronic pain.

Redirecting attention, however, should not be accomplished through suppression of the pain sensation by an act of will. Attempts to suppress pain, at least during intense flare-ups, may delay recovery from the flare-up and decrease self-efficacy for dealing with future episodes of pain (Cioffi & Holloway, 1993). On rational grounds, **dissociation** as a pain coping strategy may similarly be a risk factor for chronicity, by allowing nociception and sensitization of the dorsal horn to go on unimpeded.

On the other hand, suppression of pain *behaviors* seems to be an effective approach, for potentially reducing pain disability, sensation, and autonomic impact. This efficacy can be very helpful clinically. When an individual feels that they have no control over the pain, they can at least have control over their facial expression, or their topic of conversation, and this is a start.

Of course to change behavior, it is helpful to have the reinforcement contingencies arranged accordingly. Moreover, we have seen evidence that neurons subserving nociception can learn to fire in response to a **discriminative stimulus**. Thus, it is helpful if a friend or spouse can work with the patient to identify some do-able, enjoyable non-pain activities consistent with good pacing, and then deliberately partake of the shared enjoyment rather than reacting to the pain.

Involvement in non-pain behaviors has another advantage as well: It tends to take a person out of their "sickroom," that is, out of an environment that may be saturated with reminders of the pain, or with conditioned stimuli for, perhaps, eliciting a learned hyperalgesia.

Turning attention away from pain can be impeded by pain-related anxiety, and hence such anxiety should be aggressively treated. One source of anxiety is a concern that the pain signals physical harm. Once it develops, this anxiety tends to become self-sustaining through **confirmatory bias**. Such concerns are usually dealt with medically by reassuring the patient. Yet seeking reassurance may be similar to other types of avoidance behaviors in inadvertently perpetuating anxiety by preempting habituation (Salkovskis & Warwick, 1986). On the other hand, we might expect that education, by giving the patient the tools to rationally reevaluate their pain, would be beneficial. This should extend to other bodily reactions as well, including the stress response generated by pain. Of course one's ability to rationally reappraise anxiety is enhanced by cognitive therapy, and for some people this may be the focus of pain coping skills training.

If the anxiety is due to catastrophization, a fear of being overwhelmed by the pain, then negative cognitions are implicated directly, and changing these cognitions is a reasonable focus of treatment. A logical example is self-instructional training, in which an individual learns to identify negative self-statements and replace them with statements that enhance coping (Meichenbaum, 1977). Similarly, focusing on the objective, sensory characteristics of the pain rather than its unpleasantness or emotional elaboration may similarly be quite helpful as a competing response to anxious somatic self-monitoring (Cioffi & Holloway, 1993; H. D. Hadjistavropoulos, T. Hadjistavropoulos, & Quine, 2000). We will consider both of these approaches further in Chapter 13.

Moreover, pacing should not be confounded with a fearful avoidance of the pain. To the contrary, **graded exposure** to pain-producing situations, combined with good pain coping skills, can provide a sense of mastery and self-efficacy that itself helps reduce pain.

The nascent science of pain **psychophysics** also has implications for pain coping, particularly in the quantitative study of counterstimulation. It appears, for example, that a vibratory stimulus is most effective when it is applied to the dermatome adjacent to the pain, or to the same dermatome as the pain but on the opposite side of the body (Yarnitsky, Kunin, Brik, & Sprecher, 1997). Moreover, we have seen that attending to the counterstimulus may be important for it to effectively compete with the pain (Longe et al., 2001).

Of course accomplishing these goals will not necessarily be straightforward. Pacing may not be achievable until a person is able to separate their self-worth from their premorbid level of productivity. Absorption in important non-pain activities may ultimately require a person to resurrect their sense of life's meaning from years of losses imposed by the pain. Therapy for pain coping may not differ drastically from psychotherapy for other goals.

Nonetheless, from a knowledge of pain processing we can form hypotheses about how pain coping tools can be optimized. For example, we might suspect that ostensibly similar pain control strategies differ in their long-term impact. We have already seen the distinction between suppressing pain awareness and suppressing pain behaviors. As another example, consider the use of ice. One person might apply the ice gently at the site of pain, and perhaps reduce sensitization by decreasing afferent input to the dorsal horn. Another person might use the ice as a counterstimulus, perhaps drawing on intracortical inhibition and building self-efficacy, by applying the ice to a dermatome adjacent to the pain. A third person may find ice painful (cold allodynia), perhaps due to sensitization of **wide dynamic range neurons** in the dorsal horn. Yet this person may use ice all the same, deliberately increasing the pain to the edge of tolerability, and then experiencing a sense of analgesia and well-being when the cold is removed. This person might be eliciting an endorphinergic response, yet putting themselves at risk for further sensitization by maximizing total pain exposure. Thus a single modality, effective in all three cases, may have different physiological implications. Again, this is speculative, but it seems a reasonable research agenda to examine empirically the long-term effects of various pain coping strategies.

We will examine these and other behavioral pain coping therapies in greater detail in Chapter 13.

PART II

Principal Types of Headaches: Physiology and Psychology

CHAPTER 4

Migraines

> *Do you know what hemicrania means? A half headache. I've been having it for a few*
> *days and it is a lovely thing. One half of my head in a mathematical line from the top*
> *of my skull to the cleft of my jaw throbs and hammers and sizzles and bangs and swears*
> *while the other half—calm and collected—takes note of the agonies next door.*
> — Rudyard Kipling, in a letter to his cousin (cited in Critchley, 1996, p. 338)

Diane has had migraines since she was 14, at first once or twice a year, but gradually they have
increased to 4 to 6 a month. The pain—an intense pulsing that usually starts at her left temple—
and nausea have gotten worse, too, and even the thought of moving around during an attack is
aversive. Lights, sounds, even slight vibrations are painful, and certain smells make her gag.
She tries to "soldier on" during an attack, but her brain is sluggish and she can't find words.
Zolmitriptan helps, but her insurance company limits her to 3 pills a month. Her only warning
is a blind spot, like a ceiling fan reflected in a gray drop of water, that drifts slowly out to the
periphery and fills her with dread. Her hands and feet are always cold, and she worries about
losing her job. At first, her menses and the letdown after stress were the only triggers, but now
even a change in the weather can bring on attacks. She avoids caffeine and a long list of foods she
learned about from her husband, coworkers, and the internet.

In the IHS diagnostic criteria, migraines involve a moderate-to-severe, pulsing or throbbing
pain. The pain is generally accompanied by an aversion to light (photophobia) and to conversational sound levels (phonophobia), by nausea, and in about one-third of the cases, by vomiting.
Migraines can be exacerbated by routine physical activity such as climbing stairs. The throbbing
pain, worsened by light, sound, and simple head movements, the gastrointestinal disturbances,
temporary cognitive impairments and mood changes, all combine into a feeling of illness seep-
ing into incapacity. A migraine is an often disabling neurological condition in which headache
is but one of the symptoms.

Although "migraine" is derived from Galen's term, "hemicrania," (McHenry, 1969) unilateral pain is not required for diagnosis. Migraines are bilateral about 25 percent of the time in
adults, and even more often in children (Silberstein, Lipton, Goadsby, & R. T. Smith, 1999).

PREVALENCE

How common are migraines? Large-scale population studies identify a lifetime prevalence of
6 percent in men and 15–18 percent in women (B. K. Rasmussen, 2001). Thus, 70–75 percent
of migraineurs are female. (By the IHS criteria the disorder requires at least 2 episodes of
migraine with aura, or 5 without. Lifetime prevalence of 1 or 2 migrainous episodes may be quite

high; Haan, Terwindt, & Ferrari, 1997.) Prevalence of the disorder rises until approximately age 40, declining gradually thereafter for both sexes. Migraine without aura is approximately 5 times more common than migraine with aura (Adams, M. Victor, & Ropper, 1997).

We will see in Chapter 6 that the prevalence of tension-type headache may be increasing, at least for adolescents. There is preliminary evidence that the same may be true of migraines. In a large-scale survey, self-reported migraine prevalence in the United States increased from 2.58 percent of the population in 1981 to 4.10 percent in 1989 (National Health Interview Survey, cited in Lipton & Stewart, 1997). A survey of 7 year old children in Turku, Finland found that migraine prevalence tripled, from 1.9 percent to 6.3 percent of boys, and from 2.0 percent to 5.0 percent of girls between 1974 and 1992 (Sillanpää & Anttila, 1996). Rozen, et al. reviewed the medical records in Olmsted County, Minnesota, diagnosing migraine when the symptoms warranted. They found a 56 percent increase in one-year incidence in women and a 34 percent increase in men, for 1989–1990 compared with 1979–1981. For pediatric migraines the rise was even more striking, with one-year incidences increasing by 46 percent in boys under 10, 89 percent in boys ages 10–19, 99 percent in girls under 10, and 68 percent in girls ages 10–19 (Rozen, J. W. Swanson, Stang, McDonnell, & Rocca, 1999). Very different numbers, but in the same direction, have been reported in a Dutch study (Bandell-Hoekstra, Abu-Saad, Passchier, Frederiks, Feron, & Knipschild, 2001). The investigators found that the prevalence of weekly headache in 10–17 year old children had increased, although by only 6 percent, since 1985.

This incease could be illusory, due to an artifact such as increased awareness of migraines or willingness to seek treatment. However, Rozen, et al. found that the proportion of their sample for whom migraine symptoms were medically documented within one year of their onset increased only from 50 percent to 57 percent. Presumably, if patients were more readily seeking treatment this percentage would have risen more dramatically. There was also an increase in the range of specialists documenting migraine symptoms, and perhaps this is a key confound. It is hard for any study using medical records as its primary data to separate increased medical diagnosis from a true rise in prevalence.

A case that migraines are *not* becoming more common has been made by Lipton et al. who administered a validated headache questionnaire to a large United States community sample in 1989 (Stewart, Lipton, Celentano, & Reed, 1992) and again in 1999 (Lipton, Stewart, S. Diamond, M. L. Diamond, & Reed, 2001). They found that migraine prevalence increased, from 5.7 percent to 6.5 percent of males, and from 17.6 percent to 18.2 percent of females. However, the amount of increase was relatively small, and was overshadowed by a larger change: The percentage of respondents with migraines who reported that they had already received this diagnosis medically, increased from 38 percent in 1989 to 48 percent in 1999 (Lipton, S. Diamond, Reed, & M. L. Diamond, 2001). Certainly more data will be helpful in separating increased prevalence, if any, from increased awareness.

If migraines are indeed becoming more common, the reason is unknown. Possibly, exposure to migraine triggers (discussed below, in Chapter 10) may be increasing. As one example, we will see evidence that trait anxiety has increased markedly over the last 50 years, at least among children and adolescents (Twenge, 2000).

A similar question is raised by the variation in migraine over geographical area. Lipton and coworkers conducted a meta-analysis of 18 migraine prevalence studies using the IHS diagnostic criteria (A. Scher, Stewart, & Lipton, 1999). They found that 51 percent of the variance among prevalence rates for women, and 42 percent for men, was explained by the continent on which the study was conducted. At age 40, estimated prevalence for women was 22 percent in North America, 16 percent in Central and South America, 15 percent in Europe, 10 percent in Asia, and 7 percent in Africa. On all continents, the prevalence in men was approximately one third that in women. There is some evidence that in the United States, Asian Americans and African Americans have lower rates of migraines than Caucasians (Stewart, Lipton, & Liberman, 1996). The difference in risk persists after controlling for education as a rough measure of acculturation and, hence, the geographic variability between continents may be an indicator of a genetic component in migraine. On the other hand, it seems difficult to explain the higher rate of migraine in America than in Europe (assuming the difference is stable) on this basis.

For migraine with aura, first degree relatives appear to have an increased probability of having the disorder (relative risk ≈ 4; M. B. Russell & J. Olesen, 1995). For migraine without aura the family studies data seem ambiguous. First degree relatives show an increased risk of migraine without aura (RR ≈ 1.9) but so do the patients' spouses (RR ≈ 1.4; M. B. Russell & J. Olesen, 1995). Twin studies show a monozygotic concordance for migraines of between 14 and 100 percent, (M ≈ 50 percent) and a dizygotic concordance of between 0 and 40 percent (M ≈ 14 percent). "The observations in twins strongly support a genetic component of migraine but are too unreliable to quantify this contribution" (Haan, Terwindt, & M. D. Ferrari, 1997). In one study, it appeared that familial aggregation (presumably genetic but perhaps reflecting early environment) was relatively more important for male migraineurs (M. B. Russell, Hilden, Sørensen, & J. Olesen, 1993).

Of course there is considerable interest in discovering what the relevant genes are, for they could be clues to pathophysiology. In theory, though, there might be dozens, or even hundreds of genes that influence risk of migraines, in the way that numerous genes governing lipid metabolism affect the risk of heart disease (Peroutka, 2002). So far, studies have focused on genes relevant to immune functioning, neural stability, vasoconstriction, and the sympathetic nervous system. We will discuss these results later in the chapter.

For people with migraines, the median frequency is 1.5 episodes per month, with a median duration of slightly under one day (Ferrari, 1998b). Taking duration and frequency into account, Ferrari notes that 1 percent of the general population averages at least one day of migraine per *week*.

IMPAIRMENT AND DISTRESS

Yet it is not prevalence so much as impact that distinguishes migraine headaches. For example, Koopmans and Lamers (2000) studied psychological distress and fatigue in a large community-based sample. After controlling for demographics, the best predictor of distress was the number of comorbid physical conditions present. Beyond this, only presence vs. absence of migraines added to the prediction. For people with a single disorder, the amount of distress caused by migraines was approximately equal to that caused by heart disease, lung disease, diabetes, arthritis, or back problems.

Not only emotional well-being but cognitive functioning as well appears to be affected by migraines. Meyer and colleagues conducted repeated assessments with Folstein's Mini-Mental Status Exam (M. F. Folstein, S. E. Folstein, & McHugh, 1975) of 77 people with migraine with aura, migraine without aura, **transformed migraine**, or cluster headache. When the subjects were not having a headache, 90 percent scored in the normative range of cognitive functioning. During a headache, this figure declined to 51 percent. With a more sensitive test, the Cognitive Capacity Screening Examination, 92 percent scored in the average range outside of a headache, while only 14 percent did so during a headache. The amount of impairment was equivalent across the four diagnoses (J. S. Meyer, Thornby, K. Crawford, & Rauch, 2000). The reasons for the temporary cognitive deficit are unclear: Interference from the pain, from symptomatic headache medications, or from some part of the headache process itself might be playing a role. Its implications for functioning seem quite profound, however, especially for individuals with frequent, severe headaches.

Fortunately, however, the impairment does indeed seem to be temporary. Sumatriptan nasal spray may reverse cognitive interference along with pain (Farmer et al., 2001). And among patients drawn from the general population, migraines, even over many years, do not appear to cause cognitive decline in between migraine episodes (Gaist et al., 2005; Jelicic, van Boxtel, Houx, & Jolles, 2000).

A more permanent effect has been proposed for the visual system. Chronicle and Mullener (1994) suggest that in migraine with aura, inhibitory neurons in the primary visual cortex may ultimately sustain cumulative damage. Fortunately, this theory has received very little empirical support. Drummond and Anderson (1992) report transient impairments in visual sensitivity the day after an episode of migraine with aura, but the deficits had resolved within 10 days. Wilkinson and Crotogino (2000) report evidence of a very slight decrement in visual sensitivity to one particular type of stimulus in volunteers who had experienced a large number of lifetime auras. However, the results are so subtle (and equivocal) that they are of no clinical importance.

We should add that these negative results are by no means trivial. We will see below that people with migraines may be susceptible to repeated but relatively mild hypoxia, or lowered brain oxygen supply, due to vasoconstriction. Moreover, in one model of migraine there is a spreading wave of activation over the cortex, involving release of higher than normal levels of the neurotransmitter glutamate. Now, a high level of glutamate under truly ischemic conditions appears to be cytotoxic—it kills the receiving cells—and hence either the hypoxia itself or glutamate toxicity could in theory cause cumulative harm. Thankfully, this theoretical harm does not actually seem to occur in migraine.

ECONOMIC BURDEN

Even reversible cognitive impairment, however, along with the nausea, vomiting, photophobia, phonophobia, and exacerbation with daily activity, can have permanent economic costs. The average migraineur loses about 4½ workdays per year due to headaches (e.g., B. S. Schwartz, Stewart, & Lipton, 1997; Steiner, Scher, Stewart, Kolodner, Liberman, & Lipton, 2003; Stewart, Lipton, Simon, Liberman, & Von Korff, 1999; Von Korff, Stewart, Simon, & Lipton, 1998), with even greater absence from household activities (Edmeads & Mackell, 2002). If we further count the partial loss of productivity from working while impaired with a headache, the total number of lost workday equivalents is approximately 11 per year (e.g., B. S. Schwartz, Stewart, & Lipton, 1997; Stewart, Lipton, Simon, Liberman, & Von Korff, 1999; Von Korff, Stewart, Simon, & Lipton, 1998). Together with the much smaller direct cost of treatment, migraines cause an estimated $10—$13 billion annual economic loss in the U.S. (Ferrari, 1998a; X. H. Hu, Markson, Lipton, Stewart, & Berger, 1999).

Nearly all of the lost worktime is accounted for by 25 percent of migraineurs, who thus carry a high disability burden (Stewart, Lipton, & Simon, 1996). And 11 percent of migraineurs do not even count in these statistics because they are unemployed (Stang, Von Korff, & Galer, 1998). Not surprisingly, then, in the United States—although not in Canada or Europe—migraines are associated with lower socioeconomic status (B. K. Rasmussen, 2001). Causality has not been proven, but the increased absenteeism and high rates of unemployment support the idea of a migraine-induced "downward drift" in standard of living. Thus, vocational, emotional, and daily functioning should be assessed clinically in migraine and kept in mind as goals during treatment.

AURA

For perhaps 15 percent of migraineurs, the headaches are preceded or, less commonly, accompanied by, an aura: a set of transient neurological impairments. Auras are most often visual, but sometimes there is a somatosensory component along with or, rarely, instead of, the visual symptoms. The classic visual aura consists of a semicircular, flickering zigzag line that starts in the center of the visual field and moves out to the periphery over a period of 10 minutes up to about an hour. In its wake it leaves a "scotoma" or blind spot (M. B. Russell, Iversen, & J. Olesen, 1994). It is called a "fortification aura" because the zigzag lines look like a schematized aerial view of fortifications.[1] However, while the fortification aura is prototypical, bright stars, white spots, flashes of light, scotomas and foggy or blurry vision may all be more common (Queiroz, Rapoport, Weeks, Sheftell, S. E. Siegel, & Baskin, 1997). These simpler auras seem to be more likely to start at the periphery (Queiroz et al.). Some investigators have reported that whether visual or somatosensory, the aura is usually unilateral, with the headache on the contralateral side (M. B. Russell, Iversen, et al.). Others have found visual auras to be more often bilateral (Queiroz et al.).

Somatosensory auras generally involve a tingling **paresthesia** and sometimes numbness (which we might call a "tactile scotoma"). The hands and mouth are most often affected, but sometimes the aura progresses over one entire side of the body. Speech problems such as dysarthria, difficulties with coordination, and weakness, may accompany a somatosensory aura (M. B. Russell, Iversen, & J. Olesen, 1994). Although the data are limited, it seems that somatosensory auras will sometimes last much longer than their visual counterparts, up to several days (M. B. Russell, Iversen, et al.). Again, the headache, when it occurs, is most often contralateral.

Note, then, that somatosensory aura may include motor and speech symptoms. In the four cases I have seen, confusion and diminished consciousness have been involved as well. This is illustrated in a case study reported by Liveing, of a 17-year-old woman: "Her sight is never disordered throughout the paroxysm, but the *right arm becomes numb*, and in consequence so useless that she will let things drop from her hand . . . But the most striking feature in this case remains to be noticed; the attack when at its height, is generally attended by a remarkable sleepiness, or stupor, sometimes so great that she is very imperfectly conscious of what is passing, and does not understand what is said to her. Sometimes, in the worst seizures,[2] this *drowsiness* is such that she is quite unable to keep awake, and sinks into a profound semi-comatose sleep; whenever this is the case she awakes worse, and the suffering is sure to be prolonged through the next day in a severe form" (Liveing, 1873, p. 14).

There is a great deal of variation between persons in their aura symptoms. Visual auras may include tunnel vision, blurred vision, or "snowy" vision (M. B. Russell, Iversen, & J. Olesen, 1994). **Vertigo**, double vision, decreased level of consciousness, and impaired hearing may also occur (B. K. Rasmussen & J. Olesen, 1992b). As always, neurological symptoms, even if they are transitory, should be evaluated medically to rule out, for example, transient ischemic attacks. Also, we should note that although somatosensory aura is by no means rare, and although the

---

[1]As most famously described by John Herschel, the 19th century British astronomer and migraineur: "[It] appeared to be a pattern in straight-lined angular forms, very much in general aspect like the drawing of a fortification, with salient and re-entering angles, bastions, and ravelins, with some suspicion of faint lines of colour between the dark lines" (cited in Latham, 1872, p. 305). As Schiller (1975) notes, however, precedent belongs to Dr. John Fothergill, whose description may likewise have been informed by his own migraines: "it begins with a singular kind of glimmering in the sight; objects swiftly changing their apparent position, surrounded with luminous angles, like those of a fortification" (Fothergill, 1784, p. 120).

[2]Liveing regarded migraine as an analogue of epilepsy.

vast majority of headaches are benign, a history of dizziness or lack of coordination, and history of subjective numbness or tingling, may increase the probability of detecting a significant abnormality on neuroimaging (C. S. Mitchell, Osborn, & Grosskreutz, 1993).

Regardless of their exact appearance, visual auras often flicker, shimmer, or scintillate (Crotogino, Feindel, & F. Wilkinson, 2001). For any given person the scintillation rate is relatively constant, but it varies widely between people. Average flicker frequencies of 9 Hz up to 37 Hz have been documented, and the rates for a few auras may be even more extreme (Crotogino et al.). We will encounter theoretical explanations for both the aura and its scintillation later in the chapter.

From the nomenclature we might assume that migraine with and without aura are two different manifestations of the same disorder. In support of this, the headache phase is described in similar terms, and the response to prophylactic and abortive medications is mostly the same, regardless of whether an aura is present (Blau, 1995; B. K. Rasmussen & J. Olesen, 1992b). Moreover, in individuals who can be diagnosed as having migraine with aura, many of the migraine episodes in fact do not seem to be preceded by an aura (Blau, 1995). On the other hand, the two diagnoses have different sex ratios (the female preponderance is higher in migraine without aura), a different relationship to female sex hormones (migraine without aura is more likely to improve during pregnancy) and, as we will see, different results on imaging of regional cerebral blood flow. Moreover, it appears from population studies that the two diagnoses are no more likely to co-occur in the same person than would be expected by chance (B. K. Rasmussen & J. Olesen, 1992b).

Other data is sometimes cited as well. Thus, M. D. Ferrari et al., comparing individuals between and within migraine attacks, found that platelet serotonin content dropped during episodes of migraine without aura, but not during migraine with aura (M. D. Ferrari, Odink, Tapparelli, Van Kempen, Pennings, & Bruyn, 1989). However, this was a relatively small study containing several within-subject contrasts; a replication would be helpful before drawing firm conclusions from it.

Perhaps the most reasonable formulation at this point is that the two forms of migraine share a final common pathway involving the headache state (B. K. Rasmussen, 1995b). In the next section, we will examine what this pathway might be.

ASPECTS OF MIGRAINE PHYSIOLOGY

Thus, migaine is an intrusive and often debilitating disorder in which the cardinal symptom, pain, is embedded in a constellation of associated symptoms including, in a minority of cases, complex neurological impairments. These symptoms, of course, call out for explanation.

The Vascular Model

In this classic model, proposed by Johann Anhalt in the eighteenth century, clarified by Peter Latham in the nineteenth and given an experimental foundation by Harold Wolff in the twentieth century, migraines were attributed to vasomotor instability (Latham, 1872; Schiller, 1975; Wolff, 1963). To Anhalt, the cranial blood vessels "dilate or contract in such a way as to excite pain" (Anhalt, 1724, cited in Schiller, 1975, p. 10). For Latham, the migraine diathesis was a weakness in the central nervous system, such that it did not properly regulate the sympathetic nerves. Then, under stress or excitement, the sympathetic nerves over-fired, constricting the intracerebral arteries, and causing an aura through the resulting ischemia. Such intense firing was thought to exhaust the sympathetic nerves, leading to the arterial distention and throbbing pain of migraine (Latham, 1872).

But the vascular model has run into problems. First, the timing between headache and vasodilation has not been in accordance with theory: The headaches may begin during the vasoconstrictive phase, and end while vasodilation is still taking place (Olesen, 1990). Second, the reduction of cerebral blood flow during the vasoconstrictive phase is approximately 20–35 percent, not enough to produce true ischemia, except perhaps in isolated pockets (Lauritzen, 1994; Skyhoj, Friberg, & Lassen, 1987). Third, ischemia does not seem to account well for the intricate, evolving visual experience of the aura. In other conditions in which blood flow to the brain is decreased (e.g., a transient ischemic attack or a vasovagal reaction[3]) the typical experience, such as faintness, is much simpler (Sacks, 1992).

And there is much more going on in migraines than simple vasoconstriction and dilation. To see this, we will turn to the neurogenic model.

The Neurogenic Model

Trigeminovascular response.   Sensory nerves, of course, convey information from the periphery to the central nervous system. But recall from Chapter 2 that when a C fiber transduces a noxious stimulus, its nerve endings also release neuropeptides at the *distal* end, the site of presumed injury. This seems to be particularly important in migraine. Thus Moskowitz (1984), in an extensive program of animal studies, noted release of vasoactive peptides around cephalic arteries by sensory neurons originating in the trigeminal ganglion. The peptides, particularly substance P and **calcitonin gene-related peptide**, seem to set up a sterile inflammation, local vasodilation, and presumably a pain sensitization. Thus, the key vascular event, vasodilation, may be secondary to neural events. And it is not simply the mechanical stretching of the blood vessel that is painful. The blood vessel has also been inflamed by the nerves that surround it. In essence, the brain creates its own migraine.

Moskowitz' general model of sterile inflammation has been persuasive, but which substance is responsible for neurogenic inflammation in people has been open to debate. The strongest evidence is for calcitonin gene-related peptide, or CGRP. The level of CGRP in jugular venous blood seems to be increased during episodes of migraine with or without aura (Goadsby, Edvinsson, & Ekman, 1990). These levels are normalized following treatment with sumatriptan, a medication which is effective in ending migraine attacks (Goadsby & Edvinsson, 1993). A caveat is that the jugular vein appears to draw only from the extracranial circulation. Thus, we would also have to postulate a disruption in the **blood-brain barrier** during migraines. There is some evidence that such a disruption in fact takes place (Goadsby, 1997a; M. Smith, Cros, & Sheen, 2002).

Meanwhile, Ashina et al. have reported evidence that levels of CGRP in systemic circulation are higher **interictally** in migraineurs, at least those without aura, compared with healthy control subjects (Ashina, Bendtsen, R. Jensen, Schifter, & J. Olesen, 2000). Elevated baseline CGRP activity might be a risk factor for migraines.

Still, other substances have been proposed, in particular **nitric oxide** (Thomsen & Olesen, 1998). Nitric oxide is a reasonable candidate because it is involved in vasodilation, inflammation, and central pain transmission (Thomsen & Olesen, 1998). A byproduct, peroxynitrite, might alter platelet function by causing subtle structural damage (Taffi et al., 2005). The bioavailability of nitric oxide appears to be increased by estrogen (Geary, Krause, & Duckles, 1998; Sarchielli

---

[3]A vasovagal reaction, or neurocardiogenic syncope, is a brief loss of consciousness when strong emotions, prolonged standing, or exercise on a hot day cause heart rate and blood pressure to drop (R. Freeman & Rutkove, 2000; Grubb, 2005). Fainting at the sight of blood is an example.

et al., 1996), which could help explain the higher frequency of migraines in women, especially perimenstrually (see Chapters 8, 10, and 14 for further discussion of hormonal factors).

Neural instability.   Now, if the brain does create its own migraines, why does it do so? In one model, migraines are preceded by a spreading wave of cortical activation that leaves a cortical depression (reduction in firing rates) in its wake. The cortical depression is accompanied by **oligemia**; when nerve cells are not firing, they do not need as much blood. It is these cortical changes, it is thought, that provoke a migraine.

Spreading cortical depression was discovered accidentally by Leão, during an attempt to create an animal model of epilepsy (Leão, 1944). In the prototypical experiment, a potassium solution is applied to a small area of the animal's exposed brain. The spreading depression can then be observed as a region of reduced blood flow propagating in a band along the cortex, at about 3 millimeters per minute. Note that the oligemia does not follow vascular or neural tracts, but extends by geographic contiguity from one neuron to its neighbors. This may represent a chain reaction: The potassium ions cause large-scale depolarization of the underlying neurons, which thus release more potassium, causing nearby neurons to depolarize as well (Bureš, Burešová, & Křivánek, 1974). The critical concentration seems to be around 10–12 millimoles of potassium (McLachlan & Girvin, 1994). Now, in theory any condition that causes a group of contiguous neurons to depolarize could set this process in motion. If this occurs, the release of glutamate into the intercellular medium might also be involved in the propagation (Welch & Ramadan, 1995), although the role of glutamate appears secondary (Bureš et al.).

Now the relevance of cortical spreading depression to human beings was quite unclear. It turns out, however, that physiological psychologist Karl Lashley had migraines. And, apparently unknown to Leão, three years earlier he had been mapping the scintillations and scotomas of his own auras. From them, he concluded that "a wave of intense excitation is propagated at a rate of about 3 mm. per minute across the visual cortex. This wave is followed by complete inhibition of activity, with recovery progressing at the same rate" (Lashley, 1941, p. 419). Of course Lashley's inferences and Leão's results sound like the same phenomenon, and in 1958, Milner earned a permanent place in the migraine literature by publishing a 1-page article that pointed this out (Milner, 1958).

What would cause cortical spreading depression in migraine? Perhaps the initial wave of activation starts when neurons in a region over-fire, releasing enough potassium and glutamate to kindle nearby neurons, which then also fire, in a chain reaction.

Spreading activation/depression seems to be a good explanation for the migraine aura. As Lashley surmised, the complex visual experiences (for example, fortification auras) may be the result of the initial wave of activation. As the wave propagates over the visual cortex, the aura moves gradually from the center of the visual field out to the periphery. Negative experiences such as scotomas may be the result of the subsequent cortical depression, following behind the wave of activation. In fact, the spreading depression model may explain why auras are often visual: Potassium ions are cleared by glial cells, and the visual cortex has the lowest ratio of glial cells to neurons (Ferrari, 1998b).[4]

---

[4]The reason that auras tend to shimmer has not been definitively established. One theory traces the shimmer to the likelihood that different columns of cells in the visual cortex encode different temporal frequencies, just as they encode different sizes or, more exactly, spatial frequencies. As the wave of activation spreads into a region of cortex, the visual image would flicker in accord with the temporal frequencies encoded by the now-activated cells. An alternative theory attributes the shimmer to lateral inhibitory connections between columns of cells. These connections produce a dynamic system that presumably is set to oscillating as the wave of activation spreads into the region (Crotogino, Feindel, & Wilkinson, 2001).

The evidence for spreading depression in humans has been indirect. There have actually been attempts to produce the depression, for example during brain surgery for epilepsy, but the attempts have been unsuccessful (McLachlan & Girvin, 1994). It may be relevant that the subjects have either been non-migraineurs, or people who have migraines without aura (Goadsby, 1995). Moreover, the subjects were undergoing brain surgery for intractable epilepsy, and repeated seizures may protect against spreading depression (Parsons, 1998), as perhaps did the anesthesia used in surgery (Somjen, 2001). On the other hand, the human brain has a lower density of unmyelinated neurons than the animal brains that have been used as models, is more convoluted, and, in general, the higher the phylogenetic standing of a species, the less susceptible it is to spreading depression (McLachlan & Girvin, 1994). Still, there is indirect evidence for spreading depression in people, in the form of xenon blood flow, SPECT, functional MRI, and possibly PET scan studies suggesting a region of oligemia[5] that spreads across the posterior cortex by geographic contiguity (Cutrer, O'Donnell, & del Rio, 2000; Welch, 1997). This evidence has been strongest for migraine with aura. However, there is a little support for spreading depression, presumably asymptomatic, in migraine without aura (Welch, 1997).

We can now describe one version of the neurogenic model. There is an initial wave of activation, followed by depression across a region of the cortex. The brain registers this state as abnormal, and institutes the migraine as a defensive reaction. More exactly, the high potassium levels in the meninges during spreading depression might be enough to depolarize the C fibers, initiating the neurogenic inflammation (Moskowitz & Macfarlane, 1993). The vasodilation and **extravasation** (leakage of plasma proteins out of the blood vessels) in migraine may serve to dilute and restrict the diffusion of potassium, or other internally-produced or exogenous toxins (Moskowitz, 1984).

It turns out, however, that the link between spreading depression and trigeminovascular activation is as yet unverified. Recently Ebersberger et al. produced spreading depression in anesthetized rats every twenty minutes for three hours. Despite this, they found no evidence of plasma extravasation, release of calcitonin gene-related peptide or prostaglandin E_2, or sensitization of neurons in the trigeminal nucleus caudalis (Ebersberger, Schaible, Averbeck, & Richter, 2001).

In any event, spreading activation suggests that in addition to vascular instability, there is neural instability. In fact, EEG differences have been noted between migraineurs, assessed between migraine episodes, and healthy controls. These include increased amplitudes of visual evoked potentials (e.g., Connolly, Gawel, & Clifford, 1982) and decreased habituation of visual, auditory, novelty, and reaction-time task evoked potentials (Schoenen, 1996a; W. Wang, Timsit-Berthier, & Schoenen, 1996). Discussing his own research, Schoenen notes that "a lack of habituation was found in every study in migraineurs with or without aura between attacks when compared to healthy controls" (Schoenen, 1996a, p. 73). Behaviorally, migraineurs show greater aversion to high contrast visual gratings (Marcus & Soso, 1989), and report greater sensitivity to environmental light stimuli (Hay, Mortimer, Barker, et al., 1994), and lower discomfort thresholds for intense visual and auditory stimuli (Main, Dowson, & M. Gross, 1997), even between migraine attacks, than do healthy control subjects. Migraineurs also show increased visual **masking**, thought to be an indirect measure of cortical excitability (McColl & Wilkinson, 2000). And Wray et al. found that

---

[5]Oligemia is a reduction in blood flow to a region. Not until the reduction becomes severe enough to threaten cell viability (for brain tissue, blood flow that is 50–60 percent below normal) does the term "ischemia" apply (Baron, 2001; Koenig, Kraus, Theek, Klotz, Gehlen, & Heuser, 2001). In the oligemia preceding migraine, blood flow seems to be 20–35 percent below normal (Cutrer, O'Donnell, & del Rio, 2000).

migraineurs, assessed between migraine episodes, were faster at simple visual tasks, such as detecting the orientation of lines, than were matched control subjects (Wray, Mijovic-Prelec, & Kosslyn, 1995). Possibly, the stronger evoked potential response may have some adaptive value.[6] (However, a failure to replicate this result has also been reported; Palmer & Chronicle, 1998.)

What causes the neural instability? Montagna and coworkers used **magnetic resonance spectroscopy** to examine the proportion of high-energy compounds (such as ATP) in the brain. They report evidence that this proportion is lower in the brains of migraineurs (e.g., Montagna, Cortelli, Monari, et al., 1994; Watanabe, Kuwabara, Ohkubo, Tsuji, & Yuasa, 1996). That is, people with migraines might have an unfavorable brain energy balance.

This idea might explain stronger and more persistent optical illusions in migraineurs. For example, if a person stares for a long time at a display of dots that drift slowly to the right, later stationary dots will seem to drift slowly to the left. This "waterfall illusion" lasts longer in migraineurs (Shepherd, 2001). Although there are several possible explanations, it is reasonable to presume that cells detecting rightward motion are fatigued by the first display, and that this fatigue lasts longer in people with migraines (Shepherd, 2001).

A similar depletion of high energy phosphates has been found in the muscles and platelets of migraineurs (Lodi et al., 1997; Sangiorgi et al., 1994), leading to speculation that a **mitochondrial**[7] dysfunction is causal (Montagna, Cortelli, Pierangeli, et al., 1994). On a practical level, this has led to the theory that coenzyme Q10 or high doses of riboflavin, used in energy production, might protect against migraines. In fact, there has been some support for the use of both (Rozen, Oshinsky, et al., 2002; Sándor, Di Clemente et al., 2005; Schoenen, Jacquy, & Lenaerts, 1998). We will discuss this evidence further in Chapter 11.

Still, in most cases, no specific mitochondrial dysfunction has been identified (Klopstock, May, Seibel, Papagiannuli, Diener, & Reichmann, 1996). Conversely, in most cases of known mitochondrial dysfunction, migraine is not the only (Sparaco, Feleppa, Lipton, Rapoport, & Bigal, 2006) or even primary clinical feature (Schoenen, 1996a). In fact, migraines do not resemble the types of diseases that have been traced to mutations in mitochondrial DNA. These diseases typically cause symptoms involving the heart, skeletal muscle, and other parts of the body that use high amounts of energy (Wallace, 1999). Symptoms often appear later in life, when mitochondrial function has begun to decline, or else are progressive over the lifespan (Wallace, 1999). In contrast, migraines generally appear early in life, may remit for long periods of time, and generally become less severe with advanced age.

On the other hand, in migraine, mutated mitochondria might occur in low concentration, or in only a few brain regions (Sparaco, Feleppa, Lipton, Rapoport, & Bigal, 2006). Or migraines may involve a different type of mitochondrial defect. Thus, Pavese et al. have found large increases

---

[6]An evolutionary advantage of migraines, or of possible associated processes (sensitivity to stimulation, avoidance of novelty, physiological defense against toxins or hypoxia) has been an object of speculation (Loder, 2002c). An alternative theory draws on the fact that migraines, in contrast to other pain conditions, have no parallel in animals. Thus, migraines might somehow be a price of our greater capacity for information processing (Loder, 2002c).

[7]Mitochondria are the parts of cells in which glucose is used to make high-energy compounds for powering the cell's chemical reactions. More formally, mitochondria are the organelles in which oxidative respiration takes place. The cells of all organisms more complicated than bacteria and blue-green algae have mitochondria. Mitochondria are unusual in that they have their own DNA, separate from the cell's chromosomes. This has led to the evolutionary theory that, in the unfathomable past, mitochondria were separate organisms, living symbiotically within cells (Wallace, 1999). And because mitochondria have their own DNA, they can give rise to their own types of genetic diseases, involving problems with the production of energy in cells (N. Lane, 2005; Wallace, 1999).

in the density of a particular type of receptor on the mitochondrial membranes of migraineurs (without aura) vs. nonmigraineurs. Presumably, the receptors play a role in how mitochondrial function is regulated (Pavese, et al., 2000).

By whatever means it is generated, an unfavorable energy balance can presumably lead to neural instability because the normal resting state of neurons is maintained through active ion transport (Welch & Ramadan, 1995). When the cells lack energy for active transport, a net leakage of ions across the membrane can cause spontaneous firing.

Another source of neural instability has been proposed: subtle variations in the structure of certain nerve cell calcium channels. This theory derives from the study of familial hemiplegic migraine, or FHM. FHM is a rare disorder in which the headaches are associated with reversible mild-to-moderate hemiparesis (weakness on one side of the body), hemisensory loss, and often by dysarthria, aphasia, confusion, and visual symptoms. Its relation to other forms of migraine is uncertain. It may co-occur with normal migraines in the same patient or family, and may evolve into normal migraine as an individual matures (Haan, Terwindt, & M. D. Ferrari, 1997). It differs from normal migraine, however, in having a clear pattern of **autosomal dominant** inheritance, which makes it easier to study genetically. In fact, probable gene sites on chromosomes 1 and 19 have been reported for FHM, and the gene sites, in turn, imply an alteration in 2 subunits of the P/Q calcium channel (Ophoff, Terwindt, Vergouwe, van Eijk, et al., 1996; Gardner, Barmada, Ptacek, & Hoffman, 1997). These channels are widespread in the brain and are found both presynaptically, where they control neurotransmitter release (e.g., serotonin; Codignola, Tarroni, Clementi, et al., 1993), and at somatodendritic sites. The subunits are important for the voltage sensitivity, calcium ion selectivity, and permeability of the channels. Which of these mechanisms, if any, leads to increased excitability of the cortex has not yet been identified. Depending on the exact mutation, there may be either an increase or decrease in the current flow through the channels, and either an increase or a decrease in the number of channels per unit area (Hans, et al., 1999). Thus, the altered calcium channel might affect excitability directly, or it might work by changing the balance of neurotransmitters, for example by inhibiting serotonin release (Hans, et al.). Regardless of the exact mechanism, however, the "**channelopathy**" may be a genetic predisposition to neural instability.

Needless to say, there is great interest in determining whether a variation in calcium channels is participating in more common forms of migraine. Circumstantial evidence has been reported by Ophoff et al. They found that siblings who are alike in having migraines also tend to be alike in the chromosome region that contains one of the calcium channel genes (Ophoff, Terwindt, Vergouwe, Frants, & M. D. Ferrari, 1997). Another approach was taken by Ambrosini and colleagues. Noting that P/Q channels are found on the neural side of the **neuromuscular junction**, they studied the efficiency of the junction in migraine. In essence, they stimulated a motor axon electrically, and then examined the effect downstream on a single muscle fiber, looking for either an occasional failure of transmission across the neuromuscular junction, or abnormally slowed transmission. In fact, Ambrosini and coworkers indeed found a greater number of abnormalities in their migraineurs than in healthy control subjects. However, the abnormalities were few, subtle, and mostly affected migraineurs who had prolonged aura, and/or who had unusual aura symptoms such as motor, language, or balance problems.[8] In essence, the more closely a migraine resembled FHM, the more likely it was that subtle difficulties at the neuromuscular junction would be found (Ambrosini, de Noordhout, & Schoenen, 2001). Lipton has remarked, and we

---

[8]Certainly these symptoms can occur as part of an aura, for example in basilar artery migraine. However, they are rare, and if present they may warrant further investigation for cerebrovascular disease.

will remember here, that migraine is likely to be a heterogenous disorder, with a variety of etiologies (Lipton, 2000).[9]

The case for neural instability is a bit stronger in a second, rarer type of familiar hemiplegic migraine. Here, the mutation affects an enzyme ("sodium, potassium-ATPase") that maintains the neuron's resting state by moving sodium ions out of the cell and potassium ions in (De Fusco et al., 2003; Vanmolkot et al., 2003). If this enzyme works less effectively, the cell would be at risk for firing spontaneously. Moreover, this same enzyme is used for clearing glutamate out of the synaptic cleft, so the mutation might also prolong excitatory neurotransmission (Sparaco, Feleppa, Lipton, Rapoport, & Bigal, 2006).

A magnesium deficiency has been suggested as a risk factor for migraine, and clinical benefit has sometimes been found for magnesium supplementation (Peikert, Wilimzig, & Köhne-Volland, 1996). Magnesium deficiency is manifested in part by an increase in neuronal excitability (Mazzotta, Sarchielli, Alberti, & Gallai, 1999). The exact mechanism is not known. However, a magnesium deficiency could lead to neural instability in several ways. Magnesium may compete with calcium for access to ion channels (Ophoff et al., 1997). Magnesium appears to inhibit certain types of cortical spreading activation (Bureš, Burešová, Křivánek, 1974; Welch & Ramadan, 1995). And, as a cofactor for enzymes used in phosphorylation, magnesium is essential in maintaining energy supplies (Welch & Ramadan, 1995). We should note, too, that a magnesium deficiency can also lead to an instability of vascular tone (B. M. Altura & B. T. Altura, 1978; Farago, Szabo, Dora, Horvath, & Kovach, 1991).

Migraines and the Brain Stem. Not all theories of migraine treat events in the cerebral cortex as primary. For it appears that the trigeminovascular response is not a simple reaction by C fibers and the trigeminal nucleus caudalis, but a coordinated action by several brain stem nuclei. In particular, the periaqueductal gray region of the midbrain seems to be involved. Now, in Chapter 2 we stated that the periaqueductal gray region is involved in the *inhibition* of pain signals, and this indeed appears to be the case. As a result, implantable electrical stimulation of the periaqueductal gray region was studied as an intervention for pain control in the late 1970's and early 1980's. Raskin and coworkers note that while the procedure was often successful, 15 of 175 patients developed intense, continuous headaches lasting for two months to five years before remitting. The headaches were generally accompanied by nausea and vomiting, and sometimes by prominent visual symptoms such as wavy or zigzag lines, flashes of light or scotomas. Now, the visual symptoms had an abrupt onset and offset; they did not evolve or march like a true migraine aura. The similarity to migraines was nonetheless striking. Moreover, the headaches usually responded to a medication used for migraine treatment, dihydroergotamine (Raskin, Hosobuchi, & Lamb, 1987).

Thus, a portion of the periaqueductal gray region, slightly dorsolateral to the **dorsal raphe nucleus**, was proposed as a "**migraine generator**". Then, a few years later, Weiller, et al. published MRI scans showing activation in roughly the same region, in the area of the dorsal raphe nucleus and **locus coeruleus** in the midbrain, throughout spontaneous migraine attacks (Weiller et al., 1995). These structures are involved not only in the control of pain, but also intracerebral

---

[9]The gene for familial hemiplegic migraine is thought to play a role in other disorders as well, such as a form of ataxia, Episodic Ataxia Type 2. The ataxia resembles migraines in a key feature: It is paroxysmal rather than continuous. It appears that the exact nature of the mutation determines whether a patient manifests familial hemiplegic migraine or episodic ataxia (Berkovic, 2000). That is, if the mutation causes a drastic compromise of the ion channel, the result seems to be episodic ataxia type 2 (Ophoff et al., 1997). Similar genes are being studied as possible factors in idiopathic generalized epilepsy (Chioza et al., 2001).

and dural blood flow. In animal studies, the region appears to be linked to α adrenoreceptors (Goadsby, 1997a). Neurons in the dorsal raphe nucleus project to the trigeminal nucleus (Y. Q. Li, Takada, Matsuzaki, Shinonaga, & Mizuno, 1993).

Other nearby nuclei have been suspected of having a role in migraine pathogenesis. Gerber and Schoenen (1998) have suggested that a stronger orienting response on EEG evoked potential testing (contingent negative variation, discussed in the next chapter) implicates the locus coeruleus. And given the prominence of gastrointestinal symptoms in migraine, it is not surprising that the trigeminal system projects to the solitary tract nucleus, which receives sensory input from the viscera and is involved in nausea and vomiting (Hargreaves & Shepheard, 1999).

There is another, less direct piece of evidence that the dorsal raphe and locus coeruleus nuclei region is involved in migraines. **Transcranial Doppler** ultrasound can be used to measure the velocity of blood flowing through large vessels in the brain, such as the middle cerebral artery. Now, ordinarily when we do this, we measure velocity over a period of time, and then reduce the data to a single number, the mean velocity or an equivalent. Because, all else being equal, velocity has to increase when an artery narrows, the mean velocity can tell us the degree of vasoconstriction or vasodilation. If instead of looking at the mean velocity, however, we look at the variability, we find that it is not entirely random. A **Fourier analysis** of the data reveals that the variability is especially pronounced at 1 cycle per minute, due to an oscillation in vessel diameter called the "B wave." Now, B waves seem to be under neural control, with the neurons in question projecting from the area of the dorsal raphe and locus coeruleus nuclei. Thus, we should not be surprised to learn that B waves seem to have higher amplitudes in migraineurs, measured **interictally**, than in nonheadache controls or people with tension-type headache (Sliwka, Harscher, Diehl, van Schayck, Niesen, & Weiller, 2001; Thie, Carvajal-Lizano, Schlichting, K. Spitzer, & Kunze, 1992). Note that the measurement of B waves may be a straightforward and noninvasive way to track the effects of pharmacological and perhaps behavioral interventions on activity in the region of the "migraine generator."

Still, the specificity of midbrain activation to migraine has been questioned (Fumal, Laureys, Di Clemente, Boly, Bohotin, Vandenheede, et al., 2006). The periaqueductal gray shows increased blood flow in non-migraineurs when capsaicin is applied to the leg (Zambreanu, R. G. Wise, Brooks, Iannetti, & Tracey, 2005). And structures just lateral to the periaqueductal gray—the cuneiform nucleus and the upper part of the red nucleus—are activated by capsaicin-pain as well (Iadarola, Berman, Zeffiro, Byas-Smith, Gracely, Max, et al., 1998). Thus, the "migraine generator" may simply be a portion of the neural network for pain in general.

THE VASCULAR MODEL REVIVED

Thus, it appears that the vasodilation in migraine is not due to exhaustion of the sympathetic nerves, as Anhalt and Latham thought, but to the direct action of sensory nerves—C fibers—in producing neurogenic inflammation. And the complex symptoms of aura do not seem attributable to vasoconstriction, but to neural instability, from an unfavorable energy balance, aberrant calcium channels, or a magnesium deficiency, leading to a wave of spreading activation.

Yet the vascular model is not without evidence. Vasocontriction seems important, at least, therapeutically. From the trigeminovascular response, in which the cranial arteries become inflamed and dilated, it is not surprising that between one-half and two-thirds of migraine patients report pain reduction from simply compressing the common carotid arteries in the neck (Brunton, 1886; Goadsby, 1997a; Graham & Wolff, 1938; do *not* try this). The serotonergic abortive migraine medications such as sumatriptan and ergotamine, also effect a vasoconstriction, particularly of the middle cerebral artery (Hatch, 1993; Thomaides, Karagounakis, Spantideas, & Kate-

lanis, 2003). And in fact, medications that block neurogenic inflammation are completely ineffective against migraines, unless the medications are also vasoconstrictive (May, Gijsman, Wallnöfer, R. Jones, Diener, & Ferrari, 1996).

In addition, vascular anomalies are not uncommon in migraine. Modern studies of cerebral
blood flow suggest regional asymmetries, large oscillations, patchy decrements, and over-respon-
siveness to 5 percent carbon dioxide and 100 percent oxygen inhalation (Friberg, 1996; Welch
& Ramadan, 1995). The evidence is primarily for **oligemia**, but localized areas of true ischemia
cannot be ruled out (e.g., Skyhoj, Friberg, & Lassen, 1987). In fact on MRI scans, between 10 and
45 percent of migraineurs show very mild white matter abnormalities (Rocca, Colombo, Inglese,
Codella, Comi, & Filippi, 2003). The lesions are subtle, but seem explicable as a reaction by
glial cells to modest levels of ischemia (Rocca, Colombo, Pratesi, Comi, & Filippi, 2000). Moreover, 5.4 percent of migraineurs, but only 0.7 percent of control subjects, have small, cerebellar
infarcts (Kruit, et al., 2004). These infarcts—miniature ischemic strokes—do not seem to have
clinical consequences, but are a sign of disrupted blood supply. And we cannot exclude that
even a highly localized ischemia might be enough to trigger a migraine.

Similarly, the comorbidity between migraines and Raynaud's disease (e.g., Smyth, Hughes,
Bruce, & Bell, 1999; Stang, Sternfeld, & Sidney, 1996) implies a vasomotor component. Recall
that in Raynaud's, vasospasms in the hands can cause numbness, pain and even tissue damage.
Smyth et al. found that 33 percent of their sample of Raynaud's disease patients, but only 7 percent of matched controls, had migraines ($p < .0001$). Moreover, Raynaud's patients who also had
a family history of Raynaud's were more likely to have migraines (47 percent) than those without a family history of Raynaud's (21 percent; $p < .02$).

And migraineurs seem to have higher levels of **endothelin**–1 in their plasma between
migraine episodes (Gallai, Sarchielli, Firenze, et al., 1994). Endothelin–1 is a **peptide** with strong
vascular effects, in which an initial vasodilation (mediated by the endothelin B receptor) is followed by vasoconstriction (mediated by the endothelin A receptor; Tzourio, El Amrani, Poirier,
Nicaud, Bousser, & Alpérovitch, 2001). There is some disagreement about what happens to the
levels during a migraine episode, but the largest study to date suggests that endothelin levels rise
still further, at least early in the attack (Gallai, Sarchielli, Firenze, et al.). Furthermore, the gene
which, so far, has the strongest evidence of being a risk factor for typical migraines, is associated with the vasoconstrictive, endothelin A receptor (Tzourio, et al.).

Similarly, the activity of angiotensin-converting enzyme (ACE), and a particular **gene polymorphism** encoding this enzyme, are both elevated in migraine without aura, as they are in cardiovascular disease. Moreover, migraineurs with the gene polymorphism have more frequent
migraines than those without the polymorphism (Paterna, et al., 2000). Angiotensin-converting
enzyme produces a chemical, angiotensin, that is directly and indirectly vasoconstrictive (E. K.
Jackson, 2001). Bianchi, et al. note numerous other vascular compounds whose concentrations
seem to be different in migraineurs than in matched non-migraine controls (Bianchi, et al., 1996).
And as we will see in Chapter 11, four different classes of blood pressure medications (**beta-
blockers**, **calcium channel antagonists**, **ACE inhibitors**, and angiotensin receptor blockers)
have shown at least modest efficacy in preventing migraines. Drugs of the last three classes in particular can modulate stress-induced vasoconstriction.

Yet for all this, the vascular model is by no means well established. Note, for example, that
the research on endothelin is still in its early stages. Thus, we do not know whether endothelin
plasma levels are a good measure of its vasoactivity. And we do not know what the endothelin
A gene polymorphism actually does, except that it is not in a region coding for the structure of the
receptor (Tzourio, El Amrani, Poirier, Nicaud, Bousser, & Alpérovitch, 2001). But the same is

true of the neural model. As we have seen, cortical spreading depression may not elicit trigemi-novascular activation.

CONNECTIONS BETWEEN NEURAL AND VASCULAR MODELS

Still, the vast majority of data seem to support the neural model of migraines. Yet the neural model need not exclude a role for factors such as vasoconstriction. Blau (1992) notes that migraines can be triggered by conditions that, in higher amounts, would be damaging to the brain: alcohol, hypoglycemia, and hypoxia. Moreover, there is now a fair amount of data connecting migraine with aura to a type of cardiac defect (Sztajzel, Genoud, S. Roth, Mermillod, & Le Floch-Rohr, 2002). The defect, called a "patent foramen ovale," is a small, congenital shunt that allows blood to pass from the right to the left atrium of the heart, bypassing the lungs. It is found in about 18 percent of people who do not have migraine, 23 percent of people who have migraine with-out aura, and 45 percent of people who have migraine with aura (Anzola, Magoni, Guindani, Rozzini, & Dalla Volta, 1999; Del Sette et al., 1998). If the shunt is closed surgically (e.g., because it is unusually large and thus a risk factor for stroke), migraine with aura tends to resolve or at least drastically improve; for unknown reasons, migraine without aura improves only minimally (Morandi, Anzola, Angeli, Melzi, & Onorato, 2003; Wilmshurst, Nightingale, K. P. Walsh, & W. L. Morrison, 2000). Ordinarily, microscopic clots in the bloodstream lyse without conse-quence when the blood passes through the lungs (Meier & Lock, 2003). A congenital shunt allows these embolisms to bypass the lungs and travel to the brain (Wilmshurst et al.), causing or threatening to cause small occlusions.

Vasoconstriction may be a similar type of trigger. Even small regions of ischemia might be enough to elicit a migraine as a defensive reaction. Indeed, a key role of the trigeminovascular system may be to prevent ischemia, with CGRP-mediated vasodilation serving to terminate excessive vasoconstriction (Edvinsson, I. J. Olesen, Kingman, McCulloch, & Uddman, 1995; McCulloch, Uddman, Kingman, & Edvinsson, 1986). This hypothesis resembles the "rebound vasodilation" of the older vascular model, but with a much more sophisticated understanding of how the vasodilation comes about.

We cannot exclude, too, that ischemia might trigger spreading activation/depression, (Friberg, 1996). An energy deficit seems to cause the release of potassium ions from glial cells (which depolarize) and neurons (which hyperpolarize; Müller & Somjen, 2000). Eventually potassium concentration in the intercellular medium might reach threshold for triggering a spreading acti-vation/depression. Not surprisingly, then, there is good evidence that severe ischemia, such as at the periphery of an infarct, does indeed cause a spreading activation/depression (e.g., Aitken, Tombaugh, D. A. Turner, & Somjen, 1998; Parsons, 1998). For spreading depression may be not simply an effect of ischemia, but a defensive shut-down of activity in preparation for threatened hypoxia (Horiguchi, Snipes, Kis, Shimizu, & Busija, 2005; Yanamoto, Hashimoto, Nagata, & Kikuchi, 1998). However, it is unclear whether all of this is relevant to the much smaller shifts in perfusion that might precede a migraine.

Aside from the question of ischemia, Dreier and colleagues point out that intracarotid injec-tion of a dye (for cerebral angiography) or Xenon–133 (for brain perfusion studies) can trigger migraine auras in susceptible people. This implies that irritation of the blood vessel lining (endothelium) is enough to trigger a cortical spreading depression. Moreover, Dreier et al. present evidence that endothelin–1, the vasoconstrictor, is a robust trigger of cortical spreading depres-sion, at least in the intact rat brain (Dreier, et al., 2002). Now, endothelin–1 was not effective when applied to brain slices, even though potassium was effective. The fact that endothelin–1 produced spreading depression only in the intact brain suggests that its vascular effects were a crucial part of the process (Dreier et al.). Thus, cortical spreading depression, the most neurogenic of all migraine features, seems to have a vascular trigger.

An integrated model.   Schoenen (1996a) and W. Wang, Timsit-Berthier, & Schoenen (1996) speculate that the EEG differences in migraineurs reflect a deficiency in serotonergic modulation of cortical activation. The serotonergic system is thus thought to regulate cortical tone or readiness. The deficient inhibition could then lead to cortical overactivation and a depletion of energy resources. We might add that chronic intermittent vasoconstriction could perhaps further set the stage for this energy depletion. The depletion would lead to neural instability, and eventually a wave of cortical activation followed by spreading depression. Finally, a compensatory trigeminovascular activation would serve as an "emergency response." In this model, the greater sensitivity to stimuli in migraineurs is at the cost of a lower stimulus tolerance. The migraine episode itself would then be homeostatic: Stimuli are avoided, the blood supply to the cortex is increased through vasodilation, and the energy balance is restored.[10]

Note that the essence of the migraine experience is in the last step of the model, the trigeminovascular response. This response, however, is likely to be the nociceptive-defensive ("nocifensive") reaction of the brain to a variety of provocations. Cluster headaches, some posttraumatic headaches, and headaches associated with meningitis can all have migrainous qualities. Migraine symptoms may thus be a "final common pathway" for a number of conditions, and not only for brain energy depletion. Again, migraine is most likely "a clinically and biologically heterogenous disorder" (Lipton, 2000, p. 280).

THE PLATELET THEORY OF MIGRAINE

Another hypothesis about the etiology of migraine has received a degree of empirical support. There is some indication that blood platelets store unusually large amounts of serotonin before a migraine, and release these stores during the migraine. Serotonin is vasoconstrictive,[11] and sensitizes pain receptors. Hence, platelet release of serotonin in the brain might cause local hypoxia and pain, setting up an episode of migraine (Gawel, Burkitt, & F. C. Rose, 1979; Hanington, Jones, Amess, & Wachowicz, 1981). Moreover, the platelets of migraineurs seem to be more likely to aggregate than the platelets of non-migraineurs (Kovacs, Herman, Filep, Jelencsik, Magyar, & Csanda, 1990), apparently due to differences in platelet metabolism. Platelets synthesize vasoconstrictive and aggregatory compounds, such as thromboxane A_2, as well as compounds that have the opposite effect: vasodilators and anti-aggregatory chemicals such as prostacyclin and prostaglandin D_2. There is evidence that in migraineurs, the platelets produce lower levels of prostacyclin and other anti-aggregatory compounds (Mezei et al., 2000). Also, as a group, migraineurs appear to have higher blood levels of von Willebrand factor, both during (Cesar,

---

[10]Given the role of neural instability, we might be tempted to ask why seizures do not induce migraines. But seizures *do* induce migraines, at least sometimes. Schon and Blau (1987) found that generalized tonic-clonic seizures were followed by migraines in approximately 25 percent of patients. For roughly another 25 percent the seizures were followed by a non-migrainous headache. A. Bernasconi and colleagues have replicated these percentages for partial epilepsy (A. Bernasconi et al., 2001).

[11]In fact, this property is the source of the neurotransmitter's unusual name. Long before its role in synaptic transmission was understood, and before it was identified chemically as **5-hydroxytryptamine**, serotonin was known simply as a factor in the serum that affected vascular tone (B. L. Jacobs & Azmitia, 1992).

Garcia-Avello, Vecino, et al., 1995) and between (Tietjen, Al-Qasmi, Athanas, Dafer, & Khuder, 2001) migraine episodes. Von Willebrand factor is a chemical, part carbohydrate and part protein (glycoprotein) that is secreted by the endothelium lining the blood vessels. Von Willebrand factor activates platelets and causes them to aggregate. Now, platelets that aggregate easily could block small vessels in the brain, and contribute to a local hypoxia, setting off a migraine.

However, the finding that injection of serotonin interrupts migraine episodes, and the success of serotonin agonists such as sumatriptan, have given ascendance to an alternate theory: that the release of serotonin is functioning as a defense against migraines (Ferrari, 1998b). In more recent investigations, platelets are more likely to be studied as models for serotonin release in the nervous system than as objects of interest in their own right (Malmgren & Hasselmark, 1988). Still, we will see in Chapter 11 that there are at least 15 different subtypes of serotonin receptors. The effects of serotonin seem to depend on which subtype is being stimulated or blocked. Thus, it is quite possible that serotonin can either inhibit or facilitate a migraine, depending on the exact site of action (G. R. Martin, 1997). For example, the endothelium that lines the blood vessels appears to contain two types of serotonin receptor, 5-HT_{1B} and 5-HT_7, that may be involved in vasodilation (Hargreaves & Shepheard, 1999). Perhaps serotonin released from platelets would cause vasodilation as its first effect. If so, this might be enough to stimulate the C fibers surrounding meningeal vessels and begin the trigeminovascular process (Hargreaves & Shepheard, 1999). Of course this would in no way contradict the finding that serotonin receptors in other locations (including 5-HT_{1B} receptors on the smooth muscle surrounding the blood vessels) seem to be involved in vasoconstriction, and in ending a migraine attack.[12]

The platelet theory has not entirely disappeared. The persistent findings of subtle differences in platelet function call out for some sort of explanation. Genes involved in platelet activity seem to be upregulated during migraines, although by itself this does not prove a causal role (Hershey et al., 2004). The platelet theory has found support in regard to menstrual migraine (Benedetto, Allais, Ciochetto, & De Lorenzo, 1997). And we will encounter the theory again, and its considerable heuristic value, when we study migraine triggers such as dietary fat, and medications such as low dose aspirin.

IMMUNOLOGICAL FACTORS

Particularly in the first half of the twentieth century, migraine was sometimes regarded as a variant of allergic disease (Vaughan, 1927). The comparison to allergy is made infrequently nowadays but, as with the platelet hypothesis, there are findings that seem to impel us to it. In particular, the comorbidity in children between migraines, asthma, eczema, and rhinitis (hay fever; see Chapter 9) seems difficult to explain without drawing on the immune system.

Moreover, recent genetic discoveries suggest that there may indeed be some physiological overlap. Rainero et al. have reported evidence that a gene polymorphism for the **cytokine**, interleukin–1α, is associated with earlier onset of migraine with aura (Rainero, Pinessi, et al., 2002). The results of this first study certainly require replication. The authors point out, however, that the same gene polymorphism has been associated with earlier onset of rheumatoid arthritis and of Alzheimer's dementia. (Of note, the polymorphism is not very common, even in migraine with aura). Conversely, migraine with aura may be less common in people with a particular immunological genotype (represented by the HLA class II DR2 antigen; Martelletti, Lulli, et al., 1999).

---

[12]Thus, we cannot assume that a medication that simply raises serotonin levels across the board, such as the SSRI's often used in psychiatry, will have efficacy in preventing migraines. We will return to this topic in Chapter 11.

This genotype seems to involve lower production of the cytokine, tumor necrosis factor alpha. And a polymorphism in another cytokine-related gene, lymphotoxin α, seems to be associated with risk for migraine without aura (Trabace et al., 2002).

Assuming these genetic associations are borne out by later research, how do immune system parameters affect risk of migraine? We have seen one possible connection in Chapter 2: the proinflammatory cytokines interleukin 1β (although not interleukin 1α) and tumor necrosis factor α seem to lower pain thresholds. Possibly, the neurogenic inflammatory response of migraine is another connection (Rainero, Pinessi, et al., 2002; Trabace et al., 2002), perhaps involving immune system components to a greater extent than we now realize. Interleukin–1 is secreted by glial cells and even neurons in response to brain injury or infection (Rainero, Pinessi, et al.), which would fit with migraine as a defensive response.

Less direct is the thought that migraine could be a form of autoimmune disease. The impetus for this hypothesis is a study by Gabrielli et al., recent and in need of replication. They found that 28 percent of migraineurs, but only 4.6 percent of matched controls, had antibodies in their blood targeting endothelial cells (Gabrielli, Santarelli, Addolorato, Foschi, Cristiana, & Gasbarrini, 2002). Endothelial cells line the blood vessels. As the authors point out, these cells produce certain vasoactive substances (endothelin–1, nitric oxide, prostacyclin) and inactivate others (serotonin, **bradykinin**). Thus, an autoimmune-generated dysfunction of endothelial cells could perhaps in some way contribute to the migraine process (Gabrielli et al.).

Certainly, more work will be needed to clarify the role of the immune system in migraine pathogenesis.

CLINICAL IMPLICATIONS

Thus, beneath the surface of clinical presentation we find a range of physiological processes: vasoconstriction, sensitivity to sensory stimuli, proneness to neural instability, over-recruitment of attention, depletion of brain energy reserves and, downstream from all of these, the trigeminovascular response as an organized defensive reaction. We are not yet certain which, if any, of the upstream processes play a causal role. And perhaps different processes are causal for different migraineurs.

We can easily picture a day when the experimental psychology and neurophysiology labs are standard parts of patient assessment, giving precision to diagnosis and guidance to treatment. Perhaps it is patients with a prolonged waterfall illusion or intense visual masking (tests easily programmed into a personal computer) who will benefit from riboflavin or coenzyme Q10. Perhaps the contingent negative variation, a type of EEG event-related potential, will indicate proneness to intense recruitment of attention, and measure success at learning cognitive relaxation. Perhaps **transcranial Doppler**, either mean velocity or the size of B waves, will be the most accurate sign of vasoreactivity, for tracking the effects of thermal biofeedback (Wauquier, McGrady, Aloe, Klausner, & B. Collins, 1995). In the physical realm, magnetic resonance spectroscopy may point to interventions to improve brain energy balance.

All this belongs to the future. Routine laboratory testing (except perhaps for serum ionized magnesium levels) cannot yet be recommended outside of a research setting. But as we will discuss at the end of the chapter, the range of physiological variables we have seen can sensitize us to the range of patients we will encounter clinically. Certainly we will want to be alert to cases of prolonged aura, or aura that includes motor, balance, or language problems, as these might suggest benefit from treatments (e.g., acetazolamide, verapamil) usually reserved for hemiplegic migraine. With the possibility that cortical spreading depression is a reaction to and/or defense against ischemia, we might want to look especially closely at vasoreactivity in migraine with aura. For all patients, we will want to understand the types of triggers, whether visual, other forms of sensory stimulation, or the intense recruitment of attention. And most of all, we will want to look at stress. For it seems that a vulnerability to stress is integral to every model of migraine physiology.

MIGRAINES AND PSYCHOLOGY

Migraines and Stress

Even the genetic findings in migraine by no means exclude environmental contributors. For example, in Tzourio, et al.'s work on the gene encoding the endothelin A receptor, 80 percent of migraineurs had adenine rather than guanine at a key location. However, this was also true of 68 percent of people who did *not* have migraines (Tzourio, El Amrani, Poirier, Nicaud, Bousser, & Alpérovitch, 2001). The association between the gene polymorphism and the phenotype (having migraines) is statistical; the gene functions as one risk factor among many. And the environmental risk that keeps turning up is stress. Indeed, each of the models seems to be intertwined with stress sensitivity at some point.

In the next chapter we will review evidence that stress can bring about cerebral vasoconstriction. In particular, constriction of the anterior and middle cerebral arteries can be produced neurally, via projections from the sympathetic ganglia in the neck (Edvinsson, 1982).

More recently, elevated levels of endothelin–1 have been found in the blood plasma following an emotional stressor (Noll et al., 1996; Treiber et al., 2000). Naturally, this has led to suspicion that endothelin–1 is a mediator of stress-induced vasoconstriction and hypertension. The research is still preliminary, however, as it has not been established that higher plasma levels of this compound mean greater biological activity. And other connections are possible, for endothelin–1 is distributed throughout the nervous system. In particular, it is found in the hypothalamus and the amygdala, where it seems to play a role in catecholamine synthesis, particularly in response to stress (Y. Kurihara et al., 2000). Thus, the gene for the endothelin A receptor may affect risk of migraines by altering the magnitude of the (vascular and/or neural) stress response.

Similarly, in addition to directly constricting blood vessels, angiotensin, also implicated in migraines (Paterna et al., 2000), facilitates sympathetic neurotransmission, and thus stress-mediated vasoconstriction (E. K. Jackson, 2001).

There is also evidence linking migraine with variations in the gene for dopamine beta-hydroxylase, or DβH (Lea, Dohy, K. Jordan, Quinlan, Brimage, & L. R. Griffiths, 2000). DβH is the enzyme governing the last step in the synthesis of norepinephrine, the key neurotransmitter in the sympathetic nervous system. The enzyme also governs the next-to-last step in the synthesis of the stress hormone **epinephrine** (adrenaline; Nestler, Hyman, & Malenka, 2001). In theory, then, DβH is well positioned to influence the magnitude of sympathetic nervous system responding.

In the neural model, too, there is a role for stress. Stresses could intensify neurogenic inflammation, by priming **mast cells** to secrete histamine (Olness, Hall, Rozniecki, W. Schmidt, & Theoharides, 1999). We will examine this effect further in the next chapter. And Moskowitz and Cutrer note that for inherited ion channel disorders such as familial hemiplegic migraine, the "prototypic features include intermittent dysfunction (particularly motor control-muscle tone) often precipitated by stress" (Moskowitz & Cutrer, 1997, p. 1195). "A patient thus inherits a *headachey diathesis*" (Goadsby, 1997a, p. 28; italics in original).

Moreover, the brain stem nuclei in the region of the **migraine generator** (the periaqueductal gray, **locus coeruleus**, and the solitary tract nucleus) are interconnected (Van Bockstaele,

Bajic, Proudfit, & Valentino, 2001). The locus coeruleus in particular is sensitive to levels of **corticotropin-releasing factor** (a key stress hormone) and helps to coordinate the body's stress response (Lehnert, Schulz, & Dieterich, 1998). Indeed, the locus coeruleus is an important part of the within-brain portion of the sympathetic nervous system (Van Bockstaele et al.). Similarly, the solitary tract nucleus helps regulate sympathetic and parasympathetic cardiovascular outflow (Berntson & Cacioppo, 2000).

Now, a high degree of cortical readiness appears analogous to the orienting reflex (Schoenen, 1996a). Thus, we are not surprised that, through its connections with the forebrain, the locus coeruleus increases cortical arousal in response to stress (A. L. Curtis, Florin-Lechner, Pavcovich, & Valentino, 1997). The stress from pressure to perform well is especially effective at increasing brain arousal (Siniatchkin, Averkina, & Gerber, 2006).

Meanwhile, acute stress combined with a marginal deficiency can deplete brain magnesium levels (e.g., Chutkow, 1981). And the differences observed by Pavese et al. in receptor density on the mitochondrial membranes is essentially a marker for stress. The differences would follow if migraineurs had recently experienced an acute stressor (Droogleever Fortuyn, van Broekhoven, Span, Backstrom, Zitman, & Verkes, 2004), or had an unusually strong stress response (Pavese et al., 2000).

Even platelets seem to be stress-linked, for there is reasonably strong evidence that stress increases their aggregability (Rozanski, Blumenthal, & Kaplan, 1999). This makes sense biologically, as fight-or-flight scenarios surely include risk of injury and blood loss. The increased aggregability seems to be fostered by circulating epinephrine (Cannon & H. Gray, 1914; Kjeldsen, Weder, Egan, Neubig, Zweifler, & Julius, 1995; Spalding, Vaitkevicius, Dill, MacKenzie, Schmaier, & Lockette, 1998; Vosburgh & Richards, 1903), and by the elevation in blood lipids that accompanies stress. Thus, if migraineurs are already predisposed towards platelet activation, stress may compound the risk by providing still further activation.

Affect

Depression.   In the nineteenth century, "megrims," then plural for "migraine," was synonymous with "the blues," especially when the dysphoria was caused by feeling physically unwell (Century Dictionary, 1890, p. 3692). Of course, it is not surprising that developing a benign but severe headache disorder, or indeed any medical condition, can lead to depression. And indeed Breslau et al. found that individuals with migraines were, over a 3½ year study period, 3.2 times more likely to develop a major depressive disorder. However, the reverse was also the case: Individuals who had major depression at the start of the study period were 3.1 times more likely to develop migraines (Breslau, G. C. Davis, Schultz, & Peterson, 1994). As this was a longitudinal observational study, it cannot be used to distinguish between two competing hypotheses: that depression in some sense causes migraines, or that some unknown process is manifested first in depression and then in migraines. However, the finding, and its approximate magnitude, are robust (Breslau, Lipton, Stewart, Schultz, & Welch, 2003).

Anxiety.   Migraine also seems to increase the risk of panic disorder, perhaps as much as 13-fold (Breslau & G. C. Davis, 1993). Moreover, an important feature of severe headaches is often the anxiety they arouse. For example, Jamner and Tursky (1987) presented pain-descriptive words to migraineurs and to pain-free subjects. The migraineurs had a much stronger and longer-lasting stress reaction to the words, measured as skin conductance response. Moreover, the migraineurs' responses were stronger to words that applied to migraines than to words that characterized other types of pain.

Pain-related anxiety can be important clinically if it adds to the aversiveness of the disorder, if it leads a person to curtail their activities in anticipation of a migraine, if it helps to trigger headaches via stress, and if it leads to excessive medication use.

Indeed, negative affect is likely to be an important clinical consideration. There is evidence that in headaches and orofacial pain (e.g., temporomandibular dysfunction), disability is much better predicted by depression and anxiety than by pain severity (K. A. Holroyd, Malinoski, M. K. Davis, & Lipchik, 1999; Holzberg, Robinson, Geisser, & Gremillion, 1996; Passchier, Helm-Hylkema, & Orlebeke, 1985).

Personality

In clinical lore, migraineurs were often described as over-controlled: perfectionistic, rigid, and moralistic (Friedman, von Storch, & Merritt, 1954). However, this early literature used unstandardized methods (chiefly clinical interview) and cross-sectional designs that did not allow a distinction to be made between the causes and effects of migraines. Subsequent efforts using psychological tests generally did not identify personality factors consistently associated with migraines (Harrison, 1975). There appears to be little reason to believe that migraines derive from personality.

This is not to say, however, that there is no association between migraines and personality. In a number of carefully designed epidemiological studies, researchers have found a moderate relationship between migraines and "neuroticism", that is, susceptibility to negative affect (Brandt, Celentano, Stewart, Linet, & Folstein, 1990; Breslau & Andreski, 1995; note that "neuroticism" refers to a dimension of normal personality, and does not imply a "neurosis," Asghari & Nicholas, 1999). Importantly, this relationship has been demonstrated prospectively, at least in women. Breslau and coworkers followed a community sample of 972 people for 5½ years (97 percent retention rate). Women who scored in the highest quartile of neuroticism on the Eysenck Personality Inventory at baseline, were 4.0 times more likely than women in the lowest quartile to develop migraines over the study period. After controlling for history of major depression and any diagnosable anxiety disorder, the prospective neuroticism-migraine relationship was attenuated but still statistically significant (Breslau, Chilcoat, & Andreski, 1996).

Although a similar relationship has not been found prospectively in men, the most likely explanation is low statistical power due to small sample sizes. In men, migraines are rarer, and usually have first onset in adolescence (Lipton, Silberstein, & Stewart, 1994). Thus, men who are susceptible to migraines tend to have already developed the disorder by the time they enter into a study. In retrospective reports, the migraine-neuroticism link is generally found in both genders (Brandt, Celentano, Stewart, Linet, & Folstein, 1990; Breslau, Chilcoat, & Andreski, 1996).

Note that we are a long way from the psychoanalytic concept of migraine as a physiological expression of a particular type of psychological make-up. The migraine-neuroticism relationship is statistical rather than deterministic. Moreover, vulnerability to negative affect is, as the name implies, a risk factor for other conditions besides migraine, particularly major depression (Boyce, Parker, Barnett, Cooney, & F. Smith, 1991; Kendler, Neale, Kessler, Heath, & Eaves, 1993). It is easy to imagine how neuroticism could increase one's probability of developing migraines. Neuroticism appears to reflect **autonomic nervous system** lability, and to have a significant genetic component (Eaves, Eysenck, & Martin, 1989; Viken, R. J. Rose, Kaprio, & Koskenvuo, 1994). If one had a migraine diathesis, say for vasoreactivity or impaired brain energy metabolism, high autonomic reactivity could contribute chronic stress, producing a clinical disorder.

In theory, then, a proneness to negative affect could change the clinical course of migraine. And in fact, in a prospective study, Mongini et al. found that baseline elevations on a psychological test (the **MMPI**), and especially on the test's depression scale, predicted ongoing migraines at 7-year follow-up. Moreover, patients who had met the diagnostic criteria for major depression at baseline were half as likely as non-depressed patients to have a 50 percent reduction in migraine frequency. In contrast, neither initial frequency nor immediate response to 2–6 months of migraine treatment predicted the long-term course of the pain (F. Mongini, Keller, Deregibus, Raviola, T. Mongini, & Sancarlo, 2003).

Other traits, too, may generate stress and negative affect (e.g., **Type A Behavior Pattern**; P. R. Martin, Nathan, & Milech, 1987) or provide indications of cortical tone (W. Wang, Y.-H. Wang, Fu, Sun, & Schoenen, 1999). Thus, the role of personality in migraines continues to attract interest.

Psychodynamics and Migraine

Alfred Adler, an early psychoanalyst, traced migraines to a striving against inferiority, or more exactly, to two emotions that accompany the effort, and which increase blood flow to the head: anger and shame. "Some people when they are angry have stomach trouble at the same time, or grow red in the face. Their circulation is altered to such a degree that a headache ensues" (A. Adler, 1931, p. 42). These emotions were felt to be especially pernicious when not inwardly acknowledged or dealt with openly. Theorists who followed Adler elaborated on both themes: unadmitted emotions and the striving for achievement.

For some people with migraines have tremendous difficulty pacing themselves, even when the link between stress, lifestyle factors and pain is clear to them. In extreme cases, they seem to have adopted a level of work that is nearly unfeasible, treating sleep, regular meals, leisure, and recreation as unnecessary constraints on their time. Why would they do this to themselves? (Why do we?) Why would a person choose a lifestyle that contributes to pain?

In the older migraine literature, psychodynamic therapists proposed an answer to these questions, based primarily on clinical experience. Here, we will summarize the formulation given by C. S. Adler and S. M. Adler. Our summary will be very cursory, however, and I strongly encourage reading the original source (C. S. Adler & S. M. Adler, 1987).

The authors suggest that as children, the migraineurs often tried to perform precociously. It might be that their parents rewarded signs of being a prodigy, or that the household routines were strict, parent-centered, and left little room for being a child. Alternatively, the parents might have been undependable enough that the child concluded it was safer to grow up in a hurry. But whatever the reason, the child ended up trying to achieve beyond their level of cognitive and emotional maturity. The result would be an understandable feeling of insecurity, of not being adequate to the task (C. S. Adler & S. M. Adler, 1987).

Now, the sense of inadequacy and the efforts to overachieve may subside as the child matures and gains more life experience. However, they may also become ingrained, and even into adulthood tasks may be approached with a vague sense of dread and inadequacy. This does not mean that the person is actually inadequate. For example, Russell Elkinton, a physician, professor at the University of Pennsylvania, and the editor of the *Annals of Internal Medicine*, attributed his migraines to the stress of trying "to do well professionally while endowed with relatively modest abilities, i.e., I was playing under tension in the big league of academic medicine" (Elkinton & Graham, 1985, cited in C. S. Adler & S. M. Adler, 1987, p. 160). Of course the rest of us would feel honored to have such modest abilities.

In adulthood, avoiding this anxiety might seem to be an easy matter: Set low standards, and do not try to achieve beyond one's perceived limitations. However, the individual may have learned early to enjoy the rewards of precocious achievement, or to internalize strict standards from the pressures to meet parental demands. Note that in the theory, it is not the parental standards themselves that are internalized, but the child's idea of what the standards are. The greater the pressures, the earlier the standards may be internalized, when they are still poorly understood. Thus, the internalized standards may be more inflexible and unreasonable than what the parents had been requiring. In any case, the result is a strong need to achieve, coupled with a sense of inadequacy to achieve. It is in the efforts to solve this dual problem that the individual sacrifices rest and pacing (C. S. Adler & S. M. Adler, 1987).

Further complicating matters is the (often unconscious) resentment that can develop out of these sacrifices, and the conflict between the resentment and the efforts to be "good." In psychodynamic theory, this intrapsychic conflict produces an autonomic tension that itself can trigger migraines (C. S. Adler & S. M. Adler, 1987).

Note that an overcontrolled person with high internal standards may, in the theory, turn anger inward rather than expressing it openly. The result would be depression. Thus, psychodynamic theorists explain the comorbidity of migraines and depression as resulting from a similar intrapsychic structure (Furmanski, 1952). In this theory, depression in migraineurs would be expected to have a strong intrapunitive component, that is, guilt (C. S. Adler & S. M. Adler, 1987). In psychodynamic theory, guilt can lead to pain as a form of self-punishment and expiation (Fromm-Reichmann, 1937; Pilowsky, 1978).

Now, is any of this true? On the simplest level, Alfred Adler's formulation has support: Anger (Materazzo, Cathcart, & Pritchard, 2000) and especially its suppression (Nicholson, Gramling, Ong, & Buenaver, 2003) are likely headache triggers.[13] However, the later, more elaborate psychodynamic theories are harder to test. Certainly in the clinic, some migraineurs recount episodes of guilty rumination that culminate in a migraine. For others, an intense, poignant self-anger seems as intrinsic to the migraine attack as photophobia. But it is hard to draw firm conclusions from such single-case studies.

As a somewhat firmer basis, Passchier and coworkers used a structured projective test, the Defense Mechanisms Inventory, to measure levels of self-aggression in 23 people with frequent migraines and 23 matched control subjects. The subjects were young female college students, and were not undergoing or seeking treatment. The migraineurs showed higher levels of self-aggression. Moreover, for the migraineurs, level of self-aggression was associated with headache frequency on a headache diary and with baseline headache intensity during a psychophysiological assessment (Passchier, Goudswaard, Orlebeke, & Verhage, 1988).

There are hints, too, of linkage between migraines and aggression in the physiological literature. At least two of the brain stem nuclei in the migraine generator region, the **dorsal raphe nucleus** and the periaqueductal gray, are involved in aggression, at least in experimental animals (Gregg & A. Siegel, 2001; Koprowska & Romaniuk, 1997; Korzan, T. R. Summers, Ronan, Renner, & C. H. Summers, 2001).[14] And a subtype of serotonin receptor important in stopping migraines (the $5-HT_{1B}$ receptor) also seems to be important in regulating aggression. Migraine

---

[13]A link between migraines and anger was postulated well before psychoanalysis. For example, Ménuret de Chambaud, writing in Diderot's 18th century encyclopedia, cited "frequent but suppressed anger and rage" as a predisposing factor ("des colères fréquentes mais réprimées;" translated in Isler, Agarwalla, Würth, & Agosti, 2005, p. 1174; original French text 1765). We will see in Chapter 10 that foods eliciting bile were thought to be migraine triggers in Galenic medicine. Here, we see another connection, to the yellow bile of a choleric temperament.

[14]Of course we are familiar with the periaqueductal gray from Chapter 2, where we encountered it as an important part of the endorphinergic descending pain control system. There, it was tempting to anthropomorphize the periaqueductal gray as a benign nucleus that inhibits pain. But it has reasons for inhibiting pain and presumably one of them is so that we can fight without distraction.

abortive medications that cross the **blood-brain barrier** (e.g., zolmitriptan) appear to be highly specific for blocking aggressive behavior in animals (de Almeida, Nikulina, Faccidomo, E. W. Fish, & Miczek, 2001).

Of course a connection between migraines and self-aggression requires replication and, additionally, explication. A behavioral mediator, poor pacing, is plausible but unproven. More generally, defining the nature, mechanism, and probable biological rationale for an association between migraines and self-aggression would undoubtedly keep us well supplied with research topics for years to come.

I know of no other research on this topic, however. Thus, most of the evidence is simply the experience and clinical impressions of psychodynamic therapist-authors. Even if we accept their impressions at face value, the conclusions would necessarily be limited to the sample of people who were in psychodynamic treatment for migraines when the works were being written. Needless to say, this is a very select group, likely to be more educated, introspective, and financially well off than the general population. Migraines are more common in lower socioeconomic strata (although not in minorities), and the reasons for stress and pacing difficulties might or might not generalize to this group. Moreover, clinical samples may contain a higher proportion of individuals who are depressed, and thus might show higher levels of self-aggression than community samples. (Note, however, that the subjects in the Passchier et al. study of self-aggression were from a non-clinical sample).

But in real life we are not working with a population, but with the person before us in therapy. There, broadly speaking, psychodynamic therapists listen for the cognitive and emotional connections in the person's inner world, and they try to identify those connections that trap the person in an unhealthy and self-defeating lifestyle. By making these connections and their effects clear in a nonthreatening way, the therapist can give the person new choices, and perhaps make the behavioral tools more effective. Psychodynamic writings are not like medical research; they are not designed to produce a database about a disorder. Rather, they are the session notes of therapy that worked, and are designed to sensitize the reader to the types of themes to keep in mind when listening to the individual.

And we should not conclude from the psychodynamic description that people with pacing difficulties are particularly maladjusted. Indeed, they are not; the defense mechanisms involved are rather sophisticated and "high level." Moreover, a person's strengths and weaknesses are often the same. If the approach to life is a poor match to the diathesis of migraines, it may still be a fine road to success. "These are often, after all, the very individuals we would select as our attorney, physician, accountant, or neighbor; indeed, a recent survey showed 21 percent of the British parliament are migraineurs" (C. S. Adler & S. M. Adler, 1987, pp. 158–159). The challenge in therapy is to preserve the strengths, while promoting greater flexibility, confidence, and self-care.

CLINICAL IMPLICATIONS

We have seen that underlying all of the theories of migraine—vascular, neural, platelet, immunological—is a vulnerability to stress. Thus, a reduction in sympathetic tone is a key element of behavioral treatment. Behind this broad but effective strategy, however, the theories imply a diverse web of physical vulnerabilities, psychological predispositions, and environmental triggers. Together with our knowledge of chronic pain, the complexity can give us therapeutic leeway in even seemingly intractable cases.

Although we are not yet at the point of testing for brain energy depletion clinically with magnetic resonance spectroscopy, or neural excitability with evoked potentials or visual **masking**, we might suspect these factors when visual stimulation and mental fatigability are the primary triggers. We might then focus in treatment on pacing in mental work and exposure to sensory triggers, and consider a medication that normalizes evoked potentials or a supplement thought to improve brain energy resources. We will discuss triggers further in Chapter 10, medications and supplements in Chapter 11, and pacing in Chapter 13.

When routine psychological testing indicates hand temperature values well below the population mean, we may particularly consider a vascular response to stress as a key underlying process. Then, we might want to look especially closely at stress as a trigger, use falling hand temperature as a early warning sign for a migraine, and teach a reduction in sympathetic tone (relaxation to increase hand temperature) as a self-management skill. We will discuss hand temperature in Chapter 5 and biofeedback in Chapter 13.

The platelet model has no likely symptoms to my knowledge, but might be considered whenever migraine with aura has not responded sufficiently to other interventions. A reduction in sympathetic tone and a low fat diet are the primary self-management strategies suggested by it. We will examine dietary factors in migraine in Chapter 10.

As we have seen, the immune model is not well developed for migraine, but it comes to mind when the migraines coexist with asthma, eczema, and hay fever. Heuristically, we might focus then on assessing whether allergens are triggers, on managing trigger exposure—and on relaxation, because of its connections with decreased histamine response. We will explore this connection further in the next chapter.

A focus on the trigeminal nucleus caudalis might be considered when there are signs of heightened pain sensitivity: a constant tender, bruised feeling at the scalp, comorbid fibromyalgia (Peres, W. B. Young, Kaup, Zukerman, & Silberstein, 2001), very frequent migraines, or a plethora of unrelated triggers. Then, the variables from Chapters 2 and 3 might be brought to bear in a treatment plan. Particularly important will be developing a sense of control over the migraines, by identifying triggers, making the attacks more predictable, and teaching skills such as relaxation and mental hand warming for preventing individual migraines and reducing their overall frequency. For patients often arrive with their lives dominated by the migraines, living in the corners of time between attacks, shadowed by their unpredictability. Then, building self-efficacy must be a continuous theme running beneath our treatment efforts. We will discuss this process further in Chapters 12 and 13.

It is helpful to assess for major depression, and panic or other anxiety disorder, because of their high comorbidity with migraine, and because they can presumably trigger attacks, contribute to disability, interfere with learning behavioral skills and, in the case of depression, portend a deteriorating course of pain. For some patients, it may not be feasible to teach relaxation skills or pacing through mental work until major depression or generalized anxiety, uncontrolled worrying, is first brought under control. For others, addressing the vocational and emotional impact may be as important as reducing the migraines themselves. And although an exploration of individual dynamics, including guilt and aggression turned against the self, is not usually necessary in migraine treatment, we must be prepared to do so (or to refer out) when acquisition of behavioral skills would not be possible otherwise.

Still, all this implies a greater subtlety and specificity of intervention than the outcome literature will yet bear. At this point, the great majority of behavioral migraine treatment involves simply bringing the stress response under control. This response, however, has its own diversity. To appropriately measure and treat physical stress it is useful to know its facets in depth. This is the realm of migraine psychophysiology, linking physiological theories of migraine to psychological stress and to self-management skills such as biofeedback. It is this topic to which we will turn next.

CHAPTER 5

Psychophysiology of Migraine

I was suffering very severely with a sick headache, and stopped at a farm house on the road some distance to the rear of the main body of the army. I spent the night in bathing my feet in hot water and mustard, and putting mustard plasters on my wrists and the back part of my neck, hoping to be cured by morning.
—Ulysses S. Grant, diary entry, April 8, 1865, the day before Lee agreed to surrender (cited in Friedman, 1972, p. 666)

We have seen that nearly every physiological process thought to be involved in migraine is affected by stress. Thus, to augment stress tolerance would seem the key psychotherapeutic task, and it is true that a great deal can be accomplished by addressing the psychological mediators of stress. But historically it has not been by *emotional* self-regulation that the psychological treatment of migraine has been defined, but by biofeedback, which draws on the capacity of the human mind to influence, sometimes with remarkable subtlety, physiological functioning. Biofeedback techniques are still a mainstay of treatment, and as we will see in Chapter 13, they have accrued considerable support in controlled outcome studies. But to understand these tools, to refine them, to match them to patients, and to develop their successors, we must examine more closely the mechanisms by which stress influences migraine. That is, we must delve into the complex and murky realm of migraine **psychophysiology**.

We will begin with a natural assumption: that migraineurs as a group tend to have higher baseline levels of stress, that is, higher sympathetic tone.

MIGRAINE AND AUTONOMIC TONE

Drummond, focusing on the eye, found that the pupil is ever so slightly (.08 mm) constricted on the usual side of head pain after 30 seconds in the dark, during and between migraine headaches (subclinical **miosis**; Drummond, 1990b). Pupillary dilation is mediated by sympathetic nerves, and hence the slight constriction suggests *lower* sympathetic activity.

If this result were restricted to the eye, we could attribute it to local damage to the sympathetic nerves, perhaps from compression when the internal carotid artery wall swells during migraines (Drummond, 1990b). Alternatively, the findings at the pupil might be an aspect of trigeminovascular activation, as the eye is supplied by the trigeminal nerve (Drummond, 1990b). But there have been similar findings using other measures.

For example, in migraineurs heart rate may increase less during isometric exercise (Pogacnik, Sega, Pecnik, & Kiauta, 1993). And systolic and diastolic blood pressure may drop when a migraineur arises from a recumbent position, causing a subclinical degree of orthostatic hypotension

(Gotoh, Komatsumoto, Araki, & Gomi, 1984; R. Martin, Ribera, Moltó, Ruiz, Galiano, & Matías-Guiu, 1992; Mikamo, Takeshima, & Takahashi, 1989). It is as if, in migraineurs, the sympathetic nerves were not firing sufficiently.

Moreover, in some studies lower levels of circulating norepinephrine have been found in migraineurs, at baseline (Gotoh, Komatsumoto, Araki, & Gomi, 1984; Mikamo, Takeshima, & Takahashi, 1989), upon arising after lying supine (i.e., on one's back; Gotoh, et al.; Mikamo, et al.), or during isometric contraction (Mikamo, et al.). Norepinephrine is the neurotransmitter used to execute sympathetic responses.

Still other studies have looked at heart rate variability. We often think of heart rate as a single number, say 65 beats per minute, but of course heart rate is never exactly constant. There is beat-to-beat variability, and this variability itself can be studied (Berntson, Bigger, et al., 1997). When we subject it to a spectral analysis, we find that the variability can be divided into three frequency bands: low (.001–.05 Hz) and middle (.05–.15 Hz), both thought to reflect a mixture of sympathetic and parasympathetic activity, and high (.15–.45 Hz) thought to be purely parasympathetic (Pogacnik, Sega, Pecnik, & Kiauta, 1993). Pogacnik, et al. found that, when arising from a supine position, migraineurs showed less increase in the middle frequency bands than did nonmigraine control subjects, consistent with a lower degree of sympathetic activation (Pogacnik, Sega, Pecnik, & Kiauta, 1993).

Results for parasympathetic function have shown less of a trend, with some researchers finding evidence for hypofunction (Micieli, Tassorelli, Magri, Sandrini, Cavallini, & Nappi, 1989; Thomsen, Iversen, & Olesen, 1995a), and others finding hyperfunction (Gotoh, Komatsumoto, Araki, & Gomi, 1984) or no difference.

Now, all of this paints a much clearer picture than is justified. Heart rate variability, cardiac reflexes, and circulating catecholamines have all generated notable conflicting results and failures to replicate (see Cortelli, Pierangeli, Parchi, Contin, Baruzzi, & Lugaresi, 1991 for a review; also, Pierangeli, Parchi, Barletta, Chiogna, Lugaresi, & Cortelli, 1997). But there seems to be a mild trend in the literature towards sympathetic hypofunction.

Thus, the hypothesis of greater sympathetic tone in migraineurs appears to be wrong. From one perspective, this could be logical. Recall from Chapter 2 that fight-or-flight responding lowers pain sensitivity. The source of this stress-induced analgesia is presumably the locus coeruleus in the midbrain, through its connections to the periaqueductal gray. The locus coeruleus is part of the sympathetic nervous system; we arrive at the locus coeruleus if we follow the sympathetic nerves into the brain. Not surprisingly, then, norepiphrine is an inhibitory neurotransmitter in the spinal and brain stem pain pathways.

In Chapter 4, we encountered a theory that the locus coeruleus is part of a "migraine generator" system. But the opposite theory has also been proposed: that the locus coeruleus, by inhibiting pain, helps prevent headaches. Then a global deficit in sympathetic tone would be important because it would reflect a local deficit in this pain inhibitory system (J. W. Lance, G. A. Lambert, Goadsby, & Duckworth, 1983).

But if this theory is true, shouldn't stress protect against migraines? Not necessarily. When sympathetic function is chronically low, the receptors for epinephrine and norepinephrine may compensate by becoming more sensitive. Then conditions of true stress, when large amounts of epinephrine are released, would produce an unusually strong sympathetic response in migraineurs ("adrenergic supersensitivity;" Drummond, 1990b). During migraines themselves, levels of epinephrine and norepinephrine are not low—in fact they may be as high as in patients awaiting surgery, and are correlated with pain severity (Martínez, Castillo, Pardo, Lema, & Noya, 1993). Thus, a deficit in baseline sympathetic tone might make migraineurs less physiologically adaptable to stress (Martínez et al.). There is some evidence for this. Gotoh et al. found that in migraineurs, blood pressure was slower to return to normal after injection of norepinephrine (Gotoh, Komatsumoto, Araki, & Gomi, 1984). A similar slowness to adapt has been found at the eye after instillation of epinephrine (Fanciullacci, 1979), and at the intracranial blood vessels (Yamamoto & J. S. Meyer, 1980). Even worse, reduced tone at the locus coeruleus might be slightly uncomfortable, and lead migraineurs to seek out stimulation, inadvertently precipitating a migraine episode (Gerber & Schoenen, 1998).

In all of this, however, we have been looking at general trends in the literature. Although apparently in the minority, there have also been well conducted studies showing sympathetic *hyper*function, or no results. Whether this is due to differences in methodology, differences among migraineurs, or a more general **autonomic instability** that can produce results in either direction, is unclear (Kuritzky, 1997).

Our patients are faced with the same ambiguity. Was the migraine caused by relaxation, or was it a delayed effect of stress? Did they sleep too little, too much, or at the wrong time? Our capacity to intervene behaviorally will be stronger when we have a better sense of how (or whether) migraines fit into the chronology of autonomic events.

Still, in most studies of the psychophysiology of migraine, the focus has not been on global sympathetic tone, but on specific processes thought to be of particular relevance to the disorder. Moreover, we are often interested more in responses to psychosocial stresses than in simple autonomic reflexes. Hence, we will delve deeper into the psychophysiological realm. Here, studies have been patterned after the vascular, cortical, and trigeminovascular theories of migraine.

VASCULAR ASPECTS OF MIGRAINE
AND THERMAL BIOFEEDBACK

Extracranial measures.   A number of studies have been founded on the vascular model. Early investigations focused on the reactivity of the large extracranial cephalic arteries, particularly the superficial temporal artery. This approach was based on the belief, developed by Peter Latham and Harold Wolff, that dilation of the extracranial arteries was an important source of pain in migraines.

Given the hypothesis noted above, that migraineurs adapt more slowly to autonomic challenges (Martínez, Castillo, Pardo, Lema, & Noya, 1993), we might expect a more gradual return to baseline following psychosocial stresses. In fact, this question has been examined in 18 studies, shown in Table 5–4 and summarized in Tables 5–1 and 5–2, below. Let us briefly review their implications.

First, a box-score tabulation suggests that if post-stress recovery is different in migraineurs, it is only on cardiovascular measures. Other indices of arousal such as respiration, EMG, and electrodermal responding, show virtually no effect of migraine diagnosis. Moreover, among the cardiovascular measures, temporal pulse amplitude seems to have the greatest likelihood of an abnormal recovery, followed by pulse amplitude or temperature at other pericranial sites, and by diastolic blood pressure. Thus, migraineurs seem to differ in recovery specifically on vascular measures.

Alternatively, if we partition the cardiovascular measures into those affected primarily by alpha adrenergic mechanisms (the effects of vasoconstriction on finger temperature, pulse volume amplitude, diastolic blood pressure and, to some extent, total peripheral resistance) and those that are largely beta adrenergic (heart rate, vasodilation; Cacioppo, Berntson, Binkley, Quigley, Uchino, & Fieldstone, 1994; Ring, Harrison, Winzer, D. Carroll, Drayson, & M. Kendall, 2000) recovery differences are seen primarily for alpha adrenergic processes.

TABLE 5–1
Post-stress Recovery in Migraine as a Function of Physiological Measure

Measure	Number of Studies Employing	Number (%) Showing Abnormal Recovery in Migraineurs
Temporal Pulse Amplitude	13	8 (62%)
Pericranial Pulse Amplitude	3	1 (33%)
Forehead/Head Temperature	3	1 (33%)
Diastolic Blood Pressure	3	1 (33%)
Heart Rate	12	3 (25%)
Digital Pulse Amplitude	4	1 (25%)
Finger or Hand Temperature	5	1 (20%)
Electrodermal	6	1 (17%)
Systolic Blood Pressure	3	0 (0%)
Respiration Rate	3	0 (0%)
EMG, Other Sites	6	0 (0%)
Frontalis EMG	11	0 (0%)

But even for vascular measures, the studies are about evenly divided as to whether an effect was obtained. What accounts for this? Note that the studies differ explicitly in the type, duration, and combination of stresses, the length of initial adaptation to the laboratory, the length of recovery period, and the density of time sampling within this period. Among these method variables, the type of stressor seems particularly important.

Shown in Table 5–2 are the types of standardized laboratory stresses used to study migraine psychophysiology. Of these, brief exercise and CO_2 rebreathing seem to reliably elicit differences between migraineurs and non-headache control subjects in post-stress recovery. Loud noise and performance stress (public speaking, mental arithmetic under pressure) similarly seem to be effective.

In contrast, noise at lower volume showed no group differences, presumably because it elicited an orienting rather than a defensive response. Stressful imagery had equivocal effects, which perhaps depended on the nature or vividness of the image, or the ability of the subject. In migraines, being viewed on a video monitor produces differences only in number of skin conductance responses rather than in cardiovascular recovery (Kröner-Herwig, Dirk Diergarten,

TABLE 5–2
Post-stress Recovery in Migraine for Various Types of Stressor

Type of Stressor	No. of Vascular Studies Employing[1]	Number Showing Abnormal Recovery
Noise, 95 dB	1	1 (100%)
Public Speaking	1	1 (100%)
Mental Arithmetic	7	5 (71%)
Physical Stressor (Exercise, CO_2 rebreathing)	3	2 (67%)
Pain (Ischemia, Cold Pressor)	5	3 (60%)
Stressful Imagery	2	1 (50%)
Achievement Testing ≥40 minutes	4	1 (25%)
Noise, 80–85 dB	2	0 (0%)
Standing	1	0 (0%)

[1]Studies with at least one vascular measure: temporal pulse amplitude, earlobe pulse amplitude, forehead temperature, finger temperature, and/or digital pulse volume.

Dagmar Diergarten, & Seeger-Siewert, 1988), which fits with the general psychophysiology literature on social observation (Cacioppo, Rourke, Marshall-Goodell, Tassinary, & Baron, 1990).

Long duration intelligence tests and course examinations, although presumably quite stressful, had virtually no differential effects in the post-stress interval. Delayed recovery may be apparent only after brief stresses, those that more closely resemble a bolus injection of adrenaline. Indeed, in two of the four studies there was a long interval, around 10 minutes, before recovery measures were taken. In contrast, the half-life of epinephrine and norepinephrine in the bloodstream is only 2–3 minutes (M. G. Ziegler, 1989).

The marginal effect of ischemic and cold pressor pain is surprising. In the psychophysiology literature, the cold pressor test tends to be somewhat more effective than mental arithmetic, and much more effective than simply standing up, in eliciting a cardiovascular stress response (Mills, Berry, Dimsdale, Nelesen, & M. G. Ziegler, 1993). Moreover, as a stimulus to be endured rather than actively solved, the cold pressor tends to elicit changes in vascular parameters (alpha adrenergic) more than in heart rate (beta adrenergic; Waldstein, Bachen, & Manuck, 1997). Perhaps the effectiveness of these stressors was high enough to swamp group differences in recovery.

Overall, then, the evidence from post-stress recovery seems mildly supportive of an alpha adrenergic, that is, vascular, effect of suitable stresses in migraines. Consistent with this, there is a small amount of evidence that pharmaceutical blockade of alpha-adrenergic receptors might help prevent migraines (Ghose, Coppen, & D. Carrol, 1977), and may perhaps contribute to the effects of the classic anti-migraine drug, ergotamine (Bonuso et al., 1994).

We might also surmise that migraineurs respond differently during, and not simply after, a stressor. In the chapter appendix a summary is given of 31 studies in which this question was examined.

As in post-stress recovery, the probability of a positive result depends on the specific physiological variable, as shown in Table 5–3.

Differences between migraineurs and various control groups are seen to some degree in a number of measures. However, results are found most frequently for three measures of cephalic blood flow: head temperature, pulse amplitude at the temple, and pulse amplitude at other pericranial sites.

Whether the temporal artery abnormally dilates or constricts seems to depend on the nature of the stressor. Stressful imagery (Arena, Blanchard, Andrasik, Appelbaum, & Myers, 1985) and short-duration mental arithmetic (Drummond, 1982, 1984) seem to increase the caliber of the temporal artery, even when the mental arithmetic is combined with noise (Drummond, 1985). On the other hand, noise by itself (Ellertsen & Hammerborg, 1982; Ellertsen, Nordby, Hammerborg, & Thorlacius, 1987; but see Morley, 1985 for conflicting results), the cold pressor task (Arena, Blanchard, et al.), and long-duration achievement tests (Haynes, Gannon, Bank, Shelton, & Goodwin, 1990; Passchier, Goudswaard, & Orlebeke, 1993) seem to cause abnormal constriction. Thus, the distinction between stresses that require active coping (e.g., mental arithmetic) and those for which coping is passive (e.g., enduring noise or pain) may be important. The difference between long and short duration testing suggests that the direction of the response varies over time (Kröner-Herwig, Fritsche, & Brauer, 1993; Morley, 1985).

An unusual stress response involving finger temperature or digital pulse amplitude was found in only a fraction of the studies (22 percent and 29 percent, respectively). However, in clinical practice migraineurs often seem to have unusually cold hands under stress, including the stress of presenting for treatment. Thus, Blanchard and coworkers collected normative hand temperature readings from 221 headache patients, 105 hypertensives, 45 patients with irritable bowel syndrome, and 56 control subjects. In the published norms, patients with migraines or mixed

TABLE 5–3
The Stress Response in Migraine as a Function of Physiological Measure

Measure	Number of Studies Employing	Number (%) with Significant Difference, Migraine vs. Control
Forehead/Head Temperature	5	4 (80%)
Temporal Pulse Amplitude	22	11 (50%)
Pericranial Pulse Amplitude	4	2 (50%)
Respiration Rate	5	2 (40%)
Systolic Blood Pressure	6	2 (33%)
Digital Pulse Amplitude	7	2 (29%)
Heart Rate	23	6 (26%)
Frontalis EMG	21	5 (24%)
Finger or Hand Temperature	9	2 (22%)
Diastolic Blood Pressure	6	1 (17%)
EMG, Other Sites	13	2 (15%)
Electrodermal	13	0 (0%)

migraine and tension headaches had the lowest hand temperatures prior to biofeedback training (Blanchard, Morrill, Wittrock, Scharff, & Jaccard, 1989).

Thus, the psychophysiological studies seem to point to a stress sensitivity of the blood vessels in migraine. When we try to define this vascular effect, however, it is the variability of results that stands out. The nature of the stressor seems to be important. In addition, three other sources of variability may play a role.

First, there is likely to be considerable heterogeneity among migraineurs. For example, Drummond and Lance found that among 63 migraineurs, only 23 had full or partial relief of pain with compression of the superficial temporal artery. This subset of patients also had a significantly greater temporal pulse amplitude on the affected side during migraine, and higher skin temperature at the ipsilateral temple and upper forehead (Drummond & J. W. Lance, 1983). Drummond and Lance termed this subset as having "extracranial migraines," corresponding to Latham's and Wolff's classic views on the importance of the extracranial arteries in migraine. Moreover, Drummond found that during mental arithmetic, temporal pulse amplitude increased by 29 percent in patients with "extracranial migraine," but by only 5 percent in migraineurs whose headaches were not "extracranial." Similar results were found when the stressor was brief physical exercise (Drummond, 1984).[1]

Secondly, the measurement process is likely to introduce variability among studies. For example, "superficial temporal artery" may not be a specific enough recording site. Thus, Drummond and Lance found distention only of the frontal branch of the superficial temporal artery in migraineurs. The main trunk of the artery was not distended—in fact, numerically it was slightly constricted on the headache side (Drummond & J. W. Lance, 1983).

Thirdly, we should note that in the original studies by Graham and Wolff, distention of the superficial temporal artery was only one of the findings for the interictal period. The other finding was a greater *variability* in pulse amplitude, a variability which began to increase 3–4 days

---

[1]"It is not unreasonable that in some the meninges around the brain are affected, in others, the pericranium. . . . Even among those who feel the pain in one half of the head, usually called hemicranics, some get the feeling that the pain is on the outside of the skull, and others, deep within the head." (Galen, "On the Affected Places," 2nd century AD, cited in Isler, 1992).

before the migraine itself (Tunis & Wolff, 1953; Wolff, 1963).[2] Indeed, "The striking modifications in cranial-artery function characteristic of the headache attack merely punctuated the more or less continuous series of physiological changes that comprised part of the particular life adjustment of these persons" (Tunis & Wolff, 1953, p. 556). Three decades earlier, Crookshank had surmised as much: "the vaso-motor system is, with them, in unstable rather than in stable equilibrium, however self-contained and reserved may be their apparent attitude towards events" (Crookshank, 1926, p. 74).

I know of only one attempt to replicate Tunis and Wolff's results. Feuerstein and colleagues studied twelve subjects, measuring psychophysiological variables on the four days leading up to a migraine, and on the migraine day itself. Sure enough, temporal pulse amplitude showed higher variability three days before a migraine, although only on the right. Even more telling, the variability in right temporal pulse amplitude three days before a migraine could be predicted from state anxiety level four days before a migraine ($r = .62; p < .02$). In contrast, digital pulse amplitude, finger temperature, frontalis EMG, heart rate, and blood pressure did not change systematically in the days leading up to a migraine (Feuerstein, Bortolussi, M. Houle, & Labbé, 1983).[3]

Now, if the superficial temporal artery is a key source of pain for only a subset of migraine cases, what processes are involved for the rest? Some migraineurs who do not obtain relief from compression of the superficial temporal artery do have a reduction in pain with pressure to the common carotid arteries in the neck (Drummond & J. W. Lance, 1983; do *not* try this). Perhaps, then, distention of some other vessel fed by the carotids, such as the middle meningeal or the middle or anterior cerebral arteries plays a role (Drummond & J. W. Lance, 1983). This possibility, and advancing technology, has brought psychophysiological investigation to the intracranial arteries. We will review these studies in the next section.

We should note that a demonstration of abnormal psychophysiological reactivity in migraine leaves open a further question: What sort of role does the reactivity play in the migraine process? For example, Drummond suggests that the repeated swelling of the internal carotid artery by vasoactive peptides compresses the surrounding sympathetic nerves, compromising them, and causing a reduction of local sympathetic outflow. Sympathetic nerves primarily constrict the artery, and hence the dilation seen in migraineurs may actually be a local failure of constriction (Drummond, 1991). A local deficit of this type would not necessarily be benign. Drummond suggests that sympathetic vasoconstriction helps to buffer the trigeminovascular response. When the vasoconstriction is compromised, dilation can add to the pain from arterial swelling and sensitization, intensifying and prolonging a migraine. In theory, this could be one explanation for a deteriorating course of the disorder. We might suspect, then, that biofeedback training to constrict the superficial temporal artery may be helpful even if it is targeting an event fairly late in the migraine process. Note that such training would most likely involve increasing local sympathetic tone, and hence would not be a form of relaxation.

Intracranial measures.   In more recent studies, the investigations of vasoreactivity and abnormal blood flow patterns have been extended to the intracranial arteries (Mirza et al., 1998; Valikovics et al., 1996). To understand the results, let us first consider how cerebral circulation is regulated.

---

[2]In the published results, mean and standard deviation seem to be proportional. This would arise, for example, if pulse amplitude had a log-normal distribution.

[3]In fact, Morley has speculated that certain forms of biofeedback, which were designed to reduce blood flow to the superficial temporal artery, may actually work by reducing the variability in blood flow (Morley, 1985).

Intracranial arteries receive at least three types of innervation:

- sympathetic fibers that mediate vasoconstriction,
- parasympathetic fibers that mediate vasodilation, and
- sensory fibers from the trigeminal nucleus (Edvinsson, 2001).

The sensory fibers, of course, are precisely those responsible for the trigeminovascular response that we learned about in the last chapter. Along with vasodilation, these fibers produce the swelling, sterile inflammation, and pain sensitization that underlie migraine headaches.

The sympathetic fibers travel from the hypothalamus, through the spinal cord to the superior cervical ganglion in the neck, and from there back up to the intracranial vessels (Edvinsson, 2001). These sympathetic fibers use norepinephrine and neuropeptide Y as their primary neurotransmitters, and innervate the anterior and middle cerebral arteries, more than the basilar and vertebral arteries (Edvinsson, 1982). (We should add here that plasma epinephrine, although certainly a part of the stress response, does not cross the blood-brain barrier; R. J. Mathew, W. H. Wilson, D. Humphreys, Lowe, & Wiethe, 1997.) The parasympathetic fibers run alongside the VIIth cranial nerve. They primarily use **acetylcholine** and vasoactive intestinal peptide as transmitters, but other peptides are involved as well, as is presumably nitric oxide (Edvinsson, 2001). Meanwhile, the trigeminal nerve, as we have seen, sends pain signals to the trigeminal nucleus caudalis, and uses calcitonin gene-related peptide, substance P and glutamate as its primary neurotransmitters.

The sympathetic fibers, of course, are important in the stress response. It appears that in normal subjects, mild anxiety tends to increase cerebral blood flow, presumably reflecting an increase in general arousal via the reticular activating system. Severe anxiety, however, seems to introduce a modest vasoconstrictive effect (R. J. Mathew et al., 1997), with a 5–15 percent reduction in cerebral blood flow (Edvinsson, 1982). This vasoconstriction—a clamping down on the arteries—may serve to protect the brain from hemorrhagic stroke in the event of a sudden spike in systemic blood pressure (Edvinsson, 1982). In non-migraineurs the constriction of the large conducting arteries is offset by a compensatory dilation of the small arteries downstream (Faraci & Heistad, 1998). But perhaps migraineurs show an enhanced vasoconstriction in response to direct sympathetic stimulation. In turn, too much vasoconstriction might elicit a compensatory vasodilation (Edvinsson, I. J. Olesen, Kingman, McCulloch, & Uddman, 1995; McCulloch, Uddman, Kingman, & Edvinsson, 1986).

Now logically, we might presume that a sympathetic vasoconstriction would be countered when necessary by a parasympathetic vasodilation. However, from animal studies it appears that the parasympathetic nerves cause dilation in response to excess local carbon dioxide, not excess vasoconstriction. Under stress, the actual opponent process is between the sympathetic and the *sensory* fibers (Edvinsson, 2001). Thus, a compensatory vasodilation would actually involve the full trigeminovascular response—neurogenic inflammation, leakage (extravasation) of plasma, and pain sensitization. In this model, then, the migraine is a response by the sensory fibers to an overly intense, sympathetically mediated vasoconstriction (Edvinsson, I. J. Olesen, Kingman, McCulloch, & Uddman, 1995). The parasympathetic system may then play a secondary role, by further dilating the inflamed blood vessels, by directly stimulating sensory nerves, and by releasing additional inflammatory mediators such as histamine (Yarnitsky, Goor-Aryeh, et al., 2003).

The predominant means of testing this hypothesis has been to look at blood flow velocities in the large arteries of the brain using transcranial Doppler. If total blood flow remains constant, and an artery constricts, then of course the blood flow in the artery has to speed up. Thus, blood flow velocity can be used to measure relative artery diameter, provided we have a good sense of total blood flow.

A number of investigators have found higher blood flow velocities in migraineurs than in non-migraineurs, when assessed at rest, between migraine episodes (Thie, Fuhlendorf, K. Spitzer, & Kunze, 1990; Valikovics, et al., 1996). For example, Thie and coworkers, studying 61 patients who had migraine without aura, 39 who had migraine with aura, and 40 matched control subjects, found no differences between the two groups of migraineurs. However, the migraineurs showed higher velocities than the control subjects in all of the intracranial arteries (anterior cerebral artery, middle cerebral artery, posterior cerebral artery, and basilar artery) but not in the internal carotid artery, which is extracranial (Thie, Fuhlendorf, et al.). Similarly, there is suggestion that downstream resistances were lower in the migraineurs. These findings could imply a higher base-line sympathetic tone. In this area, too, however, results have not been entirely consistent, and the primary impression across studies is one of instability of vascular tone.

Harer and von Kummer (1991) studied vasodilation of the middle cerebral artery to 5 percent CO_2 inhalation (hypercapnia). They found much greater reactivity in migraineurs v. nonmigraineurs, provided that the migraineurs were assessed between attacks. During a migraine episode, migraineurs tended to show less reactivity to the CO_2, perhaps because the artery was already dilated. Similar findings have been reported by other investigators. However, vasodilation is not sympathetically mediated. The results with hypercapnia would suggest an exaggerated parasympathetic responsiveness.

The most directly relevant study seems to have been conducted by Micieli and coworkers (Micieli, Tassorelli, Bosone, et al., 1995). They examined the effects of a painful cold pressor task, in which subjects immersed their non-dominant hand in ice water for five minutes. Not surprisingly, blood pressure and heart rate increased, but the migraineurs did not react differently than healthy controls on these measures. No hyperventilation or breath holding seems to have occurred, as the amount of carbon dioxide in the exhaled air did not change for either group. However, the effects of the stressful task on the middle cerebral artery were very different for the two types of subjects. The control subjects showed a clear drop in blood flow velocity, suggesting vasodilation. The migraineurs, in contrast, showed an increase in blood flow velocity, consistent with vasoconstriction. There was indirect evidence of compensatory changes in resistance downstream. Migraine with and without aura were alike in showing vasoconstriction.

Now, this is exactly the pattern we would expect if migraineurs showed an enhanced sympathetic response. However, the case is by no means closed. The authors note that the response of the migraineurs resembled that of non-migraineurs administered clonidine before the test (Micieli, Tassorelli, Bosone, et al., 1995). Clonidine is an α_2-adrenergic agonist that probably blocks signals from the locus coeruleus. Thus, the authors conclude that the migraineurs were characterized by too little adrenergic activation from the locus coeruleus, rather than too much from the sympathetic ganglia.

Recall, however, that in normal subjects the stress response is a U-shaped function: vasodilation at mild levels of stress, followed by vasoconstriction at high levels. An absence of vasodilation could thus mean either an attenuated or an exaggerated stress response. Clearly, more research is needed.

Note that vasoconstriction of the large intracranial arteries need not cause a diminution in blood supply to the brain, for there may be a compensatory vasodilation of the arterioles downstream. Thus, if we hypothesize that it is a threatened drop in brain perfusion, and not simply vasoconstriction, that elicits the migraine, then we must measure the actual amount of blood reaching brain tissue.

(text continued on page 137)

TABLE 5–4

Studies of Post-Stress Adaptation in Migraine

Source	Subjects	Stressor	Measures	Time-Sampling During Recovery	Results
Anderson, Stoyva, & Vaughn, 1982	10 Hypertension; 10 Rheumatoid Arthritis; 10 Tension Headache; 10 Migraine; 10 Controls	2–3 min step-up exercise; 16 min recovery; 8.4 min silent serial 7's; 16 min recovery	Heart Rate Systolic Blood Pressure Diastolic Blood Pressure L Finger Temperature R Finger Temperature Electrodermal Frontalis EMG Wrist Extensor EMG Wrist Flexor EMG	15 64-second trials	Migraineurs' diastolic blood pressure continued upward trend throughout 16 min recovery after mental arithmetic, vs. decline for non-migraine
Arena, Blanchard, Andrasik, Appelbaum, & Myers, 1985	8 Migraine; 12 Chronic Tension Headache; 8 Combined Migraine, Tension Headache; Groups matched for demographics	Variable duration mental arithmetic; 6 min recovery; 1 min stressful imagery; 6 min recovery; 7 min cold pressor; 6 min recovery	Heart Rate R Temporal Pulse Amplitude Finger Temperature Electrodermal Frontalis EMG R Upper Trapezius EMG Wrist Flexor EMG	10-second blocks over the 6 minute recovery periods	Migraine and combined migraine-tension HA patients had slower return to baseline for finger temperature and temporal pulse amplitude; Complex but significant differences in heart rate recovery
Drummond, 1982	20 Migraine 20 Controls	2 min CO_2 rebreathing; 3 min recovery; 1 min cold pressor; 8 min recovery; 2 min mental arithmetic with noise; 3 min recovery; (Nonstress tasks not listed here.)	Heart Rate Systolic Blood Pressure Diastolic Blood Pressure Temporal Pulse Amplitude Forehead Temperature Respiration Rate	1 average for each trial/recovery period	After mental arithmetic: Migraineurs had lower heart rate and less elevated forehead temperature. After CO_2 rebreathing: Temporal pulse amplitude suppressed in migraineurs, elevated in controls; facial temperature remained elevated in migraineurs on side contralateral to usual migraine site.

Study	Sample	Task	Variables	Sampling	Results
Drummond, 1984	16 Migraine with temporal artery pain; 14 Migraine without temporal artery pain	2 min mental arithmetic; 4 min recovery; 1 min standing; 30–60 sec step-up xercise; 4 min recovery	Temporal Pulse Amplitude	1 average for each trial/recovery period	After physical exercise, temporal pulse amplitude is higher in "extracranial" than in other migraineurs.
Drummond, 2003	23 Migraine; 22 Controls	3 30-second cold pressor trials at 4 minute intervals	L Temporal Pulse Amplitude R Temporal Pulse Amplitude	30-second block beginning 7.5 minutes after last cold pressor trial	Temporal pulse amplitude elevated in migraineurs vs. controls; statistically significant only on side contralateral to immersed hand
Ellertsen & Hammerborg, 1982	8 Migraine; 8 Controls; Groups matched for gender, age and education	2 min baseline; c. 15 min of 95 dB, 1000 Hz tones at irregular intervals; 2 min recovery	Heart Rate L Temporal Pulse Amplitude R Temporal Pulse Amplitude	Variables sampled twice during the 2 min recovery period	Temporal pulse amplitude increased in migraine group during recovery, and decreased in controls
Ellertsen, Nordby, Hammerborg, & Thorlacius, 1987	16 Migraine (6 Classic, 10 Common); 8 Headache-Free Controls; All subjects female	2 min rest; 80 dB, 1000 Hz tones at irregular intervals	Heart Rate L Temporal Pulse Amplitude R Temporal Pulse Amplitude Hand Temperature Frontalis EMG	Heart Rate and Temporal Pulse Amplitude were sampled at 0.5 sec intervals over the 8 sec after each stimulus offset	No differences between migraine and control. However, recovery in temporal pulse amplitude is faster after thermal biofeedback training (right side). Also, migraineurs with greatest reduction in headaches at 2-year follow-up had had the fastest temporal pulse amplitude recoveries pre-treatment (left side).
Gannon, Haynes, Cuevas, & Chavez, 1987	8 Migraine; 8 Near-Daily Tension Headache; 8 Controls; Groups matched for gender and age	1 hour of speeded arithmetic with loud buzzer and failure feedback interspersed; 10 min recovery	Heart Rate Earlobe Pulse Amplitude Frontalis EMG Splenius Capitis EMG L Wrist Extensor EMG	1 minute averages every other minute during recovery	No recovery differences in migraineurs

(continued)

TABLE 5–4 (Continued)

Source	Subjects	Stressor	Measures	Time-Sampling During Recovery	Results
Gannon, Haynes, Safranek, & Hamilton, 1981	16 Migraine; 13 Chronic Tension Headache; 15 Controls; Groups matched for gender and age	1 min mental arithmetic; 90 seconds arm ischemia; 10 min recovery after each stressor	Heart Rate Earlobe Pulse Amplitude Frontalis EMG L Wrist Extensor EMG	3 45-second averages over each 10 minute recovery period	Migraineurs showed more vasoconstriction than headache-free control subjects during post-stress recovery
Goudswaard, Passchier, & Orlebeke, 1988	37 Common Migraine; 37 Non-Headache Controls; Groups matched for age, gender and likely were similar in SES.	Psychology course examination; 1.5 hour intelligence test; 10 min recovery after each stressor	Frontalis EMG Temporalis EMG Corrugator EMG (Absolute values, and as proportion of maximum voluntary contraction)	1 minute average at end of 10-minute recovery period	No recovery differences in migraineurs
Hassinger, Semenchuk, & O'Brien, 1999	26 Migraine; 26 Control; All Female; M_{age} = 18.5 years; Students	3 min cold pressor; 5 min recovery; 3 min serial 7's; 5 min recovery	Heart Rate Systolic Blood Pressure Diastolic Blood Pressure Stroke Volume Cardiac Output Total Peripheral Resistance	Average over 5 minute recovery period	Migraine group had higher total peripheral resistance, lower stroke volume and lower cardiac output after mental arithmetic
Haynes, Gannon, Bank, Shelton, & Goodwin, 1990	5 Migraine; 17 Chronic Tension Headache; 14 Mixed Migraine-Tension Headache	1 hour of speeded arithmetic with loud buzzer and failure feedback interspersed; 10 min recovery	Blood Volume Pulse Amplitude at 6 Pericranial Sites	1 minute average at end of 10-minute recovery period (i.e., average of minute #10)	No recovery differences in migraineurs

134

Study	Sample	Stressor	Measures	Recording Intervals	Results
Holm, Lamberty, McSherry, & P. A. Davis, 1997	30 Migraine; 39 Chronic Tension-Type Headache; 35 Control Subjects	12 min baseline; 4 min speech preparation; 2 minute speech; 12 minute recovery	Heart Rate Finger Temperature Frontalis EMG	?Single mean for 12-minute recovery	Heart rate in migraineurs did not fully recover; heart rate in other two groups did recover.
Kröner-Herwig, Dirk Diergarten, Dagmar Diergarten, & Seeger-Siewert, 1988	37 Migraine (M_{age} = 42 years); 44 Control Subjects (M_{age} = 35 years)	8 min industrial noise; 8 min of being viewed on a video monitor; 4 min recovery after each stressor	Temporal Pulse Amplitude Thumb Pulse Amplitude Temporal Temperature Thumb Temperature Electrodermal	2–8 readings (depending on variable) over 4 minute recovery	Number of skin conductance responses increased in migraineurs during post-stress recovery and decreased in control subjects
Kröner-Herwig, Fritsche, & Brauer, 1993	33 IHS Migraine without Tension-Type Headache; 32 Control Subjects matched for age and gender	40 min achievement testing; 20 min recovery	Temporal Pulse Amplitude Digital Pulse Amplitude R Frontalis EMG Electrodermal	1st minute, middle 3 minutes and last 3 minutes of 20 minute recovery	Control subjects constricted temporal pulse amplitude during stress, recovered quickly afterwards; Migraineurs dilated during initial stresses, then constricted to later stresses and throughout recovery
McCaffrey, Goetsch, J. Robinson, & W. Isaac, 1986	1 Migraine; 8 Non-Headache Control Subjects	10 min baseline 1–3 minute stressor: drinking 1% of body weight in ice water 20 min recovery	B Temporal Pulse Amplitude	5 minute blocks	For the control subjects, temporal pulse amplitude was lower post-stress than at baseline. For the single migraineur, temporal pulse amplitude was higher throughout post-stress than at baseline.

(continued)

TABLE 5-4 (*Continued*)

Source	Subjects	Stressor	Measures	Time-Sampling During Recovery	Results
Passchier, Goudswaard, & Orlebeke, 1993	37 Common Migraine; 37 Control Subjects; Groups matched on age and gender, from same student body	Psychology course examination; 1.5 hour intelligence test; 10 min recovery after each stressor	Heart Rate Temporal Pulse Amplitude Digital Pulse Amplitude Forehead Temperature Frontalis EMG Anterior Temporalis EMG Corrugator EMG Respiration Rate Skin Conduct. Level # Skin Conductance Responses	1 minute average at end of 10-minute recovery period	No recovery differences in migraineurs
Passchier, van der Helm-Hylkema, & Orlebeke, 1984	59 Migraine; 32 Tension Headache; 26 Controls Groups equivalent in gender, education level and ? age	10 min baseline; 4 min personally relaxing imagery; 2 min rest; 4 min personally stressful imagery; 2 min rest; 6 min silent mental arithmetic; 5 min recovery	Heart Rate Temporal Pulse Amplitude Temporal Blood Volume Digital Pulse Amplitude Digital Blood Volume Frontalis EMG Respiration Rate Skin Conductance Level	Average for the last (5th) minute of recovery	Digital blood volume lower in migraineurs than in control subjects during recovery (but only for male subjects)
Rojahn & Gerhards, 1986	20 Migraine; 20 Control Subjects; Groups matched on age and gender	57 seconds of aversive noise (85 dB); 5 min recovery	Heart Rate Temporal Pulse Amplitude Frontalis EMG	Five consecutive 1-minute averages	No difference in recovery slope between migraine and control subjects

Note. B = Bilateral; L = Left; R = Right

This is generally done by introducing a bolus of radioactive tracer that can cross the blood-brain barrier, and then measuring the amount of radioactivity around the head. In early migraine studies, the tracer was radioactive xenon (^{133}Xe), that was either inhaled or, for more precise administration, injected into a carotid artery. The radioactivity was then recorded from specialized detectors, often embedded in a helmet that the patient wore. This made the equipment expensive, special-purpose, and rather imprecise if only a few detectors were used. Moreover, the resulting output was in the form of a map, showing the level of radioactivity recorded over the skull surface, a rather superficial image.

A more recent technology, used often in migraine studies, is SPECT—single photon emission computed tomography. It relies on isotopes whose emissions can be detected by a gamma ray camera. The camera rotates around the head, taking pictures. A computer then uses the pictures to reconstruct views of two-dimensional slices ("computed tomographs") through the brain (Krasuski, Horwitz, & Rumsey, 1996). (Actually, ^{133}Xenon emits gamma rays too, but its decay time is so short that the camera could only take a few pictures. Hence the use of specialized simultaneous detectors.)

Even more precise techniques are PET (positron emission tomography) scans, and fMRI-BOLD (functional magnetic resonance imaging—blood oxygen level dependent).

Positron emission tomography resembles SPECT, except that the radiotracers emit positrons—antimatter electrons—rather than gamma rays. Now, positrons do not travel very far, about 0.4 to 1.4 mm, before they collide with an electron. Both particles are annihilated in the collision, producing two high energy gamma ray photons, which shoot away from each other at an approximately 180° angle. Now, the fact that two gamma rays are produced is an advantage, because it tells us that if two bursts of radiation are detected 180° apart, an annihilation probably occurred somewhere along the line of sight connecting the two detectors. And the fact that these gamma rays are of high energy is also an advantage, because then there is less attenuation from tissue absorption, and less ambiguity from scattering, than in the SPECT and xenon techniques (Krasuski, Horwitz, & Rumsey, 1996; Reiman, R. D. Lane, Van Petten, & Bandettini, 2000).[4]

PET gives a fairly direct measure of neural activity, but with the drawback of radioactivity, which limits the number of scans, and therefore the number of experimental conditions, in which a person can participate (A. K. P. Jones, Kulkarni, & Derbyshire, 2003). We can avoid this limitation by using functional MRI, which has at its core a very different process.

To understand fMRI, note that the nuclei of atoms—say, the proton that is at the center of hydrogen—are in a sense tiny magnets. In the body the atoms are oriented randomly, however, canceling each other out, so as a whole we have no magnetic field. Now, an MRI machine contains a strong magnet field, which lines up our protons in parallel to the field. Then, pulses of radio waves are aimed at the body, from a direction perpendicular to the magnetic field, lining up the protons in this new, perpendicular direction. However, in the context of the magnetic field, the perpendicular direction is a higher energy state. The protons need to absorb energy from the radio waves in order to achieve it. Now, turn off the radio waves and the protons again become parallel to the magnetic field, dropping back to the lower energy state, and releasing the stored radio wave energy. The released energy is picked up by an antenna in the MRI machine. Now, to look at brain structure, we tune into the protons (hydrogen nuclei) in water. Thus, conventional MRI images tissues in proportion to their density of water. But other nuclei with magnetic

---

[4]One sometimes hears also that SPECT allows only the determination of relative blood flow among brain regions, whereas PET provides true quantification. However, this is not an essential difference between the two methods, for in principle, SPECT can become a quantitative methodology with further refinement.

properties could be used instead, and an obvious choice is the iron found in hemoglobin. Not surprisingly, then, MRI can be adjusted to give readings of cerebral blood flow (Krasuski, Horwitz, & Rumsey, 1996; ; Reiman, R. D. Lane, Van Petten, & Bandettini, 2000).

High resolution studies at the onset of migraine with aura tend to show a wave of hyperperfusion spreading forward from the posterior cortex, followed by an area of hypoperfusion. These images seem congruent with spreading cortical depression as a model for migraine aura, as described in the last chapter. When blood flow is measured between migraine episodes, the results have been inconsistent across studies. However, Friberg, et al. report that for people whose diagnosis is either migraine with or without aura, regional blood flow shows numerous patches of asymmetry between the two hemispheres. This patchy distribution, not present in healthy control subjects, might indicate an unstable vascular tone between migraine episodes (Friberg, Nicolic, et al., 1991).

Implications for behavioral treatment.   The idea that there is a subset of patients with extracranial migraines (Drummond & J. W. Lance, 1983; Shevel & Spierings, 2004), in which dilation of the superficial temporal artery contributes significantly to pain, can be useful clinically. Often, patients in this group will have measurable heat and visible darkening and distention of the superficial temporal artery at the affected temple. For these patients, reduction in temperature at the temple may be a useful intermediate endpoint for relaxation skills, and even a direct object of biofeedback training. So too may training to constrict the superficial artery be helpful in reducing pain intensity and imparting a sense of control over the migraines.

Studies of the superficial temporal artery are linked to Tunis and Wolff's classic finding that migraines are often a 3–4 day delayed effect of stress. This insight sometimes helps migraineurs make sense of seemingly inexplicable attacks, and allows them a great deal of time to pre-empt, blunt, or prepare for the migraine.

More generally, the vascular results emphasize the psychophysiological aspect of stress and of self-management training. Subjective relaxation, which may signify only a positive affective tone, may not be sufficient for full prophylactic benefit. Rather, we may need to train relaxation to a physical criterion. Specifically, the classic application of the vascular model has been thermal biofeedback—the use of hand temperature, a type of vascular stress response—as the criterion for self-management training.

We will describe thermal biofeedback in the behavioral treatment Chapter, 13. For the moment, we will note simply that it involves learning to increase blood flow to the hands through a mental change that overlaps with deep relaxation. Patterns of extracranial and intracranial blood flow have been studied for an explanation of how this mental change is able to ameliorate migraines.

Physiology of temperature biofeedback.   Early studies, true to the model of migraines then in favor, looked at the impact of thermal biofeedback on distension of the large extracranial arteries. Thus, Dalessio, et al. trained 12 migraineurs and 5 healthy controls to volitionally increase finger temperature. All of the control subjects and all but two of the migraine subjects learned the technique. Eight of the ten migraine subjects who learned the technique had improvements in headache frequency and intensity. For the normal controls and improved migraine subjects, the volitional hand warming was associated with decreased pulse volumes at the supraorbital and superficial temporal artery beds. In the two migraine subjects who did not improve there was no decrease in superficial cephalic pulse volume with the handwarming. Even the successful migraineurs, however, had a far lower pulse response at the finger than the control subjects, as shown in Table 5–5 (Dalessio, Kunzel, Sternbach, & Sovak, 1979).

TABLE 5–5
Effects of Thermal Biofeedback on Pulse Volume in Extracranial Arteries

Subject Type	% Change In Pulse Volume During Biofeedback		
	Finger	*Supraorbital*	*Superficial Temporal*
Control	386 ± 37	−19 ± 6	−12 ± 8
Successful Migraine	127 ± 21	−14 ± 11	−11 ± 12
Unsuccessful Migraine	62 ± 12	2 ± 13	−3 ± 17

Note. Adapted from "Conditioned Adaptation-Relaxation Reflex in Migraine Therapy," by D. J. Dalessio, M. Kunzel, R. Sternbach, and M. Sovak, 1979, *JAMA, 242,* p. 2103. Copyright 1979 American Medical Association. Reprinted with permission.

Later studies turned to the intracranial arteries, using xenon-inhalation regional cerebral blood flow measurements to examine the effects of mental hand warming and hand cooling in migraineurs and comparable control subjects (Claghorn, R. J. Mathew, Largen, & J. S. Meyer, 1981). In people without migraines, hand warming and hand cooling both produced small decreases in cerebral blood flow. By contrast, hand *warming* in migraineurs was associated with an *increase* in cerebral blood flow, especially at the left hemisphere, and hand *cooling* with a *decrease* at the right hemisphere. Thus, hand warming and hand cooling had opposite effects in migraineurs in terms of cerebral circulation. Interestingly, both groups had an improvement in migraines, a phenomenon we will discuss later. Nonetheless, the hand warming group showed more improvement, and Claghorn, et al. report a correlation of −.78 ($p < .01$) between the change in left hemisphere cerebral blood flow and the self-reported mean duration of headaches. That is, increases in blood flow correlated with a reduction in headache duration. This early study is hampered by a small sample size (11 migraineurs, 9 control subjects), and I am not aware of any attempts to replicate its findings.

Sumatriptan (Friberg, 1991) appears to reverse pain associated with middle cerebral artery dilation during an episode of migraine. Thermal biofeedback may work preventively by reversing interictal middle cerebral artery (MCA) constriction. McGrady, et al., in a study of 23 migraineurs, found a significant decrease in blood flow velocity at the MCA with biofeedback training (McGrady, Wauquier, A. McNeil, & Gerard, 1994). Wauquier, et al., in a study of 25 migraineurs, found that successful biofeedback outcome was associated with lowering an elevated MCA blood flow velocity (lowering vasoconstriction) at the MCA. Blood flow velocity at other sites (ophthalmic, basilar, and carotid arteries) did not change and was not predictive of outcome (Wauquier, McGrady, Aloe, Klausner, & B. Collins, 1995). However, the mediating role of blood flow velocity has not always replicated (Vasudeva, Claggett, Tietjen, & McGrady, 2003).

It should be noted that the psychophysiology of mental handwarming is not fully understood. When it is combined with relaxation training, the handwarming is assumed to reflect a reduction in overall sympathetic tone. However, subjects can readily learn to warm just one hand, switching hands at will (Roberts, Kewman, & MacDonald, 1973; Roberts, Schuler, Bacon, Zimmerman, & Patterson, 1975). Unless it is combined with relaxation training, mental handwarming is generally accomplished without changes in heart rate, blood pressure, frontalis muscle tension, or in plasma levels of epinephrine or norepinephrine (Freedman, 1993). The volitional handwarming response can be maintained after sympathetic block and infusion of the extremity with epinephrine, suggesting that a local change in sympathetic tone is not crucial to the phenomenon. Handwarming is attenuated, and possibly eliminated, by simultaneous efferent block and infusion of the extremity with epinephrine and propranolol, suggesting that an as-yet-unidentified non-neural, beta-adrenergic ligand plays a role in the effect (Freedman, Sabharwal, Ianni, et al., 1988). Thus, there may be three or more mechanisms (circulating catecholamine, local sympathetic tone, circulating beta-adrenergic ligand) by which a person can mentally warm their hands. This raises the possibility that differences in training protocol could influence clinical or research results.

Moreover, there are almost certainly large individual differences in psychophysiology, even among people who share the diagnosis of migraine. For example, Kröner-Herwig and colleagues found that pulse volume amplitude at the superficial temporal artery increased in migraineurs during a stressor, but decreased in matched control subjects. The interaction of diagnosis by stress vs. nonstress condition was significant. However, on closer inspection, only 7 of the 33 migraine subjects responded with vasodilation; twelve showed vasoconstriction and in fourteen the pulse volume amplitude essentially did not change (Kröner-Herwig, Fritsche, & Brauer, 1993). The group differences appear to have been heavily influenced by a few migraine subjects showing large dilations. In migraine, as in other chronic pain conditions, research is needed to take into account individual differences in response pattern (see Flor & D. C. Turk, 1989).

And of course we must remember that sympathetically mediated vasoconstriction is one step removed from a migraine. The more directly relevant effect is the vasodilation produced by the trigeminovascular system. We may presume that the trigeminovascular system is responding to vasoconstriction, but perhaps, too, the system has simply become sensitized, and produces migraines with very little provocation. This possibility leads us back to the consideration of psychological factors in pain, discussed in Chapter 3.

Then, too, perhaps it is not vasoconstriction—a reduction in energy supply to the brain—that is important, but the level of energy demands on the brain. We will follow this thread in the next section.

NEURAL ASPECTS OF MIGRAINE AND EEG BIOFEEDBACK

Electroencephalographic (EEG) studies.   Recall that in one version of the neurogenic model, migraines are initiated by a wave of neural activity that spreads geographically over the cortex. The wave is thought to be a result of cortical over-firing: Neurons in a particular region (especially visual cortex, where they are packed tightly) fire quickly, releasing potassium and glutamate faster than glial cells can clear them. Potassium and glutamate concentrations rise in the intercellular medium, triggering other nearby neurons to fire in a growing chain reaction. This model implies that certain brain regions fire more strongly in people who are prone to migraines.

The primary means of studying this hypothesis has been with EEG event-related potentials. The EEG, or electroencephalogram, is a recording of electrical voltages generated by the brain (and especially by the cortex and thalamus) at the scalp. Event-related potentials are subtle perturbations in this voltage, induced by a stimulus characteristic such as novelty, a task demand such as vigilance, or a psychological process such as attention (Fabiani, Gratton, & M. G. H. Coles, 2000). The perturbations show up as a series of negative and positive peaks in voltage. The amplitude of the perturbations, that is, the depth and height of the voltage peaks, has generally been taken to reflect the degree of neural recruitment.

Three apparently related phenomena have been reported in migraineurs, assessed between migraine episodes:

- Intensity dependence in the auditory evoked potential (W. Wang, Timsit-Berthier, & Schoenen, 1996). As the loudness of a tone increases, say from 40 to 70 decibels, the amplitude of the evoked potential (measured as the height difference between N1, the negative peak at c. 100 msec post-stimulus, and P2, the positive peak c. 60 msec later) increases sharply in perhaps 45 percent of migraineurs. In contrast, only around 20 percent of nonmigraineurs show this pattern (Siniatchkin, Kropp, Neumann, Gerber, & Stephani, 2000). For the vast majority of non-migraineurs, the amplitude of the evoked response shows little change as the tone gets louder.

- Failure of habituation in the visual evoked potential. Thus, with repeated presentation of a rapidly alternating black-and-red checkerboard, the amplitude of the visual evoked potential response tends to increase over hundreds of trials in migraineurs, while decreasing in people without migraines (Afra, Cecchini, DePasqua, Albert, & Schoenen, 1998).

- Increased amplitude of the early component (c. 650 msec post-stimulus) of contingent negative variation (CNV; Kropp & Gerber, 1998; Maertens de Noordhout, Timsit-Berthier, Timsit, & Schoenen, 1986). Contingent negative variation is an event-related potential that follows the warning or "get ready" signal in a reaction-time test.

What do these results mean? The intensity dependence and the failure of habituation are sometimes interpreted as signs of brain hyperexcitability, perhaps leading to a negative energy balance through high energy demands. In particular, the intensity dependence in the auditory evoked potential may be a sign of deficient serotonergic inhibition (Hegerl & Juckel, 1993), although dopamine has also been implicated (Von Knorring & Perris, 1981). Thus, the results are theoretically as well as empirically linked to migraines. It should be noted, however, that intensity dependence, studied in years past under the term "augmenting" (versus reducing), has also been reported in relatives of people with schizophrenia, bipolar disorder, and major depression (Gershon & Buchsbaum, 1977). That is, its specificity for migraines is not high (Siniatchkin, Kropp, et al., 2000).

The increase in contingent negative variation has been interpreted to mean that migraineurs tend to "mobilize their attentional system excessively during information processing" (Siniatchkin, Kropp, et al., 2000, p. 252). The increase in contingent negative variation is not seen during the migraine episode itself (Kropp & Gerber, 1995), or for c. 3 days thereafter (Kropp & Gerber, 1998). Possibly, this could imply that migraine episodes serve a homeostatic function.

Still, the evoked potential results do not require us to conclude that the brain is hyperexcitable, incurring higher-than-normal energy demands. The results could mean that baseline cortical tone is too *low* in migraineurs. In that case, the intensity dependence and lack of habituation might occur because there is more room for the magnitude of the evoked response to grow (Schoenen, 1996b).

Transcranial Magnetic Stimulation (TMS).   Thus, the EEG data leaves unresolved the question of whether brain activation is, on average, higher or lower in migraineurs, or perhaps both higher and lower in a cyclical pattern. Therefore, the question has been approached in other ways.

In theory, we can assess brain excitability more directly by using strong magnetic pulses, from a coil held near the head, to induce currents in the underlying brain tissue. This approach is termed **transcranial magnetic stimulation** (Boylan & Sackeim, 2000; Currà, Modugno, Inghilleri, Manfredi, Hallett, & Berardelli, 2002). Excitability can be operationalized as the strength of magnetic field at motor cortex required to cause a twitch in the contralateral hand (Currà et al.), or as the threshold at visual cortex needed to elicit phosphenes—bright dots, patches, or shapes (Battelli, K. R. Black, & Wray, 2002).

For visual cortex, this seemingly straightforward process has given remarkably contradictory results, with some studies showing a reduced threshold in migraineurs (Aurora, Ahmad,

Welch, Bdardhwaj, & Ramadan, 1998; Battelli, K. R. Black, & Wray, 2002; W. B. Young, Oshinsky, A. L. Shechter, Gebeline-Myers, K. C. Bradley, & Wassermann, 2004), and others showing an increased threshold (Afra, Mascia, Gerard, Maertens de Noordhout, & Schoenen, 1998; V. Bohotin, Fumal, Vandenheede, C. Bohotin, & Schoenen, 2003). So far, the only area of agreement for visual cortex has been that thresholds in migraine with and without aura are largely the same. The excitability of motor cortex seems to be lower in migraineurs (Afra, Mascia, et al.), even those prone to sensorimotor aura (Maertens de Noordhout, Pepin, Schoenen, & Delwaide, 1992).

The discrepancies between studies may have several sources. First, migraine is most likely an etiologically heterogenous disorder: There may be different subsets of migraineurs with different thresholds for brain activation. Second, the simplicity of TMS may be deceptive. The magnetic field seems to induce currents in the facilitory interneurons that run parallel to the surface of the skull (V. Bohotin, Fumal, Vandenheede, C. Bohotin, & Schoenen, 2003). This is straightforward in motor cortex, where the representation of the hand is near the brain surface, but for visual cortex, extending deep into the cleft between hemispheres, the physiological events are less understood (V. Bohotin, Fumal, Vandenheede, C. Bohotin, et al., 2003). Indeed, the direct stimulatory effects of TMS may not extend more than 2 cm beneath the outside of the skull (Rudiak & Marg, 1994). Technical differences in magnetic coil size and shape, and the nature of the magnetic pulse, might also affect results in unknown ways (V. Bohotin, Fumal, Vandenheede, C. Bohotin, et al., 2003). As might be expected, the practice of holding the coil in place by hand does not seem to direct the field very accurately (Herwig, Padberg, J. Unger, M. Spitzer, & Schönfeldt-Lecouna, 2001). A third possibility, suggested by the CNV results above, is that migraineurs oscillate between hyper- and hypoexcitability in relation to migraine episodes (V. Bohotin, Fumal, Vandenheede, C. Bohotin, et al., 2003), but the evidence so far has been negative (W. B. Young, Oshinsky, A. L. Shechter, Gebeline-Myers, K. C. Bradley, & Wassermann, 2004).

Thus, in standard TMS our intention is to stimulate the cortex, but whether we do so, and to what degree, depends on the geometry of the underlying cortex in relation to the coil. We can gain further control over the intervention by shifting from single magnetic pulses to long trains of pulses. When the pulses are presented at high frequency, c. 10 Hz, they elicit progressively stronger responses—even seizures, in experimental animals—and regional cerebral blood flow is increased. Thus, high frequency presentation seems to stimulate cortex. The same pulses at low frequency, c. 1 Hz, cause reductions in blood flow and progressively weaker responses, suggesting inhibition (A. A. Gershon, Dannon, & Grunhaus, 2003; R. E. Hoffman & Cavus, 2002). Thus, it appears that we can activate or inhibit a brain region by varying the time between successive magnetic stimuli.

Combining this method with the type of EEG study discussed above, Schoenen and colleagues found that high frequency, excitatory trains normalized the visual evoked potential in migraineurs. Conversely, when healthy volunteers were given inhibitory trains, their visual evoked potentials showed the deficient habituation characteristic of migraine (V. Bohotin, Fumal, Vandenheede, Gérard, C. Bohotin, Maertens de Noordhout, & Schoenen, 2002). Thus, in this stillnew stream of research, migraine is a disorder of cortical underarousal.

The matter, however, is far from settled, for different methodologies give different results. For example, after a brief physical stimulus—say, a non-painful electric shock to the wrist—the evoked potential to a second shock will be smaller for a few tens of milliseconds. This fatiguelike effect is briefer in migraine (or at least in pediatric migraine without aura), suggesting overarousal at the cortex and even at the dorsal horn (Valeriani, Rinalduzzi, & Vigevano, 2005). Perhaps arousal level depends on stimulus modality—lower in the visual and auditory system, higher in the somatosensory system, setting the stage for central sensitization to pain (de Tommaso, 2005). At this point, however, we simply do not know.

Notice, then, that the same controversy about under- vs. over-arousal that we saw for the peripheral **autonomic nervous system** carries over into the central nervous system. As in the periphery, it is possible that chronic underarousal sets the stage for an over-response to certain stimuli.

Implications for behavioral treatment.   The EEG differences can refocus our efforts on known migraine triggers, as alcohol, emotional distress, and lack of sleep can increase the amplitude of event-related potentials (Siniatchkin, Gerber, Kropp, & Vein, 1999). Alternatively, the EEG differences in migraineurs might themselves constitute a target for behavioral intervention. Intuitively, bringing attentional focus under voluntary control seems at least as feasible as mentally changing finger temperature.

Is there evidence that migraineurs can change the magnitude of their evoked responses? The field of EEG biofeedback in migraines is at its earliest stages. In a recent study, Siniatchkin and coworkers gave children with migraines (approximately age 10) ten sessions of feedback on the magnitude of their contingent negative variation. In this study, "magnitude" meant the average amplitude over the period from 500 ms after the warning tone until the test tone 2500 ms later. Feedback was given visually 5 seconds after the test tone. In each session, there were trials for increasing the amplitude, trials for decreasing it, and trials without feedback to test skills acquisition. Several results were suggested: (1) Compared with matched controls, the children with migraines had higher baseline CNV amplitude, and took longer to acquire independent control over it. (2) Training led to a gradual reduction in baseline CNV amplitude, down to normal levels. (3) Compared to matched waiting-list control subjects, the children receiving biofeedback training showed a reduction in migraine frequency, and in total migraine activity. However, this reduction did not correlate with either the improvement in baseline level of CNV amplitude or with the degree of CNV control seen in the last training session, and hence might have been due to nonspecific factors (Siniatchkin, Hierundar, Kropp, Kuhnert, Gerber, & Stephani, 2000).

So far, visual or auditory evoked potential biofeedback does not appear to have been investigated. However, Panjwani et al. describe a study of Sahaja Yoga meditation, in which practitioners experienced a state of "thoughtless awareness." The study participants all suffered from idiopathic epilepsy, and were on antiseizure medication throughout the research. Over six months the meditation led to an increase in the height difference between two relatively early components of the auditory evoked potential—Na (a negative fluctuation at about 19 msec after stimulus presentation) and Pa (a positive fluctuation at c. 30 msec; Näätänen & Winkler, 1999). Moreover, although visual evoked potentials were not measured, practitioners were better able to detect very faint test stimuli. These test stimuli, low contrast sine-wave gratings, are similar to fuzzy alternating light and dark gray bars. We know from other research that the evoked potentials these gratings elicit depend on contrast[5] (Ellemberg, Hammarrenger, Lepore, M.-S. Roy, & Guillemot, 2001), so presumably the greater visual acuity implies a stronger evoked response. A no-treatment control group, and a group practicing placebo meditation (placing one's hands in a series of positions and then sitting quietly) did not show these changes. (Panjwani, Selvamurthy, S. Singh, Gupta, Mukhopadhyay, & Thakur, 2000). Thus, a meditation approach might increase rather than lower visual and auditory evoked potentials. However, we clearly need to have more

---

[5]Specifically the N1 and P1 components, approximately 70 and 110 msec post-stimulus, respectively (Ellemberg et al., 2001).

than just these two studies if we are to properly gauge the potential of EEG biofeedback as a clinical intervention for migraines.

Underneath EEG biofeedback is the hint of a larger question: Is brain hyperexcitability a *learned* state? Little is known about this. It appears, however, that exposure to stress can alter the subsequent stress sensitivity of the locus coeruleus. That is, firing rates in the locus coeruleus are increased by **corticotropin-releasing factor** (a key stress hormone) but the dose-response curve depends on prior stress exposure (A. L. Curtis, Pavcovich, & Valentino, 1999).[6] Similarly, a nurturing environment during infancy seems to decrease the number of corticotropin-releasing factor receptors in the locus coeruleus, presumably lowering stress sensitivity (Caldji, Tannenbaum, Sharma, D. Francis, Plotsky, & Meaney, 1998). As the locus coeruleus is in the presumed "migraine generator" region of the midbrain, and as the locus coeruleus helps to increase cortical arousal in response to stress (A. L. Curtis, Florin-Lechner, Pavcovich, & Valentino, 1997), its stress tuning could in theory affect susceptibility to migraines.

Meanwhile, there has been relatively little work examining whether migraineurs show exaggerated EEG changes as a short-term response to stress. An exception is a study by Rainero et al. on the effects of causing ischemia at the arm. When the ischemia was of long duration, and hence quite stressful, control subjects showed a reduction of EEG power in the alpha range (8–12 Hz). Alpha waves increase with mental relaxation, and hence electrical power in the alpha region is an inverse measure of brain activation. Migraineurs showed a reduction in alpha power to even short duration arm ischemia, suggesting an exaggerated stress response on the EEG (Rainero, Amanzio, Vighetti, Bergamasco, Pinessi, & Benedetti, 2001).

Thus, in both the neural and vascular models, mechanisms linking stress and migraine can be delineated, each suggesting an opportunity for therapeutic intervention. But as we saw in Chapter 2, exposure to nociceptive stimuli may induce a progressive sensitization of pain pathways. This is likely to be true in migraine as well, and may play an increasing role as migraines become more frequent, intense, and chronic. Over time, neural and vascular processes may fade in importance. The disorder may become defined not by the provoking stimuli, but by the readiness of the system to be provoked. And here in the trigeminovascular system we find, built-in, a new type of stress sensitivity.

INFLAMMATION, MIGRAINE, AND SELF-HYPNOSIS

We saw in the last chapter that migraines seem to involve a sterile inflammation orchestrated by the trigeminovascular system. The main features of this inflammation—sensitization of sensory nerves, vasodilation, and leakage of proteins through blood vessel walls—are similar to those found in allergic inflammation. In allergies, the inflammation involves mast cells—cells of the immune system that reside in the skin, lungs, intestines, and other tissues. When mast cells are stimulated by antibodies, they release stores of histamine and other chemicals, in a process called "**degranulation**" (under a microscope, the histamine vesicles look like granules). These chemicals produce the inflammation (Galli & Lantz, 1999).

---

[6]The effect on the curve is complex. Stress exposure seems to increase the sensitivity of the locus coeruleus to normal physiological levels of corticotropin-releasing factor, which should raise the excitability of the sympathetic nervous system. However, locus coeruleus sensitivity to high levels of corticotropin-releasing factor is *lowered* by prior stress exposure. This would presumably cause a paradoxical drop in sympathetic responsiveness to highly stressful conditions. Behaviorally, this paradoxical drop seems to correlate with a changeover from active to passive responding. Speculatively, the increases and decreases in stress sensitivity have been compared to the high level of arousal in posttraumatic stress disorder, and the behavioral inhibition of learned helplessness, respectively (A. L. Curtis, Pavcovich, & Valentino, 1999).

Not surprisingly, then, mast cells may be part of the machinery of the trigeminovascular response. Recall that in trigeminovascular activation, substance P and calcitonin gene-related peptide are secreted, causing distension, swelling, and irritation of cranial blood vessels. Of these effects, only a portion of the vasodilation is caused by the vasoactive peptides directly. Although not yet proven, it seems likely that a part of the dilation, and all of the irritation, at least in the dura mater, are mediated by histamine. Substance P and calcitonin gene-related peptide stimulate mast cells, which in turn release histamine, affecting the blood vessels (Ottosson & Edvinsson, 1997).

Now, corticotropin-releasing hormone CRH, which is secreted under stress, seems to cause intracranial mast cells to release histamine. In fact, the corticotropin-releasing hormone may actually be causing the secretion of substance P and calcitonin gene-related peptide and through them, mast cell degranulation (Theoharides, et al., 1995). The **triptans**, anti-migraine drugs which we will describe later, seem to block the changes in mast cells (Buzzi, Dimitriadou, Theoharides, & Moskowitz, 1992), which may account for the drugs' effectiveness.

Thus stress, via corticotropin-releasing hormone, may contribute directly to the trigeminovascular response. Olness and coworkers found that children who learned self-hypnosis techniques and reduced their migraine frequency, also had a decrease in a mast cell enzyme, tryptase. Because tryptase is found only in mast cells, its concentration in bodily fluids serves as a marker for mast cell activation (Galli & Lantz, 1999). Children in a waiting list control condition and children who did not practice relaxation or reduce migraine frequency had tryptase levels that held steady or increased. This fits with the idea that activation of mast cells and release of histamine may be a mechanism by which stress contributes to migraines (Olness, Hall, Rozniecki, W. Schmidt, & Theoharides, 1999).

We may note in passing that mast cells are found close to neurons in the skin, gastrointestinal tract and bladder, which may explain the role of stress as a risk factor in some cases of eczema, peptic ulcers, irritable bowel syndrome, and interstitial cystitis (Theoharides et al., 1995).

Another feature of the study by Olness, et al. deserves mention. Children who were successful in reducing migraines through self-hypnosis had higher baseline levels of tryptase (mean ≈ 1.82 ng/mL) than children who were unsuccessful (mean ≈ 0.86 ng/mL; $p < .02$). Moreover, the successful children also had a higher baseline tryptase level on average than the waiting list control group (mean ≈ 1.02 ng/mL; $p < .005$). Perhaps it is the indication of psychophysiological stress at baseline that distinguishes those who are most likely to benefit from treatment to reduce stress. In this small study, all four non-responders had baseline tryptase levels below 1.45 ng/mL, while 7 of 10 responders had baseline levels above this cutoff.

Implications.   If the results of Olness, et al. replicate, one could picture urinary tryptase levels as part of a screening battery for migraineurs. For those with baseline elevations, especially when there is comorbid asthma, allergy or eczema, typtase level could be an intermediate endpoint for gauging the adequacy of biofeedback training. And even before this day arrives, Olness et al's results serve as reminder that for different migraineurs, different underlying psychophysiological variables may be key.

For the investigations into migraine psychophysiology, which began with the vascular model, have led us far from a simple constrict-and-dilate picture. Instead, we are confronted with complexity, heterogeneity, and hints at how behavioral treatment might be refined in the future. That urinary tryptase, contingent negative variation, visual and auditory evoked potentials, quantitative EEG, and extra- and intracranial vascular reactivity, all identify a subset of migraineurs, suggests that the category "migraine" might be parsed into groups responsive to specific types of biofeedback.

Much of this belongs to the future. In the present, the range of variables alerts us to the variability and perhaps complexity of individual cases. As we have seen, the literature impels us to take a long view of stress and autonomic reactivity, with the possibility of a 4-day delay between stressor and migraine. We may do well, too, to look at how a migraineur is "using their brain." Are there rest breaks, or a quest for continuous, high intensity work? Does a feeling of mental fatigue precede a migraine? Such "cognitive pacing" might be relevant in people with sensory intolerance or who are prone to continuous vigilance (for example, from posttraumatic stress or generalized anxiety disorder). We might look, too, for signs of a vascular stress response, such as alterations in hand and, especially, pericranial (forehead, temple, or earlobe) temperature, when discussing a personally relevant stressor. Stressors that are merely endured rather than actively solved may be particularly relevant for gauging a vascular response.

Thus, we will want to look at the life stressors themselves. For as we have seen, it may not be a continuously high arousal level that distinguishes migraineurs, but a low baseline arousal against which stresses are particularly disruptive. Even diet should not be overlooked, for a high intake of dietary fats can promote platelet aggregation, and an overemphasis on refined grains might lead to a magnesium deficiency.

We will return to these topics later, when we consider triggers, and behavioral assessment and treatment.

TABLE 5-6 CHAPTER APPENDIX
Studies of Migraineurs during Exposure to Stress

Source	Subjects	Stressor	Measures	Results
C. D. Anderson & Franks, 1981	10 Migraine 10 Tension Headache 10 Controls	c. 6.5 min baseline 1 min standing 30 sec step-up exercise 16 min recovery c. 6.5 min silent serial 7's 16 min recovery	Heart Rate Systolic Blood Pressure Diastolic Blood Pressure L Finger Temperature R Finger Temperature Skin Conductance Level Frontalis EMG Wrist Extensor-Flexor EMG[3]	No differences between groups at baseline or during stressors. Baseline diastolic blood pressure correlated −.39 with ratings of in-session pain in migraineurs.
Anderson, Stoyva, & Vaughn, 1982	10 Hypertension 10 Rheumatoid Arthritis 10 Tension Headache 10 Migraine 10 Controls	2–3 min step-up exercise; 16 min recovery; 8.4 min silent serial 7's; 16 min recovery	Heart Rate Systolic Blood Pressure Diastolic Blood Pressure L Finger Temperature R Finger Temperature Electrodermal Frontalis EMG Wrist Extensor EMG Wrist Flexor EMG	Migraineurs had higher heart rates than the other groups in the sessions overall.
Andrasik, Blanchard, Arena, Saunders, & Barron, 1982	39 Migraine 62 Chronic Tension Headche 37 Mixed Headache 58 Controls Controls matched on numerous demographics	4 min baseline 4 min "relax body" 4 min "warm hand" 4 min "relax forehead" 1–4 min mental arithmetic 0.5–3 min 2nd baseline 1 min pleasant imagery 1 min stressful imagery 0.5–3 min 3rd baseline 1–7 min cold pressor task	Heart Rate Temporal Pulse Amplitude (R side or usual headache side) Finger Temperature Frontalis EMG Wrist Flexor EMG Skin Resistance Level	Only interaction involving diagnosis during stressors was for frontalis EMG. Nature of effect could not be determined as no follow-up (Tukey HSD) tests were significant.

TABLE 5-6 Chapter Appendix (Continued)

Source	Subjects	Stressor	Measures	Results
Arena, Blanchard, Andrasik, Appelbaum, & Myers, 1985	8 Migraine 12 Chronic Tension Headache 8 Combined Migraine, Tension HA Groups matched for demographics	Variable duration mental arithmetic; 6 min recovery; 1 min positive imagery; 1 min stressful imagery; 6 min recovery; 7 min cold pressor; 6 min recovery	Heart Rate R Temporal Pulse Amplitude Finger Temperature Electrodermal Frontalis EMG R Upper Trapezius EMG Wrist Flexor EMG	During cold pressor, chronic tension headache subjects increased temporal pulse amplitude while migraine and combined headache patients did not increase. During both imagery conditions migraineurs increased in temporal pulse amplitude more than did chronic tension headache patients.
M. J. Cohen, Rickles, & McArthur, 1978	13 Migraine or Mixed Headache 13 Controls matched for age, sex, and general SES	10 min rest; 7 min 67 db tones; 8 min time estimation test; 8 min reaction time test; 10 min mental arithmetic; Balloon inflation, burst; 10 min rest.	Heart Rate Cephalic temperature (near R temporal artery) Finger pulse amplitude Finger temperature Frontalis EMG Skin Conductance Level	Over session as a whole, migraineurs had higher finger temperature and cephalic temperature, and lower frontalis EMG. Migraineurs showed significant response stereotypy.
R. A. Cohen, D. A. Williamson, Monguillot, Hutchinson, Gottlieb, & Waters, 1983	12 Classic Migraine 12 Common Migraine 12 Muscle Contraction Headache 12 Mixed Headache 11 Non-Headache Controls Groups comparable in age and sex. Headache groups had the same average frequency of headaches.	10 min adaptation 3.5 min 70 db sounds 5 min adaptation 12 min stress (answering difficult questions out loud) 3 min adaptation brief 110 db siren 2 min recovery?	Heart Rate L Temporal Pulse Amplitude Finger Temperature Frontalis EMG Skin Potential	Subjects with headache diagnosis had higher finger temperature after relaxation and lower finger temperature during stress than non-headache controls. Classic migraine more reactive than common migraine on all measures.

Study	Subjects	Stressors	Measures	Results
Drummond, 1982	20 Migraine 20 Controls	2 min CO_2 rebreathing; 3 min recovery; 1 min cold pressor; 8 min recovery; 2 min mental arithmetic with noise; 3 min recovery; (Nonstress tasks not listed here.)	Heart Rate Systolic Blood Pressure Diastolic Blood Pressure Temporal Pulse Amplitude Forehead Temperature Respiration Rate	During mental arithmetic, temporal pulse amplitude increased in migraineurs and decreased in control subjects; forehead temperature increased less in migraineurs. During cold pressor, respiration rate decreased then increased in migraineurs; showed opposite pattern in controls. During CO_2 rebreathing, forehead temperature increased in migraine, not in controls.
Drummond, 1984	16 Migraine with temporal artery pain; 14 Migraine without temporal artery pain	2 min mental arithmetic; 4 min recovery; 1 min standing; 30–60 sec step-up exercise; 4 min recovery	Temporal Pulse Amplitude	During mental arithmetic, temporal pulse amplitude is higher in "extracranial" than in other migraineurs.
Drummond, 1985	10 Classical Migraine 10 Common Migraine 10 Episodic Tension Headache 10 Controls All subjects were female	4 min rest; 5 min mental arithmetic with 100 db tone for wrong answers; 4 min rest; 5 min reaction time test with 100 db tone for slow responses	Heart Rate Systolic Blood Pressure Diastolic Blood Pressure Temporal Pulse Amplitude on R or usual pain side B cheek temperature Respiration Rate	During stressors, temporal pulse amplitude increased only in classical migraine group; cheek temperature decreased in headache groups and increased in controls; respiration rate increased more in migraine than in tension headache subjects. During the 1st session, heart rate and systolic blood pressure increased more in migraine than in tension headache subjects, and more in classical than in common migraine. During first part of each stressor, temporal pulse amplitude increased more in migraine than in tension headache subjects.

(continued)

TABLE 5-6   Chapter Appendix (*Continued*)

Source	Subjects	Stressor	Measures	Results
Drummond, 1991	38 Unilateral Migraine	Body heating; 9 mins mental arithmetic	Microvascular Pulse Amplitude at L and R forehead and L and R cheeks; Perspiration at same 4 sites.	During body heating, pulse amplitude increased more on asymptomatic side. During mental arithmetic, largest pulse amplitude increase across trials was on the asymptomatic side.
Drummond, 1997	20 Migraine 21 Controls	Pressure pain to tolerance, 30 seconds at each of 8 sites; exposure to extremely bright light, 30 seconds; pressure pain + bright light, 30 seconds at each of 8 sites; 3 min rest between trials	L Forehead Pulse Amplitude; R Forehead Pulse Amplitude	Pulse amplitude increased more in migraineurs than in controls during pain. There was no clear effect of bright light.
Drummond, 2003	23 Migraine 22 Controls	3 30-second cold pressor trials at 4 minute intervals	L Temporal Pulse Amplitude R Temporal Pulse Amplitude	Pulse amplitude increased more in migraineurs than in controls before and after (but not during) 1st 2 trials.
Ellertsen & Hammerborg, 1982	8 Migraine 8 Controls Groups matched for gender, age and education	2 min baseline; c. 15 min of 95 dB, 1000 Hz tones at irregular intervals; 2 min recovery	Heart Rate L Temporal Pulse Amplitude R Temporal Pulse Amplitude	Migraineurs, but not controls, showed brief deceleration of heart rate at noise onset, and again 5 sec after noise offset. Decrease in temporal pulse amplitude during noise more pronounced in migraineurs.
Ellertsen, Nordby, Hammerborg, & Thorlacius, 1987	16 Migraine (6 Classic, 10 Common) 8 Headache-Free Controls All subjects female	2 min rest; 80 dB, 1000 Hz tones at irregular intervals	Heart Rate L Temporal Pulse Amplitude R Temporal Pulse Amplitude Hand Temperature Frontalis EMG	Decelerations in heart rate at 0–3 seconds and 4–8 seconds after noise onset were smaller in migraineurs. Decrease in temporal pulse amplitude more pronounced in migraineurs. EMG decreased over session in controls and increased in migraineurs.

Study	Participants	Procedure	Measures	Results
Feuerstein, Bush, & Corbisiero, 1982	11 Migraine 9 Muscle Contraction Headache 11 Mixed Headache 8 Controls	2 min baseline; 2 min silent practice of mental arithmetic; 2 min baseline; 2 min personal stress imagery; 2 min baseline; up to 6 min pressure pain; 1 min post-baseline	Heart Rate Temporal Pulse Amplitude Digital Pulse Amplitude Frontalis EMG Neck EMG # Skin Resistance Responses	No effects of diagnosis for mental arithmetic or pain tolerance. For stress imagery: diagnosis main effect for heart rate, post hoc tests could not locate source.
Gannon, Haynes, Cuevas, & Chavez, 1987	8 Migraine 8 Near-Daily Tension Headache 8 Controls Groups matched for gender and age	1 hour of speeded arithmetic with loud buzzer and failure feedback interspersed; 10 min recovery	Heart Rate Earlobe Pulse Amplitude Frontalis EMG Splenius Capitis EMG L Wrist Extensor EMG	Splenius capitis EMG higher in migraineurs during the stressor.
Gannon, Haynes, Safranek, & Hamilton, 1981	16 Migraine 13 Chronic Tension Headache 15 Controls Groups matched for gender and age	1 min mental arithmetic; 90 seconds arm ischemia; 10 min recovery after each stressor	Heart Rate Earlobe Pulse Amplitude Frontalis EMG L Wrist Extensor EMG	Migraineurs had slightly higher heart rates and slightly smaller change scores than the other two groups.
Goudswaard, Passchier, & Orlebeke, 1988	37 Common Migraine 37 Non-Headache Controls Groups matched for age, gender and likely were similar in SES.	Psychology course examination; 1.5 hour intelligence test; 10 min recovery after each stressor	Frontalis EMG Temporalis EMG Corrugator EMG (Absolute values, and as proportion of maximum voluntary contraction)	Corrugator EMG (as proportion of maximum voluntary contraction) higher in migraineurs during stress and post-stress.
Hassinger, Semenchuk, & O'Brien, 1999	26 Migraine 26 Control All Female Students	3 min cold pressor; 5 min recovery; 3 min serial 7's; 5 min recovery	Heart Rate Systolic Blood Pressure Diastolic Blood Pressure Stroke Volume Cardiac Output Total Peripheral Resistance	Significant main effect for diagnosis on MANOVA. Nature of effect unclear as no follow-up ANOVAs were significant.

(continued)

TABLE 5-6 Chapter Appendix (Continued)

Source	Subjects	Stressor	Measures	Results
Haynes, Gannon, Bank, Shelton, & Goodwin, 1990	5 Migraine 17 Chronic Tension Headache 14 Mixed Migraine-Tension Headache	1 hour of speeded arithmetic with loud buzzer and failure feedback interspersed; 10 min recovery	Blood Volume Pulse Amplitude at 6 Pericranial Sites	Migraineurs showed vasoconstriction and muscle contraction and mixed headache patients showed vasodilation at 3 sites (L frontal, R temporal, and R upper cervical)
Holm, Lamberty, McSherry, & P. A. Davis, 1997	30 Migraine 39 Chronic Tension-Type Headache 35 Control Subjects	12 min baseline; 4 min speech preparation; 2 minute speech; 12 minute recovery	Heart Rate Finger Temperature Frontalis EMG	No differences between groups during speech preparation. No measures were taken during the speech itself.
Kröner-Herwig, Dirk Diergarten, Dagmar Diergarten, & Seeger-Siewert, 1988	37 Migraine (M_{age} = 42 years) 44 Control Subjects (M_{age} = 35 years)	8 min industrial noise; 8 min of being viewed on a video monitor; 4 min recovery after each stressor	Temporal Pulse Amplitude. Thumb Pulse Amplitude Temporal Temperature Thumb Temperature Electrodermal	No between-group differences during the stressors. (Electrodermal not studied during the stressors.)
Kröner-Herwig, Fritsche, & Brauer, 1993	33 IHS Migraine without Tension-Type Headache 32 Control Subjects matched for age and gender	40 min achievement testing; 20 min recovery	Temporal Pulse Amplitude Digital Pulse Amplitude R Frontalis EMG Electrodermal	Temporal pulse amplitude: Control subjects constrict during stress, migraine subjects dilate during initial stresses and constrict during later stresses. Digital pulse amplitude: Coping self-statements decrease constriction in migraineurs and increase constriction in controls.

Study	Subjects	Procedure	Measures	Results
Leijdekkers & Passchier, 1990	26 Migraine without Aura 11 Migraine with Aura 34 Controls All subjects female; groups matched for age, education, social background.	1 min baseline c. 1 hour intelligence test post-stress interval	Heart Rate Temporal Pulse Amplitude from usual pain side, or random if no usual side Temporalis EMG from same side as pulse amplitude Skin Conductance	No main effects or interactions involving diagnosis.
P. R. Martin, Marie, & P. R. Nathan, 1992	19 Migraine 23 Tension Headache 13 Mixed Headache 14 Controls	10 min baseline 10 min anxiety/pain anticipation 10 min recovery 10 min listening to upbeat music	Heart Rate Temporal Artery Activity[1] Pulse Transit Time[2] Systolic Blood Pressure Diastolic Blood Pressure Frontalis EMG	Across study, migraineurs had highest diastolic blood pressure; migraineurs and mixed headache subjects had lowest pulse transit time.
Morley, 1985	12 Migraine 12 Control (patients from dental clinic) 75% Female	5 min baseline Reaction time Noise (96 db tones, 1 kHz, severely distorted) Safety-signal trials Personal stressful imagery Personal relaxing imagery Standard stressful imagery Standard relaxing imagery 3 min recovery	Heart Rate B. Temporal Pulse Amplitude Digital Pulse Amplitude Respiration Rate	Temporal pulse amplitude: More variability and different pattern on usual pain vs. non-pain side during baseline and reaction time tasks. Less constriction and more variability on pain side during noise task. Digital pulse amplitude response during reaction time task habituated more slowly in migraineurs.
Passchier, Goudswaard, & Orlebeke, 1993	37 Common Migraine 37 Control Subjects Groups matched on age and gender, from same student body	Psychology course examination; 1.5 hour intelligence test; 10 min recovery after each stressor	Heart Rate Temporal Pulse Amplitude Digital Pulse Amplitude Forehead Temperature Frontalis EMG Anterior Temporalis EMG Corrugator EMG Respiration Rate Skin Conductance Level # Skin Conductance Responses	Migraineurs had lower temporal pulse amplitudes than control subjects. Migraineurs had higher forehead temperature than controls during the intelligence test, and during the baseline for the intelligence test.

(continued)

TABLE 5–6 Chapter Appendix (Continued)

Source	Subjects	Stressor	Measures	Results
Passchier, van der Helm-Hylkema, & Orlebeke, 1984	59 Migraine 32 Tension Headache 26 Controls Groups equivalent in gender, education level and ? age	10 min baseline; 4 min personally relaxing imagery; 2 min rest; 4 min personally stressful imagery; 2 min rest; 6 min silent mental arithmetic; 5 min recovery	Heart Rate Temporal Pulse Amplitude Temporal Blood Volume Digital Pulse Amplitude Digital Blood Volume Frontalis EMG Respiration Rate Skin Conductance Level	Digital blood volume lower in male migraineurs than in control subjects during mental arithmetic. During stress imagery, male migraineurs did not show increase in digital blood volume; other 2 groups did.
Philips & M. S. Hunter, 1982	10 Psychiatric/Migraine 23 Psychiatric/Tension Headache 10 Psychiatric/Non–Headache 20 Non–Psychiatric/Non–Headache	4 min baseline 30 sec stress imagery 30 sec rest 30 sec neutral image 1 min rest 2 5-sec 85 db tones 1 min rest 6 60-db reaction time tones	R Temporal Pulse Amplitude* Frontalis EMG Temporalis EMG on R or usual pain side.	Stress imagery increased frontalis tension in headache subjects more than in controls. Repeating the image increased reactivity in tension headache and decreased reactivity in migraine.
Rojahn & Gerhards, 1986	20 Migraine 20 Control Subjects Groups matched on age and gender	57 seconds of aversive noise (85 dB); 5 min recovery	Heart Rate Temporal Pulse Amplitude Frontalis EMG	Temporal pulse amplitude response during stressor was stronger for people with migraines.
Stronks, Tulen, Verheij, Boomsma, Fekkes, Pepplinkhuizen, Mantel, & Passchier, 1998	23 Migraine 18 Tension-Type Headache 22 Non–Headache Controls	5 min baseline 3 15-min periods of mental arithmetic 20 min recovery	Heart Rate Systolic Blood Pressure Diastolic Blood Pressure Temporal Pulse Amplitude Frontalis EMG Plasma Catecholamines Plasma Serotonin Plasma 5-HIAA Platelet Serotonin	Migraine group had higher overall frontalis EMG and systolic blood pressure, with trend for higher diastolic blood pressure. No group differences on temporal pulse amplitude, but much data loss on this measure.

Study	Sample	Conditions	Measures	Results
Thompson & Adams, 1984	8 Migraine 8 Muscle Contraction Headache 8 Controls	½ min baseline 2 min thinking of personal stress imagery 1 min baseline 2 min feeling personal stress imagery 1 min baseline (similar conditions for personally relaxing scene, and then imagining a typical day)	Heart Rate L Temporal Pulse Amplitude R Temporal Pulse Amplitude Electrodermal Frontalis EMG L Temporalis EMG R Temporalis EMG	No differences between migraine and control groups.
D. E. Williams, Raczynski, & Domino, & J. P. Davis, 1993	24 Migraine 24 Muscle Contraction Headache 24 Controls All groups matched on gender and age. The two headache groups were also matched on number of headaches per week.	3 min baseline 3 min silent serial 7's during exposure to 70 db tone.	Heart Rate B Temporal Pulse Amplitude B Frontalis EMG B Upper Cervical Paraspinal EMG	No main effects or interactions involving migraine diagnosis.

Notes.
*Could not be scored during 85 db tone due to artifacts.
[1]Minimum, maximum, and average distension of temporal artery.
[2]Time interval between EKG R-wave and pulse; inversely related to systolic blood pressure and, less so, to diastolic blood pressure.
[3]EMG read from forearm as a whole. One active site was placed over the wrist extensors, and one over the wrist flexors.

CHAPTER 6

Tension-Type Headaches

> *In every case of unexplained persistent pain, the proper scientific and therapeutic tactic is to search the periphery for some undiscovered source and, if this proves negative, to proceed centrally and to question the state of the [pain] control mechanisms.*
> —Melzack and Wall (1996, p. 189)

Brian used to have "regular" headaches that would go away with aspirin or acetaminophen, but for the last 11 years the dull pressure pain has been continuous. When his boss comes in to work, Brian feels the tight, achy fatigue spreading from the base of his skull, which is always tender and uncomfortable, up the back of his head, and over the vertex to the front. His brain feels tired, too, and although he has never missed work for a headache, it is hard for him to concentrate when there is so much pain. Hunger, fluorescent lights, and the computer screen all seem to make it worse. Narcotics help a little, and he takes them daily, but he is mostly immune to them now. At night, he rests while his wife plays quietly with the children. That's all his life has been for years—going through the motions at work, and sleeping.

In the IHS diagnostic criteria, tension-type headaches are, broadly, everything that migraines are not. The pain of tension-type headaches is usually bilateral, mild in intensity, continuous, pressing or tightening in quality, and not aggravated by routine physical activity. Nausea, vomiting, photophobia (light intolerance), and phonophobia (intolerance for conversational sound levels) are rarely present. At least ten such episodes must have occurred over a person's lifetime to warrant the diagnosis. When the headaches take place on at least 15 days of the month, the disorder is termed "chronic tension-type headache;" otherwise the diagnosis is of "episodic tension-type headache." The episodic category is further divided into "infrequent episodic" (averaging less than one headache day per month) and "frequent episodic" (averaging 1–14 headache days per month).

With the transition from episodic to chronic, the frequent, pressing pain also seems to become more intrusive, oppressive, inescapable. Although patients usually continue to function at work and at home, most of their thoughts may be with the pain. The toll on quality of life can be severe. In the clinic, depression and anxiety are common (K. A. Holroyd, Stensland, Lipchik, Hill, O'Donnell, & Cordingley, 2000). It may have been years since the patient felt that they were emotionally present in their own lives.

PREVALENCE

The societal importance of tension-type headaches derives in part from their sheer number for, by any measure, they are extremely common. Lifetime prevalence in men has been estimated at 70 percent, and in women 90 percent (B. K. Rasmussen, R. Jensen, Schroll, & J. Olesen, 1991).

One-year prevalence for episodic tension-type headache appears to be 36.3 percent in men and 42.0 percent in women, and for chronic tension-type headache 1.4 percent in men and 2.8 percent in women (B. S. Schwartz, Stewart, Simon & Lipton, 1998). Even point prevalence of headaches ("do you have a headache today?") is high, estimated at 11 percent for males and 22 percent for females by Rasmussen et al. (1991).

Moreover, there is no requirement that tension-type headaches be occasional or mild. In a population survey, the proportion of respondents indicating lost work days due to tension-type headache was 8.3 percent of those with the episodic form, and 11.8 percent of those with the chronic form, of the disorder (B. S. Schwartz, Stewart, Simon & Lipton, 1998). For people with chronic tension-type headache, health-related quality of life as measured with the SF–36, seems to be as low as it is for migraineurs, even after controlling for anxiety, depression, and number of comorbid chronic illnesses (S.-J. Wang, Fuh, S.-R. Lu, & Juang, 2001).

In episodic tension-type headache, there is no detectable influence of genes; the concordance rates for monozygotic and dizygotic twins are nearly identical (Ulrich, Gervil, & J. Olesen, 2004). A gentic loading for chronic tension-type headache is more likely, as first degree relatives of sufferers have a three-fold higher risk of the disorder than do spouses or members of the general population (Østergaard, M. B. Russell, Bendtsen, & J. Olesen, 1997).

For reasons that are quite unclear, education seems to be a risk factor for episodic tension-type headache. Prevalence rates for the headaches increase steadily with amount of schooling, so that men with post-college education have 2.6 times the risk as men who stopped at grade school. Women who went beyond college had 1.9 times the risk of episodic tension-type headache as women with a grade school education (B. S. Schwartz, Stewart, Simon & Lipton, 1998). Presumably, education is serving as a marker for socioeconomic status, but it is just as unclear why a high SES would confer risk.

In Chapter 4, we saw evidence that there has been a recent, sharp increase in the prevalence of migraine in adolescents. Fewer studies shed light on tension-type headache but these, too, may be consistent with a rise in cases. Specifically, Linet and coworkers interviewed a large community-based sample of young adults in 1986 and 1987. Among subjects who were 12–23 years old, 11 percent (6 percent of the males and 13 percent of the females) reported at least 4 headaches in the previous month (Linet, Stewart, Celentano, D. Ziegler, & Sprecher, 1989). This includes migraines, but presumably the majority of headaches were tension-type. Rhee (2000) analyzed data from a similar large-scale study conducted in 1995, and found that a full 30 percent of her sample aged 11–21 had reported headaches occurring at least weekly over the past year. Certainly much more research is needed. The larger recall period in the data Rhee examined (1 year vs. 1 month) may have invited higher, more impressionistic estimates from subjects. It is possible that a high incidence of migraines may have inordinately influenced the results. If tension-type headaches are increasing in frequency, we do not know why. With all its shortcomings, the data are a reminder that prevalence of headaches, like the prevalence of an infectious disease, need not be static.

PATHOPHYSIOLOGY

Muscle pain is usually dull, aching, and cramping in quality. Thus, tension-type headaches are subjectively similar to myofascial pain. Moreover, when a headache can be unambiguously attributed to myofascial pain of the neck, it is defined as a tension-type headache under IHS criteria. Nonetheless, the outcome of controlled studies has been more complex than this. It appears that tension-type headache can be due to myofascial pain, or to a disruption of central pain regulatory systems.

Palpation of Muscles

As a starting point, consider the findings of Rigor Jensen, Jes Olesen and coworkers on muscle tenderness. Jensen found that individuals with infrequent, episodic tension-type headache (≤ 14 days per year) had far greater pericranial tenderness to palpation ($p < 10-5$) than controls (R. Jensen, 1995). The tenderness increased still further during a headache. Moreover, tenderness correlates with the frequency and severity of tension-type headaches (R. Jensen, 1999b).

Which muscles are affected? In a similar study of 14 pericranial sites, greatest tenderness to manual palpation was shown by (for females, in descending order): the trapezius (at the top of the shoulder), the hamulus pterygoid, the **sternocleidomastoid** (at the side of the neck, used for cervical rotation), the posterior neck muscle insertions, and the lateral pterygoid (used for chewing). For males the muscles showing greatest tenderness were the same, although in a slightly different order. For both genders, the least tender muscles (out of the 14 tested) were the frontalis, the posterior and anterior temporalis, and the posterior rectus capitis (at the base of the skull; R. Jensen, B. K. Rasmussen, Pedersen, Lous, & J. Olesen, 1992). Lous and J. Olesen (1982) report similar results, but with greater tenderness at the temporalis. Again, no tenderness was found at the forehead. (The location of major pericranial muscles is shown in Figure 6–1.)

Now, people often experience tension-type headaches at the forehead and temples—the least tender sites in the two palpation studies. This contrast requires explanation, and we will return to it shortly.

In the Jensen (1995) study, pressure and heat pain thresholds at the hands did not differ between controls and individuals with tension-type headache, even when the latter were having a headache. This suggests that a central mechanism, if present, is not global but restricted to head pain. However, this restriction is probably not true of all headache-prone individuals. Peres et al. report that 36 percent of their tertiary care patients with transformed migraine, especially those with depression, insomnia, and disabling headaches, had fibromyalgia as a comorbid condition (Peres, W. B. Young, Kaup, Zukerman, & Silberstein, 2001). And Okifuji and coworkers found that in their tertiary-care chronic pain program, 40 percent of headache patients (most with migraine or migraine plus tension-type headache diagnoses) showed tenderness to palpation at 11 or more of the 18 classic **tender points** for fibromyalgia (Okifuji, D. C. Turk, & Marcus, 1999). Fibromyalgia tender points are found in such disparate locations as the upper and lower back and the inside of the knees (Wolfe, et al., 1990). The headache patients did not actually have fibromyalgia, because they did not have widespread pain outside of palpation. However, they were clearly evincing a non-localized hyperalgesia. It is not known whether the condition would evolve into fibromyalgia over time. It is also not known whether these individuals, who have both headaches and widespread tenderness, require different treatments than individuals whose pain sensitivity is restricted to the head (Okifuji et al.).

The finding of pericranial muscle tenderness seems to point, of course, to the muscles. However, tenderness is also found in fibromyalgia, which is almost certainly a disorder of the *central* processing of sensory information from the muscles (Goldenberg, 1999) or of aversive stimulation in general (McDermid, Rollman, & McCain, 1996; Quimby, S. Block, & Gratwick, 1988). Moreover, in the tenderness of tension-type headache, pain intensity is a linear function of pressure. This suggests that signals from low threshold mechanosensitive neurons in the dorsal horn have been re-routed through pain pathways (Bendtsen, R. Jensen, & J. Olesen, 1996b; also see Chapter 2 above). Further, when nitric oxide synthesis is blocked in tension-type headache, possibly disrupting sensitization in the trigeminal nucleus, pericranial muscle hardness declines (Ashina, Bendtsen, R. Jensen, Lassen, Sakai, & J. Olesen, 1999). Thus, muscle hardness and tenderness may be central and not peripheral phenomena.

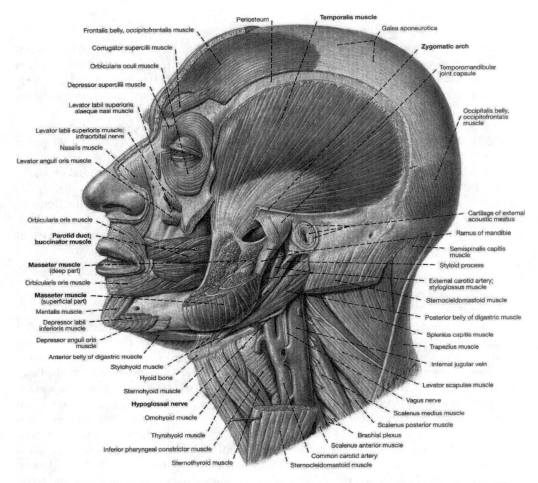

FIGURE 6–1.   Pericranial muscles. From *Anatomy: A Regional Atlas of the Human Body* (4th ed., plate 467) by C. D. Clemente, 1997, Baltimore: Williams and Wilkins. From Putz/Pabst: Sobotta, Atlas der Anatomie des Menschen, 22nd edition. Copyright Elsevier GmbH. Reprinted with permission.

Surface EMG

A more direct measure of muscle involvement is provided by surface EMG. Active muscle contraction is accomplished through the propagation of action potentials down the muscle fibers. These muscle action potentials are self-replicating spikes in voltage that are similar to the action potentials that propagate along the axons of nerve cells. As the surrounding tissue is mostly water, a conductor of electricity, the voltage spikes can be detected at the skin (Basmajian & De Luca, 1985). In surface EMG, the voltage change as measured at the skin is roughly the sum of motor action potentials taking place in a given area of nearby muscle, over a given period of time. The more forcefully a muscle is contracting, the greater the number of muscle cells taking part in the contraction, and the greater the frequency with which those muscle cells fire. As a result, surface EMG readings increase along with the force of contraction (Basmajian & De Luca, 1985).

In fact, as we will see in Chapter 12, surface EMG at the upper trapezius is a *linear* function of the force of contraction, provided that surface EMG and force are both measured as a percent of their maximum attainable values.

Not all muscle contraction is active in this way. In contractures, for example after a stroke, acetylcholine leaks slowly across the **neuromuscular junction**, causing a gradual shortening of the muscle fibers, rather than action potentials. Unlike active contractions, contractures are electrically silent to surface EMG.

Schoenen has suggested that studies conducted before 1985 are about evenly divided between those finding an EMG abnormality, and those which do not, while in more recent studies EMG elevations have generally been found (Schoenen, 1997). This shift may be due to improved instrumentation, greater diagnostic clarity since the 1988 IHS criteria, or more appreciation of the need to check posterior cervical muscles and the upper trapezius, and not simply the frontalis and temporalis. But the relationship between surface EMG and tension-type headache is far from clear, and hence we must delve more deeply into the literature.

I have found only one meta-analysis on the role of EMG. This will be supplemented by several well-designed recent studies by R. Jensen and coworkers.

Meta-analysis.   Wittrock (1997) analyzed 28 studies in which subjects with tension-type headache were compared with those without a headache diagnosis on baseline frontalis surface EMG levels. He found a moderate and statistically significant effect size for headache diagnosis ($d \approx 0.4$). There was a suggestion in the data that the effect was due to subjects who were having a headache at the time of the assessment. The best discrimination between subjects with and without a headache diagnosis seemed to come from studies in which the subjects had their eyes closed, were sitting (versus reclining) and were not anticipating a stressor (studies of effects of position versus effects of stress).

Episodic.   Jensen (1995) found that, compared with age- and sex-matched healthy controls, individuals with frequent ($>$14 days/year) episodic tension-type headache had higher pericranial EMG readings even when not having a headache. The readings did not further increase during a headache.

Chronic.   Jensen et al. (1994), in a large-scale population study, found that individuals with chronic tension-type headache had greater pericranial muscle tenderness to palpation, lower maximal voluntary contraction, and a lower mean frequency in the surface EMG power spectrum, compared with episodic tension-type headache, and with healthy controls. Resting surface EMG amplitude did not differ between the two groups. Jensen et al. interpret the results as being consistent with muscle fatigue.

Nonetheless, in both studies the EMG changes appear relatively small, and hence may not characterize many of the headache subjects. Moreover, Schoenen (1997) notes that in individual patients, EMG changes often do not correlate with level, location, or timing of pain, or with pain threshold.

Yet we cannot discount the role of muscular factors. Muscle pain is hard to localize and is often referred. Hence it may not be important for EMG elevations to correlate spatially with the pain. The forehead and temple are areas to which myofascial **trigger points** often refer pain, but they are rarely the locus of trigger points (Jaeger, 1994; Simons & Mense, 1998). Similarly, it seems noteworthy that the overwhelming majority of EMG studies (including treatment studies) in psychology have focused on the frontalis (Arena & Blanchard, 1996) which, as noted above, appears to be one of the *least* sensitive of the pericranial muscles to palpation.

When different sites have been compared empirically for their ability to distinguish people with tension-type headache, results have been mixed. Philips, for example, studied four muscles at rest (frontalis, temporalis, neck, and trapezius), and found that only the frontalis and temporalis showed elevated surface EMG readings (C. Philips, 1977). It may be relevant that many of the subjects had the chronic form of tension-type headache, as a minimum of two headache days per week was required for entry into the study. On the other hand, the results were not replicated by Hudzinski and Lawrence (1988), who studied people with at least 3 tension headaches per week. Hudzinski and Lawrence found better discrimination with electrodes at the cervical paraspinals than at the frontalis. The best discrimination, however, was achieved with the Schwartz-Mayo placement, designed to measure muscle tension from the pericranial region as a whole.

For clinical work, a sensor placement that reads broadly from the head and neck region may allow us to sidestep questions of exactly which muscles to read. For basic research, a further comparison of individual muscles seems reasonable. But before investing too much energy in this line of investigation we should first step back and ask a more basic question: Should the extent of EMG elevation correlate at all with the amount of pain? For there are at least six broad theories about the cause of muscle pain, each with its own implications for surface EMG.

SURFACE EMG AND MUSCLE PAIN

The first theory is of global muscle fatigue. Muscles cannot sustain loads of greater than 8–10 percent of maximum voluntary contraction (MVC; Westgaard, 1999a). Hence, sustained readings above, say, 25 microvolts in a muscle whose MVC is 250 microvolts implies fatigue as a source of pain. Still, although this theory is intuitively plausible, it must contend with the observation that muscle fatigue leads to an increase in pressure pain thresholds, at least short term, in healthy individuals, at the upper trapezius and deltoid muscles (Persson, Hansson, Kalliomäki, Moritz, & Sjölund, 2000). Similarly, Nakata and coworkers found that over a two hour work task, EMG levels and pressure pain thresholds were positively correlated: Research participants with higher muscle tension also had greater resistance to pain from palpation ($r = 0.62$; Nakata, Hagner, & Jonsson, 1993). This study, too, included only healthy participants and this may be key. As we have seen, people with fibromyalgia show an increase in sensitivity to pressure pain after muscle contraction (Kosek, Ekholm, & Hansson, 1996).

Moreover, studies of pain thresholds during muscle fatigue have indeed been short-term: The contraction may be sustained for only 1½ minutes (Persson et al., 2000). Hence, in a second theory, muscle pain is derived from contraction that is sustained. Possibly, the long-term contraction leads to a gradual sensitization of nociceptive pathways, or a gradual wearing down of inhibitory controls. Thus, in a study of female keyboard operators, whose job presumably involves maintaining some degree of upper trapezius tension, pressure pain thresholds decreased over the workday and over the work week (Onishi, Sakai, & Kogi, 1982). A decline was not seen in a similar study that lasted for only two hours (Nakata et al., 1993).

The third model combines aspects of the "fatigue" and "sustained contraction" theories. Motor units in a muscle are thought to have characteristic thresholds. A low amplitude contraction will involve few motor units and hence give only a weak reading on surface EMG. However, the contraction will always involve the same, low-threshold motor units. Thus, in a sustained, low-grade contraction, a few chronically activated motor units can fatigue and cause considerable pain without producing a strong electric field to surface electrodes (R. Jensen, 1999a; Westgaard, 1999b). Consistent with this, shoulder and neck discomfort in office workers correlates positively with static (i.e., sustained levels of) surface EMG, over the range of 0–5 percent of maximum voluntary contraction (Westgaard, 1999b).

On surface EMG, overuse of a few motor units may show up as a constant level of activation without very brief gaps in the signal. Westgaard and coworkers found that brief gaps (to below 0.5 percent of MVC) at times correspond to a switching of activation between motor units (Westgaard & De Luca, 1997) and appear to confer some resistance to the development of upper trapezius pain among workers (Veiersted, Westgaard, & Andersen, 1993).

The power spectrum in surface EMG—the distribution of energy across frequencies—may also be relevant. Van Boxtel (2001) notes that for a lightly contracting muscle, the power spectrum depends in part on the firing rates of the individual motor units. If a motor unit is firing at 32 Hz., it will contribute to the power spectrum at 32 Hz. Now, if a lot of motor units are firing at different rates, or if the rate of each motor unit keeps changing (such as during a dynamic contraction), the influence of firing rate washes out. But if just a few units are firing at a constant rate, then this rate will show up as a sharp peak in the power spectrum, generally somewhere between 20 and 45 Hz. Of course if just a few motor units are firing, they will presumably be the low threshold units. And while Van Boxtel did not find such peaks at the temporalis, the masseter, or the splenius capitis, they were the rule at the frontalis and the corrugator supercilii (Van Boxtel, 2001). These are also the muscles that tend to show spontaneous activity during mental effort (Van Boxtel & Jessurun, 1993; Waterink & Van Boxtel, 1994). Now, Van Boxtel was not looking for switching of activation between motor units. However, the fact that the frontalis and corrugator are susceptible to sustained, low level contractions sets the stage for isolated fatigue as an explanation for muscle pain there.

A fourth theory is based on a series of studies by Larsson and coworkers on blood circulation in painful muscles. Using Laser-Doppler flowmetry, for example, they found that microcirculation is reduced in trapezius myalgia (e.g., R. Larsson, Öberg, & S.-E. Larsson, 1999). The muscle was not contracting strongly enough for the internal pressure to impair blood flow. Rather, they suggest that the reduction is under neural control, and causes muscle fatigue and a compensatory increase in surface EMG readings. Even though the muscle tension is secondary to the circulation disturbance, however, it is not necessarily benign. The extra load on an already tired muscle could aggravate the pain (R. Larsson, Öberg, et al., 1999).

In the fifth theory, muscle pain in tension-type headache is due to myofascial trigger points, especially in the trapezius, sternocleidomastoid, masseter, and posterior cervical muscles (Jaeger, 1994; Simons & Mense, 1998). Trigger points are only c. 1–2 mm in diameter (Hubbard & Berkoff, 1993) and hence their signal on a surface electrode would be very small. On needle electrodes, trigger points may show brief spikes of activation (Travell & Simons, 1983) and possibly a very fortuitously placed surface electrode might pick this up. Alternatively, Donaldson and coworkers report 80 percent correct classification of muscles for presence versus absence of trigger points using dynamic surface EMG: During what would be an otherwise symmetrical motion (i.e., cervical flexion and extension), a muscle with a trigger point (upper trapezius at C4–5–6 level, sternocleidomastoid) showed a much stronger contraction than the contralateral side (Donaldson, Skubick, Clasby, & Cram, 1994). Note, however, that in neither approach to trigger points is the resting surface EMG level assumed to be diagnostic. In contrast, Kraft et al. do report higher resting levels, but I believe the amount of elevation is small (Kraft, Johnson, & LaBan, 1968).

A sixth possibility is that the experience of muscle pain and tension in tension-type headache derives not from the activation of the main, extrafusal fibers read by surface EMG, but from the activation of **intrafusal fibers** within the **muscle spindle**. Muscle spindles are sensory organs in the muscle that appear to detect length and velocity, i.e., stretch. Hubbard and Berkoff (1993), using needle EMG for precisely localized recordings, found muscle spindles showed spontaneous activity, and that the activity was higher in individuals with chronic tension-type headache than in control subjects. The idea that pain derives from muscle spindles may turn out to be the same as the trigger point hypothesis. The anatomical nature of trigger points has not been definitely established, and muscle spindles are a reasonable guess (Hubbard & Berkoff, 1993). However, Simons (1996) argues that trigger points are a dysfunction of the neuromuscular junction, and that Hubbard and Berkoff's recordings are actually indications of such dysfunctional motor endplates.

OTHER STUDIES OF MUSCLE TENSION

Other evidence suggests that muscle tension plays a role. For example, injection of botulinum toxin into pericranial muscles may (this is controversial; Schulte-Mattler, Krack, & BoNTTH Study Group, 2004) reduce a tension-type headache (Cheshire, Abashian, & Mann, 1994). Botulinum toxin works at the neuromuscular junction to induce a local paralysis—an extreme form of muscle relaxation.

In an experimental study of headaches, Jensen and Olesen asked volunteers to clench their back teeth lightly for 30 minutes. Over the next 24 hours, 69 percent of those having tension-type headache at least 14 days per year, and only 17 percent of control subjects, developed a headache. Increased tenderness 90 minutes after the jaw clenching was a good predictor of which subjects would go on to have a headache (Jensen & Olesen, 1996). Thus, relatively low levels of muscle tension may play a causal role for people who are already susceptible to tension-type headache. (Of course an additional implication of the study is that clenching one's teeth as a behavioral response to stress may cause tension-type headaches; Jensen, 1999b). A branch of the trigeminal nerve, called the zygomaticotemporal branch, passes through the temporalis muscle, and in theory could be become compressed when the muscle is taut (Guyuron, Tucker, & J. Davis, 2002). Thus, tension at the temporalis could irritate the trigeminal nerve, and perhaps this is enough to incite a sterile inflammatory response (Guyuron et al.).

Yet these studies are by no means conclusive. Botulinum toxin could have additional, previously unsuspected mechanisms of action. For example, there is some evidence that it can block the secretion of substance P, a neurotransmitter involved in pain pathways (Göbel, Heinze, Heinze-Kuhn, & Austermann, 2001). Moreover, it is sometimes difficult to separate the treatment and placebo effects of botulinum toxin because subjects notice that their muscles have been weakened. And jaw clenching, too, is in part a cognitive intervention because research participants may believe (and informed consent procedures may require that they be told) that jaw clenching can cause a headache. In fact, K. A. Holroyd and coworkers found that a placebo condition, holding a toothpick lightly between one's lips while watching a stress management video, produced as many headaches as prolonged jaw clenching (Neufeld, K. A. Holroyd, & Lipchik, 2000).

We may be on safest grounds if we assume that peripheral and central factors may both be present. Hu et al., studying rats, found that prolonged stimulation of craniofacial muscle nociceptive afferents produces a long-lasting facilitation of trigeminal nociceptive neurons (J. W. Hu, Sessle, Raboisson, Dallel, & Woda, 1992). That is, a central hyperalgesia specific to the trigeminal tract may follow sustained myofascial pain. Once sensitization has developed, even very low frequency nociceptive input may help to maintain it (J. Li, Simone, & A. Larsson, 1999). Thus, the categories "with" and "without disorder of the pericranial muscles" may actually be the two ends of a peripheral—central continuum. As tension-type headaches become more frequent, central sensitization may become a more important contributor (Jensen 1999b).

Exteroceptive Suppression Reflex

Central pain sensitivity in tension-type headache has been studied in several ways, among them the EMG **exteroceptive suppression reflex** (Schoenen, 1993). A subject, attempting to maintain continuous muscle tension in the masseter or temporalis by biting down, will show two, brief, reflexive lapses in activation following a very mild electrical shock near the lips. Exteroceptive suppression is a jaw-opening reflex in response to pain, a form of withdrawal from the painful stimulus, and appears to be centrally-mediated through nociceptive pathways. Although findings have been mixed, the second of the two lapses (ES2, or second exteroceptive suppression period) seems to be abbreviated or missing in some subjects with *chronic* tension-type headache (Schoenen, Jamart, Gerard, Lenarduzzi, & Delwaide, 1987). An absence of suppression implies hyperexcitability of the muscle, or of the associated motor neurons (Sharav, 1999). Thus, it is not surprising that EMG biofeedback may normalize the ES2 response (Schoenen, 1993). In one biofeedback study, the degree of improvement in the ES2 correlated across subjects with the degree of improvement in headaches (Schoenen, 1993). This could be important, as a way of studying control of temporalis muscle activity, and as a way of researching inhibitory processes in the brain stem, in tension-type headache (Schoenen, Jamart, et al.).

Having said this, we should note that the ES2 literature is clouded by conflicting findings. There have been both replications (e.g., Schepelmann, Dannhausen, Kötter, Schabet, & Dichgans, 1998; Wallasch, Reinecke, & Langohr, 1991) and failures to replicate (e.g., Aktekin, Yaltkaya, Ozkaynak, & Oguz, 2001; Bendtsen, R. Jensen, Brennum, Arendt-Nielsen, & J. Olesen, 1996) Schoenen's results. Among the explanations that have been considered are: (1) The effect may be sensitive to small changes in methodology. For example, it might be apparent only when the eliciting shock is quite weak, or when subjects remain relaxed. (2) The attenuation in ES2 might be apparent only in older subjects, and might be due to long-term medication use. And (3) the attenuation may be due to factors that are comorbid with tension-type headache, such as depression (Aktekin, et al.; Tataroglu, Kanik, Sahin, Özge, Yalçinkaya & Idiman, 2002). Also, amitriptyline, a commonly prescribed medication for chronic tension-type headache, itself seems to reduce the exteroceptive suppression reflex, and may cloud the results of some studies (Bendtsen, R. Jensen, & J. Olesen, 1996a). Moreover, it is not clear whether the shortening of the ES2 is specific to tension-type headache. Some investigators have found similar results in migraineurs during a migraine episode, and in patients with temporomandibular dysfunction (De Laat, P. Svensson, & Macaluso, 1998; Tataroglu, et al.).

DESCENDING PAIN INHIBITION

If tension-type headaches indeed involve an increased sensitivity to muscle pain, the sensitivity could be due to lower levels of descending pain inhibition. In chronic tension-type headache, it appears that diffuse noxious inhibitory controls, in which pain at one location blocks perception of pain elsewhere in the body, is impaired (Pielsticker, Haag, Zaudig, & Lautenbacher, 2005). And because diffuse noxious inhibitory controls are mediated by endorphins, a person with tension-type headache might show lower endorphin levels in the descending pain pathways. Now, currently we do not have a way to measure these levels. However, endorphins are also found in a type of white blood cell called the mononuclear cell, and hence perhaps the endorphin levels in these mononuclear cells could be used as a surrogate measure.

Now it is not at all intuitively obvious that levels of a neurotransmitter in a type of white blood cell should reflect the levels in a particular neural pathway. However, there is indeed some evidence that the amount of a particular endorphin, beta-endorphin, are markedly lower in the mononuclear cells of people with tension-type headache, measured between headache episodes (Battistella, Bordin, et al., 1996; Mazzotta, Sarchielli, Gaggioli, & Gallai, 1997). For example, in the study by Mazzotta et al., 73 percent of the patients with episodic tension-type headache had a beta-endorphin level that was at least two standard deviations below the control group mean.

In the study by Battistella et al., of children, the endorphin levels in tension-type headache were less than half the level found in healthy controls. Even more, Mazzotta et al. found that the level of beta-endorphin in mononuclear cells correlated highly with pressure pain threshold in both the headache patients ($r = 0.77, p < .0001$) and in the controls ($r = 0.81, p < .0001$). There is a little bit of evidence, at least for migraines, that behavior therapy increases endorphin levels (Helm-Hylkema, Orlebeke, Enting, Thijssen, & van Ree, 1990).

Another finding might fit with a loss of pain inhibition. In chronic tension-type headache, there may be loss of gray matter in numerous pain processing regions. Medications do not seem to be the culprit, because the loss is not seen in medication-overuse headache (Schmidt-Wilcke et al., 2005). Whether this structural change plays a role in the pathophysiology of the pain has not yet been established. Both regions that represent pain (e.g., Brodmann Area 24 of anterior cingulate cortex) and those that inhibit it (the periaqueductal gray) show the same, subtle atrophy. However, the evidence that circulating endorphins, diffuse noxious inhibitory controls, and tissue volume in the periaqueductal gray are all reduced, seems to converge on a loss of endorphinergic tone in at least a subset of patients with chronic tension-type headache.

PSYCHOPHYSIOLOGY OF MUSCLE PAIN

The IHS criteria reflect the potentially key etiologic role of emotional stress, anxiety and depression. These factors may potentially influence both peripheral and central aspects of pain.

Peripheral aspects.   **Trigger points**, at least in the upper trapezius, appear to receive direct sympathetic innervation, via alpha-adrenergic fibers (Hubbard, 1996; Rivner, 2001). In humans, McNulty and coworkers report that a mental arithmetic task that was stressful enough to raise people's **skin conductance level** also caused an increase in needle EMG readings from a trigger point in the upper trapezius. A nearby control site outside of the trigger point did not show a differential response to stress (McNulty, Gevirtz, Hubbard, & Berkoff, 1994). Conversely, the band of muscle in which a trigger point occurs loses its tautness after blockade of the (sympathetic) stellate ganglion (A. Bengtsson & M. Bengtsson, 1988). Moreover, Banks et al. found that trigger point needle EMG activity declined sharply with brief autogenics-type relaxation training (Banks, D. W. Jacobs, Gevirtz, & Hubbard, 1998). During the autogenics, finger temperature (a measure of relaxation) was negatively correlated with trigger point activity ($r = -0.55, p = .012$). It seems likely, then, that myofascial pain has a stress-linked component, at least in the upper trapezius.

The functioning of muscle spindles, possibly the anatomic basis of trigger points, is also affected by sympathetic activity (Roatta, Windhorst, Ljubisavljevic, Johansson, & Passatore, 2002). This could allow stress to participate indirectly in muscle pain, by altering how signals from the muscle are processed (Arezzo, 2002) or by disrupting proprioceptive feedback, causing abnormal patterns of muscle use (Roatta et al.).

In other studies, cognitive stress such as sustained vigilance seems to lead to increased trapezius activation, with a monotonic dose-response curve (Waersted, Bøjrklund, & Westgaard, 1994; Waersted & Westgaard, 1996). This effect seems to be potentiated when the muscle is simultaneously handling a physical task (Lundberg et al., 1994). Single motor units may remain active continuously over a 10-minute cognitive task (Waersted, Eken, & Westgaard, 1992).

Strong emotions such as anger and fear appear to increase trapezius muscle activation, perhaps through brain stem mechanisms (Westgaard, 1996). Moreover, people may show voluntary, habitual tensing of certain muscles during stress, as a learned behavior (e.g., jaw clenching; Gramling, Grayson, Sullivan, & Schwartz, 1997).

And psychosocial stress may be a risk factor, albeit small, for reduced upper trapezius microcirculation (R. Larsson, Zhang, Hongming, Öberg, & S.-E. Larsson, 1998).

Central aspects.   Workers who report higher levels of psychosocial stress also report greater neck and shoulder discomfort, particularly subjective tension. We might assume that this is mediated through higher trapezius surface EMG readings. Actually, however, psychosocial stress and static surface EMG readings appear to make separate, additive contributions to neck and shoulder symptoms. Moreover, subjective tension and actual EMG readings do not correlate (Westgaard, 1999b).

Compared with pain from cutaneous receptors, muscle pain is regulated to a greater degree by descending inhibitory controls (Mense, 1993). It seems possible, then, that muscle pain could be particularly susceptible to changes in descending inhibition, for example by psychological factors.

Now, we might presume that looking at a brain stem reflex, such as the second exteroceptive silent period (ES2), would allow us to examine an aspect of pain sensitivity separately from psychological variables. Yet we saw in Chapter 2 that descending pathways help to regulate the degree of sensitivity in the dorsal horn of the spinal cord, suggesting that even early levels of pain processing are under the control of higher brain centers. And in fact, Scott and Cadden found that the anticipation of receiving a painful shock to the leg was enough to reduce a jaw reflex similar to the ES2 (A. J. Scott & Cadden, 1996). This appears to have been a stress effect, as the degree of reduction in the reflex was correlated with the change in heart rate ($r \approx 0.50$). Other nociceptive reflexes similarly appear to be attenuated by psychological factors, such as absorption in hypnotic imagery (Kiernan, Dane, Phillips, & D. Price, 1995; Sandrini, Milanov, Malaguti, Nigrelli, Moglia, & Nappi, 2000) or other competing tasks (Bathien, 1971; Willer, Boureau, & Albe-Fessard, 1979).

Psychological Factors

Personality.   In clinical samples, tension-type headache is associated with proneness to negative affect (Cao, Zhang, K. Wang, Y. Wang, & W. Wang, 2002), and with two long-term psychiatric conditions: dysthymia and generalized anxiety disorder (Puca et al., 1999). The associations may pertain to treatment-seeking specifically, as they do not seem to be present in population samples (Merikangas, D. E. Stevens, & Angst, 1994; Waldie & Poulton, 2002). Alternatively, the association may be moderated by headache frequency: Among individuals having more than eight tension-type headaches a month, clinical depression approximately doubles the risk of developing a headache after a laboratory stressor (Janke, K. A. Holroyd, & Romanek, 2004). Consistent with the lab results, psychiatric comorbidity in the clinic seems to be a negative predictor of long-term remission (Guidetti, Galli, et al., 1998), and hence on rational grounds may require more comprehensive treatment. (We will discuss treatment matching a bit further in Chapter 16.) The combined presence of anxiety and depression may be especially important to address, as it seems to be associated with particularly high levels of pericranial muscle tenderness (F. Mongini, G. Ciccone, Deregibus, Ferrero, & T. Mongini, 2004).

In clinic and community samples, chronic tension-type headache appears associated with the tendency to experience (Blaszczynski, 1984; Materazzo, Cathcart, & Pritchard, 2000) and suppress (Arena, Bruno, Rozantine, & K. J. Meador, 1997; Materazzo et al.) anger. Whether this affects headache activity is unclear, but anger, and especially its inward suppression, are related to dysphoria (Duckro, Chibnall, & Tomazic, 1995; Tschannen, Duckro, Margolis, & Tomazic, 1992; Materazzo, et al.), and may be important to treat for restoring quality-of-life.

In addition to its relationships with negative affect, tension-type headache may by influenced by a specific cognitive style, directly suggesting a psychological approach to treatment.

Stress appraisal and coping.   There is some evidence that people with chronic tension-type headaches, compared with people who do not have headaches, experience stressful events as more undesirable, as having more impact, and as less controllable (Ehde & J. E. Holm, 1992; J. E. Holm, K. A. Holroyd, Hursey, & Penzien, 1986). Of course this could be the result of having frequent headaches, which might indeed make stressful events less desirable, more impactful, and harder to control in their consequences. However, these types of appraisals can themselves increase the effects of stress and hence there are rational grounds for postulating a self-sustaining, vicious cycle. If so, then one effect of behavioral treatment might be to interrupt this cycle by increasing patients' sense of mastery over their headaches, and therefore over stresses.

In fact, there is indeed some evidence that behavioral treatment fosters a change in expectancy and in how the stress of having a headache is appraised. Ter Kuile et al. (1995a) assigned 144 patients randomly to receive either autogenics training (a form of relaxation instruction) or explicit training in cognitive coping strategies. The acquisition of specific coping skills during treatment did not correlate with success at 6 month follow-up. However, developing a sense of mastery over pain was predictive of long-term success. Ter Kuile et al. found that the autogenics training produced approximately the same increase in coping self-efficacy as the explicit cognitive training. As measured psychometrically, at the end of the 7 sessions of treatment, subjects in both groups "were less inclined to catastrophize, they perceived themselves as more effective in controlling and decreasing their pain, expected more reinforcement [success] in controlling their pain to come from their own behaviour and less to come from physicians, medication or chance factors and they expected more pain reduction in the long term" ($p < .000005$; ter Kuile, Spinhoven, Linssen, & van Houwelingen, 1995a, pp. 261–262). The decrease in catastrophizing was associated with a decrease in global psychological distress as measured by the Symptom Checklist 90.

In Chapter 15, we will examine process studies of behavioral therapies in more detail. There, we will see that even biofeedback may work through primarily cognitive means.

As described in chapters 13 and 15, below, behavioral interventions are generally used to increase a patient's control over pericranial muscle tension (surface EMG biofeedback), increase resistance to stress (relaxation and cognitive coping skills training), or augment central pain modulation (relaxation, biofeedback, and increased self-efficacy).

ON THE RELATIONSHIP BETWEEN MIGRAINE AND TENSION-TYPE HEADACHE

> . . . nothing is more helpful to clear understanding, prompt recognition and sound memory than a well-ordered arrangement into classes, primary and subordinate. . . . [Yet] Nature, as the saying goes, makes no jumps and passes from extreme to extreme only through a mean. She always produces species intermediate between higher and lower types, species of doubtful classification linking one type with another and having something in common with both . . .
>
> —John Ray, who invented the concept of species, 1682,
> cited in Boorstin, 1983, p. 434

Thus far, we have discussed migraines and tension-type headaches as if they were easily separable pure types. Yet in the clinic, patients whose experience seems to blend the two disorders are the norm. At least three general models have been advanced to describe the relationships between migraine and tension-type headache (Takeshima & Takahashi, 1988): (1) The two forms of headache differ along a quantitative dimension of intensity (e.g., Bakal, 1982; M. Smith & N. Jensen, 1988). In this model, migraines are the form that headaches take as they become severe. (2) The two types of headaches are the end-points of a qualitative dimension, e.g., of muscle contraction vs. vascular sources of pain. In this model, a headache can derive from any proportional mixture of muscle contraction and vascular sources; tension-type and migraine are simply the prototypical extremes of the dimension (e.g., Raskin, 1982). (3) Migraines and tension-type headaches are distinct disorders. In any given person, diagnosis may be complicated because both conditions, in varying severity, may be present simultaneously (IHS, 2004 criteria).

Similarities.   The presence of muscle pain in migraines has been given as evidence for the first two models. For example, in a survey of 50 migraineurs at a headache clinic, 32 (64 percent) reported neck pain or stiffness during migraine episodes (Blau & E. A. MacGregor, 1994). Now, muscle tension could be a reaction to the migraine, much as tension of the abdominal muscles is a reaction to pain in an internal organ (Moskowitz, 1993). But on the other hand, S. Diamond (1993) and Travell and Simons (1983) note that pain referred to the orbit, tinnitus, vertigo, and lacrimation, can be elicited by pressure to trigger points or contracted, tender muscles.

And indeed approximately 50 percent of migraineurs appear to have myofascial trigger points (R. Jensen, Tuxen, & J. Olesen, 1988). Trigger point injections can improve migraine symptoms within an hour in more than half of such cases (Tfelt-Hansen, J. Olesen, & Krabbe, 1980). Blau, et al. (1994) and Tfelt-Hansen (1981) also report improvements in migraines with treatments directed to the neck muscles. And Marcus, et al. found that patients with migraines, tension-type headaches or both, were more likely than controls to have abnormal head posture and trigger points in the neck. However, the three headache groups did not differ from each other (Marcus, Scharff, Mercer, & D. C. Turk, 1999). Thus, pericranial myofascial pain may be a component of migraines as well as of tension-type headaches.

Other similarities are suggested as well. In cross-sectional studies, parafunctional oral behaviors (e.g., jaw clenching) are reported often by migraineurs (Moss, 1987), indeed as frequently and perhaps more frequently than by individuals with temporomandibular dysfunction (Moss, Ruff, & Sturgis, 1984). Conversely, it appears that the most reliable psychophysiological findings in tension-type headache are not of increased muscle tension, but of vascular abnormalities such as distension of the superficial temporal artery (P. R. Martin and Seneviratne, 1997; P. R. Martin, J. Todd, & Reece, 2005). Now, most of these studies took place before the 1988 International Headache Society criteria. A minimalist explanation would attribute the results to misdiagnosis under the 1962 system: Perhaps some migraineurs were placed in the tension-type headache category, and vice versa. However, the results of these studies seem too strong to attribute to a mild diagnostic fuzziness. Moreover, recent studies seem confirmatory. Thus, Hannerz and Jogestrand (1998), using modern criteria, report that when placed on a tilt-table with the head downwards, people with chronic tension-type headache showed greater common carotid artery distention than age- and sex-matched controls, a vascular finding in tension-type headache.

In the biochemical realm, cerebrospinal fluid levels of an antinociceptive peptide, Met-**enkephalin**, are reported to be elevated in people with chronic tension-type headache and those with migraines (Langemark, Bach, Ekman, & J. Olesen, 1995) when compared with normal controls. This may be a reaction to peripherally-generated pain, or an indication of abnormal pain regulation. Total platelet serotonin level appears to be reduced chronically in tension-type headache, and episodically during migraines (S. Diamond, 1993).

Moreover, no differences were found on measures of autonomic functioning between migraineurs and people with episodic tension-type headache (Mikamo, Takeshima, & Takahashi, 1989).

Differences.   Weighing against a connection between migraine and tension-type headache are several streams of evidence. Rasmussen et al. note that in their large, random community sample, 13 percent of migraineurs had no history of tension-type headache. This should be unlikely if migraines develop out of tension-type headaches (B. K. Rasmussen, R. Jensen, Schroll, & J. Olesen, 1992). Multivariate analyses, in which the intercorrelations between headache symptoms are displayed, show two, very distinct, non-overlapping clusters corresponding to migraine and tension-type (especially occipital-area) headaches (Takeshima & Takahashi, 1988).

Moreover, studies using the 1988 IHS diagnostic criteria appear to show a good separation between the two forms of headache. For example, patients' average descriptions of tension-type headaches are shown in Table 6–1 (Ulrich, M. B. Russell, R. Jensen, & J. Olesen, 1996).

Wöber-Bingöl and colleagues report a very similar pattern in a clinic sample of children and adolescents with tension-type headache. After excluding patients having both migraines and tension-type headache, and those whose tension-type headaches did not meet IHS criteria, very few of the headaches involved any migraine-like symptoms (Wöber-Bingöl et al., 1996). And in a large-scale ($N = 4000$) random sample, Ulrich, et al. found that the one-year prevalence, characteristics, and sex-ratio of tension-type headaches did not differ between people who also had migraines with auras, migraines without auras, or no migraines. This suggests that migraines and tension headaches are separate disorders (Ulrich, M. B. Russell, R. Jensen, & J. Olesen, 1996).

Syntheses.   Three types of synthesis have been suggested to account for the similarities between the ostensibly distinct disorders. First, the same multivariate analyses that show a clear demarcation between clusters of headache symptoms do not show a clear demarcation between headache patients (Takeshima & Takahashi, 1988). Rather, headache patients appear to be distributed along a continuum, between purely tension-type and purely migraine symptoms. Thus, the epidemiological data point towards model 3 above: that migraines and tension-type headaches are distinct disorders, but that any given patient may have both.

Second, there is data to suggest that *for migraineurs*, tension-type headaches and migraines may have a similar pathophysiological mechanism. For example, Ulrich, et al. found that migraineurs sometimes report that their tension-type headaches have dietary triggers. People with-

TABLE 6–1.
Patients' Descriptions of Tension-type Headaches

Pain severe:	3%		Nausea present:	3%
Pain not severe:	97%		Nausea absent:	97%
Bilateral:	89%		Photophobia present:	18%
Unilateral:	11%		Photophobia absent:	82%
Pressing/tightening:	77%		Phonophobia present:	18%
Pulsating:	23%		Phonophobia absent:	82%
Aggravated by routine physical activity:		17%		
Not aggravated:		83%		

Note. Adapted from "A Comparison of Tension-type Headache in Migraineurs and in Non-Migraineurs: A Population-Based Study," by V. Ulrich, M. B. Russell, R. Jensen, and J. Olesen, 1996, *Pain, 67,* p. 503. Copyright 1996 by the International Association for the Study of Pain. Adapted with permission.

out a history of migraines never reported dietary triggers in this study (Ulrich, M. B. Russell, R. Jensen, & J. Olesen, 1996). Also, Lipton et al. found that in people with migraines, moderate and severe tension-type headaches responded just as well to 50 mg oral sumatriptan as did migraines. For both tension-type and migraine headaches, sumatriptan outperformed a placebo (Lipton, Stewart, Cady, et al., 2000). Now, sumatriptan should not work for tension-type headaches, and hence its efficacy implies that the headaches were actually some sort of migraine variant.

Third, note that in the Ulrich, et al. study, tension headaches lasted longer in migraineurs, and were more likely to be chronic (>180 days/year), possibly suggesting sensitization of a common central pain pathway such as in the trigeminal nucleus. Similarly, Rasmussen et al. found that tension-type headaches tend to be more severe and frequent in people who also have migraines (B. K. Rasmussen, R. Jensen, Schroll, & J. Olesen, 1992). Thus, central sensitization has been proposed as a link between the two forms of headache disorder.

Olesen (who was also chair of the committee that developed the 1988 IHS criteria) cites evidence that in the trigeminal nucleus, and perhaps even more so in the thalamus, there may be cells that respond to more than one type of nociceptive input (Olesen, 1991). He suggests that these cells may effectively summate noxious input from myofascial and vascular sources. Moreover, he suggests that the activity of these cells is susceptible to modulation, both inhibitory and excitatory, by higher brain centers, allowing psychological variables such as stress to play a role in the generation of headaches. In this model, the primary irritant giving rise to migraines is vascular. However, myofascial and/or psychological processes can provide enough additional input to push vascular processes into a full-blown migraine. Similarly, vascular changes can play a strong supporting role to the myofascial and psychological processes thought to be involved in tension-type headaches (Olesen, 1991).

An implication of this model is that assessing and treating muscle tension and parafunctional oral behaviors may be as important in migraine as in tension-type headache. Conversely thermal biofeedback, which is presumably a vascular intervention, may have a role to play in the treatment of tension-type headaches.

CHAPTER 7

Other Primary Headaches:
Chronic Daily and Cluster Headaches

But, to the patient, it [pain] is the thing; it is the malady. . . . Further, persistent pain impairs vitality; in this sense [too] a pain is a disease.
—Costaeus (1595 or 1608) in Avicenna(1930/11th century)[1]

CHRONIC DAILY HEADACHE

The distinctive feature of chronic daily headaches is, of course, their daily or near-daily occurrence. We might suspect, then, that underlying this clinical presentation is a rather heterogenous collection of disorders (Silberstein, Lipton, & Sliwinski, 1996). And, indeed, there is some evidence for heterogeneity, with subtypes thought to include:

1. Transformed migraine, in which episodes of tension-like headache occur at first occasionally, and then with increasing frequency, between the migraine paroxysms. In time, the boundary between the two types of headaches may blur, leaving a nearly continuous pain that clinically resembles a chronic tension-type headache, but with migrainous exacerbations (N. Mathew, 1997a). Transformed migraine is different from status migrainosus, in which a migraine, with its full complement of autonomic symptoms, becomes continuous.

2. Chronic tension-type headache, in which a pure tension-type headache occurred on more than half the days of the preceding three months. Chronic tension-type headache may evolve from the episodic form (N. Mathew, 1997a).

3. Medication-overuse headache, a diffuse pain that can develop with frequent use of analgesic or acute migraine drugs. Some apparent cases of transformed migraine are actually medication overuse headaches.

4. Hemicrania continua, an unusual disorder of continuous, unilateral head pain, with intermittent autonomic symptoms, that always responds to a sufficiently high dose of indomethacin.

5. Chronic daily headaches that arise from pathology of the neck, or from a head injury.

---

[1]The lead for this quote was found in C. S. Adler, S. M. Adler & A. P. Friedman (1987)

6. New daily persistent headache which, unfortunately, as its name implies, is understood at present only on a clinical, descriptive level (D. Li & Rozen, 2002). The sole etiological hypothesis so far, with a small amount of evidence behind it, is that the headache is an accompaniment of active Epstein-Barr infection (Diaz-Mitoma, Vanast, & Tyrrell, 1987).

The distinctions among these categories are not always clear, however, clinically or conceptually. We will examine the literature on them in the pages that follow.

PREVALENCE

The prevalence of chronic daily headache in the general population is uncertain, but has been estimated at around 3 percent to 5 percent (Evers, Suhr, Bauer, Grotemeyer, & Husstedt, 1999; Pascual, Colás, & Castillo, 2001; S.-J. Wang, Fuh, S.-R. Lu, C.-Y. Liu, Hsu, P.-N. Wang, & H.-C. Liu, 2000). For specific subtypes, prevalence seems to vary from 2.5–3 percent for chronic tension-type headache and 1.5–2 percent for transformed migraine, to 0.1 percent for new daily persistent headache (Pascual, et al.).

Among patients who present to headache clinics, chronic daily headaches are much more common, although prevalence estimates vary. N. Mathew (1997a) found that 35–40 percent of clinic patients had chronic daily headaches. At the other end of the spectrum, Evers et al. (1999) found that approximately 7.5 percent of patients at their clinic in Germany met the criteria for analgesic abuse/ergotamine-induced headache.

MIGRAINE AND TENSION-TYPE HEADACHE: THE TRANSITION FROM EPISODIC TO CHRONIC

The prototypical daily headache appears to have started as episodic migraines, and maintains intermittent exacerbations having migrainous features (N. Mathew, 1997a). Such headaches have traditionally been termed "transformed migraine," with diagnostic criteria as shown in Table 7–1.

The exact proportion of daily headaches that start off as migraines is unknown, having been estimated at 80 percent in one clinical sample (N. Mathew, 1997a) and 35–49 percent in another (Evers, et al., 1999). In a population-based study, S.-J. Wang et al. found that 70 percent of chronic daily headache was in fact chronic tension-type headache, with another 25 percent having migrainous features. This suggests that the higher proportion of transformed migraine seen in the clinic is due to its greater severity than tension-type headache (S.-J. Wang, Fuh, S.-R. Lu, C.-Y. Liu, et al., 2000). In this chapter, we will focus on the unique aspects of chronic daily headache and medication overuse headache. However, as we have seen, many cases of chronic daily headaches are simply particularly bad cases of chronic tension-type headache (Goadsby, 1999). Hence, in actual practice, the clinician will want to clarify the diagnosis as much as possible.

There is some evidence that tension-type headache leads somewhat more quickly to drug-induced headache (Evers et al., 1999), and is associated with greater relapse after the daily headache has been successfully treated (Diener et al., 1989).

Evers et al. (1999) found that in their sample of 257 patients with drug-induced headache, the primary headache disorder had been present for an average of 17.2 *years* before onset of the drug-induced headache. The exact interval showed considerable variation among patients. This strongly suggests that more proximal triggering factors are important in the transformation of episodic into daily headache.

TABLE 7–1
Diagnostic Criteria for Transformed Migraine (Proposed)

A. Daily or almost-daily (>15 days/month) head pain for >1 month.
B. Average headache duration of >4 hours/day (if untreated).
C. At least one of the following:
   1. History of episodic migraine meeting any IHS criteria 1.1 to 1.6.
   2. History of increasing headache frequency with decreasing severity of migrainous features over at least 3 months.
   3. Current headache meets IHS criteria for migraine 1.1 to 1.6 other than duration.
D. At least one of the following
   1. There is no suggestion of one of the disorders listed in groups 5 to 11 [of the IHS diagnostic system; see Chapter 1 of this book].
   2. Such a disorder is suggested but is ruled out by appropriate investigations.
   3. Such a disorder is present, but first migraine attacks do not occur in close temporal relation to the disorder.

Note. In the Silberstein, Lipton and Sliwinski system, a diagnosis of transformed migraine, when present, supercedes diagnoses of episodic migraine and chronic tension-type headache. From "Classification of Daily and Near-Daily Headaches: Field Trial of Revised I.H.S. Criteria," by S. D. Silberstein, R. B. Lipton, and M. Sliwinski, 1996, *Neurology, 47*, p. 874. Copyright 1996 by the American Academy of Neurology. Reprinted with permission.

TABLE 7–2
Suspected Factors in the Transformation from Episodic to Chronic Daily Headache

Risk Factor	Percent Reporting
Analgesic drug abuse	24.0%
Stressful family situation	21.3%
Stressful working conditions	16.0%
Menopause	15.6%
Arterial hypertension	4.0%
Use of oral contraceptive	1.3%
Unknown	32.0%

Note. Adapted from "An Epidemiological Approach to the Nosography of Chronic Daily Headache," by G. Sandrini, G. C. Manzoni, C. Zanferrari, and G. Nappi, 1993, *Cephalalgia, 13*(Supplement 12), p. 74. Copyright 1993 by the International Headache Society. Adapted with permission.

What are these factors? N. Mathew (1997a) notes that primary suspicion has fallen on stress, overuse of analgesic or abortive medications, and possibly affective distress. In one retrospective study, patients recalled the following events in the six months preceding onset of chronic daily headache (Sandrini, Manzoni, Zanferrari, & Nappi, 1993), as shown in Table 7–2.

We will encounter similar studies, with similar results, below.

A related category, *chronic migraine*, is included in the second edition of the IHS diagnostic criteria (see Chapter 1). Chronic migraine resembles the episodic form, except that the migraine attacks occur at least 15 days a month, for 3 months or more. Now, in transformed migraine, the frequent, interval headaches tend to lack migrainous features. Thus, chronic and transformed migraine seem to be somewhat different entities (M. Levin, 2004).

MEDICATION REBOUND HEADACHES

In population surveys, the one-year prevalence of probable medication-overuse headache is approximately 1 percent (S.-R. Lu, Fuh, W. T. Chen, Juang, & S.-J. Wang, 2001; Zwart, Dyb, K. Hagen, Svebak, Stovner, & J. Holmen, 2004). The frequency in clinic samples, where people often have more severe or refractory disorders, is probably much higher.

Von Korff et al., in repeat surveys of 662 headache patients at the Puget Sound Group Health Cooperative, found that 21 percent reported using analgesic or abortive medications frequently (>14 days/month) and chronically (on at least 2 of 3 interviews conducted over a 2 year period). In about two thirds of cases the medications were over-the-counter analgesics. Older subjects and those with headaches >90 days in the preceding 6 months were most likely to be high users of symptomatic headache medications (Von Korff, Galer, & Stang, 1995).

At the Second International Workshop on Drug-Related Headache (1986, described in Silberstein & Saper, 1993) the following characteristics of drug-related headache were defined:

1. More than 20 headache days per month;
2. Daily headache duration exceeding 10 hours;
3. Intake of analgesic or migraine drugs on more than 20 days/month;
4. Regular intake of analgesics and/or ergotamine preparations in combination with barbiturates, codeine, caffeine, antihistamines, or tranquilizers;
5. Increase in the severity and frequency of headaches after discontinuation of drug intake (rebound headache); and
6. The nature of the underlying headache (e.g., migraine, tension headache, cluster headache, posttraumatic headache, or **cervicogenic headache**) is not related to the syndrome.

The current IHS criteria are given in Table 1–2.

Mathew and coworkers report that in a clinical series of 200 patients, the most frequently overused medications were, in descending order, butalbital compounds (e.g., Fioricet, Fiorinal; 42 percent of sample), codeine (40 percent of sample), aspirin plus caffeine or acetaminophen plus caffeine 25 percent), ergotamine (22 percent) and acetaminophen (17 percent). Patients commonly used more than one medication (N. Mathew, Kurman, & F. Perez, 1990). Chronic daily headache from **triptan** overuse has also been reported (Kaube, May, Pfaffenrath, & Diener, 1994; Limmroth, Kazarawa, Fritsche, & Diener, 1999).

Kudrow (1982) reported that, in 200 patients with chronic daily headache, amitriptyline brought improvement to 72 percent of those who discontinued use of analgesics, but to only 30 percent of those who continued the analgesics. It seems to be accepted in clinical practice that success with preventive medications is blocked by overuse of symptomatic medications. In Chapter 14 we will see evidence that high medication use can similarly impede the effectiveness of behavioral interventions (Michultka, Blanchard, Appelbaum, Jaccard, & Dentinger, 1989).

How much medication is too much? Rebound headaches have been associated with any of the following: 2 mg oral or 1 mg rectal ergotamine per day, 15 grams of caffeine per month, or 14 analgesic pills per week (Haase & Diener, 1998). Ferrari (1998b) suggests limiting sumatriptan use to an average of 2 or fewer days per week, or ergotamine to 1–2 days per week, to prevent rebound headaches. There is even some evidence for rebound headache from simple over-the-counter aspirin or acetaminophen (Rapoport, Weeks, Sheftell, et al., 1985), with a threshold dose of roughly 1000 mg per day (Sholz, Diener, & Geiselhart, 1988). The appropriate level for butalbital does not seem to have been determined yet. However, even for those medications for which safe intake levels are known, one sometimes encounters patients with apparent rebound headache at much lower doses (Schoenen, Lenarduzzi, & Sianard-Gainko, 1989). Of course, dietary caffeine is also a risk factor for chronic daily headache (Scher, Stewart, & Lipton, 2004).

Headache patients may have a specific susceptibility to rebound effects. Lance, et al., report that nonheadache patients taking high doses of NSAIDS for arthritis did not develop headaches (F. Lance, Parkes, & M. Wilkinson, 1988). Conversely, headache patients may have an increase in headaches when prescribed analgesics for other conditions (Isler, 1982). For example, S. Wilkinson, Becker and Heine (2001) studied 28 women who had been prescribed opioids to decrease bowel motility following surgical treatment of ulcerative colitis. None of the women who lacked a history of migraines developed a chronic daily headache, even with daily opioid use, while both migraineurs who used daily opioids went on to develop a chronic daily headache. Neither of the migraineurs reported using the opioids or any other daily medications for pain control, and the opioid doses were low for analgesia.

HEMICRANIA CONTINUA

The vast majority of chronic daily headaches seem to be chronic tension-type headaches, or chronic migraines with symptoms resembling tension-type headache in between the migraine episodes. However, "chronic daily headache" is a heterogenous category and before discussing further its more common forms, which are difficult to treat, we should mention hemicrania continua, which can yield readily to intervention.

Hemicrania continua, as its name implies, is a continuous headache affecting one side of the head. It is moderate in intensity, at least sometimes, but its severity generally fluctuates without clear triggers. Flare-ups are often associated with migrainous (e.g., throbbing pain, nausea, photophobia and phonophobia) and cluster headache-like (e.g., lacrimation, nasal stuffiness, **ptosis**, conjunctival injection) symptoms (M. F. P. Peres, Silberstein, et al., 2001). Perhaps half of the patients with this diagnosis have brief (<1 minute), sharp, stabbing pains superimposed on the continuous pain (M. F. P. Peres, Silberstein, et al.). Now, hemicrania continua was not discovered until 1984 (Sjaastad & Spierings, 1984), and still virtually nothing is known about its pathophysiology. What makes the diagnosis important, however is this: It nearly always responds to a **nonsteroidal anti-inflammatory medication**, indomethacin, although the dose may need to be high (M. F. P. Peres, Silberstein, et al.). In fact, as originally proposed, the diagnosis requires this response to indomethacin. The IHS diagnostic criteria may be found in Table 1–2. Because the IHS criteria are still new and untried, earlier, alternative criteria are given in Table 7–3 (Goadsby & Lipton, 1997). In Chapter 11, we will discuss indomethacin further.

As with all cases of headaches that seem easy to diagnose on clinical criteria we must be careful that the patient has received medical consultation. Although rare, cases of hemicrania due to a tumor, and cases thought to be associated with HIV infection, have been reported (Antonaci & Sjaastad, 1992; Brilla, Evers, Soros, & Husstedt, 1998).

Hemicrania continua is presumed to be rare, but in fact we do not know, because it resembles other forms of chronic daily headache, and because responsiveness to indomethacin is very difficult to include in a population-based survey. Thus, Peres et al. suggest that indomethacin be tried empirically in all cases of unilateral chronic daily headache (M. F. P. Peres, Silberstein, et al., 2001).

NEW DAILY PERSISTENT HEADACHE

New daily persistent headache is much as its name implies: daily from the outset. In Vanast's initial description, patients had no prior history of headache, and no apparent precipitating cause such as a physical trauma or psychosocial stress (Vanast, 1986). More recent diagnostic criteria due to Silberstein, et al. are less restrictive, but maintain the clear distinction between new daily persistent headaches and those that develop out of migraines or episodic tension-type headaches (Silberstein, Lipton, S. Solomon, & N. Mathew, 1994).

TABLE 7–3
Earlier Diagnostic Criteria for Hemicrania Continua

A. Headache present for at least 1 month
B. Strictly unilateral headache
C. Pain exhibits the following three features:
    1 Is continuous but fluctuating
    2. Is moderate in severity, at least some of the time
    3. Lacks precipitating mechanisms
D. Absolute response to indomethacin
E. May have associated stabbing headaches
F. At least one of the following
    1. There is no suggestion of one of the disorders listed in groups 5 to 11 [of the IHS diagnostic system; see Chapter 1 of this book]
    2. Such a disorder is suggested but is ruled out by appropriate investigations
    3. Such a disorder is present, but first headache attacks do not occur in close temporal relation to the disorder

D2. One of the following autonomic features is present with severe pain exacerbation:[a]
    1. Conjunctival injection
    2. Lacrimation
    3. Nasal congestion
    4. Rhinorrhea
    5. Ptosis
    6. Eyelid edema

Note. From "Classification of Daily and Near-Daily Headaches: Proposed Revisions to the I.H.S. Criteria," by S. Silberstein, R. B. Lipton, S. Solomon, and N. Mathew, 1994, *Headache, 34*, p. 6. Copyright 1994 by the American Headache Society. Reprinted with permission. And from "A Review of Paroxysmal Hemicranias, SUNCT Syndrome and Other Short-Lasting Headaches with Autonomic Features, Including New Cases," by P. J. Goadsby and R. B. Lipton, 1997, *Brain, 120*, p. 204. Copyright 1997 by Oxford University Press. Reprinted with permission.

[a]Goadsby and Lipton (1997) permit criterion D2 to be used in place of D.

In Vanast's sample, 58 percent of the patients were female (Vanast, 1986). In a study by Li and Rozen, 71 percent were female (D. Li & Rozen, 2002). Onset often seems to be in adulthood for men (20s, 30s, 40s) and a bit earlier for women (teens, 20s, 30s; D. Li & Rozen, 2002; Vanast, 1986). In both studies the samples were of patients presenting for treatment; demographics in the community is largely unknown.

The main clinical features include those of migraine and tension-type headache. Thus, pain is steady in about half the cases and throbbing in half. Nausea is present in one-half to two-thirds of cases. Photophobia and phonophobia are accompaniments for one-third to two-thirds of patients. Of note, a significant minority has other neurological symptoms, such as tinnitus or dizziness (c. one-third of patients) or **paresthesia** (one-third to one-seventh; D. Li & Rozen, 2002; Vanast, 1986). The new IHS criteria are given in Table 1–2. The earlier, research criteria are given in Table 7–4.

Onset, although sudden, is not always without etiological clues. Vanast and coworkers found that 84 percent of their patients (vs. 25 percent of controls) had evidence of an active infection with Epstein-Barr virus (Diaz-Mitoma, Vanast, & Tyrrell, 1987). Li and Rozen found that in 30 percent of their patients the headache began at the time of an infection or flu-like illness, at the time of surgery not involving the head in 12 percent, and at the time of a life stressor in 12 percent (D. Li & Rozen, 2002). Psychological distress and a low energy level have also been reported (Bigal, Sheftell, Rapoport, Tepper, Weeks, & Baskin, 2003).

Tricyclics, muscle relaxants, and anticonvulsants are occasionally effective for new daily persistent headache (Takase, Nakano, Tatsumi, & Matsuyama, 2004). To my knowledge, no other

TABLE 7–4
Earlier Diagnostic Criteria for New Daily Persistent Headache

A. Average headache frequency of >15 days/month for >1 month.

B. Average headache duration >4 hours/day (untreated). Frequently constant without medication but may fluctuate.

C. No history of tension-type headache or migraine that increases in frequency and decreases in severity in association with the onset of NDPH (over 3 months).

D. Acute onset (developing over <3 days) of constant unremitting headache.

E. Headache is constant in location.

F. Does not meet criteria for hemicrania continua.

G. At least one of the following
   1. There is no suggestion of one of the disorders listed in groups 5 to 11 [of the IHS diagnostic system; see Chapter 1 of this book]
   2. Such a disorder is suggested but is ruled out by appropriate investigations
   3. Such a disorder is present, but first headache attacks do not occur in close temporal relation to the disorder

Note. From "Classification of Daily and Near-Daily Headaches: Proposed Revisions to the I.H.S. Criteria," by S. Silberstein, R. B. Lipton, S. Solomon, and N. Mathew, 1994, *Headache, 34,* p. 5. Copyright 1994 by the American Headache Society. Reprinted with permission.

treatments have been studied. Vanast suggests that spontaneous remission is common: In his clinical sample, 86 percent of men and 73 percent of women were headache-free within two years (Vanast, 1986). However, other investigators report a more refractory course (R. W. Evans & Rozen, 2001; Takase, et al.).

PATHOPHYSIOLOGY

What mechanisms underlie a chronic daily headache? An answer to this question might allow us to identify and intervene with headache patients at risk for a deteriorating course (Loder & Biondi, 2003).

With chronic daily headache especially, it is important at the outset to be sure that we are, in fact, dealing with a primary headache, and not the result of a physical disorder. In tertiary care clinics, 4–14 percent of treatment refractory, chronic daily headaches are associated with elevated pressure in the cerebrospinal fluid that had escaped detection because it did not cause a swelling of the optic disc in the eye (papilledema; Quattrone, Bono, R. Oliveri, Gambardella, Pirritano, Labate, et al., 2001; S.-J. Wang, Silberstein, S. Patterson, & W. B. Young, 1998). Clinically, the headaches were indistinguishable from a primary headache, usually transformed migraine, even in such details as overuse of medications, perimenstrual exacerbation, response to dihydroergotamine, and family history of migraine (S.-J. Wang, Silberstein, S. Patterson, & W. B. Young, 1998). Thus, a neurologist may perform a lumbar puncture (to measure the pressure) or magnetic resonance venography (to look for a blood clot blocking the venous outflow from the brain). Still, the other 86–96 percent of refractory daily headaches have other causes, and these too are becoming less mysterious.

Thus, Welch and colleagues found that as the number of years with migraine increased, so too did the amount of non-blood iron in the periaqueductal gray region of the midbrain. We have seen that the periaqueductal gray is a key part of descending pain inhibitory pathways. The authors speculate that over time, repeated activation of the periaqueductal gray during migraines causes iron accumulation, **oxidative stress**, and progressive failure of the pain control system (Welch, Nagesh, Aurora, & Gelman, 2001). Similar models, in other brain regions, have been proposed for Alzheimer's and Parkinson's diseases (Zecca, Youdim, Riederer, Connor, & Crichton, 2004) and, much more speculatively, normal brain aging (Suh, Moreau, Heath, & T. M. Hagen,

2005). Still, Welch's interpretation is preliminary and does not seem to account for the progression to chronic daily headache: Individuals with daily headache had no higher concentration of iron than those with episodic migraine (Welch, et al.).

Along a somewhat different tack, Fusco et al. studied central sensitization as a candidate. Specifically, they administered electric shocks to the dorsal surface of the forearm in 20 healthy controls, 10 people with (episodic) migraine without aura, 10 with episodic tension-type headache, 8 with transformed migraine, 7 with chronic tension-type headache, and 5 with new-onset chronic daily or near-daily headache. All of the people with transformed migraine were overusing symptomatic medications, and the 5 who successfully tapered were re-tested 25 days after discontinuing the medications (Fusco, Colantoni, & Giacovazzo, 1997).

Now, what makes this a test of central sensitization is that all of the subjects were taught to distinguish the immediate pain from the shock, and a second pain which arises shortly after the immediate pain. The second pain is produced by central excitatory circuits.

Visual analogue scale ratings of the intensity of the immediate pain elicited by the shocks did not differ between groups. However, ratings of the second pain were higher in the patients with transformed migraine and in those with new-onset daily or near-daily headache. After tapering, the people with transformed migraine had a renormalization of second pain ratings. People with chronic tension-type headache and people with episodic headaches did not differ in their ratings from the control subjects. Thus, for two groups of chronic daily headache there is evidence for central sensitization, and there is evidence that in transformed migraine, drug rebound is involved.

On a physiological level, several models have been advanced for rebound pain. Using transcranial Doppler, Haase and Diener (1998) found that patients with chronic daily headache showed rebound vasodilation after withdrawal from vasoconstrictive medications. Thus, the medications might temporarily disrupt autoregulation of cerebral blood flow.

Nicolodi, Del Bianco and Sicuteri (1997) note that increased availability of a neurotransmitter can lead to a compensatory decline in receptor sensitivity. Thus, chronic daily use of the migraine abortives sumatriptan (a serotonin agonist specific to the $5HT_{1B/D/F}$ receptor subtypes) and ergotamine (a broad spectrum agonist of serotonin and other neurotransmitters) seems to lead to decreased sensitivity of the relevant receptors, increased frequency of migraines, and escalating dosage. Conversely, propranolol and methysergide are serotonin antagonists (of course propranolol also antagonizes beta-adrenergic sites) and help prevent migraines, perhaps by increasing the sensitivity of serotonin receptors (Nicolodi, Del Bianco, & Sicuteri, 1997).

Markedly lower platelet serotonin levels have been reported in patients with analgesic abuse headaches compared with migraine patients and nonheadache controls. Moreover, in patients with analgesic-induced headaches, the platelets had numerous, large vacuoles along the secretory pathways, giving a visual impression that the platelets had been depleted. Possibly, this may be a model for the neural effects of analgesic overuse (Srikiatkhachorn et al., 1998).

A fourth possible mechanism has been proposed by Fields (1997, 2001), and draws on what is known about tolerance to opioid medications. Recall from Chapter 2 that the descending pain modulatory system can facilitate as well as inhibit pain transmission. At least part of the facilitation is by way of "on" cells in the rostral ventromedial medulla. Of course, we would not be surprised to learn that opioids inhibit "on" cells. More specifically, the mu opioid receptor opens potassium channels, causing a rapid hyperpolarization of the cell, so that the cell is less likely to reach firing threshold (Ingram, 2000).

However, opioids set in motion a second process as well: They inhibit adenylyl cyclase, an enzyme that produces cAMP in the cell (Ingram, 2000). The production of cAMP is the first step in a cascade of chemical reactions that leads to the opening of sodium channels (Nestler,

Hyman, & Malenka, 2001). As more of its sodium channels close, the neuron becomes less likely to fire. In fact some anti-seizure medications (e.g., Dilantin, Tegretol) and topical anesthetics (e.g., lidocaine) work by partially inactivating or blocking sodium channels (Nestler et al.).

Now, to open potassium channels is a fairly simple process. However, the closing of sodium channels occurs indirectly, by inhibition of adenylyl cyclase. And enzymes are often embedded in feedback loops, so that when the enzyme is inhibited, the cell simply makes more of it (Nestler, Hyman, & Malenka, 2001). This "**enzyme induction**" is a common source of drug tolerance, and opiates are no exception. The "on" cells appear to increase the concentration of adenylyl cyclase (and also another enzyme, protein kinase A, which is downstream in the same reaction cascade) to make up for the inhibition by the opiate. Then when the opiate wears off, not only are the two enzymes no longer inhibited; they are present in higher-than-normal concentrations (Nestler et al.). As a result, the "on" cell becomes more likely to fire, giving rise to rebound. Now, if the rebound pain is treated with more opioids, this "opponent process" can presumably lead to further enzyme induction, pain sensitivity, and chronic pain.

In fact, opiates can cause pain under conditions of continuous administration, without any withdrawal or rebound ("opiate-induced abnormal pain sensitivity;" Mao, 2002).[2] One culprit may be chronic facilitation of "on" cell firing, which in turn seems to increase sensitivity of the dorsal horn (Vanderah, Ossipov, J. Lai, Malan, & Porreca, 2001; Vanderah, Suenaga, Ossipov, Malan, J. Lai, & Porreca, 2001). A second culprit may be an increase in dynorphin levels in the spinal cord. Dynorphin is one of the endorphins. Presumably it inhibits pain, but it also causes incoming C fibers to over-secrete transmitters such as calcitonin gene-related peptide (Gardell, et al., 2002). There is even evidence that neuronal cell death from glutamate toxicity can be hastened by narcotic pain medications (Mao, Sung, Ji, & Lim, 2002).

In terms of rebound specifically, another type of opponent process may be operative as well. When people or animals are repeatedly exposed to morphine, they develop tolerance, of course. It turns out that part of this tolerance is specific to the situation in which the exposure occurred. That is, part of the tolerance is a classically conditioned defensive response by the organism, termed "**associative tolerance**" (S. Siegel, Baptista, J. A. Kim, McDonald, & Weise-Kelly, 2000). This conditioning may take place in the amygdala, which has inputs into the pain-modulating circuitry (Mitchell, Basbaum, & Fields, 2000). Now, after associative tolerance has developed, it is not unreasonable to suppose that exposure to the environment alone, without the morphine, would produce hyperalgesia, and indeed there some evidence that this occurs (Grisel, Wiertelak, L. R. Watkins, & Maier, 1994). There is an important caveat, however, for it is clear that classical conditioning can also cause pro-opioid rather than anti-opioid effects. Indeed, this is one of the mechanisms thought to underlie the placebo response (Ader, 1997). Ader suggests that when morphine is used for pain control, it supports rather than disrupts homeostasis, and therefore does not elicit a defensive response as would, say, morphine used as a drug of abuse. Alternatively, Ramsay and Woods note that the direction of response in drug conditioning experiments can be changed by altering cognitive expectancies (Ramsay & Woods, 1997). Whether the expectancies

---

[2]In transformed migraine and rebound headache, tapering from the inciting medications is generally the appropriate clinical course. But notice the quandary that opiate-induced hyperalgesia creates when we treat other conditions, say, chronic low back pain. If an opiate is losing effectiveness because of ordinary tolerance, then increasing the dose would be a reasonable strategy, provided there are no contraindications (Mao, 2002). But if the opiate is losing effectiveness because it is heightening one's sensitivity to pain, then *lowering* the dose would be appropriate (Mao, 2002). In the future, psychophysics (quantitative sensory testing for widespread hyperalgesia or allodynia) will probably be helpful clinically for distinguishing between these two aspects of opiate tolerance (Compton, Charuvastra, & Ling, 2001).

help direct the classical conditioning or simply override it seems unclear. To my knowledge, the discussion remains in the realm of theory. At this point we do not yet know the circumstances under which one or the other type of conditioned response predominates.

With associative tolerance, we have transitioned from a physiological to a psychological model of rebound. One could also propose a more general psychological model of chronic daily headache. The frequent medication use may be a marker for a felt loss of control over the headaches, and a fear of being overwhelmed by them. This in turn would lead to vigilance to pain (see Chapter 3), an expectation of pain, and hence to further sensitization to headaches. In fact, the medications may contribute to this process. Rapid pain relief from an analgesic or migraine preparation would constitute negative reinforcement for attending to pain (Fordyce, 1976; Gerber, Miltner, & Niederberger, 1988). As an external means of controlling pain, the medications could also undermine self-efficacy: Pain coping would be attributed to the medication and not to one's own ability. In time, the pattern of anticipating pain, attending to it, and fearing it would become progressively overlearned, strengthened by the negative reinforcement from pain medications (Gerber, et al.).

To my knowledge, there has been relatively little fine-grained research to support or disconfirm this model. In contrast, there have been studies suggesting more generally that psychological factors play a role in the development of chronic daily headache.

PSYCHOLOGICAL FACTORS

In a retrospective study, Mathew et al. (1982) compared 61 patients whose migraines evolved into chronic daily headaches, to 82 age- and sex-matched patients with episodic migraines. Variables that distinguished the two groups are given in Table 7–5.

Stress and medication overuse are also reported by Giglio et al. (1995) and Sandrini et al. (1993).

The retrospective studies, of course, cannot distinguish between cause and effect. However, an association with stress seems to persist as methodology improves. Thus, in a retrospective, population-based study, people with chronic daily headache were more likely than those with episodic headache to recall significant **life events** in the year that the chronic headache began, or in the year immediately preceding onset. People with episodic and chronic headache did not report different levels of life stresses for subsequent years, suggesting that the stress was causal (Stewart, Scher, & Lipton, 2001). Moreover, people who are divorced, widowed, or separated seem to be more likely to have chronic daily headache than those who are single or currently married. Similarly, being divorced, widowed or separated reduces the probability that chronic daily

TABLE 7–5
Patient Characteristics in Chronic Daily Headache vs. Episodic Migraine

Variable	Daily Headache %	Episodic Migraine %
MMPI Scale Elevations	70.5%	12.2%
Identifiable Stressors	67.2	30.5
Medication Overuse	52.4	6.0
Hypertension	16.3	2.4
Traumatic Life Events	13.1	0.0

Note. Adapted from "Transformation of Episodic Migraine into Daily Headache: Analysis of Factors," by N. T. Mathew, E. Stubits, and M. P. Nigam, 1982, *Headache, 22,* p. 67. Copyright 1982 by the American Headache Society. Adapted with permission.

headache will remit over 1-year of follow-up (Scher, Stewart, Ricci, & Lipton, 2003). And in a Norwegian population selected for initial absence of analgesic use, a low socioeconomic status at baseline was associated with chronic daily headache 11 years later (K. Hagen, Vatten, Stovner, Zwart, Krokstad, & Bovim, 2002). Possibly, both low socioeconomic status and divorce, separation, or death of a spouse, are demographic markers for a high level of life stress.

All of the variables noted by N. Mathew et al. (1982), except perhaps for hypertension, are likely to have a strong psychological component, suggesting that psychological treatment may be an important part of recovery. For example, Ferrari and Sternieri (1996, cited in N. Mathew, 1997a) reported the key reasons given by patients for daily analgesic use, shown in Table 7–6.

In a small study, Gerber, et al. found that 91 percent of patients with daily headaches felt that the pain would be unbearable without medications to control it, and that 57 percent believed that they would not be able to function adequately on their jobs (Gerber, Miltner, & Niederberger, 1988).

In my own experience, however, these results suggest an unusually high level of dependence on the medications. Many patients seem to fall into daily analgesic use simply because they do not know that medication overuse headaches are a possibility.

CAVEATS

The studies so far, then, imply that chronic daily headache overlaps considerably with medication rebound, and with other forms of chronic pain syndrome. But how strong, actually, are these associations? For we should note that nearly all of the studies have involved patients at tertiary care headache clinics, and thus may not characterize chronic daily headache in the population at large.

Blanchard, et al. found that among their research participants, who had been drawn from the surrounding community, only about 10 percent of those with continuous high-intensity headaches were also high medication consumers. Moreover, although the patients with continuous headaches indeed had higher average scores on most of the MMPI clinical scales (specifically, scales 1, 2, 3, 7, 8, and 9) the differences were not impressive. Further, in most cases the high medication consumers did not have scores that were high enough to suggest a clinical syndrome (Blanchard, Appelbaum, Radnitz, Jaccard, & Dentinger, 1989). And as a group, patients who were using high amounts of medications showed no differences at all on the MMPI, **Beck Depression Inventory**, State-Trait Anxiety Inventory, a psychosomatic inventory, or the Holmes

TABLE 7–6
Reasons Given for Daily Analgesic Use

Reason	% Reporting
Inability to cope with the pain	68%
Apprehension about a headache developing if drug is not taken	62
Ability of the analgesic to make headache more bearable, enabling the patient to function at work	62
Belief that there is no other cure	61
Medical advice to take med PRN	58
To reduce tension and anxiety	41
Recurrence of pain soon after previous consumption	30
To aid sleep	19

Note. From "Chronic Headache and Analgesic Abuse," by A. Ferrari and E. Sternieri, 1995, *Ten Years of Headache Research in Italy*, p. 49. Copyright 1995 CIC Edizioni Internazionali. Reprinted with permission.

and Rahe Life Events Scale, from controls matched for diagnosis and gender[3] (Michultka, Blanchard, Appelbaum, Jaccard, & Dentinger, 1989).

Thus, we have seen several versions of what chronic daily headache looks like. Depending on the study, it may involve medication rebound, a high amount of life events stress, and/or psychopathology, or it may simply be a chronic tension-type headache. In practice, then, it seems best to take an empirical approach, and not assume too much from headache frequency alone.

TREATMENT

In Chapter 14 we will see that the efficacy of behavioral treatment, at least for the cognitive and psychophysiologic therapies studied so far, depends on how literally the term "daily headache" is to be taken. The prognosis for patients whose headaches occur 5–6 days a week is nearly as good as for those with more episodic forms. However, for those whose headaches are nearly continuous, efficacy drops off drastically (Blanchard, Appelbaum, Radnitz, Jaccard, & Dentinger, 1989).

For the most refractory headaches, then, what are our options? N. Mathew et al. (1990) report that, for CDH patients who are overusing symptomatic medications, improvement is seen when the medications are tapered. This does not happen immediately, however. Abrupt termination of use can provoke a severe rebound headache lasting for 5 to 7 days (N. Mathew, 1993). In practice, the prescribing physician will generally taper the medication gradually. After the first week, the headache will typically continue to subside in frequency and severity. This improvement generally occurs within 4 (Haase & Diener, 1998) to 6 weeks (Evers et al., 1999), although the "analgesic washout period" can be as long as 12 (N. Mathew et al., 1990) or even 16 weeks (Warner & G. M. Fenichel, 1996).

Based on clinical experience, Warner and Fenichel report that the amount of medication used before the taper does not seem to predict the duration of the washout period. Similarly, the original type of headache (migraine vs. tension-type vs. mixed) does not seem predictive of the washout period. However, the length of withdrawal does seem to be a function of the type of medication. Post-withdrawal headaches tend to last only 3–7 days after triptan overuse, more than 7 days after ergots, and more than 2 weeks (albeit with gradually decreasing intensity) after simple or compound analgesics (Katsarava, Fritsche, Muessig, Diener, & Limmroth, 2001). Not surprisingly, then, analgesics are also associated with a higher relapse rate than are triptans or ergots (Katsarava, Limmroth, Finke, Diener, & Fritsche, 2003).

Mathew reports an approximately 67 percent success rate with multidisciplinary treatment. "Concomitant behavioral intervention, including biofeedback therapy, individual behavioral counseling, family therapy, physical exercise, and dietary instructions, is imperative for successful management of patients with CDH" (N. Mathew, 1997a, p. 182). Even so, one third of patients eventually relapse. Several characteristics seem to distinguish these patients from those who remain improved (N. Mathew, 1993), as shown in Table 7–7. In the table, DST is the dexamethasone suppression test, which indicates hyperactivity of the hypothalamic-pituitary-adrenal axis. A positive dexamethasone suppression test tends to indicate a mood disorder, and in fact the other distinguishing variables in Table 7–7 are psychosocial. What can be said about them? Most of the MMPI abnormalities were elevations on scales 1, 2, and 3, as is found in chronic pain syndrome. Associations between childhood abuse and chronic pain were discussed in Chapter 3, and tend to be fairly strong. Thus, chronic daily headache, at least in the most refractory subset

---

[3]Patients in the high medication group tended to be older, to have had headaches for longer, and to have greater total headache activity than other patients. Hence, complete matching on these variables was not feasible (Michultka et al., 1989).

TABLE 7–7

Risk Factors for Relapse after Treatment for Chronic Daily Headache

	Relapsed (N = 140)	Sustained Improvement (N = 311)
Abnormal MMPI	100%	48%
Alcoholism in Parents	58%	17%
Abuse in Childhood	52%	8%
Positive DST[a]	30%	11%

Note. Adapted from "Intractable Chronic Daily Headache: A Persistent Neuro-Biobehavioral Disorder" by N. T. Mathew, R. Kurman, and F. Perez, 1989. *Cephalalgia, 9*(Supplement 10), p.182. Copyright 1989 International Headache Society. Adapted with permission.

[a]DST is the dexamethasone suppression test, which indicates hyperactivity of the hypothalamic-pituitary-adrenal axis

of Mathew's sample, seems to share features with other types of chronic pain syndrome, and presumably would benefit from chronic pain treatment.

On the other hand, Blanchard et al., whose continuous-headache patients appear to have fewer psychological difficulties, speculate that a 3–4 month course of behavioral treatment for tension-type headache, with a strong component of cognitive stress-management therapy, might be effective (Blanchard, Appelbaum, Radnitz, Jaccard, & Dentinger, 1989).

CLUSTER HEADACHES

> *Some recur exactly every second day, once a week, or once a month. It is common for the attacks to increase around equinoxes and solstices, often in subordinate periods during which they actually infest at certain fixed hours within the space of every day and night.*
>
> —Thomas Willis, 1672 (cited in Mendizabal, 1999)

For weeks at a stretch, a few hours after falling asleep, Richard has awakened with an intense drilling pain just above his right eye. He rocks or paces in agony, and sometimes bangs his head on the dresser, as if to counter one pain with another. Oxygen works partway. Sumatriptan injections work very well, but the tightness at his throat scares him. His daughter wishes he would stop smoking, and he has tried repeatedly. He avoids alcohol like the plague, though— it's a big trigger. Sometimes an unexpected stressor also seems to set off a headache, like the computer going down again at work. His coworkers wondered if he was feigning the headaches to get narcotics until he got a headache once at work, and they saw his right eye—bloodshot, tearing, and half-closed.

The cardinal features of cluster headaches are (1) their strong periodicity; (2) the pattern of brief, intense, recurrent pain; and (3) the involvement of local parasympathetic overactivity such as tearing, injection of the conjunctiva, and a congested or runny nose, all on the same side as the headache (N. Mathew, 1997b). It appears that approximately 10 percent of the time, cluster headache is preceded by an aura, such as black-and-white flashing lights, a loss of color vision, or a bad smell (Matharu & Goadsby, 2001; Silberstein, Niknam, Rozen, & W. B. Young, 2000).

PREVALENCE

Cluster headaches are thought to be rare, with a prevalence of 7 per 10,000 (S. Solomon, 1997). Men appear to be five or six times more likely than women to have cluster headaches (Rasmussen, 1995a). First-degree relatives of cluster headache patients have a much higher probability of having the disorder themselves, with the increment in risk estimated as 14-fold (Haan et al., 1997) or even 39-fold (Leone, M. B. Russell, et al., 2001).

PATHOPHYSIOLOGY

In the absence of more definitive knowledge, there have been several theories of the pathophysiology of cluster headaches. Needless to say, given the periodicity, one theory is of a disorder involving the biological clock, which is probably found in the suprachiasmatic nuclei of the hypothalamus. In fact, alterations are found in the circadian pattern of a number of hormones during, but not outside of, cluster periods (Leone & Bussone, 1993; Leone, Maltempo, Parati, & Bussone, 1994). There appears to be an annual rhythm as well, as noted above by Willis. In a prospective study of 900 cluster periods recorded by 400 male patients, there was a marked increase in period onset 2 weeks after the summer and winter solstices (Kudrow, 1994).

Like the periodicity, the parasympathetic symptoms have been interpreted as having a hypothalamic origin. This is supported by evidence that diurnal heart rate is lower during cluster periods (Micieli, Cavallini, et al., 1994; for reasons that are unclear, this finding is stronger for individuals whose headaches are exclusively on the right side).

All told, then, it is not surprising that PET scans show a region of increased cerebral blood flow in the gray matter of the hypothalamus on the same side as the headache (May, Bahra, Büchel, Frackowiak, & Goadsby, 1998). The increased blood flow was found after cluster headaches had been induced by inhaling nitroglycerine, but there was no similar result when the nitroglycerine was inhaled by people who were not in a cluster period, and who therefore did not develop a headache. And the only gene so far found to convey risk for cluster headache encodes a receptor for *hypocretin*, a hypothalamic neurotransmitter involved in pain, stress, and the sleep-wake cycle (Rainero, Gallone, et al., 2004).

Now, the hypothalamus projects to regions of the brain stem involved in pain facilitation (dorsal reticular nucleus; Almeida, Cobos, Tavares, & Lima, 2002) and inhibition (periaqueductal gray; Lumb, 2002) and, not surprisingly, is involved in descending pain control (Hori, T. Oka, Hosoi, M. Abe, & K. Oka, 2000). Thus, the hypothalamus could perhaps cause head pain as a central hyperalgesic state (van Vliet, Vein, Le Cessie, M. D. Ferrari, & van Dijk, 2003).

Cluster headaches are almost always unilateral, and in fact they almost always occur on the same side of the head in each attack. This calls to mind, if somewhat vaguely, the possibility of a structural lesion. If so, the most likely site would be the cavernous sinus because of the confluence there of nociceptive, sympathetic and parasympathetic nerves (Moskowitz, 1988). There have been a few studies suggesting that there is indeed an inflammation there (Gawel & Ichise, 1994; N. Mathew, 1997b). Hardebo (1991) has proposed a model in which sterile inflammation and swelling of the internal carotid compresses the surrounding sympathetic fibers. This temporarily impairs their functioning, shifting the balance of activity locally to the parasympathetic system.

The effectiveness of subcutaneous sumatriptan suggests that cluster headaches involve the trigeminovascular system. In fact, Goadsby and Edvinsson (1994) have reported increased levels of two substances, calcitonin gene-related peptide and vasoactive intestinal polypeptide, that are thought to be a part of the sterile inflammatory response. Alternatively, sumatriptan may be effective simply as a vasoconstrictor (Hardebo, 1994).

Now, a trigeminovascular response suggests that there is, in fact, a vascular component to cluster headaches. Indeed, alcohol, nitroglycerin, histamine, and increased body temperature (from exertion or a warm environment) all of which are vasodilators, can provoke cluster headaches in individuals with the disorder (Blau & H. O. Engel, 1999). Conversely, oxygen inhalation, which produces vasoconstriction of cerebral arteries, is an effective treatment (N. Mathew, 1997b). Some authors have felt, though, that oxygen saturation itself is the key variable. Nitroglycerin can produce a mild drop in blood oxygen levels, while sleep apnea and exposure to high altitudes, which similarly reduce blood oxygen, can induce cluster headache attacks in people with the disorder (N. Mathew, 1997b).

Note, then, that the theories can be broadly grouped as neural (hypothalamic), vascular, and as structural/inflammatory. Pursuing the neural track, Evers and colleagues asked whether people with cluster headaches show differences in visual event-related EEG potentials the way migraineurs do. Evers et al. indeed found ERP differences, but not of the type seen in migraine. Compared with age- and gender-matched nonheadache controls, people with episodic cluster headache showed increased latencies of P2, N2, and P3 (measured at Pz) during but not outside of a cluster period. The latencies were normalized by effective prophylactic medication, even though in most cases the medications themselves would not be expected to reduce ERP latencies. In individuals with chronic cluster headache the latencies were even greater than in episodic cluster periods, and returned only partway to normal with successful prophylactic medication. Unlike in migraines, there were no differences between groups in the amplitude or habituation of ERP components (Evers, Bauer, Suhr, Voss, Frese, & Husstedt, 1999).

BEHAVIOR

Biobehavioral factors have rarely been studied for cluster headaches. Presumably, the strong periodicity of cluster headaches is taken to indicate a more purely endogenous source, and, as we have seen, there may be a significant genetic component. Nonetheless, there are a few pieces of evidence to suggest that environmental factors may play a role. First, as noted, vasodilators, and alcoholic beverages in particular, seem to function as triggers (S. Solomon, 1997). Some investigators, although not all, have found that alcohol use and misuse are higher in patients with cluster headache. Manzoni, for example, examined the records of 374 males with cluster headache who had attended the University of Parma Headache Centre. He found that 87.5 percent of patients with the episodic form of cluster headache, and 97.6 percent of those with the chronic form, were regular drinkers. By comparison, 59.2 percent of the general Italian population, matched for age and gender, drink regularly (Manzoni, 1999). Tobacco use was also high: current or former smokers comprised 88.8 percent of those with the episodic form and 95 percent of those with the chronic form of the disorder.

The difficulty with these studies, of course, is their correlational, observational nature. Alcohol and tobacco use could be manifestations of, or be genetically linked to, cluster headache. This perhaps is made more likely by the fact that cluster headache has been associated with structural differences in the hypothalamus.

There are, however, two further indications that environmental factors may be important. First, in contrast to migraine, which is described in Sumerian, Greek, Roman, medieval, and modern texts (McHenry, 1969), a description of cluster headaches does not appear until 1650 (Mendizabal, 1999)—despite the dramatic and unmistakable characteristics of the disorder. It is as if cluster headache emerged de novo in post-Renaissance Europe. Of course tobacco is not an Old World crop, and was not introduced to Europe until approximately 1500.

A second finding that, if corroborated, would implicate environment in a fairly strong way pertains to the gender ratio of the disorder. The overwhelming majority of those with cluster headache are male, with male:female ratios of 5:1 and 8:1 reported in the literature. However, when Manzoni computed the ratio for patients at the University of Parma, broken down by year of onset, he obtained the results shown here in Table 7–8 (Manzoni, 1997).

TABLE 7–8
The Changing Gender Ratio in Cluster Headache

Year of Onset	N	Male:Female Ratio
Before 1960	29	6.2:1
1960's	46	5.6:1
1970's	158	4.3:1
1980's	184	3.0:1
1990–1995	65	2.1:1

Note. From "Male Preponderance of Cluster Headache is Progressively Decreasing over the Years," by G. C. Manzoni, 1997, *Headache, 37*, p. 588. Copyright 1997 American Headache Society. Reprinted with permission.

A similar trend has been reported by second group (Ekbom, D. Svensson, Traff, & Waldenlind, 2002). Manzoni (1997) suggests that referral patterns and awareness of cluster headache in women remained stable during the period of his study, and that rates of the headache did not decline in men, implying that cluster headache is becoming steadily more common in women. Of course, this would seem to require a lifestyle or other environmental explanation. Manzoni (1998) draws the natural (but unproven) inference that the changing role of women is a factor. He noted that during the 1950–1995-study period, male predominance in smoking and employment declined, while there was no significant change in gender ratios for alcohol and caffeine use. Thus, the data seem to point especially towards smoking as a risk factor.

IMPLICATIONS FOR BEHAVIORAL TREATMENT

If cluster headache involves the hypothalamus, we would not be surprised to find emotions involved as well. And, indeed, L. Kudrow (1993) suggests that "bursts of anger, prolonged anticipatory anxiety, and excessive physical activity should be avoided because cluster attacks are apt to occur during the relaxation period that follows," and that "prolonged experience of anger, hurt, rage, or frustration during cluster periods often is associated with a new onset of a cluster period" (L. Kudrow, 1993, p. 187).[4] This seems to suggest that stress-management and anger-management interventions could be helpful in reducing the frequency of cluster headaches.

Still, so much of cluster headache seems endogenously generated. Surely the mood swings could be endogenous as well. Note, however, that the hypothalamus, like the rest of our body, is designed to respond to the environment in a way that maximizes our fitness. At least in animals, social stress changes catecholamine and **endothelin** levels in the hypothalamus. By analogy, we may note the effects of vasodilators. Peres, et al. suggest that they exert their effects by changing body temperature, forcing the hypothalamus to respond to restore homeostasis (M. F. P. Peres, Seabra, Zukerman, & Tufik, 2000). Somehow in the course of the response, a cluster headache is set off. Perhaps the same is true with strong emotions.

Cluster headaches seem to involve a sterile inflammation produced by the trigeminovascular system. We saw in Chapter 5 that in this inflammation, calcitonin gene-related peptide causes mast cells to release histamine, and that this process may be potentiated under stress by

---

[4]For many years, Lee Kudrow has been renowned as an international expert on cluster headaches, having written the classic text on the subject (Kudrow, 1980). Nowadays, however, what he is *really* famous for is being the father of Lisa Kudrow, who played Phoebe on TV's *Friends*. Lisa Kudrow joined her father on a research project, and hence she, too, is published in the cluster headache literature (H. B. Messinger, M. I. Messinger, L. Kudrow, & L. V. Kudrow, 1994).

corticotropin-releasing hormone (Theoharides, et al., 1995). In children, successful reduction in migraines with relaxation training was accompanied by a decrease in urine levels of tryptase, a mast cell enzyme (Olness, Hall, Rozniecki, W. Schmidt, & Theoharides, 1999). Thus, it is possible, albeit speculative, that relaxation training would confer some resistance to a trigemino-vascular response in cluster headaches as it may in migraines.

The most useful type of evidence, of course, would be a demonstration of the efficacy of behavioral treatment. We will return to this topic in Chapter 14. There we will see that the behavioral outcome literature for cluster headache is remarkably sparse, but that the little that is available offers modest encouragement.

CHAPTER 8

Benign Secondary Headaches: Cervicogenic, Temporomandibular Dysfunction, Trigeminal Neuralgia, and Posttraumatic Headache

So if the pain be expressed, the cause must assuredly be connected with the great or small occipital nerve, and in all probability depends on disease of the spine between the first and second cervical vertebrae.

—John Hilton, c. 1860, cited in Pearce (1995)

Tension-type headache is regarded as a primary headache disorder with, as we have seen, a probable component of central sensitization. In contrast there are two related disorders that historically have been thought to involve headaches secondary to a mechanical malfunction: cervicogenic headache and temporomandibular dysfunction (TMD).

CERVICOGENIC HEADACHE

As the name implies, cervicogenic headaches are those definitely traceable to neck pathology. Recent diagnostic criteria include (Sjaastad, Fredriksen, & Pfaffenrath, 1998):

1. unilateral head pain that is always on the same side;
2. neck pain on the same side as the head pain;
3. objective and subjective restriction of neck range of motion;
4. reproduction of the head pain with palpation of the neck or occipital area of the head; and
5. relief of pain after greater occipital nerve or C2 nerve block.

The 1988 IHS diagnostic criteria, in contrast, require neck pain, aggravated by neck movement or sustained posture; altered range of motion, tone or tenderness of neck muscles; and radiologic evidence of an abnormality in structure (e.g., fracture or rheumatoid arthritis), movement, or posture (Headache Classification Committee, 1988). In the 2004 revision, even such broad radiographic signs are dispensed with, in favor of "clinical, laboratory and/or imaging evidence of a disorder or lesion within the cervical spine or soft tissues of the neck known to be, or generally accepted as, a valid cause of headache" (Headache Classification Subcommittee, 2004, p. 115). Clearly, this is a diagnosis based more on clinical feel than crisp delineation.

Yet the somewhat vague criteria seem to work, for the prevalence of cervicogenic headache in tertiary care centers and among those with frequent headaches is relatively stable at 14–18 percent (Anthony, 2000; Nilsson, 1995; Pfaffenrath & Kaube, 1990). Translating this into prevalence rates for the general population is less certain, and values of ¼–4 percent have been proposed (Haldeman & Dagenais, 2001).

Pathophysiology

As we learned in Chapter 2, the trigeminal nucleus caudalis, which processes pain signals from the head, is functionally integrated with the dorsal horns of the upper cervical vertebrae, which handle pain signals from parts of the neck (Edmeads, 1988; Goadsby, 1995). Moreover, in the trigeminal nucleus, the somatotopic representation of the head is "upside down," with the encoding area for the top of the head (ophthalmic division of the trigeminal nerve) being closest to the encoding area for the neck (Edmeads, 1988). Not surprisingly, then, pathology in the neck can cause head pain. Moreover, Edmeads notes three other pathways by which pathology in the upper cervical structures can refer pain to the head:

1. The back of the head is innervated by the occipital nerve, which is an extension of the C2 nerve root.
2. The trigeminal nerve and C2 are connected indirectly through the tentorial nerves.
3. The C1 sensory nerve root refers pain to the eye, forehead, and vertex.

Against this anatomic backdrop, three broad processes in particular have been implicated in the genesis of headaches.

Myofascial trigger points are identified clinically, usually by a physiatrist or physical therapist. Trigger points are small and firm, exquisitely tender, occur in characteristic locations, and refer pain in characteristic distributions (Travell & Simons, 1983). Generally the trigger points occur in a taut band of muscle that twitches when the trigger point is firmly palpated (Travell & Simons, 1983).

Several neck muscles receive sensory innervation from the C1, C2, and C3 levels, and thus can generate head pain (Davidoff, 1998). Specifically, trigger points in the splenius capitis refer pain to the top of the head, those in the splenius cervicis refer pain to the ipsilateral eye, and those in the multifidus refer to the suboccipital region. Trigger points at the base of the skull can also generate headaches. Thus, the semispinalis capitis refers pain to the ipsilateral temple, while the semispinalis cervicis refers pain to the occipital region (Graff-Radford, Jaeger, & Reeves, 1986; Travell & Simons, 1983). The **sternocleidomastoids**, i.e., the large muscles at the side of the neck, are also innervated by the upper cervical segments. The sternocleidomastoids refer pain to the forehead, and can cause the eyes to become teary and red (Davidoff, 1998; Travell & Simons, 1983). A summary of the muscles relevant to head pain is given in Table 8–1. Note that the referral patterns do not follow a dermatomal distribution the way, say, a radiculopathy would. The anatomical basis for the referral patterns is unknown, but presumed to be due to convergence of pain pathways in the dorsal horn (Davidoff, 1998).

Now, there is some doubt about whether trigger points can be identified with adequate inter-examiner reliability. Marcus and coworkers found coefficient kappas of 0.74 for trigger points in the neck, 0.81 for those in the head, and 1.00 for trigger points in the shoulder (Marcus, Scharff, Mercer, & D. C. Turk, 1999). Coefficient kappa is the proportion of times two raters agree, corrected for the level of agreement that would be expected by chance (J. Cohen, 1960). Thus, values between 0.74 and 1.00 are quite good. However, in other studies much lower values have been obtained.

TABLE 8–1
Typical Trigger Point Referral Patterns for Muscles Relevant to Head Pain

Muscle	Location	Pain Referral To:
Digastric	Underside of chin, deep at side of upper neck	Upper side of neck, sometimes extending to occiput; throat under chin; sometimes 4 lower incisor teeth and alveolar ridge
Frontalis	Forehead, extending up towards vertex	Spreads upwards and over the forehead
Lateral Pterygoid	Inside mouth, at back of upper jaw	Deep into the TMJ and to region of the maxillary sinus
Masseter	Back of jaw, in front of ear	Eyebrow; deep in ear; top or bottom molars; side of lower jaw; mid-cheek
Medial Pterygoid	Inside mouth at back of lower jaw	Diffusely to tongue, pharynx, and hard palate; also below and behind TMJ including deep in ear
Multifidus	Very deep cervical paraspinal area, especially at base of neck and upper back	Suboccipital Region
Occipitalis	Back of head	Diffusely over top of head; intense pain deep in orbit and sometimes in eyelids
Orbicularis Oculi	Around the eyeball	Eyebrow and down nose
Semispinalis Capitis	Very deep cervical paraspinal area	Just below occipital ridge; temple and forehead
Semispinalis Cervicis	Very deep cervical paraspinal area	Occiput, towards vertex
Splenius Capitis	Posterolateral neck, esp. upper neck	Vertex
Splenius Cervicis	Posterolateral neck, esp. lower neck	Diffuse pain through inside of head, esp. behind eye, sometimes cap-like over the occiput
Sternocleidomastoid	Side of neck, from behind ear (mastoid process) to sternum and medial clavical	Forehead; over and around eye; deep behind eye; occiput; behind and in ear
Suboccipitals	Deep beneath skull	Poorly defined, internal head pain
Temporalis	Temple, side of head anterior to and above ear	Temple, eyebrow, behind eye, upper teeth, sometimes maxilla and TMJ
Upper Trapezius	Proximal upper shoulder, back of neck	Temple, suboccipital and posterolateral neck, back of eye, sometimes angle of jaw
Zygomaticus Major	Cheek	Arc from mid-forehead, down side of nose to cheek just beyond outer edge of upper lip

Note. Information on referral patterns is from "*Myofascial Pain and Dysfunction: The Trigger Point Manual. Volume I: The Upper Extremities,*" by J. G. Travell and D. G. Simons, 1983, Baltimore: Williams and Wilkins.

Moreover, even if they can be found reliably, most of the evidentiary basis for trigger points resembles that of psychodynamic concepts thirty years ago: clinical reports by therapists steeped in the particular model. Thus, it can be unclear whether the reports should be treated as straightforward descriptive data, or as perceptions so colored that they resemble deductions from theory. Moreover, even if the reports were entirely correct, they would not get beyond the level of description. Thus, for example, we would not know the pathophysiology of a trigger point, their specificity and sensitivity for diagnosing various disorders, whether they play a causal role, or the specific efficacy of treating them (versus clinical benefit from nonspecific effects). Not surprisingly, then, the myofascial literature is controversial. Bogduk, for example, whose careful researches we will encounter shortly, points out that the myofascial literature is "declarative but not scientific" (Bogduk, 1997, p. 370). Still, we will continue to refer to trigger points. The concept has permeated the practice of physical therapy and related disciplines, and it has worked its way into the literature on tension-type headache, migraine, cervicogenic headache, and posttraumatic headache. A few blinded studies have begun appearing (e.g., Marcus, Scharff, Mercer, & D. C. Turk, 1999). And my own bias is to attend carefully to clinical reports, because their authors are generally very close to the subject matter, and presumably, however steeped in theory, are attempting to describe what they see. Ultimately, however, progress will require that the literature mature. Very similar comments can be made about many of the other entities in this chapter (Bogduk, 1997).

The *greater occipital nerve* runs from the C2 sensory root up to the back and top of the head (Anthony, 1992). Presumably, it can become irritated anywhere along its course, referring pain to the head. There is some controversy about the nature of the pain, but as a neuralgia it should involve brief paroxysms of jabbing, lancinating pain (Bogduk, 1997).

Anthony suggests that many cases of transformed migraine are actually migraines that had been triggered by greater occipital nerve irritation. Over time, the migraines subside, but the nerve irritation remains, causing the chronic daily headache. Thus, Anthony (1992) reports that in 98 of 383 migraineurs, the headaches were consistently on one side of the head and there was marked tenderness of the greater occipital nerve as it crossed the superior nuchal line on that side. Moreover, for the majority of these patients, injection of local anesthetic or steroid to the area of the nerve eliminated their headaches. It is important to remember that this research was not blinded or controlled, and that all examination and outcome evaluation was by the person who conducted the injections. As is often the case, however, a loss of internal validity is a gain in ecological validity. After all, clinical practice isn't blinded either, and the patients who were headache free were probably quite pleased regardless of the research design.

Now, myofascial pain and greater occipital neuralgia are very similar in pain location and quality, in their response to palpation of the neck and occiput, and in their response to injection. Thus, they can be very difficult to distinguish from each other (Graff-Radford, Jaeger, & Reeves, 1986). In fact, the greater occipital nerve passes through the semispinalis capitis muscle. Travell and Simons (1983) suggest that if the muscle is taut, as may be the case in myofascial pain, the nerve can become entrapped by the muscle, causing the neuralgia. Now, severe cases of greater occipital neuralgia are sometimes treated by severing the nerve, and, hence, Graff-Radford, et al. suggest that a careful examination for trigger points be conducted first, before considering the surgical option. Psychologists conducting biofeedback should beware as well: Not everything that can compress the greater occipital nerve is as benign as a taut muscle. Again, it is imperative that the physical diagnosis be made by a physician or similar healthcare provider.

C2 neuralgia is thought to arise from compression of the C2 spinal nerve or the C2 dorsal root ganglion. It involves attacks of lancinating occipital area pain superimposed on a dull pain in the occipital, frontal, temporal, and orbital areas (Bogduk, 1997). C2 neuralgia resembles cluster headache in that the attacks are accompanied by lacrimation (watery eyes) and conjunctival and ciliary injection on the same side as the pain, and sometimes by dizziness, blurred vision, or a runny nose. Moreover, the attacks generally occur as often as 4–5 times per day or as seldom as 2 times a week, with pain-free intervals of days to months (Bogduk, 1997). The distinction from true cluster headache is the complete relief of pain following a C2 nerve block (Bogduk, 1997).

The *zygapophyseal joints*[1] in the spine, also called the *facet joints*, are richly innervated (S. Lord, Barnsley, Wallis, & Bogduk, 1996). In particular, when the **zygapophyseal joint** at C2–3

---

[1]These are the "hinges" between adjacent vertebrae, allowing the spine to flex.

is irritated, it refers a deep, aching pain to the back of the upper neck, as far forward as the ear, and to the lower occipital region on the same side as the joint (Dwyer, Aprill, & Bogduk, 1990). With more severe irritation the pain can apparently spread to the forehead as well (Bogduk & Marsland, 1986).

In addition to its characteristic referral pattern, the joint may become suspect from manual exam (Treleaven, Jull, & Atkinson, 1994) or through the elimination of pain when the joint is anesthetized (S. Lord, Barnsley, Wallis, & Bogduk, 1996). In a manual exam, the physical therapist or chiropractor is generally looking for hypomobility of the vertebrae—a feeling of abnormal stiffness or resistance to passive movement, also called segmental dysfunction—together with reproduction of the patient's clinical pain. This sounds rather subjective, but Jull et al. report *complete* concordance with diagnostic injections of local anesthetics (Jull, Bogduk, & Marsland, 1988). That is, a manual therapist was able to detect whether joint dysfunction was the source of neck pain, and if so, which joint was relevant, with perfect sensitivity and specificity. The only flaws in this remarkable study are the fairly small number of patients (20) and the fact that only one therapist was assessed. Because "a feeling of abnormal resistance" by definition depends on clinical experience, it is unclear how far the results can be generalized.

Of course we might also assume that degenerative changes on x-ray are an indication that the pain can be attributed to the zygapophyseal joints. However, from the limited data so far available, cervicogenic headache and degenerative changes in the cervical spine seem to be uncorrelated (Fredriksen, Fougner, Tangerud, & Sjaastad, 1989).

Inflammation.   In the search for characteristics specific to cervicogenic headache, Martelletti et al. have noted high levels of proinflammatory cytokines (interleukin–1β and tumor necrosis factor-α) in the extracranial (jugular) circulation (Martelletti, Stirparo, & Giacovazzo, 1999). Cervicogenic headache is often preceded by a whiplash injury, and Martelletti et al. suspect that the injuries might be inducing long-term inflammatory changes (Martelletti, Stirparo, & Giacovazzo, 1999). In support of this theory, the investigators found that infusions of infliximab (Remicade), a chimeric[2] monoclonal antibody that inactivates tumor necrosis factor-α (Mikuls & Moreland, 2003), produced rapid and sustained reductions in cervicogenic headache (Martelletti, 2002). Of course we must be cautious in interpreting the results of this non-blinded trial, given the high rate of placebo responding for which headaches are known.

Joint pain versus myofascial pain.   The interrelationship of joint hypomobility and myofascial pain is still a matter of controversy. One theory, of course, is that tension in the muscles around the spine is the source of resistance to vertebral movement. An alternative view has been proposed by Maigne, who founded the program in manual therapy at the University of Paris. He suggested that pain originating from the joint causes changes in the associated soft tissues as a local sympathetic reaction (Meloche, Bergeron, Bellavance, Morand, Huot, & Belzile, 1993). Specifically, he reports that the skin in the associated dermatome is thick and painful when pulled from the underlying tissues and rolled between the fingers. The muscles in the myotome associated with the joint develop taut bands or spasms. The tendon insertions in the relevant sclerotome are painful to palpation; for example, the insertion of the levator scapula at the upper medial corner of the shoulder blade is in the C4 sclerotome. Moreover, the posterior parts of the facet joints develop a painful swelling (Meloche, et al.). Thus, in Maigne's system, joint dysfunction can have a broad effect. If the soft tissue changes disappear when the joint is anesthetized,

---

[2]A mouse antibody that has been engineered to more closely resemble an antibody from a human being.

Maigne's conceptualization is supported for that patient. However, whether this is the only or the most common type of interaction between joint and soft tissue does not appear to have been resolved in the literature.

A step back.   Now, there is little debate that pathology involving the neck can cause headaches. However, the diagnosis of cervicogenic headache has been controversial because it does not require demonstrated neck pathology or trauma, and because its criteria have not been rigorously studied (Leone, D'Amico, Grazzi, Attanasio, & Bussone, 1998). Leone, et al. note that in their samples, pain that is always on the same side ("sidelocked pain" or "fixed unilaterality") is usually due to migraines. The reason, it seems, is that migraines are so frequent in their headache clinic population, that if only a small proportion of migraineurs have sidelocked pain, their absolute numbers are still greater than the number with cervicogenic headache. And sidelocked pain may not be uncommon in migraine. Lipscombe and Prior found that for 45 percent of the migraineurs in their practice, the pain localized to one side of the head consistently (Lipscombe & Prior, 2002). Moreover, the high base rates of tension-type headache and neck problems assure that the two sets of symptoms will co-occur in a significant number of patients who do not have cervicogenic headache (Leone, D'Amico, Grazzi, et al.). There is even evidence that successful nerve blocks, which would seem to directly implicate the neck, can work through nonspecific factors, such as by decreasing input to the trigeminal nucleus (N. Mathew, 1997b).

TEMPOROMANDIBULAR DYSFUNCTION

Temporomandibular disorders are a class of problems affecting the temporomandibular region (in front of the ear) and functionally related areas such as the temple and the angle of the lower jaw. The cardinal feature of TMD is pain that occurs or worsens with activity such as chewing (S. F. Dworkin, 1999). Not surprisingly, given the involvement of the temporal region, people with TMD often have tension-type headache as well. In fact, the pain from temporomandibular dysfunction and tension-type headache can be very difficult to distinguish, except that temporomandibular pain is usually unilateral (Sharav, 1999). Besides pain, other features which may be present include: (1) Crepitus or other signs of degeneration in the temporomandibular joint, where the lower jaw meets the temporal bone, and (2) Jaw locking in the open or closed position, limited jaw opening, or other signs of displacement of the articular disk. (The disk is made of fibrous material and is inside the joint. In its proper position, it cushions between the temporal bone and the lower jaw, and facilitates joint mobility; Glaros & Glass, 1993).

Temporomandibular pain has been associated most frequently with damage or degenerative changes in the joint, displacement and reduction of the articular disc, and muscle pain and dysfunction (Glaros & Glass, 1993). Of these, pain involving the muscles of mastication seems to be present in the majority of cases (S. F. Dworkin, 1999). Particularly important muscles are the masseter (in front of the ear, used in closing the jaw), and the lateral and medial pterygoids (inside the cheek, used for jutting the jaw forward, or sliding it from side to side; Glaros & Glass, 1993). There is pain with use of the muscles and when they are palpated. In the dental literature this is often referred to as myofascial pain but not necessarily with the implication of trigger points. The muscle tenderness and pain may be due to central sensitization, and strong similarities and overlapping symptoms with fibromyalgia have been noted (Aaron, M. M. Burke, & Buchwald, 2000; Widmer, 1991). When the temporomandibular joint is involved it is usually as an arthralgia (pain on palpating the joint) and not as an arthritis or arthrosis, which would involve frank degenerative changes (S. F. Dworkin, 1999).

As this description implies, TMD is a potentially complex set of disorders in which pain of both central and peripheral origin may play a role. Moreover, it has been argued that TMD symptoms are rather common in the general population (Sharav, 1999), with a waxing and waning course (Egermark, Carlsson, & T. Magnusson, 2001; T. Magnusson, Egermark, & Carlsson, 2000). Thus, for the subset of individuals with severe and chronic TMD and the resulting lifestyle disruption, issues of chronic pain and pain coping are often important (Glaros & Glass, 1993). It seems that with TMD, as with other chronic pain syndromes, we must consider psychosocial factors (S. F. Dworkin, 1999). In fact, this principle is embedded in the current research diagnostic criteria for TMD. The criteria involve a two-axis system, in which Axis I is for the physical pain generating process, and Axis II is for measures of pain intensity, functional impairment, depression, and somatic focus (S. F. Dworkin & LeResche, 1992).

In the rest of this section, we will focus on temporomandibular dysfunction as a pain disorder, rather than as a structural problem involving the joint or disc. Hence, this section applies primarily to those instances of temporomandibular disorder in which muscle pain and dysfunction, or a painful but otherwise undamaged joint, predominate. This subset appears to contain the great majority of cases (S. F. Dworkin, 1999).

Prevalence

Among children and adolescents, the prevalence of TMJ-area pain at rest is around 2–6 percent, with slightly higher estimates, 3–8 percent, for pain during jaw function. Among adults, population-based surveys suggest an overall prevalence of 4–12 percent for pain at rest, and 2–6 percent for pain with use of the jaw (Drangsholt & LeResche, 1999). Temporomandibular disorders are more prevalent in women than in men, and are specifically more frequent in women of childbearing age. In the community, the female preponderance is 1.5 : 1.0 or 2 : 1, and among those seeking treatment it is 4 : 1 (S. F. Dworkin, Huggins, et al., 1990). The higher rate of treatment seeking by women may indicate greater symptom severity, as more intense pain is a predictor of whether someone consults a healthcare practitioner for TMD (Von Korff, E. H. Wagner, S. F. Dworkin, & K. W. Saunders, 1991).

Pathophysiology

Estrogen.   Now, the association with childbearing years suggests a role for reproductive hormones, and indeed there is evidence to support this. In a study by Dao, et al., women reported more intense pain from TMD during the three days before menstruation (Dao, Knight, & Ton-That, 1998). LeResche and coworkers have provided additional evidence. Specifically, they used a large insurance company database to cross-tabulate prescriptions for female hormones and referrals for TMD treatment. They studied two groups of women: those above age 40 who were on hormone replacement therapy for menopause, and those age 15–35 who were taking oral contraceptives. When compared with non-TMD cases, women on estrogen replacement therapy had an increased risk of TMD (**odds ratio** = 1.64, $p < .001$) that remained significant after correcting for overall healthcare utilization (odds ratio = 1.32, $p = .002$). Moreover, there was a positive dose-response relationship, with cumulative estrogen intake of greater than 185 mg/year showing the strongest increment of risk. The association between progestin and TMD was weak or nonexistent. The use of oral contraceptives caused an increment in risk, even after controlling for total healthcare utilization, but it was not as strong as for hormone replacement therapy (odds ratio = 1.19, $p < .05$; LeResche, Saunders, Von Korff, W. Barlow, & S. F. Dworkin, 1997).

At this point, the mechanism by which estrogen influences TMD is not known. It could work peripherally by affecting joint laxity or inflammation, or centrally by altering pain transmission and modulation (LeResche, Saunders, Von Korff, W. Barlow, & S. F. Dworkin, 1997). We will encounter a similar question in Chapter 10, when we study migraine triggers.

Still, we should add that while estrogen use predicted referral for TMD treatment, overall healthcare utilization was a stronger predictor. Thus, even in this study, individual psychological differences appear to be important.

Central sensitization.   As in tension-type headache, it is likely that central factors heighten pain intensity in at least certain cases of TMD. Maixner and coworkers, comparing female patients with chronic TMD to age- and gender-matched controls, found lower pressure pain thresholds at the left and right wrists, and more rapid pain increase to repetitive heat pulses at the right index finger, in the patients (Maixner, Fillingim, Sigurdsson, Kincaid, & Silva, 1998). Moreover, patients with chronic TMD had lower thresholds and tolerance for thermal pain at the forearm, and were less tolerant of forearm ischemia, than were matched controls (Maixner, Fillingim, Booker, & Sigurdsson, 1995).

Psychophysiology, Psychology, and Implications for Behavioral Treatment

Psychophysiology.   A number of authors have found higher masseter surface EMG readings when thinking of a personally relevant stressor. The effect seems specific to TMD (it is not found in patients with low back pain) and specific to the masseter (in patients with TMD it is not found at the biceps; Flor, Birbaumer, Schulte, & Roos, 1991). The classic experimental stressor, mental arithmetic, is not necessarily sufficient to bring out stress-related differences. In a number of studies, elevations in masseter EMG have been found at baseline. However, these studies have generally lacked a sufficient adaptation period, and hence the authors may have been inadvertently reporting the stress reaction to being in a laboratory (Flor, Birbaumer, Schulte, et al.).

In Chapter 6 we noted that people with chronic tension-type headache may show a deficit in a reflex that inhibits muscle tension at the masseter (second exteroceptive silent period; Schoenen, 1993). This decreased inhibition implied greater excitability of the muscles of mastication, or of the associated motor neurons. Not surprisingly, similar findings have been reported in patients with temporomandibular dysfunction, although the results seem to depend on the details of method and subject selection (Sharav, 1999).

TMD patients may be less able to discriminate levels of muscle tension at the jaw than are pain-free controls (Flor, Schugens, & Birbaumer, 1992; Glaros, 1996, 1997), placing the patients at greater risk for maintaining high levels of tension in daily life. Now, this result requires explanation. Why wouldn't ambient pain sensitize a person to small fluctuations in muscle tension?

Recall that in Chapter 2 we encountered evidence that muscle tension inhibits subsequent pain perception, even at a different muscle than the one that was tensed (Persson, Hansson, Kalliomäki, Moritz, & Sjölund, 2000). Similarly, Knost and coworkers found that when individuals with chronic back pain tensed either their back or their forearm, their EEG response to electric shock was dampened. Specifically, the size of the difference between the N150 and P260 peaks in the somatosensory evoked potential decreased. Moreover, if it decreased enough, pain ratings also went down (Knost, Flor, Birbaumer, & Schugens, 1999). Now, in Chapter 2 we interpreted results like these as showing that descending inhibitory pathways had been activated. An alternative explanation is that muscle tension and pain compete for the same processing resources. (There is a third possible explanation as well, that the pain reduction is due to an increase in blood pressure, through the mechanisms discussed in Chapter 2. However, blood pressure did not emerge as a mediating variable in Knost et al.'s data.)

Competition for central processing resources may take place in temporomandibular disorders (Hollins, Sigurdsson, L. Fillingim, & Goble, 1996). Thus, individuals with chronic TMD tend to have higher thresholds for perceiving vibration. Moreover, the effect is specific to those individuals for whom pain on palpation is considerably greater than their ambient pain (Hollins et al.). Presumably, processing resources have been reallocated from sensing vibration to sensing pressure pain.

Knost et al. point out that the decrease in pain can then reinforce increased muscle tension, potentially leading to a vicious cycle in which, ultimately, the muscle tension itself becomes the primary problem and source of pain.

Muscle tension is not the only psychophysiological variable to show an association with TMD. Jones and coworkers found that TMD patients tended, on average, to show higher levels of **cortisol** secretion in response to the stress of public speaking and mental arithmetic than did pain-free controls (Jones, Rollman, & Brooke, 1997). Further, a small subset of TMD patients showing normal levels of secretion nonetheless showed a different pattern of cortisol response than the controls. For this subset of TMD patients, reported level of stress was inversely rather than directly related to cortisol secretion, implying that the secretory process had been down-regulated, perhaps from chronic overstimulation. As we saw in Chapter 3, evidence for down-regulation of cortisol secretion has been reported in fibromyalgia (Crofford et al., 1994) and many other pain conditions (Heim, Ehlert, & Hellhammer, 2000).

Behavior has also been implicated. Patients with TMD often engage in parafunctional oral behaviors such as gum chewing and **bruxism** (Moss, Ruff, & Sturgis, 1984). Bruxism includes jaw clenching, which appears to be related to stress, and rhythmic jaw grinding, which generally occurs in sleep and for which the role of stress has some evidence (Hicks & Conti, 1991) but is less certain (Glaros & Glass, 1993). Other risk factors for nocturnal bruxism include snoring, obstructive sleep apnea, cigarette smoking, and high intake of alcohol or coffee (Ohayon, K. K. Li, & Guilleminault, 2001). Jaw clenching is a strong risk factor for TMD (Velly, Gornitsky, & Philippe, 2003), but does not appear to be necessary or sufficient (Glaros & Glass, 1993). In fact, people who are edentulous and who therefore cannot brux, may still develop TMD (Sharav, 1999). Still, when parafunctional behaviors are present they presumably play a contributing role, and their remediation would be part of TMD treatment. Behavioral techniques of habit change can thus be of benefit.

Why would people with TMD engage in behaviors that can perpetuate their pain? Some behavioral theorists have noted that not only people, but animals too, engage in "adjunctive behaviors" when placed in frustrating circumstances (e.g., Gramling, Grayson, T. N. Sullivan, & S. Schwartz, 1997). Most of the adjunctive behaviors are oral: in animals, biting, pecking, eating, drinking, licking the airstream, etc., and in people, eating, drinking, biting one's fingernails, hair or pen, thrusting the jaw, pulling one's lips, and so on. It may be that the behaviors, even though they do not change the situation, help to relieve boredom or frustration. Then they would be maintained by short-term reinforcement, even if their long-term effect is pain. Alternatively, the behavior may be a hard-wired response to stress, sharpening the teeth and strengthening jaw muscles to prepare for primitive combat. Rhythmic clenching might even help blood flow to the brain by increasing venous drainage from the head, just as walking helps keep blood from pooling in the legs (H. S. Bracha, Ralston, A. E. Williams, Yamashita, & A. S. Bracha, 2005). Gramling et al. found that people with TMD reported more oral parafunctional behaviors in general, were seen to engage in them more often on videotape analysis, and during onset of a frustrating task had higher masseter surface EMG readings than age- and sex-matched controls (Gramling,

Grayson, et al.). In this study, the higher EMG readings may be indicative of greater amounts of covert parafunctional behaviors during the start of frustrating circumstances.

Note that muscle tension need not be elevated to very high values to have an impact. Glaros and coworkers taught pain-free subjects to maintain masseter EMG values below 2.0 μVolts for ten 17-minute sessions spread over two weeks. Subjects then increased EMG values above 10 μVolts for another eight 17-minute sessions during weeks three and four, and then again reduced readings below 2.0 μVolts for the last ten sessions, during weeks five and six. Note that the 10 μVolt threshold used in weeks three and four corresponds to a very light clench, albeit maintained for 17 minutes. By contrast, maximum voluntary contraction can be as high as 100 μVolts (Fogle & Glaros, 1995). Despite the fact that this was a relatively mild intervention, two of the five subjects discontinued the study because they developed TMD during the 10 μVolt condition (Glaros, Tabacchi, & Glass, 1998). Now, the study was not blinded, and it is possible that expectancies on the part of the experimenter or the subjects contributed to the pain. However, it is doubtful that further studies should be conducted of a procedure that seems to induce TMD.

Depression, anxiety, and other psychological disorders.   Now, in 50–80 percent of cases, TMD symptoms appear to be self-limiting. Rarely does the disorder worsen from one year to the next. At this point, the best predictors of chronicity are high scores on scales measuring depression and somatic focus (Drangsholt & LeResche, 1999; S. F. Dworkin, 1996).

Interviews of patients with acute TMD tend to show higher rates of anxiety disorders, and to a lesser extent, mood and substance abuse disorders, than in the general population. For patients whose TMD has become chronic, the rate of psychological disorders again appears elevated, with anxiety, depression, and somatic focus predominating (Gatchel, Garofalo, Ellis, & Holt, 1996; Velly, Gornitsky, & Philippe, 2003). The meaning of this, however, is not certain. The association may be accounted for by symptoms of posttraumatic stress disorder (De Leeuw, Bertoli, J. E. Schmidt, & C. R. Carlson, 2005), suggesting that emotional trauma may be causal, possibly through the mechanisms dicussed above, in Chapter 2. Technically, however, the studies do not shed light on cause and effect, because they focus on current psychological disorders in patients with TMD, or retrospectively look for past disorders. I am aware of only one prospective study on TMD. In it, there was indeed a tendency for depression at the start of the study to predict later development of TMD, but the association was not statistically significant (Von Korff, Le Resche, & S. F. Dworkin, 1993).

The relationship between psychological disorders and TMD seems to be specific to myofascial pain. Signs of disc displacement, and of joint changes such as arthralgia, osteoarthritis, and osteoarthrosis, were not related to psychopathology (Kight, Gatchel, & Wesley, 1999). S. F. Dworkin (1996) explains this type of data by noting that myofascial pain depends on subjective report, and hence should be more vulnerable to cognitive or emotional factors than disc or joint diagnoses, which involve more objective signs. It is also quite possible that pain is a more distressing symptom than, say, limited jaw opening, and may tax a person's coping resources more. Alternatively, Kight et al., point out the role of muscles in emotional expression. Possibly, long-term negative affect leads to frequent activation of facial muscles, and ultimately to muscle pain (Kight et al.). To distinguish between these hypotheses, it may be helpful to study people whose pain is restricted to the temporomandibular joint (arthralgia).

We should add that the relationship between myofascial pain and psychopathology, although statistically significant, is quite weak, with phi correlation coefficients of approximately 0.165 (Kight et al., 1999). Certainly one would not be justified in assuming psychopathology based on a TMD muscle pain diagnosis.

Implications for behavioral treatment.   We saw in Chapter 6 that trigger point needle EMG readings are negatively correlated with finger temperature as a measure of relaxation (r = –0.55; Banks, D. W. Jacobs, Gevirtz, & Hubbard, 1998). Thus, autogenics training to a high finger temperature criterion seems reasonable. Also reasonable is reducing bruxism through a combination of oral habit change, progressive muscle relaxation, and learning to discriminate tense from relaxed states with surface EMG. Comorbid anxiety and depression may need to be treated as well. Perhaps even more than with other disorders, good pain coping skills seem crucial in TMD to maintain functioning and limit emotional distress. Thus, many of the factors reviewed in Chapter 3, and many of the therapies discussed in Chapter 13, may be relevant.

Not surprisingly, then, Goldstein notes in a recent review of the dental literature that the "current standard of care for common chronic nonstructural TMD is management with multidisciplinary cognitive behavioral therapy and muscle relaxation measures" (B. H. Goldstein, 1999, p. 382).

TRIGEMINAL NEURALGIA

We cannot cover secondary headaches without mentioning trigeminal neuralgia, for a practitioner specializing in headaches will receive an occasional referral with this diagnosis. True trigeminal neuralgia is characterized by paroxysms of brief, intense stabbing facial pain. So intense is the pain, in fact, that people with the disorder may wince, giving rise to the now antiquated diagnosis "tic douloureux," that is, "painful tic" (Kitt, Gruber, M. Davis, Woolf, & Levine, 2000). The pain is often elicited by light touch to "trigger zones" around the mouth or cheek, although these may not be present early in the disorder, and are too unreliable to be a diagnostic criterion (P. Rasmussen, 1991). Trigeminal neuralgia is rare, with an incidence of approximately .004 percent, and primarily affecting those of late middle age or older. The disorder appears to be slightly more common in women, but this may simply reflect the fact that fewer men live to reach old age (Kitt et al.).

The cause of trigeminal neuralgia is unknown, but is thought to include compression of the trigeminal nerve by blood vessels as it approaches the trigeminal ganglion. This is supported by intra-operative findings, the rapid relief of pain by surgery to separate the blood vessel and nerve ("microvascular decompression"), and by recent imaging studies (Kitt et al., 2000). The evidence is far from certain: The disorder is uncommon, the imaging technology is new, the surgical results are not proof (surgery can be a very powerful placebo; Finneson, 1969; Wall, 1999), and no one yet knows the frequency of trigeminal nerve compression in asymptomatic individuals (Kitt et al.). Still, nerve compression of vascular origin remains the most important theory. Ominous causes, however, need to be excluded. Imaging studies, to check for a tumor or other lesion, are generally appropriate in trigeminal neuralgia (Zakrzewska, 2002).

The standard first-line treatment for trigeminal neuralgia is anticonvulsant medication, especially carbamazepine (Tegretol; Fields, 1996; Zakrzewska, 1999). If the medication loses its effectiveness and if other anticonvulsants or baclofen do not work, then the physician may recommend a neurosurgical consult for consideration of microvascular decompression (Fields, 1996). P. Rasmussen (1991) reports his clinical experience that injections of steroids or anesthetics to the temporomandibular joint brings temporary improvement, presumably by reducing proprioceptive signals functioning as triggers.

So far, in few studies has trigeminal neuralgia been examined for behavioral aspects. Other types of neuralgia, however, show clear exacerbation by stress ("sympathetic-sensory coupling;" see Chapter 2) and when this is the predominant trigger it may be possible in some cases to control the pain through effective **stress management** skills. Moreover, there seem to be cases in which not just TMD but also myofascial pain of the neck is a key aggravating factor. Thus, surface

EMG, and relaxation skills as an adjunct to physical therapy, may also help manage the condition. And psychological work in pain coping can be a useful complement to medication (Zakrzewska, 1999), for medications generally do not eliminate the pain completely. Thus, the patient will have to choose between adapting to the residual pain, and undergoing a delicate operation. Or patients may find medication side effects (especially disruptions in attention and alertness) aversive in themselves. Moreover, 76 percent of individuals with this disorder report that chewing and talking trigger the pain bursts (P. Rasmussen, 1991), and hence avoidance behaviors can have considerable impact (Zakrzewska, 1999). The neuralgia can also lead to background pain, between the paroxysms, suggesting central sensitization. And as we saw in Chapter 3, intense paroxysms of pain may make other sensations more aversive, perhaps contributing to somatic focus and pain-related anxiety. Skills for adapting to pain and for ending a pain-stress-avoidance cycle may thus be of utility.

Having said this, in my experience few if any of the patients referred with a trigeminal neuralgia diagnosis actually have paroxysmal stabbing pain with trigger zones. Rather, the diagnosis seems to be used in practice as a synonym for "chronic idiopathic facial pain." Patients with chronic idiopathic facial pain may indeed benefit from chronic pain treatment just as may individuals with other types of chronic pain. However, I would recommend that the psychologist request evaluation by a neurologist, if one is not already on the case, before embarking on behavioral treatment of any individual who carries a diagnosis of trigeminal neuralgia.

POSTTRAUMATIC HEADACHES

> *It has justly been said by one of the greatest masters of the Art of Surgery that this or any other country has ever produced—Robert Liston—that no injury of the Head is too trivial to be despised.*
>
> —John E. Erichsen (1866, p. 1)

Michael was a driven, successful teacher until two car accidents in one winter. Since then, he has had a continuous dull ache encompassing his entire head, mental fatigue, irritability, and difficulty concentrating and remembering. He prepares for class in brief, unsatisfactory scraps of time, and checks and rechecks his work. The stress only intensifies the pain. His face seems frozen in consternation and worry.

The International Headache Society criteria distinguish between those posttraumatic headaches for which there are strong confirmatory signs of a head trauma (e.g., loss of consciousness greater than 30 minutes, or imaging demonstration of a traumatic brain lesion), and those headaches for which the confirmation is much weaker ("symptoms and/or signs diagnostic of a concussion"). As a hint of the difficulties in this field, we may note that the majority of patients seen clinically for posttraumatic headache do not have strong confirmatory evidence that a head trauma took place (M. Hines, 1999). Tests, such as the neurological examination, skull x-rays, other CNS imaging studies, evoked potential EEG, cerebrospinal fluid, and tests of vestibular function, may be normal. Indeed, Hines has argued that reliance on these tests would be premature for clinical work, because they imply that the headaches should be related to the test results, when in fact we usually do not know what the mechanism of headache is (M. Hines, 1999).

Incidence

The overall yearly incidence of head injury in the developed world seems to be approximately 0.25 percent (Kraus, McArthur, & Silberman, 1994). It is likely that four-fifths of these individuals have headaches afterwards (M. S. Elkind & A. H. Elkind, 1999), for a yearly incidence of posttraumatic headache of about 0.20 percent. In 80–90 percent of cases, however, the headaches resolve within a few months (M. S. Elkind & A. H. Elkind, 1999), and thus the incidence of *chronic* posttraumatic headache appears to be an order of magnitude lower, c. 0.02–0.04 percent.

More recent data have been supportive. Thurman, et al., analyzing hospital discharge data and death certificates, found that the yearly incidence of head injury in the US has dropped to around 0.09 percent, (0.07 percent if deaths are excluded), presumably due to air bags, child safety seats, and greater use of seatbelts (Thurman, Alverson, Dunn, Guerrero, & Sniezek, 1999). However, only one-quarter of head injuries result in hospitalization or death (Sosin, Sniezek, & Thurman, 1996), and so the actual incidence is presumably four times higher, or 0.36 percent. By correcting for deaths and applying the assumptions of Elkind and Elkind we arrive at a yearly incidence of chronic posttraumatic headache of around 0.04 percent.

Pathophysiology and Psychology

Although not uncommon as long-term sequellae of head injury (Triplett, Hill, Freeman, Rajan, & Templer, 1996), little is known about posttraumatic headaches. In the absence of more definite knowledge, five broad models have been suggested, and these perhaps may be of some use in guiding treatment.

Mechanical aspects.   The rapid deceleration that often causes a head injury (for example, in a motor vehicle accident) can also give rise to trigger points in the cervical muscles (Travell & Simons, 1983). Thus, in one view, posttraumatic headaches may represent referred pain from a chronic myofascial dysfunction, similar to the presumed muscular aspects of tension-type headache. Of course muscles are not the only structure that can be injured in whiplash. Thus, for example, chronic referred pain from upper cervical joints could play a role (Treleaven, Jull, & Atkinson, 1994), as could an injury-induced temporomandibular dysfunction (Kolbinson, J. B. Epstein, & Burgess, 1996; Steed & Wexler, 2001). Soft tissue factors are consistent with the finding that long-term headaches are more likely if the head was rotated or inclined at the time that whiplash injury occurred (Radanov, Sturzenegger, & Di Stefano, 1995; Sturzenegger, Radanov, & Di Stefano, 1995).

Not surprisingly, then, Duckro et al. found that the vast majority of their subjects with posttraumatic headache had localized or widespread tenderness to muscle palpation (Duckro, Chibnall, & Greenberg, 1995). The muscle tenderness was correlated with scores on the **Beck Depression Inventory**, the Spielberger Anger Expression Inventory, and the Pain Disability Index. Duckro et al. suggest that the muscle tenderness represents a primary myofascial problem that is producing secondary emotional effects, but the direction of causality has not been settled empirically.

In other work, more subtle problems have been detected. Using a manual examination, Treleaven and coworkers found that patients who had headaches following a concussion were more likely to also have painful dysfunction at their upper cervical joints. Decreased endurance in the neck flexor muscles and increased muscle tightness were also found, but such mainstays of the physical exam as posture and active neck range of motion did not differ from controls (Treleaven, Jull, & Atkinson, 1994).

Support for the role of the upper cervical joints comes from another direction as well. Bogduk and coworkers first used nerve blocks to identify symptomatic zygapophyseal (facet) joints in patients with chronic neck pain from a motor vehicle accident. On later days, they then used either a local anesthetic or a placebo (saline) "nerve block" in a double-blind, crossover design. They found that in 49 percent of patients, neck pain was eliminated by the anesthetic but not the placebo. Now, for patients whose primary symptom was headache, a true placebo-control was not possible because the nerve block for the relevant joint, C2–3, also causes numbness of skin, which the patient would be able to detect. Therefore, to help rule out placebo responding, either a long-acting or a short-acting anesthetic was injected in a double-blind, crossover design. For 50 percent of patients, the long-acting and the short-acting anesthetic each eliminated the headache for the expected duration of action (S. Lord, Barnsley, Wallis, & Bogduk, 1996). All of this would seem to commend a close examination of the zygapophyseal joints in posttraumatic headache.

Vascular aspects.   SPECT and xenon 133 inhalation studies in people with chronic post-traumatic headaches show areas of hypoperfusion, suggesting that regulation of cerebral blood flow is disrupted (Abdel-Dayem, et al., 1998; Gilkey, Ramadan, Aurora, & Welch, 1997). In this second model the headaches, like migraines, have a vascular component. Moreover, a number of biochemical similarities have been reported between migraine and posttraumatic headache (Packard & Ham, 1997a). Thus, in a random sample of 1,950 36-year-old males living around Zurich, Switzerland, a reported history of a severe head trauma increased the probability of reporting a history of migraine by a factor of 4.7. Mild head injury also increased the probability of migraine, but not to a statistically significant extent. The retrospective, questionnaire nature of the data is a drawback, but the investigators tried to corroborate the reports with medical records wherever possible (Merikangas & Angst, 1996). Now, it seems unlikely that migraines or a predisposition to migraines would cause a head injury, and thus we are left with the opposite causality: Head injuries, at least severe ones, seem to increase the probability of developing migraines.

Doubts and controversies.   Nonetheless, any purely mechanical theory of posttraumatic headaches must contend with the fact that severity of injury is at least uncorrelated and perhaps *inversely* correlated (Couch & Bearss, 2001; Yamaguchi, 1992) with the probability of developing a chronic headache. (As we have seen, this is not true of posttraumatic migraines, but the vast majority of posttraumatic headaches do not seem to be migrainous). Yamaguchi's patients were a series of 121 consecutive disability claimants presenting for independent medical evaluation. Among the patients who had sustained a mild head injury, 72 percent reported severe posttraumatic headaches. In contrast, among those who had had a severe head injury, only 33 percent reported chronic posttraumatic headaches. Couch and Bearss' data are from a retrospective chart review of 87 patients seen at a hospital neurology clinic. Of those patients with mild head injury, 80 percent went on to have a chronic daily headache; this was true of only 24 percent of patients with severe head injury.

And there are stronger caveats. Chronic headaches are thought to be rare among professional athletes, despite a relatively high rate of minor head injuries (Duckro & Chibnall, 1999). Analogously, Berry reports that in a retrospective study of 20 drivers in the Demolition Derby, averaging 1900 lifetime collisions per driver, there were *no* reports of chronic whiplash or disability (Berry, 2000). These data seem to compel us to look beyond the mechanics of the accident, to consider individual differences and/or the psychosocial context of the injury.

Still, we must be careful. The results, of course, are qualified by the select nature of the samples (M. D. Freeman, 2001). Professional athletes and drivers are most likely younger, better prepared for collision, in better physical condition, and perhaps more sensation-seeking than the population as a whole. Perhaps the ability to withstand repeated blows without sustaining physical disability is one of the features separating athletes who attain a professional career from those who do not. And the actual data on sports-related headaches are remarkably sparse.

Sallis and Jones, for example, surveyed 320 college and 123 high school football players, and found that 21 percent had had a football-related headache during their most recent game (Sallis & K. Jones, 2000). Junge et al. studied 588 soccer players by questionnaire and found that 28 percent reported problems with headaches (Junge, Dvorak, Chomiak, Peterson, & Graf-Baumann, 2000). Now, because the incidence of headaches in the general population is so high, and because the questionnaire studies do not distinguish between acute and chronic head pain, it is hard to know how to interpret these figures. However, three aspects of the data seem noteworthy. First, Sallis and Jones found that 24 percent of defensive backs, 19 percent of defensive linemen, and 19 percent of offensive linemen reported football-related headaches, while only 10 percent of receivers and 2 percent of kickers did so. This implies that the headaches were due to tackling, although perhaps tackling merely led players to attribute their headaches to football. Second, of those football players who had had a headache during their most recent game, only 19 percent had reported it to the team coach, trainer, or physician (Sallis & K. Jones, 2000). Thus football players might not be resistant to headaches, so much as resistant to reporting headaches. Third, lest we assume that sports injuries are necessarily benign, Matser et al. note that performance of soccer players on neuropsychological tests is inversely correlated with the number of concussions they have sustained, and with the number of times they have headed the ball (Matser, Kessels, Lezak, et al., 1999; Matser, Kessels, Jordan, et al., 1998). Now, none of this data truly answers our question, which is of the prevalence of chronic posttraumatic headache in athletes. The data do, however, give us pause before accepting the sports analogy too readily.

Moreover, data on the relationship between severity of head injury and probability of having a chronic headache may simply be an artifact of sampling bias (Couch & Bearss, 2001). After all, if you had a minor head injury, what else would bring you to a neurologist besides "soft" symptoms such as headaches? People with severe head injuries presumably have many reasons to see a neurologist, even if they do not have headaches.

Another type of argument is given by Berry (2001), when he points out the "common clinical experience" (with which my own experience agrees) that chronic disability is *not* usually seen in the driver who caused the accident. Thus, for example, it is generally the occupants of the car that is rear-ended, and not the people in the car that did the rear-ending, who present for treatment. Against this, we may juxtapose clinical observations from the 19th century, when the motor vehicles were railroads. Erichsen (1882) observed that when a train was struck from behind, passengers facing forward seemed to have the more severe injuries, while when the train was struck from the front, it was the passengers facing backwards who seemed to suffer more injury. Now the potential for compensation would be the same regardless of which way the passengers were facing, so Erichsen's observation, if we accept it, brings us back to a more biomechanical explanation.

And Yamaguchi himself does not rule out a biomechanical explanation. Recall that in his clinical series, people who had sustained a severe head injury were less likely to report a chronic posttraumatic headache than people who had sustained a mild head injury (Yamaguchi, 1992). However, the people who had had a severe injury were also more likely to have normal cervical spine x-rays. Presumably, this was a coincidence, as most of the abnormalities were degenerative changes that may not have been accident-related. However, the abnormalities *were* related to the probability of reporting a posttraumatic headache. Thus, Yamaguchi raises the question of whether the degenerative changes might be a biasing factor in favor of developing a posttraumatic headache.

Attributions.   A third model is illustrated in a study by Schrader and colleagues, of car accidents in Lithuania. Lithuania was chosen because, at least at the time of the research, accident insurance and a belief that whiplash could be disabling were both rare. In the retrospective study,

Schrader et al. found that 53 percent of their accident victims had headaches, and 9 percent had headaches more than 7 days per month. However, in an age- and sex-matched control group the corresponding rates were equally high: 50 percent and 6 percent, respectively. Moreover, of those accident victims who had frequent headaches, most (85 percent) had had frequent headaches before the injury. The authors speculate that posttraumatic headaches are not consequences of the motor vehicle accidents at all, but are headaches from other sources that come to be attributed to the accidents (Schrader, Obelieniene, et al., 1996). Possible reasons for the attribution might include compensation and litigation, cultural belief that whiplash can lead to long-term disability, and even the involvement of the therapeutic community (Obelieniene, Schrader, Bovim, Miseviciene, & Sand, 1999).

A difficulty with the attribution model is that chronic posttraumatic headaches generally present as part of a constellation of postconcussion symptoms, which may include depression and irritability; fatigue, dizziness and tinnitus; and/or reports of impaired concentration and memory (Duckro & Chibnall, 1999). Thus, posttraumatic headaches do not seem to be fully interchangeable with tension-type headaches.

Rebound.   Note that we have already encountered daily headaches in Chapter 7, where they were related not to a head injury, but to frequent use of symptomatic headache medications. In fact, N. T. Mathew (1993) reports, based on clinical experience, that medication overuse headaches are usually accompanied by restlessness, fatigue, irritability, depression, and memory difficulties, and can be worsened by even small amounts of cognitive or physical effort. The resemblance to posttraumatic headaches is striking, and of course individuals diagnosed with posttraumatic headache are often consumers, and sometimes over-consumers, of headache medications. Thus, in the fourth model, head injuries are thought to be generally responsible for only acute headaches; the transformation into chronic headaches, like the transformation of migraine into daily headache, is considered to be a function of high intake of analgesic or vasoconstrictive medications.

Does this theory hold up in practice? Warner and G. M. Fenichel (1996) suggest that 9 of 11 (or 82 percent of) consecutive referrals to the Vanderbilt Headache Clinic for chronic posttraumatic headache actually had drug-rebound headache. However, their sample is small and nonrandom, and the supporting data is anecdotal and open to interpretation (P. E. Sternberg, 1997). Haas (1997) reports an unpublished clinical series in which 9 of 48 (or 19 percent of) individuals referred for posttraumatic headache were better diagnosed as having drug rebound headache. Thus, the data so far are variable and weak. They compel us to look carefully for analgesic overuse, and to treat it when it is present, but they do not seem sufficient to invalidate the diagnostic category of posttraumatic headache.

Stress, trauma and chronic pain.   In a fifth model, the focus is on stressors from lifestyle disruption, and possible cognitive limitations, and/or Posttraumatic Stress Disorder. These stressors are thought to perpetuate a chronic headache disorder through psychophysiological mechanisms (Martelli, Grayson, & Zasler, 1999). Thus, van der Naalt et al. found that in their sample of 67 patients with mild or moderate head injury, the incidence of headache at first declined, from 37 percent of patients at 1 month post injury, to 26 percent at 3 months, and on down to 19 percent at 6 months. However, at 1 year post-injury the percentage with headaches was back up to 32 percent. Now, 73 percent of patients had returned to work or school, most within the first 6 months. The authors speculate that as they settled in to their occupations, minor difficulties with concentration or fatigue may have become more apparent (van der Naalt, van Zomeren, Sluiter, & Minderhoud, 1999).

The prevalence of Posttraumatic Stress Disorder (PTSD) among patients with chronic post-traumatic headaches is unknown but thought to be quite high. Hickling and Blanchard (1992) found that 50 percent of one sample of 20 posttraumatic headache patients met the diagnostic criteria for PTSD. The prevalence was 75 percent in a second sample of 20 reported by the same investigators (Hickling, Blanchard, Silverman, & Schwarz, 1992). And Chibnall and Duckro (1994) found a prevalence of 29 percent in their sample of 41 chronic posttraumatic headache patients. Thus, the chronic stress of PTSD may be a factor contributing to the headaches. Moreover, it appears that treatment of PTSD is likely to be an important component of therapy for chronic posttraumatic headache.

For other patients, disability may become more severe and lasting. In time, a chronic pain syndrome may develop, in which catastrophizing and avoidant, maladaptive coping contribute to distress, disability, and further stress. In fact, Todd et al. noted that some of their posttraumatic headache patients seemed afraid to exert themselves cognitively, out of concern that it would worsen the headaches, or even worsen a brain injury. These patients responded to formal cognitive-behavioral treatment for phobic avoidance of cognitive effort (Todd, Martelli, & Grayson, 1998, cited in Martelli, Grayson, & Zasler, 1999).

These five competing and disparate models serve to stake out the terrain in what will hopefully be an intensively researched field. In the meantime, treatment of posttraumatic headaches is by analogy (Silberstein, Lipton, & Goadsby, 1998). If the headache is primarily migrainous in clinical presentation, suggesting activation of the trigeminovascular system, then migraine treatments are tried. If the headache appears primarily myofascial, or if it resembles a chronic tension-type headache, then treatments appropriate to this comparison are brought to bear. Regardless of the type of headache physiology, treatments for chronic pain syndrome may be relevant, particularly if the headaches are causing significant emotional distress or disruption of psychosocial functioning. Thus, Martelli et al. suggest that a multicomponent approach, including cognitive-behavioral and medical treatments, and broader psychotherapy if needed, is the appropriate intervention for chronic posttraumatic headache (Martelli, Grayson, & Zasler, 1999).

CHAPTER 9

Headaches in Children

"boo-boo head."

—2 year old boy with a migraine, quoted in C. F. Barlow (1994, p. 93)

During a migraine, Pam seems wan, sensitive, and weak, with big dark eyes. She gets dizzy and nauseated and buries her head in her mother's arms, where it's dark. Her head hurts a lot, towards the front, on both sides. Running around seems to bring them on, especially if she gets sweaty or it's a bright sunny day. But an hour later she's out running around again.

It would be bad enough if chronic headaches were an affliction of adults only. As we will see, however, children and even infants can have migraines and perhaps other types of headaches as well. Thus, as we study these disorders, better positioning ourselves to assess and treat, it behooves us to consider the data on pediatric headaches specifically.

There is no separate diagnosis for a headache occurring in a child or adolescent. In general, young people are susceptible to the same types of headaches as are adults, most commonly migraines and tension-type headaches, but also cluster headache (Del Bone, 1987), chronic daily headache (Gladstein, Holden, Winner, Linder, et al., 1997; Holden, Gladstein, Trulsen, & B. Wall, 1994), analgesic rebound (Abu-Arefeh, 2001; Vasconcellos, Pina-Garza, Milan, Ernesto, & Warner, 1998), and headache that follows head trauma (Callaghan & Abu-Arefeh, 2001). Thus, quite a bit of material relevant to children can be found throughout this book. However, because of the special nature of the population, a few findings in the empirical literature are collected here.

PREVALENCE

Several studies have bearing on prevalence. They use somewhat different case definitions, somewhat limiting the comparability of their results.

In a classic paper, Bille (1962) examined all 9000 school children, ages 7–15, in Uppsala, Sweden, in 1955. He found that 3.9 percent of the children had migraines, and that 6.8 percent had frequent nonmigrainous headaches. The prevalence of migraine increased with age, with 1.4 percent of the 7-year-olds and 5.3 percent of the 15-year-olds meeting the diagnostic criteria. A female preponderance began emerging at age 11.

Nearly 30 years later, Abu-Arefeh and Russell found a one-year migraine prevalence of 10.6 percent in Aberdeen, Great Britain, comprising a prevalence of 7.8 percent for migraine without aura and 2.8 percent for migraine with aura (Abu-Arefeh & G. Russell, 1994). Thus, Abu-Arefeh and Russell obtained a rate that was nearly three times higher than that reported by Bille. Now, as Bille used the classic diagnostic criteria of Vahlquist (1955), and Abu-Arefeh and

Russell used those of the International Headache Society (Headache Classification Committee, 1988), their results are not strictly comparable. However, shifting from the IHS criteria to those of Vahlquist seems to increase reported migraine prevalence by only one-third (Mortimer, Kay, & Jaron, 1992). Hence, Abu-Arefeh and Russell suggest that the 172 percent increase they found over Bille reflects a true change in migraine prevalence.

Even more telling are the results of Laurell, et al. who, in consultation with Bille, repeated his study of Uppsala, with comparable questionnaire and sampling, and using the Vahlquist criteria (Laurell, Larsson, & Eeg-Olofsson, 2004). They found that by 1997, the one-year prevalence of pediatric migraine had increased by 69 percent, to 6.6 percent. The one-year prevalence of *any* headache had also increased, from 59 percent to 84 percent, despite the exclusion of headaches due to fever or illness in the later survey (Laurell et al.).

In the United States, a large-scale population study by Linet, found a *4 week* migraine prevalence of 3.8 percent in boys ages 12–17, and 6.6 percent in girls (Linet, Stewart, Celentano, D. Ziegler, & Sprecher, 1989). Note that these figures, too, are higher than Bille's, despite the fact that Bille was asking about one year prevalence. In the Linet et al. study, 57 percent of boys and 76 percent of girls had experienced a headache of some type during the preceding four weeks.

Another particularly definitive study of childhood headache was conducted by Aromaa et al. in a province in southwestern Finland (Aromaa, Sillanpää, Rautava, & Helenius, 1998). They defined a representative cohort of 1278 births, of whom they were able to examine 968 at age 7 years. In all, in the preceding 6 months, 15 percent of the children had experienced a headache severe enough that it interfered with their daily activities. There were no sex differences.

MIGRAINE

Diagnosis

Compared with diagnoses by pediatric neurologists, the 1988 IHS migraine criteria seemed to have poor sensitivity. In one study, only 27 to 39 percent of children diagnosed as having migraines met the IHS criteria (Maytal, M. Young, Shechter, & Lipton, 1997), and similar results have been reported by others (e.g., Gallai, Sarchielli, Carboni, Benedetti, Mastropaolo, & Puca, 1995; Gladstein, Holden, Peralta, & Raven, 1993). The main culprit seemed to be a much briefer headache duration in children. For patients under 15 years old, the IHS criterion were 2 to 48 hours, vs. 4 to 72 hours in adults, but the reduction probably wasn't enough. In empirical studies, a duration of 1 hour is quite typical of childhood migraines (Maytal, et al.). This 1-hour minimum duration was accepted in the 2004 revision, provided it is corroborated in a prospective diary (Headache Classification Subcommittee, 2004).

Maytal et al. report that the IHS criteria fare considerably better when they are modified to reflect a 1 to 72 hour duration (Maytal et al., 1997), but controversy remains. In a study by Rossi, et al, of 320 children with chronic and/or recurrent headaches, 12.2 percent of attacks had a duration of less than one hour. Not surprisingly, then, Rossi et al. suggest eliminating duration altogether as a criterion (L. Rossi, Cortinovis, Menegazzo, Brunelli, Bossi, & Macchi, 2001). On the other hand, Abu-Arafeh and Callaghan (2004) found only 3 children out of 246 (1.2 percent) whose migrainous headaches were consistently shorter than one hour. For these few individuals, however, otherwise typical migraines could be as short as 5 or 10 minutes.

Other criteria have also been called into question. For example, in the study by Rossi et al., pulsatile pain was not present in the majority of migraineurs until ages 10–15. In children below the age of 6, less than 40 percent had a pulsating pain. Whether this age-dependence reflects a true change in migraine experience, or whether it is simply too difficult for young children to describe a pulsating pain, is not known (L. Rossi, et al., 2001). Meanwhile, in a population-based study by Aromaa et al., approximately ¾ of the children had headaches that were bilateral and frontal or supraorbital in location, and felt like a "gnawing" or "tightening" pain, despite the fact that 55 percent of the children with headaches met IHS criteria for migraine specifically (Aromaa, Sillanpää, Rautava, & Helenius, 1998). Similarly, Gallai et al. found that 57 percent of their pediatric migraineurs had bilateral pain (Gallai, Sarchielli, Carboni, et al., 1995), while for Guidetti, et al. the figure was around 80 percent (Guidetti, Bruni, Cerutti, et al., 1991). Thus, for many children with migraines, unilateral location was similarly non-diagnostic. Some have even argued that a clear distinction between migraine and tension-type headache cannot be made in children (L. Rossi et al.), or that characteristic types of headache should be identified separately in each age group (Gallai, Sarchielli, Carboni, et al.; Gladstein, Holden, Peralta, et al., 1993).

Age at Onset

The two year old whose quote begins this chapter is not the youngest child with migraine reported by C. F. Barlow. One boy seemed to have migraines beginning at 4 months, and two other children by 9 months of age. On the uncertain foundation of published clinical series, Barlow estimates that 1–2 percent of migraineurs have first onset by age 2.

How do we know if a very young child has migraines? Technically we do not, as we cannot ask them about the diagnostic criteria. However, certain symptoms are strongly suggestive of migraine: A disorder that occurs in discrete episodes, with complete recovery in between; associated with vomiting, pallor, abdominal pain, irritability, lethargy, vertigo and/or ataxia; sometimes with communication of head pain; relieved by sleep; in a child with a family history of migraine (C. F. Barlow, 1994; Elser & Woody, 1990).

Elser and Woody report on several preschool children with severe headaches who seemed to improve significantly with very low dose amitriptyline or imipramine. In some cases the medication was gradually withdrawn after 2–3 months without the headache returning. Children with ophthalmoplegic migraines (headaches accompanied by unilateral **ptosis** and oculomotor nerve paresis) had poorer outcomes, however (Elser & Woody, 1990).

Comorbidity

Allergies.   There is a small but persistent literature suggesting that allergic conditions such as asthma, eczema, and rhinitis (hay fever), are more common in children who have headaches. Conversely, Mortimer et al., studying 1,077 children ages 3–11 in a general medical practice, found that among those with allergic condition, the risk of headache was increased. Although this was statistically significant for "headache" as a general category, the increased risk was numerically strong specifically in migraine. The percent ratio (relative risk) of migraine diagnosis was 1.78 for children with asthma, 1.86 for eczema, and 2.88 for rhinitis (Mortimer, Kay, Gawkrodger, Jaron, & Barker, 1993).

Now, the drawback of using medical patients is that the comorbidity may be a result of selection bias. That is, patients who have more than one condition might be more likely to seek treatment, giving the illusion that the conditions are correlated. Presumably, this confound would most affect settings in which patients are a highly select group, such as a tertiary care specialty clinic, and be less of a problem in a general medical practice. Still, it would be far preferable to have data from a large prospective cohort study. And as it turns out, in this case we do. Specifically, Chen and Leviton examined the relationship between asthma in children, and a history of migraine, asthma or allergies in the mother, among 2510 children from the Collaborative Perinatal Project.

They found that if the mother had a history of migraines, the child was 1.9 times more likely to have asthma. By contrast, if the mother had a history of asthma or allergies, the child was 2.1 times more likely to have asthma. And if the mother had both a history of migraines and a history of asthma/allergies, the asthma risk in the child was 3.6 times higher than if the mother had neither condition. All of these associations were statistically significant of course, given their magnitude and the large sample size. There were no sex or racial effects, and cigarette smoking did not interact with the maternal history variables (T. C. Chen & Leviton, 1990).

These results are noteworthy. We saw in Chapter 4 that migraines may be becoming more prevalent in western counties but that the evidence is not iron-clad. In this chapter we have seen somewhat stronger evidence that migraines are becoming more common in children specifically. Stronger still is evidence that the prevalence of asthma is increasing in the western world (Grant, R. Wagner, & Weiss, 1999; Woodruff & Fahy, 2001), and the same may be true for rhinitis and eczema. For example, Titus K. Ninan and George Russell found that the prevalence of asthma and eczema approximately doubled, and that of hay fever nearly quadrupled, among 8–13 year old children in Aberdeen Scotland between 1964 and 1989 (Ninan & G. Russell, 1992). Thus, the comorbidity between asthma and migraines lends some circumstantial evidence to the idea that migraines may be becoming more prevalent.

Why would migraines and allergies be connected? Speculation has focused on histamine, which is vasoactive, released in allergies, and a likely mechanism through which calcitonin gene-related peptide dilates and inflames blood vessels (Ottosson & Edvinsson, 1997). Others have focused on a possible role of platelet activating factor in bronchial constriction and the possible increase in platelet aggregation during migraines (Mortimer, Kay, Gawkrodger, Jaron, & Barker, 1993). However, we must be careful not to infer too much from correlational data. For example, there is a little bit of data suggesting that acetaminophen could be a risk factor for asthma, at least in adults (Shaheen, Sterne, Songhurst, & Burney, 2000), and of course migraineurs can be high consumers of acetaminophen.

Periodic syndrome.   Another condition that has been associated with childhood migraines is referred to as the "periodic syndrome of childhood" (Wyllie & Schlesinger, 1933). The periodic syndrome is a group of symptoms that, like migraine, occur in discrete episodes, lack a simple physical cause, and appear to have a psychological or stress-related component. The classic symptoms in this group, together with their typical age of onset, are (Lanzi, Zambrino, Balottin, Tagliasacchi, Verrcelli, & Termine, 1997): motion sickness (1 year old), cyclic vomiting (2 years), limb pain (growing pains; 3 years), periodic fevers of unknown origin (5 years), abdominal pain (6 years), and benign paroxysmal vertigo of childhood (7 years). Lanzi et al. found that all of these components except for motion sickness were more frequent in children with migraine. Thus, we could place migraines, with an average age of onset of 7 years, as the last step in this sequence.

From the lower pain thresholds seen at the ipsilateral forearm during migraines (see Chapter 4) we might expect that *arm pain* as a migraine accompaniment would be rather common. In fact the actual prevalence is unknown, but based on a clinical series of adults and their knowledge of their cachement area, Guiloff and Fruns estimate an annual incidence of somewhat over 3 per 100,000 people (Guiloff & Fruns, 1988). At such a low rate of occurrence one wonders whether the association is anything more than coincidence. However, the authors note that in individual cases the covariation in head and hand, arm, or shoulder pain (and sometimes head and leg, knee, or foot pain) can be strong. In any event, it appears that limb pain in children is much more common than in adults (Knishkowy, Palti, Tima, B. Adler, & Gofin, 1995), and presumably some fraction of these cases fall within the scope of periodic syndrome.

Another type of periodic disorder, *benign paroxysmal vertigo of childhood*, is characterized by brief episodes in which a person feels as if their surroundings are spinning, without loss of consciousness, without auditory or neurological changes, and without known medical cause (Abu-Arafeh & G. Russell, 1995b). As in all the periodic syndromes, the episodes are separated by periods of complete remission. Now, vertigo seems to be rather common in 5–15 year old children, with approximately 18 percent reporting at least one such episode over the preceding year. However, attribution can usually be made to infection, trauma, or other medical condition. The one-year prevalence of benign paroxysmal vertigo, in which there are at least 3 medically unexplained attacks over the course of a year, seems to be only around 2.6 percent (Abu-Arafeh & G. Russell, 1995b).

An association with migraine is suggested from several directions (Abu-Arafeh & G. Russell, 1995b): "Tiredness" and "stress" are sometimes reported as triggers. Attacks are occasionally associated with phonophobia, photophobia, or anorexia, although more commonly with pallor or nausea. Also, children with benign paroxysmal vertigo are approximately 2.3 times more likely than matched control children to have at least one first-degree relative with migraine.

Cyclic vomiting syndrome involves recurrent episodes of intense vomiting (peak intensity 12.6 emeses per hour), often leading to dehydration, but occurring relatively infrequently (on average 1.9 times per month in a clinic sample), and unexplained after gastroenterological, neurological, endocrine, and metabolic work-up (Pfau, B. U. K. Li, Murray, Heitlinger, McClung, & Hayes, 1996). Pfau et al. suggest that frequent (more than nine attacks per month) and lower intensity episodes (less than four emeses per hour) do not fit the pattern of cyclic vomiting and are more likely to have a gastrointestinal cause.

The prevalence of cyclic vomiting syndrome is not known with certainty, in part because it has been little studied, and in part because it is hard to rule out transient organic causes (such as an infection) in community surveys. Abu-Arafeh and G. Russell report a prevalence of 1.9 percent among 5–15 year old public school children in Aberdeen, Scotland (Abu-Arafeh & G. Russell, 1995a). However, the true prevalence rate may be higher or lower, depending on whether the authors over- or underestimated the presence of underlying organic pathology (Abu-Arafeh & G. Russell, 1995a; B. U. K. Li, 2001). In the community, cyclic vomiting syndrome may be less severe than in clinic samples, with 8 attacks per year on average (Abu-Arafeh & G. Russell, 1995a) rather than the average of 23 attacks per year noted by Pfau et al. Attacks typically seem to last 4–48 hours. Approximately 30 percent of sufferers report comorbid travel sickness, and traveling can be a trigger of individual attacks. Rest and sleep are often reported to be helpful (Abu-Arafeh & G. Russell, 1995a).

How do we draw a connection between cyclic vomiting syndrome and migraines? The triggers for cyclic vomiting, given in Table 9–1, resemble those for migraines. For most children cyclic vomiting syndrome spontaneously remits between the ages of 9 and 14, but at least one third then go on to have migraines (B. U. K. Li, 2001). In one large clinical series, of children who meet the quantitative criteria for cyclic vomiting, 47 percent had a first degree relative with migraines (versus 14 percent of children with more frequent, low-intensity vomiting episodes). Cyclic vomiting resembles migraines, too, in occurring somewhat more frequently at night, in having associated photophobia and phonophobia, and in seeming to respond to migraine prophylactics such as propranolol or cyproheptadine (B. U. K. Li, 2001; Pfau, B. U. K. Li, Murray, Heitlinger, McClung, & Hayes, 1996). In Chapter 2 we saw that nausea can elicit hyperalgesia, and hence we are not surprised to learn that hyperalgesia can accompany the vomiting episodes (B. U. K. Li, 2001).

What accounts for the association between migraine and periodic syndromes? Lanzi et al.'s study was conducted in a medical setting and hence we cannot rule out selection bias. An attempt

TABLE 9–1
Triggers for Cyclic Vomiting Syndrome

Trigger	Percent of Children Reporting
Infections (e.g., sinusitis)	41%
Excitement or Stress	34%
Ingesting Chocolate, Cheese, or MSG	26%
Physical Exhaustion or Lack of Sleep	18%
Allergic Events	13%
Menstruation	13%
Motion Sickness	9%

Note. Data are from "Cyclic Vomiting Snydrome: Age-Old Syndrome and New Insights," by B. U. K. Li, 2001, *Seminars in Pediatric Neurology, 8* p. 13. Copyright 2001 by Elsevier. Reprinted with permission.

was made to control for this by using children at other types of clinics for comparison (psychosis, epilepsy, neuromuscular disease) and for them no association with periodic syndrome was found. However, selection bias need not affect all conditions equally. For example, a child with a severe neuromuscular disease might be brought in for treatment regardless of whether there was a comorbid condition. Thus, the association could be artifactual. On the other hand, the periodic syndrome seems to make sense. Abdominal pain and limb pain might indicate deficits in pain inhibition. Vomiting and vertigo could be early migraine symptoms.

Until recently there was little research, and we could discuss cyclic vomiting only in the descriptive clinical terms of a 19th century diagnosis. Recently, however, cyclic vomiting syndrome has begun to yield to investigation, and the emerging data suggests further parallels to migraine. Thus, there is evidence that a few children with cyclic vomiting syndrome have defects in their mitochondrial DNA (Boles, Chun, Senadheera, & L.-J. C. Wong, 1997; Boles & J. C. Williams, 1999). And heart rate variability data suggests higher sympathetic tone (To, Issenman, & Kamath, 1999). These may be the first clues to a diathesis underlying the periodic syndrome. We will seek further clues in the next section, on "defining risk."

Defining Risk

Some investigators have suggested that a proneness to severe headaches can be detected in infancy, offering the hope that preventive strategies can be devised. Thus, Guidetti and coworkers, studying a cohort of 1184 children born at Rome University, found that 15 percent could be classified as "hyperreactive" at 6 months of age. The "hyperreactive" category was defined as increased reactivity to standard stimuli (e.g., a 12 watt flashlight held 6 inches in front of the child's eyes), and spontaneous behaviors such as an absence of self-quieting behaviors or minimal spontaneous sleeping after meals. Now, this was a prospective study, and the authors were able to assess 56 percent of the hyperreactive children (and a somewhat higher proportion of matched control children) approximately 10 years later. The authors found that by late adulthood or early adolescence, 53 percent of the hyperreactive children, but only 15 percent of the matched controls, had developed "common migraine," which is an older term corresponding roughly to migraine without aura. Moreover, most of the hyperreactive children with migraine had first manifested a "periodic syndrome" such as recurrent abdominal pain, growing pain, benign paroxysmal vertigo, or cyclic vomiting (Guidetti, Ottaviano, Pagliarini, 1984).

My sense is that the use of the older diagnostic criteria (the IHS system would not be published for another 4 years) and the fact that *none* of children in either group developed tension headache, raise questions about whether the diagnosis of "common migraine" can truly be translated into "migraine without aura." If we wish, however, we can read "severe headaches" instead. Either way, the results seem quite striking and deserving of follow-up.

Other investigators have found that severe headaches can be predicted to some extent from early childhood variables. Not surprisingly, a history of suspected headache at age 3, known headache at age 5, and the mother's history of headaches prior to pregnancy, predict a child's headaches at age 6. But sleep difficulties and nocturnal confusion seizures at age 3 also predict severe headaches at age 6. Signs of depression at age 3 are predictive, too. And a variety of problems at age 5, including travel sickness, concentration difficulties, nocturnal enuresis, long-term disease, behavior problems, unusual fatigue, and gregariousness, all seem to augur severe headaches at age 6 (Aromaa, Rautava, Helenius, & Sillanpää, 1998). Perhaps just as significant are the variables that did *not* predict onset of headaches: such indicators of family environment as parental divorce, single-parent home, and number of younger siblings. Similarly, Balottin, et al. felt that the majority of very young children referred to their tertiary care headache clinic had a comorbid psychological condition, especially social or separation anxiety disorder (Balottin, Nicoli, Pitillo, Ginevra, Borgatti, & Lanzi, 2004). As with the results of Guidetti, et al., we are left with the impression that severe headaches in early childhood are part of a more general, internal vulnerability.

Given the potential role of operant factors in pain, we might suspect that the parents of children with severe recurrent headaches would be more likely than other parents to respond solicitously to their children's pain. Data relevant to this is found in a population-based study of 6 year olds in Finland (Aromaa, Sillanpää, Rautava, & Helenius, 2000). Aromaa et al. found that parents of children with severe headaches were *less* likely to report displaying negative emotion to the child's pain, compared with parents of matched control children (odds ratios 0.3–0.4, $p = 0.02$ to $<.001$; Aromaa, Sillanpää, Rautava, & Helenius, 2000). Moreover, the mothers of children with headaches were less likely to restrict the child's play out of concern the child would be hurt (odds ratio $= 0.5, p < .05$). On the other hand, the possibility of **modeling** was supported, as the fathers of children with headaches (but not the mothers, at least at the mother's report) were more likely to have high pain sensitivity themselves (Aromaa, Sillanpää, Rautava, & Helenius, 2000).

Surface EMG in Children

There have been few studies of muscle tension in pediatric migraine. In a rare exception, Pritchard (1995) conducted a surface EMG assessment of the frontalis, occipitalis, and neck muscles in 12 children with severe headaches and 12 matched control subjects. In this study, "severe headache" meant at least two headaches a week that were accompanied by at least 3 of the following: nausea or vomiting, aura, photophobia, phonophobia, disability, paleness or lethargy, or change in behavior. Clearly, most or all of these children would be diagnosed as having migraines. Pritchard found no differences in activation at the frontalis or occipitalis muscles, and no differences in stress reactivity at any of the sites. However, throughout the study, children in the headache group had higher activation at their neck muscles. Children in the headache group also had more variability in neck muscle tension, but even so 7 of the 12 were greater than 2 standard deviations above the control group mean. This is a much more striking result than is generally found in adults, and Pritchard suggests that similar studies in children might help us shed light on how primary headache disorders develop.

OTHER TYPES OF HEADACHE

Tension-Type Headache

In children, tension-type headaches are sometimes referred to as "chronic nonprogressive headaches," as opposed to migraines, which are acute-recurrent, and headaches from organic pathology, which are often chronic and progressive (Rothner, 1978). Less is known about pediatric tension-type headache than about migraines, and tension-type headache may even be less common than migraines in this age group. A few studies, however, have focused on the chronic form of tension-type headache.

In Aberdeen, Scotland, the prevalence of chronic tension-type headache among 5–15 year old public school children has been estimated at 0.9 percent (Abu-Arafeh & G. Russell, 1994).

And in one pediatric headache clinic, chronic tension-type headache was one of the most common diagnoses (20.5 percent of 356 patients), second only to migraine without aura (27.8 percent). As might be guessed, chronic tension-type headache was the most frequent cause of chronic near-daily headache in this clinic population, accounting for 63.5 percent of the cases as a sole diagnosis, and another 30.4 percent of cases as a mixed diagnosis in combination with migraine without aura (Abu-Arafeh, 2001).

For chronic tension-type headache, the IHS criteria seem to fare rather well. Abu-Arafeh reports that in 81 percent of those with the diagnosis, there was no more than one migraine-like associated symptom (nausea, photophobia, or phonophobia). Moreover, the headaches were rarely unilateral (3.5 percent of cases). Rather, they generally occurred at the forehead (53.0 percent of cases) or encompassed the entire head (29.6 percent; Abu-Arafeh, 2001). In contrast, the IHS criteria for episodic tension-type headache seem to have difficulties. Headaches that would otherwise be diagnosed as tension-type headache may be too short (less than 30 minutes per episode) or have associated autonomic features suggestive of migraine, yet without seeming to be a true mixed headache (Gallai, Sarchielli, Carboni, Benedetti, Mastropaolo, & Puca, 1995).

Abu-Arafeh suggests that stress, in the form of a health problem in oneself or one's family, or bereavement, is a frequent predisposing factor, having preceded or accompanied the onset of headache in 51 percent of cases (Abu-Arafeh, 2001). Certainly, this is consistent with the literature on chronic tension-type headache in adults. However, without knowing the rates for these stresses in the general population, and among children referred for other disorders, it is hard to draw a firm conclusion.

Posttraumatic Headache

Callaghan and Abu-Arafeh report that of 528 children and adolescents who had attended a headache clinic, 21 had posttraumatic headache specifically (Callaghan & Abu-Arafeh, 2001). In most cases, the head trauma was due to a playground or sports injury, although accidental falls, traffic accidents and, unfortunately, assaults, were also among the causes. In 62 percent of cases the headaches met the diagnostic criteria for episodic or chronic tension-type headache, which was a higher proportion than in the remaining 507 patients (37 percent; Callaghan & Abu-Arafeh, 2001). Of note, in all cases the parents were quite worried on intake about their child's medical condition. However, the course appeared to be stable over follow-ups ranging from 5 to 29 months. No significant worsening is reported, and only 2 of the 21 children became headache-free (Callaghan & Abu-Arafeh, 2001).

Medication-Overuse Headache

In population surveys, 0.3–0.5 percent of junior high school students have chronic daily headache in the context of frequent analgesic use (Dyb, T. L. Holmen, & Zwart, 2006; S.-J. Wang, Fuh, S.-R. Lu, & Juang, 2006). To shed light on whether the analgesics are a likely cause of the headaches, however, we must turn to clinic studies, in which medications can be discontinued.

Vasconcellos, et al. note that of 46 children and adolescents who came to the Vanderbilt Pediatric Headache Clinic because of daily or near daily headache, 30 were also high consumers of analgesics (Vasconcellos, Piña-Garza, Millan, & Warner, 1998). Acetaminophen and ibuprofen were the most commonly used medications, but butalbital-containing compounds, nonsteroidal anti-inflammatories other than ibuprofen, and even narcotic analgesics were reported as well (Vasconcellos, et al.). That the headaches had a strong rebound component is suggested by the results when the medications (and caffeine) were discontinued, and amitriptyline started. Average headache frequency declined from 27.5 days per month to 5.4, while average intensity on a 0–3 scale declined from 2.5 to 1.3. Symptoms began to improve about 2½ weeks after the medications were discontinued, and continued improving for another 4 weeks (Vasconcellos, et al.). Thus, being a child does not seem to confer immunity to medication overuse headache. On the other hand, this clinical series resembles those of adults, in suggesting that migraines may be a risk factor. In all, 79 percent of the children and adolescents with rebound headache had a personal history of migraines, and most of the rest had a family history of migraines (Vasconcellos, et al.).

Caffeine from soft drinks may be a similar problem. Hering-Hanit and Gadoth (2003) note that of 105 children seen for chronic daily headache, 36 were over-consuming caffeinated soda. In fact, the typical intake for these 36 children (average age, 9 years) was 1.5 liters of cola per day, or the caffeine equivalent of 2 cups of coffee. Of the 36, 33 became and remained headache-free after tapering from soda. The remaining 3 children went on to have occasional episodic migraines without aura. Family history of migraine was not particularly common in the chronic daily headache (7/36 children) but did seem to predict the subsequent episodic migraines (3/3 children).

Other Chronic Daily Headache

In the community, the one-year prevalence of chronic daily headache in junior high school students has been estimated as 1.5 percent, and is three times more common in girls (c. 2.4 percent) than boys (c. 0.8 percent). Using the Silberstein and Lipton criteria (see Chapter 7), the most common diagnoses were transformed migraine (56 percent) and chronic tension-type headache (34 percent), with no identifiable cases of hemicrania continua or new daily persistent headache. Medication overuse seemed to play a role in one-fifth of the cases (S.-J. Wang, Fuh, S.-R. Lu, & Juang, 2006).

In contrast, Gladstein and Holden report that the most common forms of chronic daily headache in their clinic were new daily persistent headache and "comorbid headache," each accounting for about 40 percent of cases (Gladstein & Holden, 1996). "Comorbid headache" refers to headaches that resemble transformed migraine, but without a prior history of episodic migraine. Thus, comorbid headache is similar to the older category of "mixed headache" in adults. Logically, people seen in specialty clinics would have more severe, unusual or hard-to-treat conditions.

Little is known of the pathophysiology of daily headaches in children specifically. In children, as in adults, daily headaches seem to be accompanied by more functional impairment and emotional distress than even episodic migraines (Carlsson, Larsson, & Mark, 1996; Metsähonkala, Sillanpää, & Tuominen, 1998).

ON PEDIATRIC HEADACHES IN GENERAL

Natural History

Several authors have investigated whether migraine disorder diagnosed in childhood persists and becomes adult migraine. A striking example is the work of Bille. From among the migraineurs in his 1955 study, he selected 73 who had a relatively high attack frequency, at least 1 per month. So far, he has followed these 73 participants for 40 years. There have been no drop-outs from the study, although 2 subjects passed away between the 30- and 40-year follow-ups. From the vantage point of 40 years, it appears that 23 percent of the childhood migraineurs became permanently migraine-free in their teens or early adulthood. However, at 40 years, 51 percent of the subjects were still having regular migraines. The remaining 26 percent had not had migraines recently, but had continued to have migraines at the time of the earlier follow-ups (Bille, 1997).

Now, 51 percent chronicity after 40 years sounds quite disheartening. However, the frequency of migraine attacks had lowered markedly by then, with many subjects having fewer than 1 per year.

Similar results were reported by Dooley and Bagnell (1995), in a 10-year follow-up of children who had been seen at a hospital-based pediatric neurology clinic. In all, 81 percent of the original sample provided follow-up data. Of 18 children with tension-type headache, 50 percent were headache free, 39 percent still had tension-type headaches, and 11 percent went on to develop migraine without aura at follow-up. Presumably, these prevalence figures are not too different from those in the general population. In contrast, of the 49 children who had migraines without aura, only 20 percent were headache free. Another 22 percent had tension-type headache, and the remaining 57 percent (after rounding error) still met the diagnostic criteria for migraine (Dooley & Bagnell, 1995). However, across all subjects, the frequency of headaches had declined from an average of 11.0 per month to 2.1 per month.

Some decline in frequency would be expected simply from regression to the mean. People are likely to seek out neurological consultation when their headaches are occurring particularly frequently. The follow-up, in contrast, takes place at an unselected time, from the point of view of the subject, and hence the headaches are likely to be less troublesome then. It seems reassuring, however, that for children presenting clinically with migraines, the prognosis is for at least a marked reduction in headache frequency.

If childhood headache tends to persist on some level into adulthood, we can also ask whether it is a harbinger of other adult disorders. This question has been examined in a population-based study in Great Britain, in which 11,407 children were followed from birth to age 33 (Fearon and Hotopf, 2001). This group comprised 69 percent of the original sample, with no identifiable confounding from subject attrition. At age seven, 8.2 percent of the children, and at age eleven, 15.4 percent, had "frequent headache or migraine." These children were more likely at age 33 to report headaches (odds ratio = 1.79) or multiple somatic complaints (odds ratio = 1.61), after controlling for potential confounds such as socioeconomic status in childhood and psychiatric symptoms in adulthood. In fact, adult psychiatric symptoms themselves were slightly predicted by childhood headache, after correction for childhood demographics (odds ratio = 1.17; Fearon & Hotopf, 2001).

The picture is by no means bleak, however. First, the risk conferred by childhood headache, even for adult headache, is rather small in absolute terms. Moreover, it is not just symptoms that may be long lasting: Equally persistent may be a tendency to use coping skills learned in childhood. Dooley and Bagnell note that the children seen in their neurology practice were taught to identify headache triggers and to use nonpharmacological tools such as relaxation. None of the children was initially prescribed medication. When contacted 10 years later, 30.3 percent reported using medications for headaches, versus use of medications by 87 percent of people with headaches in the general population (Dooley & Bagnell, 1995).

Associated Symptoms

Aromaa and colleagues found that children with headache were more likely than non-headache children to report travel sickness (52 percent vs. 25 percent) and **bruxism** (48 percent vs. 32 percent), and to have parents or grandparents (but not siblings) with a history of headaches. On physical exam, the children with headaches were more likely to be tender at the temporomandibular joint (31 percent vs. 15 percent) or at the occipital insertion areas (28 percent vs. 8 percent; Aromaa, Sillanpää, Rautava, & Helenius, 1998).

Triggers

Just as in adults, environmental stresses have been suspected in the headaches of childhood. Even in very young children, onset of the disorder or of individual attacks is thought by some to follow, perhaps 40 percent of the time, such life events as a change in nursery school, birth or illness of a sibling, and conflict or separation of the child's parents (Balottin, Nicoli, Pitillo, Ginevra, Borgatti, & Lanzi, 2004).

Other factors have been implicated as well. In the aforementioned study by Aromaa et al., headaches often began in the afternoon, with the most commonly identified triggers as given in Table 9–2 (Aromaa, Sillanpää, Rautava, & Helenius, 1998).

Ice cream (cold) and fear were more commonly triggers for the children diagnosed with migraines than with tension-type headache. The other triggers did not differ to a statistically significant extent between the two diagnostic groups (Aromaa, Sillanpää, Rautava, & Helenius, 1998).

TABLE 9–2
Triggers for Childhood Headaches

Trigger	Percent of Children Reporting
Fatigue, Sleep Deprivation	72%
Excitement	65%
Other Illness or Fever	64%
Overexposure to Sunlight	62%
Physical Exercise	49%
Mental Distress	44%
TV Watching	41%
Missed Meals	40%
Fear	27%
Ice Cream (Cold)	23%

Note. Data are from "Childhood Headache at School Entry: A Controlled Clinical Study," by M Aromaa, M. L. Sillanpää, P. Rautava, and H. Helenius, 1998, *Neurology, 50,* p. 1731. Copyright 1998 by the American Academy of Neurology. Reprinted with permission.

Similar results have been reported by others. By contrast, McGrath and Hillier give an alternative view. They note that among environmental factors, only dietary triggers have been studied prospectively in children, with studies tending to be disconfirming. Thus, the lists of potential triggers derived from questionnaire studies or interviews with parents are actually lists of attributions for or beliefs about headaches. McGrath and Hillier suggest that these beliefs become self-fulfilling prophesies. The child is taught to avoid the triggers, and when they cannot they become anxious. The anxiety, and presumably the expectation, is the true headache trigger (McGrath & Hillier, 2001).

We will examine triggers in detail, and the question of whether they should be avoided, in Chapter 10.

PART III

Clinical Guide to Headaches

CHAPTER 10

Headache Triggers

. . . during weeks of small household confusions, lost laundry, unhappy help, cancelled appointments, on days when the telephone rings too much and I get no work done and the wind is coming up. On days like that my friend comes uninvited.

—Joan Didion, 1979, p. 172

People with a long history of migraines often matter-of-factly divide their lives into before and after the advent of triptan medications. Although people with tension-type, cluster, and chronic daily headaches still await a breakthrough of such magnitude, we have seen progress on these fronts too. Yet the role of even a brilliantly conceived medication is surely not to blunt the impact of a toxic lifestyle. In headaches, as in blood pressure regulation, and the prevention of cancer and heart disease, lifestyle change is neither "alternative" nor "complementary," but the starting point of health. In the pages that follow, we will examine ways, both pharmacological and behavioral, of reducing the burden of headaches.

One approach to treating headaches is to reduce exposure to the triggers that cause them. But what are these triggers? In the nineteenth century, clinical experience suggested "gastric irritation; powerful impressions on the sensorium, as by the combined sights, sounds, and general excitement of public spectacles and assemblies; ovarian irritation and catamenial [menstrual] periods; over-taxing the sight on small objects, or straining after accommodation by the asthenopic [weak-sighted] or hypermetropic [farsighted]; strong odours; and so forth; and perhaps more certainly influential than any of them—mental emotion and excessive brain-work" (Liveing, 1872, p. 365).

More recent answers are found in large scale, retrospective studies. For example, Robbins (1994) compiled reports from 494 patients with migraines (see Table 10–1). In agreement with Liveing, stress was the primary trigger for both women and men.

Stress has also been identified as a major precipitating factor by children who had tension-type or migraine headaches (Osterhaus & Passchier, 1992), and by parents of children with migraines (Budd & Kedesky, 1989).

Similarly, Rains and Penzien (1996), in a headache clinic sample, found that stress, too much or too little sleep, skipping meals, alcohol, and exercise, as well as smoke, glare, and temperature changes, were the most frequently nominated triggers. Note that in these studies, dietary triggers, although identified, were less important than stress and several other behavioral and environmental factors. Rains and Penzien thus suggest that it is these more common triggers that should be the focus in clinical work.

TABLE 10–1
Migraine Triggers (From Patient Reports)

Trigger Factor	% Patients Reporting	% Female	% Male
During Stress	62%	64%	54%
Weather Changes*	43	47	32
Perimenstrual	—	50	—
Missing a Meal*	40	43	31
Sunlight	38	40	31
Undersleeping	31	33	23
Foods	30	31	28
Perfume*	29	34	10
Cigarette Smoke*	26	29	13
After Stress is Over	24	25	22
Oversleeping	24	26	19
Exercise	15	14	16
Sexual Activity*	5	4	9

Note. From "Precipitating Factors in Migraine: A Retrospective Review of 494 Patients," by L. Robbins, 1994, *Headache, 34*, p. 214. Copyright 1994 by the American Headache Society. Reprinted with permission.
*Denotes triggers whose occurrences differed between men and women, $p < .05$.

TABLE 10–2
Dimensions Underlying Headache Triggers

Rank	Type of Trigger	Examples	Type of Headache
1	Negative Affect	Predominantly stress Also anxiety, depression, anger	Migraine & Tension
2	Visual Disturbance	Flicker, glare, eyestrain	Migraine only
3	Somatic Disturbance	Sneezing, coughing, pollen	Migraine only
4	Environmental Stress	Humidity, high temperature	Migraine & Tension
5	Consumatory	Alcohol, food, hunger	Migraine only

Note. Adapted from "Towards a Functional Model of Chronic Headaches: Investigation of Antecedents and Consequences," by P. R. Martin, D. Milech, and P. R. Nathan, 1993, *Headache, 33*, p. 463. Copyright 1993 American Headache Society. Adapted with permission.

P. R. Martin, Milech, and Nathan used a mathematical technique, factor analysis, to condense retrospective trigger reports into five global dimensions. The predominant types of headache trigger, ranked from most frequent (rank 1) to least frequent, are shown in Table 10–2.

Let us examine individual triggers, then, from most to least common in Robbins' (1994) list.

STRESS

Given the evidence we have seen, that migraines and tension-type headaches can be stress-linked, whether through psychophysiological or cognitive mechanisms, we would not be surprised to find stress as a trigger. And in fact, the role of stress in migraines has long been noted. "Every mental irritation will add to the strength of the disease, and retard the wholesome operation of the remedies prescribed for its cure" (Mease, 1819, p. 36). More recently, stress has been implicated in prospective and laboratory studies.

In a time-series analysis of headache diary data, Mosley, et al. found that stress was most likely to have an immediate effect in precipitating a tension headache, but to have a 1–3 day lagged effect in migraine. The combination of peak intensity and duration of migraine episodes was predicted by the number of daily **hassles** in the three days before the headache (Mosley, Penzien, Johnson, Brantley, Wittrock, Andrew, & Payne, 1991). This was replicated by Sorbi, et al., who also found that sleep disturbance the night before a migraine episode was partially predicted by the incidence of daily hassles the day before (Sorbi, Maassen, & Spierings, 1996). And in Chapter 5 we saw similar results from Feuerstein's group, in which state anxiety was elevated four days before a migraine, and predicted temporal pulse amplitude three days before a migraine (Feuerstein, Bortolussi, M. Houle, & Labbé, 1983).

It seems possible that emotional changes during a migraine prodrome could lead to an increased perception of stress as a consequence of the migraine. However, Sorbi et al. found that tension, annoyance and irritability were highest in the 24–60 hours preceding a migraine, while daily hassles were highest at a later point, less than 24 hours before a migraine.

Differentiation between mood and hassles is also implied in a study by Levor, et al. There, mood and energy declined steadily over the three days preceding a migraine. Hassles, however, seemed to be higher throughout the three day period, with no apparent trend (Levor, M. J. Cohen, Naliboff, McArthur, & Heuser, 1986).

Laboratory-induced stress by itself is often enough to precipitate a migraine (e.g., Gannon, Haynes, Cuevas, & Chavez, 1987; Haynes, Gannon, Bank, Shelton, & Goodwin, 1990) or a headache of unspecified type (P. R. Martin & Teoh, 1999). In contrast, exposure to a single dietary trigger generally has little effect in laboratory studies. Lai, et al., however, exposed migraine-prone subjects to four potential triggers in rapid succession and induced headaches in 42 percent (C. Lai, Dean, D. K. Ziegler, & Hassanein, 1989).

P. R. Martin and Teoh studied 46 people with migraine, 17 with episodic or chronic tension-type headache, 12 with atypical tension-type headache, and 15 people without a headache disorder. They found that headache activity was highest 3 days after exposure to a laboratory stressor. In general, headache diagnosis (or lack of diagnosis) did not seem to affect study results.

Laboratory studies such as these are helpful as confirmation of survey results. However, for ethical reasons the informed consent for a study has to warn of the possibility and perhaps even the likelihood of provoking a headache. Presumably, this can produce a "**nocebo effect**," bringing about pain directly, or lowering pain thresholds at the head. Thus, a laboratory study of a particular trigger is really the study of the particular trigger plus the nocebo effect.

The prospective studies reviewed earlier in this chapter have focused largely on daily hassles (Kanner, Coyne, Schaefer, & Lazarus, 1981; Kohler & Haimerl, 1990). An alternative is to define stress in terms of major, negative life events such as the death of a close relative. There is some evidence that life event stress tends to precede, and hence may play a role in initiating, chronic headaches (De Benedittis, Lorenzetti, & Pieri, 1990; Stewart, Scher, & Lipton, 2001). Similarly, a relationship between negative life events and headache frequency seems to be found primarily in large samples of relatively young participants, say, 16 to 22 years old (Reynolds & Hovanitz, 2000). Presumably, in a young sample the headache disorder is likely to be of relatively recent onset. In contrast hassles, and in particular the tendency to appraise events negatively, may play more of a role in maintaining an established benign headache disorder (De Benedittis & Lorenzetti, 1992). Positive major life events, such as marriage or a promotion, do not seem to be related to headaches, even if they require adjustment (Reynolds & Hovanitz, 2000).

All of this seems to commend the value of leading a stress-free life. There may be an alternative, however. Marlowe (1998) found that the correlation between frequency of headaches and frequency of stressful events was mediated by self-efficacy. The more a person felt capable of handling stressors effectively, the lower the correlation between headaches and stress.

Changes in stress over time.   In Chapter 4, we saw evidence that the prevalence of migraine may have increased substantially over the 1980's. If this increase turns out to be real, then presumably an environmental factor is needed to explain it. Stress may be such a factor, for it appears that trait anxiety, or proneness to negative affect, has also increased, at least among children and young adults.

Specifically, Twenge (2000) located 170 studies that included trait anxiety scores for college students between 1952 and 1993, and 99 studies that gave scores for children between 1954 and 1981. For both college students and children, the average scores increased by approximately 1 standard deviation over the study period, so that the typical respondent at the end of the study was scoring at the 84th percentile of respondents from the 1950s. Put differently, the average child in the 1980–1988 dataset was obtaining higher trait anxiety scores than children at a psychiatric clinic in the late 1950s (Twenge, 2000).

What accounts for this? As with migraines, there might have simply been a change in willingness to report distress. However, Twenge also obtained significant lagged correlations between society-wide measures of social isolation and threat (e.g., divorce rate, percentage of adults living alone, crime rate) and college students' anxiety levels ten years later, suggesting that a proneness to negative affect was established in childhood by exposure to large societal trends. Moreover, because personality appears to be relatively stable after late adolescence, the increase in anxiety will presumably continue, on average, through the lifetime of the cohort (Twenge, 2000).

Still, although trait anxiety seems to have increased, we are a long way from proving that this accounts for the (possible) increase in migraines. After all, many other variables also changed over the 1980s, and stress is by no means the only putative migraine trigger.

WEATHER

Individuals with chronic pain often attribute fluctuations in their level of discomfort to changes in the weather (Jamison, Anderson, & Slater, 1995; Shutty, Cundiff, & DeGood, 1992). Given the frequency of this effect in patients' reports, it is surprising that it is all but invisible when studied empirically. For example, Diamond et al. examined the relationship between 9 meteorological variables and the headache records of 100 migraineurs, comprising 1884 migraine episodes. Despite the reasonably large dataset, no effects of weather were seen (S. Diamond, Freitag, & Nursall, 1990). Schulman et al. went even further. They showed that headache diaries of 75 patients were fit very closely by a statistical model, in which every day was the equivalent of every other day. Now, all 75 patients lived in the Boston area and kept their diaries for the same month. Needless to say, in terms of weather, every day was *not* the same as every other day, so the results essentially exclude all possible day-by-day weather fluctuations in one swoop. In a closer examination of barometric pressure specifically, there were no effects of the current or previous day's readings (Schulman, Leviton, Slack, Porter, & Graham, 1980). On the other hand, this was a highly select sample, we do not know their exact diagnoses, and I do not know the statistical power associated with Schulman, et al.'s analysis.

An exception to all of these negative results appears to be the impact on migraines of the Chinook winds in Canada's southern Alberta province. The Chinook is a brisk, warm, dry westerly wind that comes in from the Canadian Rockies. It is an intriguing candidate for study because, unlike hot dry winds in Israel or California, it is not a source of heat stress. Indeed, the Chinook winds bring moderating temperatures in winter and hence are often welcome (Cooke, M. S. Rose, & Becker, 2000).

In an initial study, Piorecky et al. correlated the occurrence of headaches in 13 migraineurs with the onset of Chinook winds in meteorological reports. In all, data was available on 369 separate headaches. Of note, the patients were keeping their headache diaries as part of a drug trial. Thus, the patients were not selected for having "weather-responsive headaches," and did not know that a weather-related hypothesis was also being studied (Piorecky, Becker, & M. S. Rose, 1997). Overall, the probability of a headache beginning on a non-Chinook day was 14.65 percent. On a Chinook day, defined as a day on which Chinook winds occurred, or the day before the wind began, the probability was 17.26 percent ($p = .042$). Moreover, the effect appears to interact with age. For the 5 migraineurs below age 42, the **odds ratio** for headache onset with Chinook weather was nonsignificant and, actually, below 1.00 (0.92, *ns*). For the 5 migraineurs between ages 42 and 45 the odds ratio was 1.24 ($p < .02$). For the 3 patients above age 50 the odds ratio was 1.84 ($p < .01$).

Cooke, Rose and Becker (2000) replicated and extended these results on a sample of 75 patients who recorded a total of 1,495 separate migraines. Again, Chinook winds increased the probability of migraine onset, with an odds ratio of 1.19 ($p < .05$). As it turns out, all of the increased risk was for days on which the maximum wind velocity was greater than 38 kilometers per hour (c. 24 mph; odds ratio = 1.41, $p < .05$). Again an interaction with age was found, with subjects at or above age 50 being particularly susceptible. Moreover, the day preceding a Chinook wind was also a risk factor, with an odds ratio of 1.24 ($p < .01$). The pre-Chinook effect did not interact with age, wind velocity, or with the effect of Chinook days. In a post-hoc questionnaire, subjects' assessments of whether they were Chinook sensitive showed essentially no correspondence to the actual findings derived from their headache diaries and meteorological records.

Now, how is it that a warm and welcome wind would cause migraines? The pre-Chinook effect is so far completely unexplained. The effect of the Chinook winds themselves contains the clue that wind velocity must be high. As wind speed increases, especially to above 38 km/hour, the concentration of positive ions in the air increases. These ions may have a number of biological effects, including on serotonin metabolism. Still, this explanation is by no means certain. In the classic theory and associated data, prolonged exposure to positive ions has *analgesic* properties, at least in rats, mediated by serotonergic pathways (Beardwood, Abrahams, & Jordi, 1986; Krueger & Reed, 1976). Surely analgesia would make a migraine less likely to occur. And as Chinook winds are accompanied by rising temperatures and falling barometer readings, there are certainly competing hypotheses that do not depend on ions (Cooke, M. S. Rose, & Becker, 2000).

HORMONES

In retrospective studies, menstruation is widely reported as a risk factor for migraines. Prospectively, a particularly careful investigation involved the analysis of 7300 daily headache records from a random sample of 74 women, ages 22–29 years, drawn from the general population, and suffering from migraine (Johannes, Linet, Stewart, Celentano, Lipton, & Szklo, 1995). Menstruation did indeed turn out to be a risk factor, although the results were only statistically significant for migraine without aura. Specifically, the probability of having a migraine without aura during the first three days of menstruation, compared with other days, was 1.66 times as great.

How can we explain this? As it turns out, estrogen has a number of effects that may be relevant to migraines. Recall that one of the signs of sensitization in the dorsal horn is that **receptive fields** for mechanical (pressure) stimuli become wider. In fact, Bereiter and coworkers found that receptive fields in the trigeminal nucleus caudalis were enlarged after estrogen injection, at least in experimental animals (Bereiter, Stanford, & Barker, 1980; Marcus, 1995). As we have seen, estrogen also increases the bioavailability of nitric oxide (Geary, Krause, & Duckles, 1998), which causes vasodilation, and which may be an excitatory neurotransmitter in pain systems (Thomsen & J. Olesen, 1998). Indeed, in women whose migraines are exclusively triggered by the onset of menses ("menstrual migraine"), platelet nitric oxide activity may be unusually high in the late luteal (premenstrual) phase (Sarchielli et al., 1996). Mast cells, which secrete histamine and probably cause the irritation and some of the dilation of dural blood vessels during migraines, contain estrogen receptors. Thus, estrogen may potentiate the effect of substance P on histamine release (Rozniecki, Dimitriadou, Lambracht-Hall, Pang, & Theoharides, 1999; Vliagoftis et al., 1992). In the cortex, neuronal excitability is enhanced by estrogen (M. Smith, L. Adams, P. Schmidt, Rubinow, & Wassermann, 2002).

It seems, then, that estrogen can have far-reaching effects. There is a catch, however: The time around menstruation is characterized by the *lowest* estrogen levels of the menstrual cycle (Silberstein & Merriam, 2000). Thus, it may be more relevant to ask what biochemical changes accompany falling estrogen levels. Again, there are many results, and we do not know which, if any, will prove to be of primary importance.

Beta-endorphin is found in the hypothalamus, where it inhibits the production of gonadotropin releasing hormone (Silberstein & Merriam, 2000). Nearly all brain beta-endorphin is found specifically in the hypothalamus and in its long axonal projections (Pomeranz, 2001). Estrogen seems to facilitate beta-endorphin production, and in the absence of estrogen, hypothalamic endorphin levels fall (Marcus, 1995; Wardlaw, Wehrenberg, Ferin, Antunes, & Frantz, 1982; Wehrenberg, Wardlaw, Frantz, & Ferin, 1982). Endophinergic nuclei in the hypothalamus project to the periaqueductal gray, and hence may inhibit the pain signal (Pomeranz, 2001). Recall, too, that endorphins inhibit firing of the locus coeruleus, in the migraine generator region (Fioroni, Martignoni, & Facchinetti, 1995).

Regardless, the change in neurotransmitter levels in the hypothalamus leads to a key question: Does the entire hypothalamic-pituitary-adrenal cortical axis change its stress sensitivity premenstrually? There indeed seems to be evidence of increased cortisol response to stress (Marinari, Leshner, & Doyle, 1976), and even an exaggerated blood pressure response to **tyramine** (Ghose & P. Turner, 1977, see below), prior to menstruation.

Declines in estrogen level appear to be associated with lowered blood and platelet serotonin, decreases in the binding affinity of platelet serotonin receptors, but with an increase in the total number of available platelet serotonin receptors (Marcus, 1995). In the nervous system, serotonin is an inhibitory neurotransmitter in pain pathways. The validity of blood platelets as an indicator of serotonin dynamics in the central nervous system has not yet been resolved, however (Marcus, 1995). A falling estrogen level also appears to affect the amount of norepinephrine and the strength of its receptor binding (Marcus, 1995) as well as the degree of sensitivity to dopamine (Gordon & B. I. Diamond, 1981). And amidst all these neurochemical theories we should mention the classic model of estrogen withdrawal, which was vascular: Estrogen was thought to cause an increase in the number of α_1 adrenoreceptors on vascular smooth muscle cells. However, this is balanced by estrogen's stimulation of inhibitory α_2 **adrenoreceptors**, inhibiting neurotransmitter release. When estrogen levels fall, it was argued, the stimulation of α_2 receptors ends immediately, while the additional α_1 receptors stay in place for awhile. The net effect would be increased sensitivity to norepinephrine by the blood vessels: a bias towards stress-elicited vasoconstriction (Benedetto, Allais, Ciochetto, & De Lorenzo, 1997).

Although hormone replacement studies suggest that estrogen withdrawal is particularly important in migraine (Somerville, 1972, 1975), progesterone levels also drop premenstrually. And this too may be relevant, as progesterone seems to suppress at least part of the sterile inflammatory response: the leakage of proteins into blood vessel walls (W. S. Lee, Cutrer, Waeber & Moskowitz, 1995). Similarly, progesterone seems to prevent the accumulation of calcitonin gene-related peptide in the trigeminal nucleus (Moussaoul, Duval, Lenoir, Garret, & Kerdelhue, 1996). This peptide seems to be the key mediator of neurovascular inflammation in migraine. Perhaps when its levels in the trigeminal nucleus are low, the intensity or probability of a migraine is also reduced. Progesterone seems to suppress cortical excitability (M. Smith, L. Adams, P. Schmidt, Rubinow, & Wassermann, 2002). And menstruation itself is associated with the entry of prostaglandins, produced in the uterine lining, into general circulation (E. A. MacGregor, 1997). Prostaglandins are inflammatory, hyperalgesic chemicals that may be the proximal cause of the sterile inflammation of migraine. And, to complete the picture, there is evidence that estrogen and progesterone by themselves have analgesic properties (Dawson-Basoa & Gintzler, 1996; Gintzler & Liu, 2001).

Thus, although we do not know exactly why hormonal changes in women trigger migraines (or why estrogen appears to be a risk factor for TMD; see Chapter 8) the numerous interactions between neurotransmitters, prostaglandins, and sex hormones provide at least a general rationale and the starting point for much future research.

BRIGHT LIGHTS, CONTRAST, FLICKER AND GLARE

As we have seen, people often report intense visual stimulation as a headache trigger. There has been little laboratory investigation of this, however. An exception is the study by P. R. Martin and Teoh, noted previously (P. R. Martin & Teoh, 1999). The investigators subjected people to a five cycle per second strobe light in a dark room, while asking them to read small print on a computer monitor in front of them. Not surprisingly, the intervention produced a rather strong increment in headache activity. Of note, although the increase was seen immediately, it seemed to peak approximately 3 days after exposure. Approximately 51 percent of their participants had a diagnosis of migraine; others had typical or atypical tension-type headache or no headache diagnosis. However, diagnosis (or lack thereof) did not seem to influence the results, and the types of headaches the subjects actually developed are not specified.

Triggering of headaches by visual stimuli is poorly understood. It seems possible that visual triggering is related to the presence of photophobia between migraine episodes. If so, then we should note that people who are prone to tension-type headache also report, interictally, more aversion to intense visual stimuli than do control subjects. However, the aversion reported in tension-type headache is not as severe as in migraineurs, and may involve sensitivity to different wavelengths. That is, the discomfort for migraineurs appears to peak at long (red) and perhaps short (blue) wavelengths, while for people who are prone to tension-type headache, middle wavelengths (green) appear to be the most uncomfortable (Main, Vlachonikolis, & Dowson, 2000). Of course this refers to group averages; for any particular person triggers may be idiosyncratic.

Not surprisingly, mild improvement has been reported with the use of tinted lenses, either rose-colored (to screen out the flicker of fluorescent lights; Wilkins, 1991), or individually selected to maximize the clarity and ease of printed text (Good, R. H. Taylor, & Mortimer, 1991;

Wilkins, Patel, Adjamian, & B. J. W. Evans, 2002). For computer monitors, it possibly may help to use the operating system to change the screen's refresh rate (Kowacs, Piovesan, Werneck, Fameli, & Pereira da Silva, 2004).

AMOUNT OF SLEEP

How changes in sleep pattern trigger migraines, and even whether they do, is not currently known. It may be relevant that certain brain stem nuclei in the migraine generator region (locus coeruleus, dorsal raphe nucleus) are also involved in sleep and dreaming (Göder, et al., 2001).

DIETARY TRIGGERS

In 1674, when Thomas Willis discussed inciting factors in "cephalalgia," he included "errata in victu"—errors in diet (T. Willis, 1674, p. 282, cited in Liveing, 1873, p. 42). Nowadays, suspected trigger foods for migraine are commonly given in texts and patient education materials (e.g., American Council for Headache Education, 1994), such as Table 10–3.

The supporting evidence for these varies widely, from double-blind placebo-controlled trials for red wine (Littlewood, Gibb, Glover, Sandler, P. T. G. Davies, & F. C. Rose, 1988), aspartame (e.g., S. M. Koehler & Glaros, 1988), and MSG (for a general MSG syndrome; W. Yang, Drouin, Herbert, Mao, & Karsh, 1997), to rare case studies for dietary nitrites (Vaughan, 1994). It is likely that only a small minority of migraineurs has dietary triggers, and within this subset the most important triggers may vary from patient to patient.

To explain dietary triggers, a number of pharmacologically active food substances have been cited.

Caffeine.   Caffeine is widely suspected as a migraine trigger, although definitive studies appear to be lacking. Still, the substance affects a striking range of biological processes. For example, by impeding the opening of potassium channels, caffeine appears to increase the excitability of neurons throughout the cortex (Fredholm, 1995; Kalmar & Cafarelli, 1999), and in fact is used to prolong the induced seizures of electroconvulsive therapy (Sawynok, 1995). Caffeine promotes the release of acetylcholine, dopamine, serotonin, and norepinephrine, and in a particular brain location it increases the binding affinity of dopamine to D_2 receptors (Fredholm, 1995). Brain serotonin levels may be increased by caffeine, at least in experimental animals (Nutrition Reviews, 1988). Moreover, caffeine raises blood levels of epinephrine (J. D. Lane, 1994), increasing heart rate and constricting arterioles in the hands and feet. Caffeine might also

TABLE 10–3
Suspected Dietary Triggers in Migraine

1. Red Wine	2. Citrus Fruits	3. MSG
Other Alcoholic Beverages	Nuts	Nitrites
Caffeine	Onions	Aspartame
4. Aged Cheese	5. Chocolate	6. Eggs
Sour Cream, Yogurt		Other Dairy
Yeast Extracts		Beans
Dried Smoked Fish		Fatty Foods
Pickled Herring		

increase levels of cortisol and norepinephrine, although the evidence for this is mixed (J. D. Lane, 1994). Furthermore, caffeine has subtle effects in promoting increased muscle tension (Kalmar & Cafarelli, 1999).

Despite all this, the mechanism by which caffeine would act as a headache trigger seems quite unclear. The fact that it causes vasoconstriction at the hands might suggest a similar effect on the cerebral arteries. Consistent with this, caffeine appears to reduce cerebral blood flow (Cameron, Modell, & Hariharam, 1990; R. J. Mathew, Barr, & Weinman, 1983). On the other hand, a transcranial Doppler study revealed only vasodilation in response to caffeine, at least in habitual consumers of caffeine (Couturier, Laman, M. A. J. van Duijn & H. van Duijn, 1997). The seizure-promoting activity of caffeine seems consistent with a neurogenic model of migraines. However, the eleptogenic activity is specifically a result of acute administration. With long-term intake, which is undoubtedly a better model clinically, caffeine has very different effects: a *decrease* in the likelihood of seizures, decreased susceptibility to ischemic brain damage, decreased locomotor activity and, remarkably, improved spatial learning ability (Fredholm, 1995). Thus, while caffeine's ability to promote migraines is something of a truism, it is perhaps the most under-researched of all putative dietary triggers.

Regardless of the effects of caffeine administration, it is clear that caffeine *withdrawal* is a significant cause of headaches. In the amounts generally consumed in America (c. 2 cups of coffee per day on average) abrupt cessation of coffee intake produces a moderate or severe headache in approximately 50 percent of people (Silverman, Evans, Strain, & Griffiths, 1992), possibly due to dilation of extracranial arteries (R. J. Mathew & Wilson, 1985). The symptoms of caffeine withdrawal peak after 1–2 days, but can last for as long as a week (Sawynok, 1995). Thus, as an ingredient in over-the-counter migraine preparations, caffeine can potentially contribute to rebound headaches.

Red wine.   Although red wine is widely regarded as a migraine trigger, with support from at least one double-blind, placebo-controlled trial (Littlewood, Gibb, Glover, Sandler, P. T. G. Davies, & F. C. Rose, 1988), it is not at all clear that alcohol is the culprit. Indeed, in the study by Littlewood, et al., the "placebo" was a heavily disguised mixture of vodka. Red wine contains many other constituents, of course, including histamine and flavonoids.

There is preliminary evidence that flavonoids can cause platelets to release serotonin (Glover, Pattichis, Jarman, Peatfield, & Sandler, 1994; Sandler, N.-Y. Li, Jarrett, & Glover, 1995). This would fit with the platelet theory of migraine. Alternatively, the effect on platelets might indicate that red wine has a similar effect in the brain. Neurons in the periaqueductal region, in the neighborhood of the suspected migraine generator, are largely serotonergic. Red wines, even of the same label, vary widely in their serotonin-releasing property. If indeed this property is important in triggering migraines, it should ultimately be possible to identify the offending compound and create migraine-free red wines (Sandler, N.-Y. Li, et al.).

Other pharmacological properties have been cited. For example, a component of red wine might impede the binding of serotonin to a subset of receptors (Sandler, N.-Y. Li, et al., 1995). Whether this is important in headaches is not known. Also, red wine flavonoids might inhibit an enzyme that detoxifies dietary phenols, phenolsulphotransferase P (Littlewood, Glover, & Sandler, 1985). We shall have more to say about this below, under "flavonoids."

Tyramine.   The human body manufactures certain important chemicals by removing a "carboxyl group" from one amino acid or another (A. White, Handler, & E. L. Smith, 1973). Now, the carboxyl group is the acidic part of the molecule, and therefore the altered amino acids are actually no longer acids. Thus, they are simply called "amines"—or "biogenic amines," because they are biologically generated. Some of them are quite well known. Dop*amine*, hist*amine*, serotonin (5-Hydroxytrypt*amine*), and norepinephrine are all examples of biogenic amines (Premont, Gainetdinov, & Caron, 2001). Other, similar chemicals are present only in trace amounts, however, and are much more poorly understood. Two of them, tyramine and phenylethylamine, have been suspected migraine triggers.

Tyramine is found in foods such as red wine, aged cheese, sour cream, and the group 4 triggers in Table 10–3. It is vasoactive and can raise blood pressure (Merikangas et al., 1995). Ordinarily, dietary tyramine is deactivated by monoamine oxidase (MAO) in the intestine, and in typical concentrations should presumably only cause problems in people who are taking MAO inhibitors (Perkins & Hartje, 1983). However, there is some evidence that migraineurs may have an unusual difficulty in metabolizing tyramine. In particular, male migraineurs appear to have naturally lower platelet MAO activity than control subjects, and an increased susceptibility to the blood pressure effects of tyramine (e.g., Peatfield, Littlewood, Glover, Sandler, & F. C. Rose, 1983; Sandler, Youdim, & Hanington, 1974). Moreover, migraineurs, at least those without aura, appear to have unusually high plasma levels of octopamine and synephrine—metabolites of tyramine—in between migraine episodes (D'Andrea, Terrazzino, et al., 2004).

As a vasoactive compound, tyramine was initially discussed within the vascular model of migraines. However, its impact could as easily be neuronal. Tyramine closely resembles norepinephrine (P. L. McGeer, Eccles, & E. G. McGeer, 1978), and seems to cause its release from cells (Rothman & M. Baumann, 2002). Thus, tyramine has been thought of as a kind of internally generated **amphetamine** (P. L. McGeer et al.). More recently, receptors for tyramine have been found in such places as the locus coeruleus and the dorsal raphe nucleus (Borowsky et al., 2001), which are in the region of the putative migraine generator. Even the platelet model can be invoked, for platelets release tyramine, a vasoconstrictive, when they are activated (D'Andrea, Terrazzino, Fortin, Cocco, Balbi, & Leon, 2003).

Still, the exact role of tyramine in the human body is not yet known, and its status as a migraine trigger is by no means definite. The higher baseline levels of its metabolites might simply be an indirect measure of a hypoactive sympathetic nervous system. That is, if less of the amino acid tyrosine is being converted into norepinephrine, then perhaps more is available to be made into tyramine (D'Andrea, Terrazzino, et al., 2004). Moreover, the ability of tyramine to induce migraines has been supported in several but not all double-blind, placebo-controlled trials (Kohlenberg, 1982; Vaughan, 1994), there is no evidence that female migraineurs have lower MAO activity, and contrary to expectation, MAO inhibitors appear to help rather than worsen migraines (Anthony & J. W. Lance, 1969).

Incidentally, tyramine as a dietary trigger should not be confused with the "tyramine challenge test." There is some evidence that tyramine conjugation, a minor pathway for tyramine deactivation, tends to be lower in migraineurs, in people with facial pain, and in people with unipolar depression (Aghabeigi, et al., 1993; K. R. Merikangas, Stevens, J. R. Merikangas, et al., 1995). That is, if people with these diagnoses are given a tyramine capsule, their urine subsequently shows lower than expected levels of tyramine sulfate. The finding does not have sufficient sensitivity and specificity to be useful for diagnosing individual cases. Of course, the fact that it is common to the three separate diagnostic groups has been interpreted as indicating a biochemical similarity between them. So far, however, this result does not seem to be related to tyramine sensitivity. Tyramine conjugation is relatively unimportant in determining tyramine levels in the body, and it has not been established that dietary migraineurs are more or less likely to show a deficit in it (K. R. Merikangas, Stevens, J. R. Merikangas, et al.).

Phenylethylamine is, like tyramine, a biologically active amine. Structurally, it closely resembles dopamine, and it can most likely potentiate neurotransmission by dopamine (P. A. Janssen,

Leysen, Megens, & Awouters, 1999) and by norepinephrine (Perkins & Hartje, 1983). In particular, phenylethylamine has a high affinity for the binding proteins used in the reuptake of norepinephrine and dopamine and thus it may be a reuptake inhibitor for these two neurotransmitters. Thus, like tyramine, it has been suspected of functioning as an internally generated amphetamine (P. A. Janssen, et al.). And it, too, has receptors in the brain—in fact the same receptors that bind tyramine (Borowsky et al., 2001).

Phenylethylamine is found in chocolate and some cheeses (Anderson, 1995) and, like tyramine, it is catabolized by monoamine oxidase (Sandler, Youdim, & Hanington, 1974). Phenylethylamine has passed some (Hanington, 1983; Vaughan, 1994) but not all (e.g., Marcus, Scharff, D. C. Turk, & Gourley, 1997) double-blind, placebo-controlled tests. In particular, Karoum and coworkers found no change in phenylethylamine concentration in blood, urine or cerebrospinal fluid after subjects consumed foods high in the substance (Karoum, Nasrallah, & Potkin, 1979).

Histamine.   Perhaps the strongest case for a dietary triggering agent can be made for histamine. Foods such as citrus, tomatoes, strawberries and egg whites, may cause the release of histamine in the body (Vaughan, 1994). Wantke, et al., studying food sensitivity rather than migraines, found that plasma histamine levels were higher at baseline and 30 minutes after ingesting red wine, in symptomatic vs. asymptomatic participants (Wantke, Gotz, & Jarisch, 1994). Similarly, in migraineurs higher levels of histamine have been reported during migraines (Haimart, Pradalier, Launay, Dreux, & Dry, 1987) and after ingesting dietary trigger foods (G. Olsen, Vaughn, & Ledous, 1989).

Some red wines contain over 13 mg of histamine per liter (Kanny, Gerbaux, et al., 2001; Wantke et al, 1994), and cheese, fish, and sausages also contain histamine (Vaughan, 1994). Still, Kanny, et al., found that red wine had no effect on plasma histamine in people who were not wine-intolerant (Kanny, Bauza, et al., 1999). In people who were wine-intolerant, red wine did indeed increase blood histamine levels, but this was unrelated to the wine's histamine content (Kanny, Gerbaux, et al.). The authors speculate that acetaldehyde may be the actual trigger.

When infused directly, histamine reliably produces headaches in nonmigraineurs, and migraines in migraineurs, in a dose-dependent fashion (Thomsen & J. Olesen, 1998). For reasons that are unknown, the immediate headache is often followed in migraineurs by a delayed-effect migraine having its peak intensity at approximately 5.5 hours after infusion. Histamine seems to up-regulate nitric oxide synthase (Thomsen & Olesen, 1998). Recall, too, that migraine pain may be due to sterile, neurogenic inflammation of cerebral blood vessels caused by activation of the trigeminal nucleus. This inflammation, in dura mater at least, seems to involve **degranulation** of mast cells and hence release of histamine (Dimitriadou, Buzzi, Moskowitz, & Theoharides, 1991).

Flavonoids comprise a broad class of polyphenols found in fruits, spices, tea, chocolate, and other plant-based foods. They have been regarded traditionally as non-nutritive, because there is no acute deficiency syndrome associated with their absence, or even anti-nutritive, because they make proteins and certain minerals harder to digest (L. R. Ferguson, 2001). But flavonoids are biologically active all the same, modulating the induction and activity of a number of enzymes, including those involved in inflammation, DNA production and repair, and cellular responses to heat- and **oxidative stress** (L. R. Ferguson, 2001). Thus, it is likely that flavonoids are responsible for at least some of the properties of medicinal plants, and perhaps some of the health benefits of a plant-based diet (Middleton, Kandaswami, & Theoharides, 2000). But then, pharmacological activity is not always benign.

Flavonoids have recently been suspected as triggers, based on circumstantial evidence. These compounds are found in high concentration in red wine (up to 1.2 *grams* per liter) and citrus fruits. Some flavonoids can inhibit an enzyme that degrades catecholamines, and one flavonoid in particular, catechin, has strong vascular effects (Littlewood, Gibb, Glover, Sandler, P. T. G. Davies, & F. C. Rose, 1988). There is some evidence that the enzyme that degrades flavonoids, the P subtype of phenolsulphotransferase,[1] is less active in migraineurs who report dietary triggers than in those who do not, and least active of all in those who report citrus fruits as triggers (Littlewood, Glover, & Sandler, 1982).

Although the evidence is less consistent, the M subtype of phenolsulphotransferase may also be less active in migraineurs vs. non-migraine controls. The M subtype deactivates serotonin, dopamine, and norepinephrine in the bloodstream and, most likely, to some extent in the brain as well (Coughtrie, Jones, & Roberts, 1994).

Besides red wine polyphenols, isoflavones, a class of flavonoids found in soy, nuts, and other plant-based foods (Mazur, 1998), have attracted attention. Isoflavones are considered a type of **"phytoestrogen"** because they act at estrogen receptors—as either antagonist or agonist, depending on concentration and other factors (Setchell, 1998). Thus, the role of reproductive hormones in migraine suggests that isoflavones could have an effect. Moreover, one particular isoflavone, genistein, by blocking tyrosine kinase, prevents serotonin from constricting the basilar artery (Kitazono, Ibayashi, Nagao, Kagiyama, Kitayama, & Fujishima, 1998), and perhaps other large cerebral arteries as well. Certain acute antimigraine medications constrict cerebral arteries by stimulating serotonin receptors. Genistein has the opposite effect, at least in this respect, and might perhaps contribute to vasomotor instability (P. A. Engel, 2002). And at least two dietary isoflavones, genistein and daidzein, inhibit $GABA_A$ receptors (Dunne, Moss, & Smart, 1998; Huang, Fang, & Dillon, 1999). Now, GABA—gamma-amino butyric acid—is an inhibitory neurotransmitter. Agonists at the $GABA_A$ receptor help prevent migraines, perhaps by reducing cortical excitability. In contrast, flavonoids that have an inhibitory effect at the $GABA_A$ receptor might raise cortical excitability and promote migraines (P. A. Engel, 2002).

Consistent with this theory, Engel describes a case of new-onset migraine with visual aura in a 57-year-old male physician after starting high dose isoflavone supplements (135–177 mg/day) for chronic prostatic discomfort. The migraines resolved when isoflavone intake was reduced to 73–115 mg/day, but occasional visual auras continued. When isoflavone use was decreased further, to around 60 mg/day, the auras resolved as well (P. A. Engel, 2002).

Of course we must be careful not to conclude too much from a case study, and this is all the more true here. For Burke, et al. have presented a double-blind, placebo-controlled trial in which phytoestrogens *decreased* the occurrence of perimenstrual migraines in women (B. E. Burke, R. D. Olson, & Cusack, 2002). We will discuss this trial below, in Chapter 11. Perhaps isoflavones can prevent the estrogen withdrawal thought to underlie perimenstrual migraines. Because isoflavones can act as either antagonist or agonist at the estrogen receptor, depending on concentration (Setchell, 1998), dosage may be crucial. Thus, it could be relevant that Burke et al. administered a mixture of phytoestrogens, in which soy isoflavones were included at 60 mg/day, the lowest dose used by Engel (B. E. Burke et al.). Also, the effects of isoflavones seem to depend on the background level of endogenous estrogen (Setchell, 1998). Thus, the impact could be different in men and post-menopausal women than in women prior to menopause.

---

[1]The enzyme's name describes its function. Phenolsulphotransferase transfers a sulphate group to phenol and related compounds. This makes the compounds less biologically active and hastens their excretion (Coughtrie, Jones, & Roberts, 1994). The P subtype specializes in dietary phenols such as flavonoids, while the M subtype works differentially on **monoamines** such as dopamine (Coughtrie, Jones, & Roberts, 1994).

And of course, Engel's results, although backed by theory, may be a coincidence, or an exceptional case.

Aspartame is the methyl ester derivative of a dipeptide—two amino acids linked together (aspartic acid and phenylalanine). Because it is approximately 200 times sweeter than an equal weight of sugar (Schiffman et al., 1987), it can be used as an artificial sweetener in amounts too small to add significant calories. In the gastrointestinal tract it is broken down into its constituent amino acids. These amino acids occur naturally in such foods as meat, milk, and vegetables, and hence there are rational as well as empirical grounds for regarding aspartame as safe (Butchko, 1997). However, reports to the FDA of adverse reactions (particularly headaches; Centers for Disease Control, 1984), and the fact that high doses can shift the balance of amino acids in the brains of mice and rats (Walton, Hudak, & Green-Waite, 1993) have led to investigations of aspartame as a headache trigger. We will focus on three studies, each examining the question from a different angle.

Koehler and Glaros (1988) studied 25 migraineurs who had responded to a newspaper advertisement, and who suspected that aspartame affected their migraines. The research used a double-blind, placebo-controlled, crossover design. After a four-week baseline, subjects took capsules of either aspartame (group 1) or placebo (group 2) for four weeks. This was followed by a one-week washout period, and then four weeks in which group 1 took the placebo and group 2 took aspartame. The subjects took the capsules at home. They did not alter their lifestyle, but they did keep a headache diary and food intake records. The aspartame dose was 1.2 grams per day, approximately equal to the amount in 2 liters of diet soda. The authors note a 56 percent attrition rate, equivalent in the placebo and aspartame conditions, apparently due to the amount of record-keeping asked of subjects. Among the treatment completers (11 subjects) the aspartame phase was associated with a greater frequency of migraines, and a trend for the migraines to last longer, when compared with the baseline and the placebo phases. The significant effect of aspartame was due to greater headache activity in about half of the migraineurs, with no change seen in the other half.

Similarly, Van Den Eeden and associates studied 44 people who responded to a newspaper advertisement, and who felt that aspartame gave them headaches. Most did not have migraines, however. As in the Koehler and Glaros study, a double-blind, placebo-controlled crossover design was used. Again, subject attrition, due to noncompliance and reported side effects, was high but equivalent in the placebo and aspartame conditions. The aspartame dose was higher, equal to approximately 4 liters of diet soda per day. For the 18 (41 percent) study completers who gave usable data, headaches were significantly more frequent, although not longer or more intense, in the aspartame condition. For those subjects who did not complete the study but for whom some data were available, headaches were numerically more frequent in the aspartame condition (Van Den Eeden, Koepsell, Longstreth, van Belle, Daling, & McKnight, 1994).

The third study, conducted by Schiffman and colleagues, focused on 40 people who had reported an adverse reaction to aspartame to either the FDA or to G. D. Searle and Company, the makers of NutraSweet. The forty people included a physician, a college professor, two corporate vice presidents, a professional pianist, a business statistician, several nurses, salespersons, administrative assistants, and so on. They were flown in from around the country to Duke University Medical Center for an intensive study of their reactions to aspartame and placebo challenges. On day 3 of the study, subjects received either 3 doses of aspartame (for a total dose equivalent to 4 liters of diet soda) or a placebo. Day 4 was for washout and on day 5 subjects received whichever treatment (aspartame or placebo) they had not received on day 3. As in the other studies we have reviewed, Schiffman et al. used a double-blind crossover design. Unlike the other studies however, there were no significant differences in headaches between the aspartame and placebo phases. Moreover, of those subjects who developed headaches, only one-fifth felt that they were like their usual headaches (Schiffman, et al., 1987).

The negative results of Schiffman et al. might be due to the very short study duration, the specific sample, or the fact that people were tested outside of their usual environments. On the other hand, the effect of aspartame, if any, may be far from robust. As Van Den Eeden and colleagues point out, the near ubiquitous use of aspartame suggests that adverse reactions are relatively rare (Van Den Eeden et al., 1994). As with other putative dietary triggers, only a small minority of people may be susceptible. Still, it seems reasonable that the possibility of aspartame as a trigger be entertained whenever aspartame consumption is high.

Dietary fat was included in early compilations of migraine triggers based on patient self-report (P. Wilson, cited in Hanington, 1968; Selby & J. W. Lance, 1960). Since then, little work has been done in the field. Yet, as Bic and colleagues point out, a connection between dietary fat and migraines is not altogether improbable. Higher dietary fat will generally lead to a higher concentration of lipids and free fatty acids in the blood stream, which in turn can increase blood platelets' tendency to aggregate and to release serotonin, both of which seem to occur during migraine episodes (Bic, Blix, Hopp, Leslie, & Schell, 1999). High dietary fat intake could also have pro-inflammatory properties because prostaglandin E2, a key inflammatory mediator, is produced from a fatty acid, namely, arachidonic acid (W. Wagner & Nootbaar-Wagner, 1997). Moreover, stress, caffeine, vigorous exercise, and oral contraceptives, all of which are suspected migraine triggers, in fact increase blood levels of lipids and free fatty acids (Bic, Blix, Hopp, & Leslie, 1998).

Not surprisingly, then, Bic et al. found that in a sample of 54 migraineurs, daily fat intake as assessed by food diary correlated 0.44 with headache frequency, measured prospectively. People who consumed at least 69 grams of fat per day had an average of 10.0 headaches over a 28 day monitoring period, while people whose daily intake was lower than 69 grams had an average of 5.4 headaches over the same period. When the subjects were placed on a low fat diet, getting roughly 10 percent of calories from fat, the correlation disappeared, presumably because intake was below the threshold for an effect. What is more, the number of migraines was drastically reduced: 65 percent of the subjects achieved at least an 85 percent reduction in total headache activity (Bic, Blix, Hopp, Leslie, & Schell, 1999).

Of course we must take care to not rely too heavily on this single, uncontrolled trial. It is quite possible that the patients' increase in self-efficacy, the investigators' enthusiasm, or some other factor accounts for the results. Moreover, the intake of many other nutrients besides lipids changed over the course of the study due to the shift to a low-fat diet. Further, caffeine consumption was purposefully discouraged, and declined by 40 percent. Still, in view of the other health benefits that have been attributed to a low fat diet, the area seems ripe for further study.

Moreover, there is historical precedent for the use of a low fat diet in the prevention of migraine. From the 1930s to the 1950s, Max Gerson, a physician and refugee from the Nazis, claimed that he could cure cancer with a curious mix of dietary strictures, coffee enemas, and liver and vitamin B_{12} injections. His program was never well studied scientifically, and ultimately came to be regarded as the quintessential quack therapy. Still, the centerpiece of his treatment, a no-salt, low-fat, plant-based diet emphasizing fruit and vegetable juices, has a modern ring as sound nutritional advice. Originally, however, he did not invent the diet with cancer in mind. Rather, he developed it as an effective self-treatment of his own disabling migraines. When he set up his medical practice in 1919, he administered the diet to other migraineurs, only later adapting it to arthritis, lupus vulgaris, and ultimately cancer (P. S. Ward, 1988, cited in M. Lerner, 1994; U.S. Congress, 1946).

Even further back, James Mease (1819)[2] seems to be recommending a low fat diet in his emphasis on foods that are easily digested: "The dinner should consist principally of vegetables. Most persons, in the United States, eat much more animal food than is necessary for health" (Mease, 1819, p. 23). And "I hold up both hands against rich pastry. It is death to a stomach subject to the derangement of nerves producing sick-headache" (p. 25).[3,4]

And in the 18th century we can find similar warnings against a high fat diet: "There are some things which, in very small quantities, seldom fail to produce the sick head-ach[e] in some constitutions. Such are a larger proportion than usual of melted butter, fat meats, and spices, especially common black pepper. Meat pies often contain all these things united, and are as fertile a cause of this complaint as any thing I know; so are rich baked puddings, and every thing of a similar nature" (Fothergill, 1784, p. 108). Fothergill believed that migraines were triggered when bile irritated the stomach. Accordingly, "bilious" and indigestion-producing foods—commonly, those high in fat—were to be avoided. The belief was apparently quite popular in the nineteenth century (Liveing, 1873, p. 44).

Fothergill had most likely been influenced by Tissot who, in 1784, had suggested that migraines arose when irritation of the stomach spread in some way to the trigeminal nerves (H. A. Riley, 1932). But the idea that headaches were due to noxious effects of bile did not originate with Tissot, but with Galen (131–201 AD), and was echoed by later writers such as Avicenna (980–1037 AD; H. A. Riley, 1932). In this day of radioconjugated monoclonal antibodies, it is hard to remember that Galenic notions held sway for nearly two millennia, and came right up to the doorstep of scientific medicine.

Arginine similarly seems to be a candidate trigger, because it is the precursor of nitric oxide, and because, at least in experimental animals, diets high in **arginine** have significant vascular effects that are mediated by nitric oxide (e.g., Phivthong-ngam, et al., 1998). Because the amino acid glutamine inhibits nitric oxide synthesis in endothelial cells, and because lysine, ornithine,

---

[2]Of James Mease's work on headaches we know very little, except that his book was popular and went through five editions (W. S. Miller, 1925). Of the man himself, we know a little more. Mease (1771–1846) was a 1792 graduate of the University of Pennsylvania medical department, where he became a student and lifelong friend of Benjamin Rush, M.D. (Horrocks, 1999; W. S. Miller, 1925). Mease's interests were broad, however, and in addition to his essay on migraines and his expertise on rabies, he authored an early geological study of the United States (Horrocks, 1999). A historian, too, he wrote to Thomas Jefferson, learning and transmitting to posterity the location of the house in which the Declaration of Independence was written (J. F. Watson, 1887). As a member of Philadelphia society, Mease helped promote the career of John Audubon by introducing him to the American artistic and scientific elite (A. Ford, 1964). And while Mease himself has become an obscure, almost forgotten figure, one of his historical works, "The Picture of Philadelphia," is in print today, almost 200 years after it was written (Mease, 1811/1970).

[3]Thus, Mease took a practical, empirical orientation. This is seen also in his approach to rabies, his primary medical specialty. Although he was opposed to Benjamin Rush's prescription of aggressive bloodletting to treat rabies, he allowed that "if a single fair case of the disease be hereafter cured by the depleting [bloodletting] plan, I will waive all theory on the subject, and adopt the practice" (cited in W. S. Miller, 1925, pp. 10–11). Nowadays, it is tempting to think of medicine before the germ theory of disease, before organic chemistry and experimental physiology, as mere dark superstition. But in the context of migraines, which have benefited little from the germ theory of disease, we can see the wisdom that developed in the practical trade of early 19th century doctors.

[4]Of course, not all of Mease's 19th century insights have stood the test of time. He describes in detail two cases in which recurrent migraines were cured by means of Fowler's mineral solution. Now, trace minerals sound healthy, but Fowler's solution was actually "arsenic dissolved in water by means of the vegetable alkali. It is perfectly safe . . ." (Mease, 1819, p. 12). Do *not* try this! Even here, though, there may have been more wisdom than it now seems—although the arsenic was undoubtedly carcinogenic. In Mease's day, the young country was riddled with infectious diseases. A half-century later, Liveing suspected that the arsenic had in fact been curing headaches that were due to undiagnosed malaria (Liveing, 1873).

and canavanine inhibit arginine transport (Wu & S. M. Morris, 1998), it may be the balance among these amino acids and not the raw amount of arginine that is important. Only three common food types have arginine as their highest amino acid constituent (Pennington, 1998), and all are generally on the standard lists of migraine triggers (citrus, nuts, onions). Nonetheless, the role of dietary arginine in migraine at this point is entirely theoretical. In terms of the role of arginine more generally, levels may be elevated in the platelets of people who have migraine with aura, but apparently not in their blood plasma, or in the platelets or plasma in migraine without aura (D'Andrea, Cananzi, Perini, & Hasselmark, 1995).

Nitrite.   Nitrites are salts used to give processed meats their red color. Nitrates are also sometimes used, and work because they are reduced in meat to the corresponding nitrites. Nitrite has been implicated as a headache trigger in single-blind case study (Henderson & Raskin, 1972) and a small double-blind placebo-controlled study (Cornwell & L. Clarke, 1991). The reason for a connection between nitrite and headache is quite unclear, and there is a general dearth of research on the subject. In one theory, nitrite is metabolized to give nitric oxide (W. Scher & B. M. Scher, 1992). However, the direction of metabolism is usually exactly the opposite: nitrite and nitrate salts are generally the end products and not the starting point of nitric oxide processing.

Dietary triggers and non-migraine headaches.   In contrast to migraines, there has been little investigation of the role of diet in tension-type headaches. Scharff, et al. note that individuals with tension-type headache were as likely as those with migraines to report dietary triggers, particularly alcohol, chocolate, and MSG (Scharff, D. C. Turk, & Marcus, 1995). However, this might have been due to the high frequency of headaches in this clinic population (Ulrich, M. B. Russell, R. Jensen, & Olesen, 1996). We have seen that chronic daily headache often evolves out of episodic migraines. In these cases, the "interval headaches" in between migraine episodes are clinically indistinguishable from chronic tension-type headache, but is noteworthy for responding to migraine abortive medication. Analogously, in a population-based study, Ulrich et al. found that only people who also had a history of migraines identified dietary triggers for tension-type headaches.

Other studies as well, however, imply a role for diet in tension-type headache. In a study by P. R. Martin and Seneviratne (1997), fasting (or possibly caffeine withdrawal) was found likely to be a trigger. And Guarnieri et al., in agreement with Scharff, found that intake of red wine correlated with the frequency and severity of tension-type headaches (Guarnieri, Radnitz, & Blanchard, 1990). There were also significant negative correlations between headache activity and the amount of fresh fruit and cooked vegetables in the subjects' diet, raising the possibility that the fruits and vegetables were functioning as protective factors (Guarnieri, et al.).

CLUSTER HEADACHES

For cluster headaches, the classic ingested triggers are vasodilators: alcohol (not only red wine), histamine, and nitroglycerine (Connors, 1995). Platelet and plasma levels of trace amines are even higher in cluster headache patients, during and between cluster periods, than in migraineurs (D'Andrea, Terrazzino, et al., 2004). To my knowledge, though, there have been no reports of triggering by tyramine-containing foods. Decreases in blood oxygen levels or increases in carbon dioxide may precipitate cluster headaches (L. Kudrow & D. B. Kudrow, 1990). Thus, apnea should be evaluated in people whose cluster headaches routinely occur in the first few hours of sleep (Chervin, Zallek, X. Lin, J. M. Hall, Sharma, & Hedger, 2000).

WEEKEND HEADACHES

These, of course, are headaches that occur exclusively or primarily on weekends. They are generally migraines or tension-type headaches (Torelli, Cologno, & Manzoni, 1999), and are found to be more common in men than women in some studies (Hering, Couturier, & Steiner, 1992) but not others (Torelli, et al.). Weekends can include a number of migraine triggers such as decreased caffeine intake, increased use of alcohol, and changes in one's sleep-wake cycle (Hering, et al.). A sudden drop in stress could perhaps be a trigger as well, as parasympathetic activity can increase secretion of histamine by mast cells (Theoharides, et al., 1995).

INFECTION

Infection has sometimes been reported clinically to be a migraine trigger. The mechanism behind this effect is unknown, but we saw in Chapter 2 that certain immune system chemicals, or cytokines, can induce hyperalgesia (L. R. Watkins & Maier, 2000), including hyperalgesia at the trigeminal nucleus. Moreover, a particular cytokine, interleukin–1, tends to increase platelet aggregability, raise levels of corticotropin-releasing hormone, and produce sustained elevations of neuronal firing in the locus coeruleus (Licinio & M.-L. Wong, 1997). Thus, there are several plausible mechanisms by which infections could lower the threshold for a migraine. If we think of migraines as a defensive response by the brain, a lower threshold in times of illness makes sense.

INTERACTIONS AMONG TRIGGERS

In migraine trigger research, double-blind, placebo-controlled trials have been criticized as lacking ecological validity (e.g., Scopp, 1992). Proponents of this view suggest that in daily life, multiple triggers can function synergistically. For example, Dalton (1975) asked 1883 women to recall, each time they had a migraine, whether they had consumed any of four trigger foods in the preceding 24 hours: cheese, chocolate, citrus, and alcohol. In the 2313 records that resulted, each trigger was found to precede perimenstrual migraines approximately 30 percent of the time. However, migraines that did not occur perimenstrually were only preceded by one of the trigger foods approximately 10 percent of the time. In another study, the vasoactive effects of tyramine were greater around the time of menstruation (Ghose & P. Turner, 1977). Similarly, Nicolodi and Sicuteri (1999) found that low doses of alcoholic beverages were much more likely to lead to migraines when consumed on stressful occasions. (However, their design does not allow determination of whether the stress itself, or the combination of stress and alcohol, was the trigger.)

There are theoretical reasons for assuming that multiple triggers will function synergistically. Thus, alcohol and tyramine inhibit diamine oxidase, which breaks down histamine, and phenol-sulphotransferase P, which catabolizes flavonoids (Littlewood, Gibb, Glover, Sandler, P. T. G. Davies, & F. C. Rose, 1988; Wantke, Gotz, & Jarisch, 1994). All four components, alcohol, tyramine, histamine, and flavonoids, can occur together in red wine. Citrus fruits contain flavonoids and **arginine**, and may cause release of histamine. Histamine appears to up-regulate nitric oxide synthase, while arginine is the raw material for producing nitric oxide. Thus, Scopp (1992) notes that tyramine and glutamate have each been found to elicit headaches in double-blind, placebo-controlled studies, but only when the substances were consumed at home vs. in a laboratory setting. We have seen similar results for aspartame. Presumably, other triggers were present simultaneously in the home.

In contrast, these interactions are sometimes purposefully excluded in double-blind, placebo-controlled trials. Thus, in a particularly well-controlled study of chocolate in migraines, subjects were placed on a diet free of tyramine, phenylethylamine, histamine, caffeine, nitrites, MSG, and aspartame for two weeks prior to and during the administration of chocolate. Moreover, the chocolate was purposely not given perimenstrually (Marcus, Scharff, D. C. Turk, & Gourley, 1997).

Still, although a case can be made that many trigger studies lack ecological validity, there is a key limitation in the evidence: We have not yet demonstrated experimentally that the effects of triggers actually do summate. A first attempt to clarify this issue was made by P. R. Martin and Seneviratne (1997), by crossing presence vs. absence of food deprivation with presence vs. absence of a laboratory stressor, in a two-by-two factorial design. That is, half of the subjects were asked to refrain from all food and drink except water for the 19 hours prior to the study. Half of the subjects were asked to solve anagrams, many of which actually had no solutions, while being given periodic negative feedback on their performance. (Of course the subjects were debriefed immediately following the study.) The food deprivation by itself did not significantly increase negative affect, suggesting that the fast was not simply another way of producing stress. Now in the study, food deprivation and the stressor each appeared to produce headaches, and there was no interaction between the two. Subjects who were exposed to both the food deprivation and the stressor did indeed have a greater probability of getting a headache, but this was simply the sum of the effects of the two triggers separately. Moreover, the triggers did not interact with diagnosis: The effects were the same in migraineurs as in subjects with tension-type headaches (P. R. Martin & Seneviratne, 1997).

A limitation of the study is that the type of headache was not determined. Headaches were assessed during and immediately after the stressor, which lasted approximately 33 minutes. The headaches were an immediate consequence of the stressor. Perhaps, then, most of the headaches were tension-type, even among the migraineurs. The study may not tell us about migraine triggers, although this is not certain. Also, we do not know which aspect of food deprivation was the culprit. As the authors point out, the food deprivation headaches might have been produced by caffeine withdrawal.

In a second study from the same laboratory, stress and noise were crossed in a factorial design. As in Martin and Seneviratne's research, both factors triggered headaches, and were additive (non-interacting), despite the fact that stress made the noise more aversive. Seventy-five percent of subjects with a migraine diagnosis and 86 percent of those with tension-type headache rated the laboratory pain as the same or similar to their usual headaches, implying but not proving that both types of headache were triggered (P. R. Martin, J. Todd, & Reece, 2005).

Although questions remain, particularly about migraine triggering, Martin's work is a valuable model for how the question of interaction can be studied rigorously.

OTHER DIFFICULTIES IN TRIGGER STUDIES

Ecological validity is not the only aspect of controlled trials that has been criticized. A second difficulty is an often high rate of placebo responding (Lipton, Newman, & S. Solomon, 1988). This has been attributed to the stress of being given a potential migraine trigger (Kohlenberg, 1982), to expectation, and to classical conditioning. Jessup (1978) has argued that the nausea accompanying a migraine, and the food cravings that can precede a migraine, are a natural set-up for **conditioned taste aversion**: a powerful, rapidly-acquired learned avoidance of the foods that preceded the nausea (Jessup, 1978). As we saw in Chapter 2, conditioned taste aversion may include a conditioned hyperalgesia, at least in rats, if the food is later consumed (Wiertelak, et al., 1994). Scharff and Marcus (1999) have noted that chocolate ingestion may be higher perimenstrually, or during stressful work periods when the office vending machine is the source of meals. It may be the stress, skipped meals, or hormonal changes that actually account for the migraines; the chocolate may be just a marker (Blau, 1992; Scharff & Marcus, 1999).

A related problem in controlled trials is subject selection. A common strategy is to restrict the study to migraineurs who indicate that their headaches can be provoked by a particular food. However, individuals may report trigger foods that actually have no pharmacological effect on their migraines. Hanington (1967, 1968), who first proposed the tyramine hypothesis, felt that a person's retrospective report was likely to be spurious, an artifact of what they had read, or of illusory correlations. She reserved the term "dietary migraineur" to individuals who had actually altered their diet to avoid headaches, and she estimated that only 5 percent of individuals with migraines would meet this definition. Approximately 5 percent of the migraineurs in a study by Nicolodi and Sicuteri (1999) appeared to have a particular sensitivity to alcohol as a trigger. Moreover, there may be different subsets of people, each having different triggers. As noted, Littlewood et al. (1982) found that phenolsulphotransferase P activity was lower in dietary vs. nondietary migraineurs, and lowest in those reporting citrus as a trigger.

Conversely, Scopp emphasizes that migraine patients may often be unaware of their triggers, because they may not know what to look for, or because the elimination of a single trigger may not be sufficient to change headache frequency. In case studies and small-scale trials in which multiple triggers have been targeted simultaneously, high rates of improvement have been reported (Blau & Thavapalan, 1988; Radnitz, Blanchard, & Bylina, 1990). However, these studies were not blinded or controlled.

The problem of identifying migraineurs with true dietary triggers pertains to clinical work as well as controlled trials. Because retrospective reports can be unreliable, it seems best in individual work to either have available a long-term dietary-and-headache record from the patient, from which triggers can be determined prospectively, or to begin by eliminating multiple triggers simultaneously. If the migraines have a temporal pattern (e.g., occurring around menstruation), then it may be possible to limit trigger elimination to those times when a headache is likely. The drawback to working without a record, however, is that for many migraineurs dietary triggers may not be significant enough to require a change.

INDIVIDUALIZED TRIGGERS

Recall that Duncan and associates demonstrated that, at least in monkeys, nociceptive neurons in the trigeminal nucleus can learn to fire in response to a discriminative stimulus (Duncan, Bushnell, R. Bates, & Dubner, 1987). Thus, we might speculate that conditioned hyperalgesia plays a role in triggering migraines. To my knowledge, this possibility has not been studied directly.

Alternatively, an originally neutral stimulus might become a migraine trigger through classical conditioning of autonomic responding. That is, the stimulus might elicit, say, vasoconstriction, because previously it had been paired with a true unconditioned trigger. This possibility at least has a strong theoretical rationale. And a similar model has been proposed to explain another disorder with discrete triggers: multiple chemical sensitivity, or idiopathic environmental intolerance (Giardino & Lehrer, 2000). However, there appears to be little direct empirical research to confirm that classically conditioned migraine triggers actually exist.

Several studies address the question indirectly. First, evidence that vasoconstriction at the hands can be classically conditioned has been reported by a number of investigators, beginning with Cytovitch and Folkman in 1917 (e.g., Cytovitch & Folkman, 1917; Lipp, Siddle, & Vaitl, 1992; Marinesco & Kreindler, 1934; Menzies, 1937; Shmavonian, 1959). Classically conditioned vasoconstriction has also been reported at the superficial temporal artery (Korn, 1949), a case study result that is quite deserving of further investigation. By and large, however, only healthy volunteers were used in these studies.

Indeed, there seems to have been only a single study in which conditioning of vasomotor responding was examined in migraineurs specifically, and its results seem ambiguous. Price and Clarke paired a soft tone at one frequency with a loud burst of white noise, while another soft tone, different in frequency, was not paired with the noise (K. Price & Clarke, 1979). The noise was a stressor and tended to produce vasoconstriction in the hands of both migraineurs and non-migraineurs. After awhile, the tone paired with the white noise began to produce vasoconstriction by itself, consistent with classical conditioning. In the nonmigraineurs, this effect was specific to the paired tone; the unpaired tone produced vasodilation. The migraineurs, in contrast, acquired a vasoconstriction response to both soft tones. Thus, the Price and Clarke study confirms previous research in suggesting that vasoconstriction can be learned through classical conditioning in nonmigraineurs. The fact that the response was more general in migraineurs perhaps might be due to greater response stereotypy, or deficient central control over autonomic responding. The long-term effects of vasoconstrictive medications (none of the subjects had taken vasoconstrictives within 48 hours of the study) also cannot be excluded (K. Price & Clarke, 1979).

MacQueen and coworkers found that secretion of histamine by mast cells, at least mucosal mast cells in the rat, can also be classically conditioned (MacQueen, Marshall, Perdue, Siegel, & Bienenstock, 1989).

Another possibility is that the neural changes associated with migraine can be reproduced through learning. This, at least, was Liveing's belief about certain cases of visual triggers: "Such a pathological *habit* indeed of disturbance through this channel may the sensorium acquire by its frequent repetition" (Liveing, 1873, p. 55, italics in original). In support of this, he notes that "the late Sir John Herschel, a sufferer from purely visual megrim, states, in a letter to Dr. Airy, that an attack was produced in him by allowing the mind to dwell on the description of the appearances. This is very interesting, showing, as it does, that the same kind of impression on the sensorium, whether arriving through channels of sense or idea, may be followed by the same result" (Liveing, 1873, p. 55). This hypothesis, of a top-down component in migraine, remains as intriguing, and as unproven, as it was in Liveing's day.

Thus, the idea that migraine triggers can come about through classical conditioning remains a plausible theory, with a degree of indirect support in the literature. However, quite a bit of further research is needed to clarify whether such idiosyncratic triggers in fact exist, and whether they are clinically significant.

TRIGGERS AND THERAPY

The question of whether triggers can be classically conditioned is important clinically. If triggers are like risk factors, then the best advice is to avoid them, for the more exposure, the greater the likelihood of a headache. But for triggers acquired through classical conditioning, the risk is incremented only for relatively brief exposures. With long exposure, the headache response would extinguish, and the trigger would lose its effectiveness (P. R. Martin, 2000, 2001).

P. R. Martin has examined this possibility, by exposing 110 people to a strobe light in a dark room. Every 15 seconds, the light was switched off for 5 seconds, providing a short break between trials. Not surprisingly, people who were exposed to the light for 20 or 33 minutes (15 or 25 minutes, respectively, not counting the breaks) were considerably more likely to develop a headache than people who simply sat quietly in normal lighting. However, the relationship was curvilinear: With an exposure time of 47 minutes (35 minutes of strobe light), the amount of headache tended to be intermediate between "no exposure" and exposures of shorter duration (P. R. Martin, 2001). This was as true for people with a headache disorder as for people who rarely get them. Presumably, if exposure time were increased and the process repeated several times, the participants would eventually desensitize to the trigger.

This area of research seems too new, for now, to recommend a sweeping change in clinical practice. We need to know first how robust the effect is, to which types of triggers it applies, and whether it produces better results in actual practice than trigger avoidance. For now, it generally seems reasonable to stay with the standard advice of encouraging patients to avoid triggers. The research path begun by P. R. Martin should be followed, however, for if he is right, avoiding triggers could be as deleterious in headaches as avoiding feared situations is in anxiety.

HEADACHES, TRIGGERS, AND THE BIRTH OF PSYCHOLOGY

Although exposure therapy for triggers is brand new as a research agenda, without it, psychology might have been slower to originate. . . .

The first work in the new science was Gustav Fechner's *Elemente der Psychophysik*, or *Elements of Psychophysics* (Fechner, 1860/1966). Psychophysics, of course, is the attempt to discover the relations between physical variables (such as the radiant energy from a light source) and psychological variables (such as perceived brightness). The fact that such relations can be described mathematically helped establish the possibility of a psychological science. And it was Fechner who invented psychophysics, on October 22, 1850. In a sense, we pay homage to him and to his followers whenever we ask patients to rate their level of pain.

Fechner's first career, however, was in physics, and through his translation of French textbooks and his own unusually careful experimentation, he helped bring rigor to its practice in Germany. In fact, by the age of 33 he had published 16 empirical studies in the hard sciences, several volumes of his own in chemistry and physics, many translations, was the editor of a pharmaceutical journal, and had become a physics professor at the University of Leipzig. He then compiled and wrote nearly a third of a roughly 8000-page encyclopedia. Then, at age 39, he collapsed (Marshall, 1969, 1982).

The nature of Fechner's collapse is unknown. It has been attributed to exhaustion (Marshall, 1969), a "nervous breakdown" (Boring, 1942), a "habit neurosis" (W. James, cited in Boring, 1950), damaged eyesight following experiments on afterimages that involved staring for prolonged periods at the sun, and eyestrain from experiments on binocular vision (Hall, 1912). In the brief descriptions of it that are available, however, it resembles status migrainosus, a continuous migraine, with pain at his head and eyes, worsened by effort, photophobia, and problems digesting his food. Remarkably, it lasted for years. During this time, he remained in a darkened room; if he moved about during the daytime his eyes were heavily bandaged. He could not read or look around. Concentration was painful, for "the muscles of the scalp, especially those of the occiput, assumed a fairly morbid degree of sensibility whenever I tried to *think*" (Fechner, 1860, in regard to "a former illness," cited in W. James, 1890/1901, p. 436). In time he stopped speaking as well, because speaking worsened his head pain, and because of his digestive problems he stopped eating. He recalled in his diary: "I do not know for how many weeks I was without meat and drink, and at the same time felt no hunger. I never had imagined that a man could hold out so long without food and drink. Meanwhile I continued to go about, although I was constantly becoming thinner and more feeble. Finally I was no more than a skeleton and had to lie down for sheer weakness. My mind remained perfectly clear, but I came near perishing from starvation, and all hope of my recovery was abandoned" (Fechner, cited in Lowrie, 1946, p. 38). Ultimately, he found a few foods that he could eat in small amounts. But by then, in addition to the burdens of boredom and pain, Fechner's thoughts were racing, and he exerted much of his effort against a vivid sense of impending insanity.

An experimentalist even near death, Fechner stumbled on a path to recovery: "It was on October 1 that as a consequence of anger I began to speak quickly and vivaciously, without paying any regard to the disagreeable sensations in my head which commonly resulted from the effort to speak. But now these sensations did not manifest themselves, in spite of the fact that not many days before the utterance of a few words seemed too much. I attributed this to the excitement I was under and was encouraged thereby to speak repeatedly, with a sort of desperate disregard for my head, and I found that it succeeded, if only I made pauses between sentences" (Fechner, cited in Lowrie, 1946, p. 41). He tried applying this discovery to his vision as well. He had previously been unsuccessful in gradually reacclimating his eyes to dim light, but now he found success by briefly exposing them to the full light of his surroundings. "Instead of being passive the action was intent and energetic" (Lowrie, 1946, p. 41).

We may wonder whether exhaustion, depression (H. Schröder & C. Schröder, 1993), and the avoidance of triggers inadvertently turned acute pain from Fechner's afterimage or binocular vision experiments into chronic pain. Certainly his recovery seems to presage modern treatment in its emphasis on active over passive coping (G. K. Brown & Nicassio, 1987; Mercado, L. J. Carroll, J. D. Cassidy, & Côté, 2005). Regardless, Fechner seemed changed by his illness. Under a pseudonym he had written philosophical treatises before his illness, but now he propounded his philosophy openly and with determination (Marshall, 1982). Psychophysics, for Fechner the relation of soul to matter, a science in the service of philosophy, was a part of this larger project (Boring, 1966). It was the beginning of experimental psychology, and although Fechner is not usually associated with clinical psychology, Freud later recalled that "I was always open to the ideas of G. T. Fechner and have followed that thinker upon many important points" (Freud, 1925/1963, p. 114). Indeed, Fechner's techniques for determining sensory thresholds are still used to this day, for example to test the strength of analgesic medications.

Now, disability benefits tend to have a bad name these days, particularly in operant psychology where they are viewed as reinforcing a pain focus. So it is a matter of fairness that we mention that Fechner was subsisting on a small disability pension from the University of Leipzig when he invented scientific psychology. In fact, he remained on disability for 45 years, never returning to formal employment, but researching and writing, propounding psychophysics, until the end of his life.

Of course the research on exposure therapy for triggers has hardly begun, and Fechner's dramatic recovery 150 years ago cannot yet lead us to recommend it for broad application.

IMPLICATIONS FOR BEHAVIORAL TREATMENT

Early in treatment, reviewing potential triggers, aided by a list such as the one shown at the end of this chapter, can be useful as patients begin to track their headaches. Identifying triggers, prodromal signs, or temporal patterns can be particularly reassuring to people for whom the attacks have felt random, arbitrary, and punishing. Even so strong a trigger as stress may have escaped notice if it has a 3- or 4-day delayed effect, or if the stresses have become so frequent that the patient no longer thinks of them. In tracking, small stresses (daily hassles) should be included. We will discuss formal headache tracking at the end of Chapter 12.

Other patients may report a set of triggers matter-of-factly at the outset of the assessment. Here, it is useful to clarify briefly whether this knowledge derives from direct experience vs. reading or previous medical advice. Some conscientious patients will avoid tyramine-containing foods for years without ever having experienced a dietary migraine.

Still other patients, for whom a plethora of environmental triggers has been vivid, may have devoted a great deal of effort to titrating exposure to those that are controllable (e.g., fluorescent lights in stores) and suffering through those that are not (such as the weather). Even here, however, formal tracking can be useful for sorting out the relative importance of the triggers, and for helping the patient bring objective, dispassionate problem solving to bear on the pain.

Once triggers have been identified, there is a range of therapeutic options. Lifestyle factors such as over- or undersleeping, caffeine and overwork, may be obvious to the patient, but require collaborative problem solving and behavioral habit change to overcome. Stresses that can be appropriately avoided or changed can also be addressed via problem solving. Otherwise, work can focus on how the stresses are appraised cognitively and on the psychophysiological responses they elicit.

The worsening of migraine without aura perimenstrually seems to call for use of exogenous hormones, but we will see in Chapter 11 that the question is not so simple. An alternative is to remove compounding factors such as stress.

Whenever there is a range of significant triggers, attempting to avoid all of them may be more disabling than beneficial. Here, too, it seems best to target a few salient triggers, especially stress, overwork, caffeine, and mental fatigue. The potential for triggers to have additive effects suggest that we do not have to address all of them to bring the headaches under control.

Especially when triggers are salient or numerous, we should try to gauge whether they are eliciting a strong psychophysiological stress response or cognitive expectation of a migraine that might be the true mechanism of action. The stress response might be apparent in-session, for example as forceful tensing of the facial muscles, or involve a striking signature on psychophysiological testing, especially **skin conductance level**. We will discuss this testing in Chapter 12, on assessment. When it is the cognitive or physical responses that seem key, and avoiding the triggers would cause lifestyle constriction, then a systematic desensitization protocol seems a reasonable option.

Odors, whether second-hand smoke, diesel or fresh asphalt when driving, or perfume at worship or in the workplace, can be particularly salient and challenging. Here, especially, it is important to judge the relative feasibility of avoiding vs. desensitizing.

Thus, identifying triggers, as part of the broader project of finding patterns and early warning signs for the headaches, can help establish both the objective mindset and the concrete agenda for behavioral treatment. We will consider this treatment in more detail in Chapter 13.

DAILY HEADACHE RECORD

Date:_____   Time Completed:_____

Headache
   Average intensity (0–10):_____   Time began:_____   Time ended:_____

Stress
   Average stress level (0–10):_____

Did the headache involve
   ___Pulsating Pain ___ Pain on One Side of Head ___ Nausea
   ___Pressing/Tightening Pain ___Worsened by Routine Physical Activity (e.g., climbing stairs)
   ___Pain on Both Sides of Head ___Aversion to Light
   ___Aversion to Conversational Sound Levels

Dietary Factors
   ___Aged cheese
   ___Dried smoked fish
   ___Sour cream
   ___Yogurt
   ___Yeast extracts
   ___Chocolate
   ___Citrus
   ___Dairy
   ___Onions
   ___Nuts
   ___Beans
   ___Caffeine
   ___Fatty foods
   ___Monosodium glutamate, Chinese food,
      hydrolyzed vegetable protein
   ___Nutrasweet

Environmental Factors
   ___Bright light
   ___Glare
   ___Fluorescent lighting
   ___Perfumes
   ___Fumes
   ___Weather changes
   ___Extended travel

Lifestyle
   ___Missed sleep
   ___Missed meals
   ___Cigarette smoking
   ___Exertion

Hormonal
   ___Menstruation

Finger Temperature

      Before relaxation_____   After relaxation_____

Adapted from *Migraine: The Complete Guide* by the American Council for Headache Education, 1994, pp. 66–67. New York: Dell. Used with permission.

CHAPTER 11

A Guide to Headache Medications

He gently prevails on his patients to try,
The magic effects of the ergot rye.
  —Attributed to Alfred, Lord Tennyson (cited in Critchley, 1996, p. 338)

In trigger avoidance and desensitization we took a self-management approach to headaches. Here, we shift strategies, and survey the sweeping range of pharmacologic options. These tools, of course, have multiplied greatly in the last fifteen years, and can be of marked clinical benefit. But utility is by no means assured; depending on the medication and the patient's history, the specific drug may be complicating or ameliorating the clinical picture, and facilitating or hindering treatment.

AHCPR AND THE U.S. HEADACHE CONSORTIUM

Over 100 drugs have shown efficacy in treating migraine, including several classes of medication that simply did not exist 15 years ago. Thus, one of the main problems in pharmacotherapy is information management: consolidating a huge literature into useable form. Fortunately, for migraines this task has been achieved in technical reviews by Duke University's Center for Clinical Health Policy Research, conducted for the United States Agency for Healthcare Policy and Research (AHCPR; later, the Agency for Healthcare Research and Quality). These technical reviews formed the basis for clinical guidelines by the U.S. Headache Consortium, a multispecialty group comprised of representatives of several organizations involved in migraine treatment[1] (Silberstein, 2000). Individual patients differ of course, and the guidelines, designed for primary care physicians, were not intended to replace professional judgment. They were, however, meant to be definitive. We will draw on them throughout the migraine sections of this chapter.

ACUTE ANTI-MIGRAINE MEDICATIONS

Ergotamine and Dihydroergotamine

Ergotamine is an alkaloid derived from naturally occurring but nonetheless dangerous sources, such as a fungus that grows on rye. Its efficacy for migraines was first noted by Edward Woakes

---

[1] The American Academy of Neurology, the American Academy of Family Physicians, the American College of Emergency Physicians, the Amercian College of Physicians—American Society of Internal Medicine, the American Headache Society, the American Osteopathic Association, and the National Headache Foundation (Silberstein, 2000)

(P. J. Koehler & Isler, 2002; Woakes, 1868), and it was rapidly added to the therapeutic arsenal (P. J. Koehler & Isler, 2002). Indeed, it remains in use to this day, generally in combination with caffeine (Cafergot, Wigraine).

Ergotamine is a broad-spectrum agent, stimulating certain classes of dopaminergic (D_2) and adrenergic (α_1 and α_2) receptors, most or all types of serotonergic receptors, and certain other receptors that have not yet been characterized (Tfelt-Hansen, Saxena, et al., 2000). Its efficacy most likely derives from its status as a serotonin agonist, through the same mechanisms of action as the triptans (M. D. Ferrari, 1998b).

Despite long clinical use, the efficacy of ergotamine has been surprisingly hard to demonstrate consistently, except with high and possibly unsafe doses. The very low oral and rectal bioavailability (possibly increased slightly with coadministration of caffeine) may account for the variable results. However, when ergotamine works it seems to produce a prolonged vasoconstriction that may be particularly useful for preventing headache recurrence (Silberstein, 2003).

The primary side effects of ergotamine are increased nausea (no small consideration in migraine), fibrosis (pulmonary, **retroperitoneal**, or involving the valves in the heart), ano-rectal ulcers or stenosis with suppository use, **myocardial infarction** (heart attack), and limb ischemia sometimes causing **neuropathy** (Meyler, 1996). The side effects usually occur with chronic daily use (ergotamine abuse) or long-term intermittent treatment, but there are occasional reports of adverse events following a single therapeutic dose (Meyler, 1996). Unfortunately, long-term intermittent treatment is the most common format for using ergotamine.

In all, oral ergotamine, with or without caffeine, is accorded Group 3 status by the Consortium: conflicting or inconsistent evidence of utility (Silberstein, 2000).

A further derivative, dihydroergotamine (DHE) has the unusual advantages of very long duration of action and, correspondingly, low rates of headache recurrence (Silberstein, 1997, 2003). In addition to the same mechanisms of action as the triptans (described below), DHE may also be active at the periaqueductal area of the midbrain (involved in transmission of pain) and the dorsal raphe nucleus (in the putative migraine generator region; Goadsby, 1997b).

Although dihydroergotamine is less vasoconstrictive than its parent molecule, ergotamine, and less prone to cause nausea, the contraindications are similar: coronary artery or cerebrovascular disease, peripheral vascular disease, impaired hepatic or renal function, sepsis, and of course pregnancy or sensitivity to ergots (Silberstein, Schulman, & M. M. Hopkins, 1990). As the ergots tend to raise blood pressure, uncontrolled hypertension would similarly be a contraindication. DHE, in all its modes of delivery (intravenous, intramuscular, subcutaneous, and intranasal) is placed in Group 1 by the Consortium: proven, pronounced statistical and clinical benefit (Silberstein, 2000).

Triptans

Sumatriptan (Imitrex; Imigran) is a serotonin agonist. By design, it is much more selective than ergotamine, binding specifically to a group of serotonin (5-HT) receptor subtypes (1A, 1B, 1D, and 1F). Indeed, the development of sumatriptan was a landmark in migraine research, not only because of its significant efficacy, but because its high selectivity shed light on migraine physiology at the level of receptor subtypes (Deleu & Hanssens, 2000). To my knowledge, none of the body's many serotonin systems is as precisely characterized as that involved in ending migraine attacks.

Four theories have been proposed to account for sumatriptan's efficacy: (1) Vasoconstriction through stimulation of 5-HT_{1B} receptors in the blood vessel wall. (2) Binding to 5-HT_{1D} sites on the terminal axons of nociceptive nerves, inhibiting the release of vasoactive peptides such as calcitonin gene-related peptide (Goadsby, 1995). (3) Attaching to vesicles in the proximal ends of nociceptive fibers, preventing the release of neurotransmitters into the trigeminal nucleus (Ahn & Basbaum, 2005). And (4) binding to sites within the trigeminal nucleus, where serotonin functions as an inhibitory neurotransmitter, presumably decreasing pain transmission (Goadsby & Hoskin, 1996; Goadsby & Knight, 1997b). The fourth of these models is perhaps the least likely, as sumatriptan, being **hydrophilic** (water- rather than fat-soluble), does not generally cross the blood-brain barrier (Ferrari, 1998b).

The efficacy of sumatriptan is quite high. In a meta-analysis, Goadsby (1998) concluded that 60 percent of patients are pain-free (vs. 18 percent on placebo), and 79 percent are at least improved (vs. 27 percent on placebo), two hours after subcutaneous injection. Generally, if sumatriptan injection works for a patient, it will do so consistently. However, the migraines reoccur in approximately one-third of patients. A second administration will often be effective, but if the headache again recurs, a third dose is not recommended. Also, the injections have a somewhat higher rate of side effects than oral triptans and, of course, patients find the mode of delivery unpleasant (Rapoport & Tepper, 2001).

Sumatriptan intranasal spray can be an alternative to injections. Its speed of onset is variable, but tends to be faster than that of oral triptans. Its efficacy can also be variable, however, and patients often dislike the taste (Rapoport & Tepper, 2001).

The efficacy of oral sumatriptan is lower than for the injections, with approximately 35 percent of patients pain-free (vs. 9 percent on a placebo) and 58 percent improved (vs. 25 percent on a placebo) after two hours (Goadsby, 1998). Sumatriptan does not appear to be effective for pediatric migraine, perhaps because the headaches are shorter (Hämäläinen, Hoppu, & Santavuori, 1997; Korsgaard, 1995).

Newer triptans. A host of new medications are, like sumatriptan, selective 5-HT$_{1B/1D}$ agonists. This burgeoning class includes *zolmitriptan* (Zomig), *naratriptan* (Amerge, Naramig), *rizatriptan* (Maxalt), *almotriptan* (Axert, Almogran), *frovatriptan* (Frova, Migard), and *eletriptan* (Relpax). These medications are "second generation triptans" and represent attempts to improve on sumatriptan with higher bioavailability (for more rapid and consistent effects), greater lipophilicity (more fat-soluble, for anti-nociceptive activity at brain stem sites) and longer half-life in the plasma (to hopefully lower headache recurrence rate).

Zolmitriptan seems to have the same effects on ciruculation, both cranial and peripheral, as sumatriptan (Rolan & G. R. Martin, 1998). However, zolmitriptan is also twice as lipophilic, crosses the blood-brain barrier, and binds at the solitary tract nucleus and the trigeminal nucleus caudalis in the migraine generator region (Goadsby & Knight, 1997a; A. Mills, P. Rhodes, & G. R. Martin, 1995). At the trigeminal nucleus, it seems to reduce activation in response to an electrical stimulus (Goadsby & Hoskin, 1996). Zolmitriptan is more bioavailable than oral sumatriptan. Its half-life in the plasma is 2.5–3.0 hours, but the effectiveness may be extended by its active metabolite, called "183C91," which is also a 5-HT$_{1B/D}$ agonist (Rolan & G. R. Martin, 1998). Whether all this translates into greater efficacy is uncertain. In my patients' experience, zolmitriptan seems to be particularly effective. However, a single large-sample head-to-head comparison produced the surprising result that zolmitriptan, sumatriptan, and placebo were equivalent (Diener & K. Klein, 1996; an inadvertent demonstration of psychological factors in migraine). Still, failure to respond to sumatriptan does not predict response to zolmitriptan, so the availability of the two triptans allows treatment to be optimized for the individual patient (Rolan & G. R. Martin, 1998).

Naratriptan is absorbed slowly, remains in the plasma longer, and dissociates less readily from its receptor binding than most other triptans (Rapoport & Tepper, 2001; Tepper, Rapoport, & Sheftell, 2002). In practice, naratriptan takes longer to work (generally 3–4 hours), but also has a lower rate of headache reccurence than most other triptans (N. T. Mathew, 1999). It has a lower efficacy for severe migraines, but also a lower rate of side effects, than sumatriptan and zolmitriptan. All of this seems to make naratriptan a reasonable choice for mild or moderate migraines (N. T. Mathew, 1999), or when headache recurrence is a significant problem. And while its slow timeframe can be a problem in acute migraine treatment, naratriptan may turn out to have a niche in preventing menstrual migraines (Newman et al., 2001), cluster headaches (Eekers & Koehler, 2001; Loder, 2002a), and perhaps even transformed migraines (Sheftell, Rapoport, & Coddon, 1999).

From early meta-analyses of Phase II and Phase III trials, it appears that zolmitriptan may have somewhat greater efficacy than sumatriptan, at the cost of a somewhat greater risk of side effects. Conversely, naratriptan appears to have a lower efficacy than sumatriptan, but to be extremely well tolerated, and with a lower rate of headache recurrence, around 20–25 percent (Goadsby, 1998; Salonen, 1999). A natural goal, of course, would be to develop a triptan that combines the high efficacy of zolmitriptan with the tolerability of naratriptan.

Rizatriptan 10 mg has been reported to give a higher probability of becoming pain free at 2 hours, when compared with zolmitriptan 2.5 mg, naratriptan 2.5 mg, and sumatriptan 25–100 mg. People who took rizatriptan were also more likely to be relieved of associated migraine symptoms such as nausea or photophobia, and (except in the comparison to sumatriptan 100 mg) to maintain most or all of their improvement for 24 hours. The studies were conducted by Merck Research Laboratories, affiliated with the manufacturer of rizatriptan (J. U. Adelman, Lipton, et al., 2001), and are among the few direct head-to-head comparisons available so far in the literature (Oldman, L. A. Smith, McQuay, & Moore, 2002). Propranolol, but not other **beta-blockers**, increases the plasma concentration of rizatriptan by 70 percent. Thus, patients who are taking propranolol should not exceed 5 mg per day of rizatriptan (Dahlöf & Lines, 1999).

Almotriptan is notable for high bioavailability during and between migraine episodes, a low incidence of side effects, and an apparently low rate of headache recurrence (Pascual, 2001). Its efficacy seems similar to that of 100 mg sumatriptan (Pascual, 2001).

Frovatriptan has two unique properties, although their clinical import is uncertain. The first is an unusually long whole-blood half-life of c. 26 hours, versus 2–6 hours for other triptans (Comer, 2002). The long half-life, however, seems to be due in part to binding of frovatriptan to red blood cells (Buchan, Keywood, A. Wade, & C. Ward, 2002), which also seems to limit bioavailability. The second property is the relative specificity of its vasoconstrictive effects to the cerebral arteries. In particular, the effect of frovatriptan on coronary arteries seems to follow an inverted-U shaped function, with a lessening of vasoconstriction at the highest concentrations (Comer, 2002). In addition to the 5-HT$_{1B/D/F}$ agonism seen with other triptans, frovatriptan also causes modest stimulation of 5-HT$_7$ sites, which seem to dilate coronary arteries (Comer, 2002). Here, too, clinical relevance is uncertain, however: No triptan is appropriate when coronary artery disease is known or suspected.

Frovatriptan is water soluble and crosses the blood-brain barrier to only a small extent (Buchan, Keywood, et al., 2002). It seems to have few side effects or drug interactions (Buchan, A. Wade, C. Ward, S. D. Oliver, A. J. Stewart, Freestone, 2002; Géraud, Spierings, & Keywood, 2002).

Eletriptan has a steep dose-response curve (Rapoport & Tepper, 2001). This contrasts with sumatriptan for which, as we will see, there is relatively little difference in efficacy between the 50 mg and 100 mg oral doses. In theory, a steep curve should allow dosages to be individually tailored (Rapoport & Tepper, 2001). Eletriptan is also the most lipophilic of the triptans so far available (Rapoport & Tepper, 2001), but this does not seem to make a practical difference. Of much greater clinical relevance is this: Because it is metabolized by the liver's cytochrome P450–3A4 enzyme system, eletriptan cannot be used with drugs that inhibit this system. The primary contraindications are for certain antibiotics (such as erythromycin) and anti-fungal agents (such as ketoconazole). However, other substances inhibit the 3A4 enzymes as well, including the migraine preventives verapamil and nifedipine (Tepper, C. Allen, Sanders, A. Greene, & Boccuzzi, 2003), and herbs such as goldenseal, cat's claw, Echinacea, wild cherry, chamomile, St. John's wort, licorice,[2] soy, and soy isoflavones (Budzinski, B. C. Foster, Vandenhoek, & Arnason, 2000; B. C. Foster, et al., 2003). A fuller list of potential drug interactions is given in Table 11–1.

All of the triptans (except technically for almotriptan, eletriptan, and frovatriptan, which are too recent to have been rated yet) fall in the Consortium's Group 1 (proven, pronounced benefit; Silberstein, 2000). Evidence is still accumulating about whether any of these newer medications is better than the others or better than sumatriptan. We will examine some of this data next.

Comparing Triptans

Because triptan studies use the same diagnostic system, outcome criteria, and rating scales (Tfelt-Hansen, G. Block, et al., 2000), they are suitable grist for meta-analyses and quantitative reviews (Ferrari, Roon, Lipton, & Goadsby, 2001; Géraud, Keywood, & Senard, 2003). To date, three such reviews have been conducted, whose combined results are given in Figure 11–1 (Dahlöf, Dodick, Dowson, & Pascual, 2002; Ferrari, Goadsby, Roon, & Lipton, 2002; Oldman, L. A. Smith, McQuay, & Moore, 2002). There are fewer studies in which two triptans are compared directly, but the results generally replicate those of the meta-analyses (Ferrari, Roon, Lipton, & Goadsby, 2001).

Speed of onset.   Speed of onset has been defined as the proportion of treated migraine episodes for which pain declines from a moderate or severe level, to mild or none, by 1 hour. For this standard, the most important characteristic of a triptan is not its chemical structure, but how it is delivered. Subcutaneous injections of sumatriptan (6 mg) provide rapid pain relief in about 70 percent of attacks; the intranasal forms of sumatriptan (20 mg) and dihydroergotamine (2 mg) achieve this outcome c. 50 percent of the time. In contrast, oral triptans are less effective, with sumatriptan (50 and 100 mg), naratriptan (2.5 mg), and eletriptan (40 mg) all at around 30 percent, and zolmitriptan (2.5 and 5 mg) at around 40 percent. Among the oral formulations, rizatriptan (10 mg) has a numerical advantage, giving 1-hour pain relief in 43 percent of migraine episodes (Oldman, L. A. Smith, McQuay, & Moore, 2002).

Thoroughness of pain relief.   As we have defined it, a good outcome can be achieved simply by reducing moderate pain (2/3 in intensity) by one point, to mild pain (1/3). This is a somewhat tepid result, and not, of course, most patients' ideal (Lipton & Stewart, 1999; Massiou, Tzourio, el Amrani, & Bousser, 1997). An alternative is to seek the proportion of moderate or severe migraine attacks for which pain is reduced to 0/3 by 2 hours post-dose. By this stringent but reasonable criterion, none of the oral triptans fares well. Rizatriptan (10 mg) comes closest, with pain-free outcomes in 40 percent of attacks. Zolmitriptan (5 mg), low dose rizatriptan (5 mg), eletriptan (40 mg), and sumatriptan (100 mg) all give pain-free outcomes about 30 percent of the time, followed by low dose zolmitriptan (2.5 mg), 25 percent, and low-dose sumatriptan (50 mg) and naratriptan (2.5 mg) at around 20 percent of migraines. As in other short-term efficacy measures, subcutaneous sumatriptan (6 mg) outperforms the oral medications: It gives pain-free outcomes in about 60 percent of migraine episodes (Oldman, L. A. Smith, McQuay, & Moore, 2002).

---

[2]Licorice the herb. Licorice the candy is usually flavored with anise oil (Fetrow & Avila, 2001).

TABLE 11-1
A Guide to Triptan Medications

Triptan	Advantages	Disadvantages	Particular Uses	Contraindications and Interactions[a]
Almotriptan 12.5 mg	Low side effect rate, Low recurrence		Use with patients who have low acceptance of triptan side effects	
Eletriptan 40 mg	High response rate	Higher potential for drug interactions	Severe migraines	Cytochrome P450 3A4 inhibitors[b] (see below); Reduce dose in cases of renal impairment
Frovatriptan 2.5 mg	Low side effect rate, Low recurrence, Few drug interactions	Slow onset	Frequent migraines; Prevention of menstrual migraines	
Naratriptan 2.5 mg	Low side effect rate, Low recurrence	Slow onset, Lower efficacy for severe migraines	Frequent, mild-to-moderate episodic migraines; Prevention of menstrual migraines; Use with patients who have low acceptance of triptan side effects	
Rizatriptan 10 mg	Rapid onset, High initial efficacy, Consistent response	Recurrence	? When migraines are typically of short duration and relatively low frequency, or in situations where uninterrupted functioning is essential; severe migraines	MAO inhibitors; Reduce dose in cases of renal impairment, If taking propranolol, rizatriptan intake should not exceed 5 mg/day
Sumatriptan 100 mg	Much clinical experience	Recurrence	Severe migraines	MAO inhibitors, Hepatic impairment
Zolmitriptan 2.5 mg	Still effective when taken late in migraine	Higher rate of side effects; Some recurrence	Severe migraines	MAO inhibitors. Reduce dose in cases of hepatic impairment; Reduce 24-hour dose if patient is taking cimetidine. Contraindicated by Wolff-Parkinson-White syndrome.

Notes. [a]All triptans are contraindicated for patients with cardiovascular or cerebrovascular disease. Triptans should not be co-administered with each other or with ergotamine or dihydroergotamine. [b] Cytochrome P450 3A4: Eletriptan should not be co-prescribed with clarithromycin, erythromycin, indinavir, itraconazole, josamycin, ketoconazole, nelfinavir, and ritonavir. Other drugs that may interact with eletriptan by inhibiting the 3A4 enzyme system include bromocriptine, clotrimazole, cyclosporine, desmethylsertraline, dexamethasone, erythromycin, fluconazole, miconazole, navelbine, nicardipine, nifedipine, norfluoxetine, progesterone, quercetin, quinidine, saquinavir, verapamil, vinblastine, and vincristine. Ergotamine and dihydroergotamine also belong on this list, but should not be co-administered with any triptan (Tepper, C. Allen, Sanders, A. Greene, & Boccuzzi, 2003)

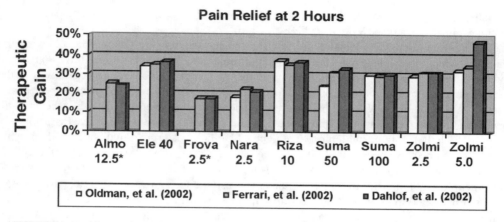

FIGURE 11–1.   Meta-analyses of comparative efficacy of triptans.

*Data on almotriptan and frovatriptan are not included in the meta-analysis by Oldman, et al.

Source: "How does Almotriptan Compare with Other Triptans? A Review of Data from Placebo-Controlled Trials," by C. G. H. Dahlöf, D. Dodick, A. J. Dowson, & J. Pascual, 2002, *Headache, 42*, pp. 99–113; "Oral Triptans (Serotonin 5-HT1B/1D Agonists) in Acute Migraine Treatment: A Meta-Analysis of 53 Trials," by M. D. Ferrari, K. I. Roon, R. B. Lipton, & P. J. Goadsby, 2001, *Lancet, 358*, pp. 1668–1675; and "Pharmacological Treatments for Acute Migraine: Quantitative Systematic Review," by A. D. Oldman, L. A. Smith, H. J. McQuay, and R. A. Moore, 2002, *Pain, 97*, pp. 247–257.

Recurrence.   Even when a triptan completely removes pain, the migraine may re-emerge, typically in about 12 hours (Géraud, Keywood, & Senard, 2003). Although a second dose can be taken, the headache can re-emerge yet again, and the risk of medication overuse is increased proportionately, particularly if the migraines are frequent (Visser, Jaspers, de Vriend, & Ferrari, 1996). Thus, minimizing recurrence has become a key goal in developing second-generation triptans.

At this point, headache recurrence is operationalized as the return of pain to a 2/3 (moderate) or 3/3 (severe) level, after having first been reduced to 1/3 (mild) or 0/3 (pain-free), within 24 hours of taking the medication. This has been a high enough bar for current medications. But as migraines can last for 72 hours, more stringent definitions of recurrence will be appropriate in the future (Tfelt-Hansen, G. Block, Dahlöf, et al., 2000).

In the data so far available, recurrence rates seem to vary between 40 percent for rizatriptan (10 mg), to around 33 percent for sumatriptan (oral, 100 mg) and zolmitriptan (2.5 mg), around 25 percent for almotriptan (12.5 mg), naratriptan (2.5 mg), and eletriptan (40 mg), to an average of 17 percent for frovatriptan (Géraud, Keywood, & Senard, 2003). Not surprisingly, the best predictor of sustained relief is a long half-life in the bloodstream; triptans whose half-lives are greater than three hours seem to fare noticeably better than the others (Géraud, Keywood, & Senard, 2003).[3] The second predictor seems to be magnitude of effect at the 5-HT$_{1B}$ receptor specifically. Binding and effectiveness at the 5-HT$_{1D}$ receptor appear unrelated to the probability of recurrence. This adds to the impression that vasoconstriction is necessary for a triptan to be clinically useful (Géraud, Keywood, & Senard, 2003). Conversely, recurrence after taking

---

[3]However, when sumatriptan is studied in depth, a given person's probability of headache recurrence does not depend on how rapidly they metabolize the drug (Visser et al., 1996). The reason for the discrepancy is not clear.

sumatriptan seems to be more frequent in people whose migraines, untreated, are severe or long-lasting (Visser, Jaspers, de Vriend, & Ferrari, 1996).

The commonsense explanation for recurrence, that triptans are temporarily blocking the migraine symptoms while leaving the underlying disorder unchanged, is supported by two types of evidence. In a positron emission tomography study, Weiller et al. showed ongoing activity in the "migraine generator" region of the brain stem even after successful treatment of an attack with suma-triptan (Weiller, et al., 1995). And patients report that before a recurrence, even when they are still pain-free, they can feel that the migraine is still present (Visser, Jaspers, de Vriend, & Ferrari, 1996).

On the balance, then, which product is best? Dodick has argued that actually there is no "best" triptan because people will differ in the mix of efficacy, speed of onset, tolerability, and freedom from headache recurrence that best suits them (Dodick, 2002a). And for unknown rea-sons, people seem to differ in which triptans they respond to. Thus, for example, patients who have not benefited in previous trials of sumatriptan may still have a high probability (c. 75–80 percent) of responding to zolmitriptan or rizatriptan (other triptans were not studied; N. T. Mathew, Kailasam, Gentry, & Chernyshev, 2000). Note that the authors are not referring to mixing triptans on the same day, a practice that is not currently recommended.

And there may be limits, in any event, to a rational choice among triptans. As Saper has noted, the variability in response among persons is greater than the variability in the literature among the molecules (Saper, 2001). For example, although frovatriptan has, on average, one of the slowest onsets, some patients' migraines resolve rapidly after taking it (Rapoport & Tepper, 2001). Thus, although rational analysis can give us a starting point, it still leaves a wide latitude for art, judgment, and trial-and-error (Saper, 2001).

Side Effects and Caveats

The primary side effects of the triptans, like those of ergotamine and DHE, are vasoconstrictive: They are contraindicated for people with heart disease, hypertension, or peripheral artery disease. Naturally, there has been considerable interest in developing triptan-like drugs that impede neu-rogenic inflammation without constricting arteries. So far, however, none of these drugs has been effective unless it has also been vasoconstrictive (Diener, Kaube, & Limmroth, 1998). For exam-ple, a trial of bosentan, which blocks neurogenic plasma extravasation into the dura mater, was stopped early because of a complete lack of efficacy (May, Gijsman, Wallnöfer, R. Jones, Diener, & Ferrari, 1996). On the other hand, an experimental 5-HT$_{1F}$ agonist, which is not vasoconstric-tive but which appears to block pain transmission in the trigeminal nucleus caudalis, has proven effective in preliminary human trials (D. J. Goldstein, et al., 2001).

Zolmitriptan, and perhaps other triptans, should be avoided in cases of Wolff-Parkinson-White syndrome, a congenital disorder involving abnormal EKG and heart arrhythmia (Rolan & G. R. Martin, 1998).

Subjective side effects for the triptans include tightness, numbness and tingling, especially in the chest, neck, or jaw, but apparently with no abnormalities on EKG; warmth, heaviness, or paresthesias elsewhere in the body; fatigue and somnolence; nausea, dizziness, or dry mouth (Rolan & G. R. Martin, 1998).

Zolmitriptan and rizatriptan do not appear to have been studied in pediatric migraine. Nara-triptan, like sumatriptan, has not proven effective for adolescents (Rothner, Edwards, Kerr, et al., 1997).

Although the triptans were developed to treat migraines, their success in resolving any given headache does not necessarily imply that the headache was a migraine. There is, of course, the ever-present possibility of placebo responding. Moreover, headaches from an organic cause, such as a tumor, may respond to sumatriptan, at least if the carotid artery is involved (Manfredi, Shenoy, & Payne, 2000).

Table 11–1 gives a summary of the triptans.

Other Acute Migraine Medications

Anti-emetics. As nausea is a common feature of migraines, it is not surprising that drugs to combat it would be included in acute migraine treatment, especially at emergency rooms. Emergency treatment may include injection of *metoclopramide* (Reglan, Maxolon), *prochlorperazine* (Compazine, Stemetil) or even *chlorpromazine* (Thorazine), whose effectiveness presumably traces to their being dopamine antagonists. Metoclopramide has also been used to enhance the effectiveness of oral anti-migraine drugs, by increasing gastric motility. Gastric motility is often low during migraine episodes (Welch, 1993). In fact, there is evidence that the anti-emetics are effective in relieving the migraine episode as a whole (Welch, 1993).

In the Consortium guidelines, intravenous prochlorperazine is in Group 1 (proven, pronounced benefit), while intravenous metoclopramide, intravenous chlorpromazine, and intramuscular or rectal prochlorperazine fall in Group 2 (moderate benefit). Intramuscular or rectal metoclopramide is in Group 3 (conflicting or inconsistent evidence; Silberstein, 2000). The most serious side effects, when they occur, are motoric: dystonia, especially in children, with metoclopramide, and risk of tardive dyskinesia with chlorpromazine and prochlorperazine.

Isometheptene compound (Midrin) consists of a sympathomimetic and smooth muscle relaxant (isometheptene), a mild sedative (dichloralphenazone), and an analgesic (acetaminophen). Isometheptene compound has been used as a migraine treatment for more than 50 years, with more recent studies continuing to support its efficacy (e.g., Behan, 1978). In the Consortium guidelines it falls in Group 2 (moderate benefit), primarily for mild or moderate headache (Silberstein, 2000). However, the reason that a sympathomimetic and smooth muscle relaxant would reduce migraines is not very clear. One recent study suggests that the isometheptene itself may constrict the external carotid arteries, via agonism at α_{2A} and α_{2C} adrenergic receptors (Willems, Valdivia, Saxena, & Villalón, 2001).

Nerve blocks and topical treatments. Injection of steroid and local anesthetic into the greater occipital nerve is a rational treatment strategy for headaches originating from certain types of neck pathology. In fact, however, the injections may also be effective for preventing cluster headaches (N. Mathew, 1997b) and migraines (Caputi & Firetto, 1997; Gawel & Rothbarth, 1992), although the latter finding has not always replicated (Bovim & Sand, 1992). How would a nerve block in the posterior cervical region help treat pain that appears to originate in the head itself? One explanation may be that the blockade reduces input to the trigeminal system, and hence helps to raise the threshold for a trigeminovascular response (N. Mathew, 1997b).

In fact, we may not need an occipital block to achieve this effect. In several studies, intranasal lidocaine has been an effective topical treatment for migraines and cluster headaches (Kittrelle, Grouse, & Seybold, 1985; Maizels, B. Scott, W. Cohen, W. Chen, 1996). Again, the active process may be a decrease in total input to the trigeminovascular system (N. Mathew, 1997b). Alternatively, intranasal lidocaine may work by lowering activity in the parasympathetic sphenopalatine ganglion, which is located above the nose (Edvinsson, 1991; Yarnitsky, Goor-Aryeh, et al., 2003). Recall that although parasympathetic fibers are not thought to have a primary role in migraines, they may contribute by dilating already inflamed blood vessels, and by sensitizing nearby sensory nerves. There is some evidence that intranasal lidocaine is particularly effective at reducing pain in migraines with prominent parasympathetic features (e.g., rhinorrhea, lacrimation, nasal congestion, or conjuctival injection; Yarnitsky, Goor-Aryeh, et al.). (Consortium Group 2: moderate benefit; Silberstein, 2000).

Analgesics.   Opioid analgesics raise pain thresholds, and correspondingly decrease pain intensity, by binding to receptors principally in the spine, medulla, and periaqueductal gray regions. There are three known types of opioid receptors. μ-opioid receptors are found chiefly in the brain, and are thought to mediate pain reduction, and such side effects as sedation, euphoria, respiratory depression, and a reduction in peristalsis (Markley, 1994). κ-opioid receptors are found primarily in the dorsal horn and are thought to mediate primarily analgesia and sedation (Markley, 1994). The function of δ-opioid receptors is uncertain. Opioid analgesics include *meperidine* (Demerol), *fentanyl* (Duragesic), *hydrocodone* (with acetaminophen: Vicodin), *oxycodone* (with acetaminophen: Percocet), and *propoxyphene* (with acetaminophen: Darvocet), as well as such long acting variants as *methadone*, MS Contin (a slow release formulation of morphine), and OxyContin (a slow release formulation of oxycodone).

Opioids, of course, are well known as drugs of abuse. Interestingly, however, patients who do not have a history of substance abuse (a potentially important caveat) appear to have almost no likelihood of developing a true addiction when treated with opioids for acute pain (Porter & Jick, 1980). That is, the patients develop a physical dependence, but are weaned off the medications successfully and virtually never become street addicts. People who abuse opioids may have an unusual vulnerability to the addiction, or there may be something in the context of pain that protects against addiction. Of course we may not know in practice whether a patient has a history of substance abuse.

There is at least one opioid designed to have low abuse potential: *Butorphanol* (Stadol) is a κ-opioid agonist and thus produces analgesia and sedation. However, it is also a μ-opioid antagonist, and thus produces dysphoria rather than euphoria. In fact, butorphanol can precipitate a withdrawal syndrome in people habituated to other opioids (Markley, 1994). The efficacy of the intranasal form is high enough to have earned it a Group 1 designation by the Consortium (proven, pronounced benefit; Silberstein, 2000). Despite this useful profile, there are three drawbacks to butorphanol. First, the abuse potential, although designed to be low (Markley, 1994), is by no means negligible. "Excessive administration, improper selection, and use for frequent headaches have led to numerous cases of physical and psychologic dependence" (Silberstein, Saper, & Freitag, 2001, p. 160). Second, butorphanol is sedating, and should not be used in situations where it would place patients at risk (Silberstein, 2000). Third, like all analgesics, the opioids are subject to overuse by patients and subsequent development of drug rebound headaches (Markley, 1994). Reports "from the field" suggest that patients may habituate to butorphanol and thus overuse it (G. Solomon, 1995).

Ibuprofen (Motrin), *naproxen* (Naprosyn, Anaprox, Aleve), *ketoprofen* (Orudis) and other nonsteroidal anti-inflammatory medications, are functionally related to aspirin. This class of medications blocks the cyclooxygenase enzymes and hence inhibits the production of prostaglandins, which play a role in inflammation and in sensitizing pain receptors. Moreover, there is some evidence that they act centrally, decreasing nociceptive transmission in the dorsal horn of the spinal cord (Kaube, Hoskin, & Goadsby, 1993; Vanegas & Schaible, 2001). When used for migraines, the nonsteroidals may function in part by impeding neurogenic inflammation, and in particular the release of calcitonin gene-related peptide (Goadsby & Edvinsson, 1991).

In the Consortium guidelines, ibuprofen and naproxen are in Group 1 (proven, pronounced benefit), while diclofenac potassium (Cataflam), intramuscular ketorolac (Toradol), and flurbiprofen (not approved in the United States) are in Group 2 (moderate benefit; Silberstein, 2000).

The nonsteroidals are generally recommended for migraines that are mild, moderate, or that have responded to similar treatment in the past. Still, ketoprofen, which was not rated when the Consortium guidelines were produced, has since been found to have the same efficacy as zolmitriptan in the acute treatment of migraine (Dib, Massiou, M. Weber, Henry, Garcia-Acosta, & Bousser, 2002).

Prostaglandins need only be present for a few minutes to cause a pain sensitization that lasts for hours. Thus, for migraines the medications may work best if taken very early in the headache (Welch, 1993).

Of course, the nonsteroidals can have significant gastrointestinal side effects, and a history of peptic ulcer or bleeding may contraindicate them.

Caffeine is a vasoconstrictive and it may improve the absorption of ergotamine (Sawynok, 1995). There is some evidence that caffeine by itself has analgesic properties for the pain from muscle ischemia (Myers, Shaikh, & Zullo, 1997) and nonvascular headaches (Ward, Whitney, Avery, et al., 1991). When added to acetaminophen, it appears to increase analgesic efficacy for tension-type headache (Migliardi, Armellino, Friedman, Gillings, & Beaver, 1994). In fact, Lipton, et al. note response rates in migraine to an aspirin, acetaminophen and caffeine combination that rival the rates seen for sumatriptan (Lipton, Stewart, Ryan, Saper, Silberstein, & Sheftell, 1998; Consortium grade 1: proven, pronounced benefit; Silberstein, 2000). Along with pain, phono-phobia, photophobia, nausea, and self-rated disability also improved. However, persons with vomiting or severe disability during migraines were excluded from the trials.

Butalbital a barbiturate, lowers neural activity by facilitating the binding of gamma-amino butyric acid, an inhibitory neurotransmitter, to GABA-A receptors. Butalbital may also impede the action of glutamate at AMPA-type receptors (Silberstein & McCrory, 2001). In the laboratory, butalbital seems to block nociceptive transmission through the trigeminal nucleus caudalis (Cutrer, Mitsikostas, Ayata, & Sanchez del Rio, 1999). In the clinic, however, short of producing uncon-sciousness, barbiturates seem to have little or no analgesic activity (Silberstein & McCrory, 2001). They might potentiate the action of opiates, however, and for headaches butalbital is generally combined with acetaminophen (Fioricet, Esgic), aspirin (Fiorinal), other non-steroidal anti-inflammatories (Optalidon), or aspirin plus codeine (Fiorinal with Codeine, Esgic Plus).

In Consortium guidelines, the combination of butalbital, aspirin and caffeine, with or with-out codeine, is accorded Group 2 status. Still, as a barbiturate with an elimination half-life of *61* hours, butalbital is not without risks. Acute overdose can cause death, daily use can bring tolerance, sometimes addiction, and abrupt withdrawal can provoke seizures (M. Raja, Altavista, Azzoni, & Albanese, 1996) and delirium tremens (Silberstein & McCrory, 2001). By far more common, however, is that use of butalbital more than 2–3 times per week is associated with rebound headaches, and transition from episodic migraine to daily headache.

Choosing an Acute Medication

Not surprisingly, patients' concern is generally for rapid, complete, and lasting relief of symptoms (Lipton & Stewart, 1999). This fits well with U.S. Consortium recommendations, to stratify care based on migraine severity and disability (Silberstein, 2000).

The reason for the recommendation is straightforward: In a large, multicenter study, only 43 percent of patients with mild disability responded to a combination of aspirin and metoclo-pramide for their migraines. The efficacy dropped even further for moderate (31 percent) and severe (26 percent) disability (Lipton, Stewart, A. M. Stone, Láinez, & J. P. C. Sawyer, 2000).

Thus, starting patients with migraine-related disability on a low intensity treatment, assessing whether it works and then switching to a triptan as necessary ("**stepped care**") in most cases simply postpones effective treatment (Lipton, Stewart, A. M. Stone, et al.[4]). Moreover, any economic advantage to minimizing use of triptans in migraine-disabled patients may be illusory. Stepped care allows greater ongoing disability (Lipton, Stewart, A. M. Stone, et al.), and may even involve higher direct costs due to frequent office visits and speciality consultations (P. Williams, Dowson, Rapoport, & J. Sawyer, 2001).

In patient surveys, route of administration is not so important, but all else being equal, traditional tablets and capsules are preferred over other routes, such as nasal spray or subcutaneous injection (Lipton & Stewart, 1999). Oral disintegrating tablets are a second choice, and perhaps a first choice if there is nausea, or if water is not usually available (Dodick, 2002b; Lipton & Stewart, 1999).

Finally, we should note three medications which have failed placebo-controlled trials in migraine: *acetaminophen*, intravenous (but not intranasal) *lidocaine*, and intravenous *granisetron* (Kytril, 5-HT$_3$ receptor antagonist; Silberstein, 2000).

MIGRAINE PROPHYLAXIS

Serotonin and Migraine Pharmacology

Thus, the triptans, the most specific of acute migraine medications, are defined by their effects on serotonin receptors. As we will see, this is equally true of most migraine prophylactics. Thus, to truly understand migraine pharmacology, we must first consider serotonin.

Serotonin, of course, is found in the central nervous system, especially the raphe nuclei of the midbrain. Through the brain stem nuclei, serotonin affects the functioning of several cortical and limbic systems (Nestler, Hyman, & Malenka, 2001). However, the vast majority of serotonin in the body is not located in the central nervous system at all, but peripherally, in such places as the skin, gastrointestinal tract, and blood platelets. Perhaps surprisingly, the most common serotonergic drugs, the tricyclics and the selective serotonin reuptake inhibitors (SSRI's), have little known anatomic or receptor subtype specificity. They simply block the serotonin reuptake mechanism, and this mechanism seems to be the same wherever serotonin is released. Thus, the SSRI's are "selective" only insofar as they affect serotonin levels specifically. In theory, they can act everywhere serotonin is found (Murphy, Andrews, Wichems, Q. Li, Tohda, & Greenberg, 1998). Given such widely dispersed activity, it seems remarkable that their side effect profile is as benign as it is.

Now, from the effectiveness of the triptans and the high comorbidity between migraine and major depression, we might be tempted to conclude that migraine is a serotonin deficiency state. Similarly, we saw in Chapter 5 evidence of reduced sensory habituation in migraine. This implies a deficit in inhibition, and thus in the inhibitory neurotransmitter, serotonin (W. Wang, Timsit-Berthier, & Schoenen, 1996).

Yet the situation is not so clear. Fenfluramine and reserpine, which release serotonin from presynaptic neurons, can bring about a migraine-like headache (Silberstein, 1998). Migraines, too, are produced by *m*-chlorophenylpiperazine (mCPP), a chemical which releases serotonin,

---

[4]Disclosure: Two of the authors of this study were employees of AstraZeneca, makers of the triptan to which aspirin and metoclopramide were compared.

blocks its reuptake, and directly stimulates 5-HT 1A, 2A and 2C receptors (Leone, Attanasio, Croci, Ferraris, et al., 1998). Conversely, chronic administration of reserpine depletes serotonin (along with dopamine and norepinephrine) and, naturally, causes depression. However, it also protects against migraines (Silberstein, 1998). And as we will see below, many of the migraine prophylactic medications are actually serotonin antagonists. Even the effectiveness of the triptans is ambiguous evidence, because the 5-HT$_{1D}$ receptor is inhibitory: It reduces net serotonergic transmission (Gonzalez-Heydrich & Peroutka, 1990).

How can this be? One explanation may lie in the timing of serotonin levels. A chronic deficiency may cause a sensitization of serotonin receptors. Then, triggers that release serotonin may produce an inordinate response, and give rise to the migraine itself (Hamel & Saxena, 2000).

A second explanation hinges on the exact serotonin receptor subtypes that are involved. Serotonin is used as a neurotransmitter throughout the animal kingdom, including in such primitive organisms as coelenterates (e.g., jellyfish), mollusks, and flatworms (D. L. Murphy, Andrews, Wichems, Q. Li, Tohda, & Greenberg, 1998). As species become more advanced, the serotonin molecule does not change, but the neuronal systems in which it is employed become more numerous and complex. Along with this increase in complexity, there is a differentiation of serotonin receptors into subtypes. Currently, there are seven known families of serotonin receptors: 5-HT$_1$ to 5-HT$_7$. Five of the families (5-HT$_1$, 5-HT$_2$, and 5-HT$_5$) are further divided into subtypes (e.g., 5-HT$_{1A}$) for a total of 15 receptor subtypes so far identified (D. L. Murphy et al.). The serotonin receptor subtypes thought to be relevant to migraine are shown in Table 11–2.

Much of the work on acute migraine drug development has focused on ever more precise determination of the relevant receptor subtypes, and ever more precisely targeted medications. Specifically, seven subtypes of serotonin receptor appear to be relevant to migraine. Two of the receptors clearly have anti-migraine effects. The role of these receptors has been delineated in the course of developing the triptans, the selective 5-HT$_{1B/1D}$ agonists, as migraine treatments. A third receptor, the 5-HT$_{1F}$ subtype, is being explored as a possible site for developing anti-migraine drugs that are not vasoconstrictive (D. J. Goldstein et al., 2001).

The role of three other receptor subtypes, 5-HT$_{2B}$, 5-HT$_{2C}$, and 5-HT$_7$ is more speculative, but may involve pro-migraine activity. The 5-HT$_{2B}$ and 5-HT$_7$ receptors have each been implicated in the vasodilation of cranial arteries (Terrón, 2002). 5-HT$_7$ receptors are found, too, on C fibers and in lamina I and II of the dorsal horn, where they seem to promote pain sensitivity (Rocha-González, Meneses, Carlton, & Granados-Soto, 2005). Similarly, 5-HT$_{2A}$ and 5-HT$_{2C}$ receptors, found widely in the central nervous system, may facilitate nociceptive transmission (Fozzard & Kalkman, 1994; Srikiatkhachorn, Suwattanasophon, Ruangpattanatawee, & Phansuwan-Pujito, 2002). Migraine prophylactics, including propranolol, methysergide, and cyproheptadine, seem to antagonize the 5-HT$_{2B}$ and 5-HT$_{2C}$ receptors (Fozard & Kalkman, 1994; G. R. Martin, 1997; Schmuck, Ullmer, Kalkman, Probst, & Lubbert, 1996), and perhaps also 5-HT$_7$ receptors (Terrón, 2002). Moreover, the higher a drug's affinity for these three receptors, the lower the dose needed to prevent migraines (Kalkman, 1994; Terrón, 2002). Conversely, beta-blockers that do not show activity at the 5-HT$_{2B}$ and 5-HT$_{2C}$ receptors do not prevent migraines.

Still, we cannot discount that the brain may use serotonin to interrupt the migraine process at an early stage (Nicolodi, Del Bianco, & Sicuteri, 1997). In this model, serotonin antagonists may help prevent migraines by producing a compensatory sensitization of serotonin receptors (Nicolodi, Del Bianco, & Sicuteri, 1997) or increasing the rate of serotonin synthesis (D. C. Chugani et al., 1999). The fact that the medications do not begin to show efficacy until several weeks have elapsed indeed seems to support some sort of compensatory process (Nicolodi, Del Bianco, & Sicuteri, 1997). And even without medication, the 5HT$_{1A}$ receptor seems to be hyper-

TABLE 11–2
Serotonin Receptor Subtypes of Potential Relevance to Migraines

5-HT Receptor Subtype	Location	Presumed Action	Representative Medication
5-HT$_{1A}$	Central	May increase nausea, reduce anxiety, and inhibit nociceptive firing in dorsal horn	Agonists: ergotamine, dihydroergotamine, buspirone, m-chlorophenyl-piperazine
5-HT$_{1B}$	Cerebral blood vessel walls; ? trigeminal nucleus caudalis	Vasoconstriction; ? blocks pain transmission	Agonists: Sumatriptan, Other Triptans
5-HT$_{1B}$[a]	Cerebral blood vessel endothelium	? Vasodilation	Agonists: Sumatriptan, Other Triptans
5-HT$_{1D}$	C fiber terminals; ? trigeminal nucleus caudalis	Prevents release of vasoactive peptides; ? blocks pain transmission	Agonists: Sumatriptan, Other Triptans
5-HT$_{1F}$	Trigeminal nucleus caudalis; substantia gelatinosa of spinal cord	? Blocks pain transmission in trigeminal nucleus	Agonists: Sumatriptan, Zolmitriptan, LY334370[b]
5-HT$_{2A}$	Unmyelinated sensory nerves; ? sympathetic nerve terminals; spine; frontal cortex	? Pro-nociceptive; ? Pro-inflammatory; ? Nitric oxide release	Agonists: D.O.I., m-chlorophenylpiperazine
5-HT$_{2B}$	Blood vessel endothelium	Possibly release of nitric oxide, causing vasodilation and facilitating sterile inflammation	Antagonists: Propranolol, Methysergide, Cyproheptadine
5-HT$_{2C}$	Widespread in central nervous system	Possibly activate cyclo-oxygenase pathways, increasing prostaglandin synthesis; ? pro-inflammatory, ? pro-nociceptive	Agonist: m-chlorophenyl-piperazine; Antagonists: Propranolol, Methysergide, Cyproheptadine
5-HT$_7$	Blood vessel endothelium; ? C fibers; ? Dorsal Horn	? Vasodilation; ? Pro-nociceptive	Agonists: Frovatriptan; Antagonists: Methysergide, Cyproheptadine, Ritanserin, SB–269970[c]

Notes. [a]Note that the 5-HT$_{1B}$ receptor subtype seems to have different actions depending on where it is located. [b]LY334370 is an experimental serotonin agonist that is highly selective for the 5-HT$_{1F}$ receptor subtype (D. J. Goldstein, et al., 2001). [c]SB–269970 is an experimental antagonist of 5-HT$_7$ receptors (Rocha-González, et al.).
Sources of information: Cassidy, E. Tomkins, Dinan, Hardiman, & O'Keane (2003); Comer (2002); Goldstein, Roon, Offen, Ramadan, Phebus, Johnson, Schaus, & M. D. Ferrari, (2001); Hargreaves & Shepheard (1999); P. Li & Zhuo (1998); G. R. Martin (1997); Rocha-González, et al. (2005); Silberstein, Saper, & Freitag (2001); Srikiatkhachorn, Suwattanasophon, Ruangpattanatawee, & Phansuwan-Pujito (2002); Terrón (2002).

sensitive in migraineurs (E. M. Cassidy, E. Tomkins, Dinan, Hardiman, & O'Keane, 2003; Leone, Attanasio, Croci, Ferraris, et al., 1998). This receptor has anti-anxiety and anti-nociceptive effects, much as we would expect if the brain were using serotonin as an antidote.

In all, then, it is unclear whether simply increasing serotonin activity will be beneficial in migraine. Depending on where the serotonin is acting, it might either increase or decrease the probability of a migraine.

PREVENTIVE MEDICATIONS

Although the advances in acute migraine drugs are impressive, there are times when the treatments fail us. They are contraindicated by coronary artery disease. Their safe use during pregnancy is yet unproven. Their regular use more than two days per week risks transition to chronic daily headache. And when migraines occur more than twice per month, cause disability more than three days per month, or are potentially dangerous (basilar and hemiplegic migraine, migrainous infarction) waiting for the next attack is unreasonable. In all of these cases, preventive treatment should be instituted (Silberstein & Freitag, 2003; V. Snow, K. Weiss, E. M. Wall, & Mottur-Pilson, 2002). And here, unfortunately, the pharmacological advances have been less impressive.

Here, too, we will take note of the evidence-based guidelines from the U.S. Headache Consortium. The category definitions differ somewhat from those for acute medications, but the general thrust is the same: decreasing evidence for efficacy as one moves from Group 1 to Group 5 (Ramadan, Silberstein, Freitag, T. T. Gilbert, & Frishberg, nd; Silberstein, 2000.)

U.S. Headache Consortium Groups for Migraine Preventives

Group 1: Medium to high efficacy, good strength of evidence, and a range of severity (mild to moderate) and frequency (infrequent to frequent) of side effects;

Group 2: Lower efficacy than those listed in Group 1, or limited strength of evidence, and mild to moderate side effects;

Group 3: Clinically efficacious based on consensus and clinical experience, but no scientific evidence of efficacy;

Group 4: Medium to high efficacy, good strength of evidence, but with side effect concerns;

Group 5: Evidence indicating no efficacy over placebo.

A summary of migraine preventives is given in Table 11–3.

Beta-Blockers

Propranolol (Inderal), a beta-adrenergic antagonist, can reduce migraine activity by about 45 percent (K. A. Holroyd & Penzien, 1990; K. A. Holroyd, Penzien, & Cordingley, 1991). There is evidence that this efficacy can be increased (Mathew, 1981), and perhaps almost doubled (K. A. Holroyd, France, Cordingley, Rokicki, Kvall, Lipchik, & McCool, 1995), by combining propranolol with thermal biofeedback. Other beta-blockers are probably effective as well (Welch, 1993). Besides propranolol, *metoprolol* is well supported (Diener, Kaube, & Limmroth, 1998), and there is similarly evidence for *timolol, nadolol,* and *atenolol* (K. E. Andersson & Vinge, 1990). In Consortium guidelines, propranolol and timolol fall in Group 1, and atenolol, metoprolol, and nadolol fall in Group 2; Silberstein & Freitag, 2003).

At this point, the mechanism by which beta-blockers work in migraine prophylaxis is entirely unknown. They may stabilize autonomic function (Zigelman, et al., 1992). Alternatively, their effectiveness may derive from antagonizing beta-adrenergic sites in the locus coeruleus (Hargreaves & Shepheard, 1999), which is in the putative migraine generator region of the midbrain. Similarly, beta-blockers appear to help normalize the interictal contingent negative variation (Schoenen, 1986) and intensity dependence of the auditory evoked potential (Sándor, Áfra, Ambrosini, & Schoenen, 2000). This would be consistent with the theory that beta-blockers

TABLE 11-3
Preventive Medications for Migraine

Medication	FDA	Group[a]	Final Dosage[b]	Advantages	Disadvantages	Side Effects	Contraindications and Interactions
Propranolol	Y	1	80–240 mg/day			Fatigue, Depression, Reduced Exercise Tolerance, Sleep Disturbance	Contraindicated by depression, diabetes mellitus, and asthma. Lower dose with concomitant fluvoxamine, fluoxetine or paroxetine
Timolol	Y	1	20–30 mg/day				Lower dose with concomitant fluoxetine or paroxetine
Divalproex Sodium	Y	1	500–1500 mg/day			Nausea, Alopecia, Tremor, Weight Gain, Menstrual Disorders, Polycystic Ovaries	Contraindicated by pregnancy, hepatic disease
Gabapentin	N	2	1200–2400 mg/day	Few drug interactions		Somnolence, Dizziness, Asthenia	
Topiramate	Y	3	100 mg/day (or lower, if limited by side effects); tritrate by 25 mg/day/week; to discontinue, decrease dose by 50 mg every 3 days	Efficacy in transformed migraine, migraine with clinical depression, and migraine for which other preventives have failed	Limited experience, Modest efficacy, Frequent side effects	Paresthesias (25–68%), Cognitive difficulties (4–15%), Dizziness (<2–4%), Nausea (<2–4%), Weight loss (M = 1.2–1.4 lbs/month)	History of kidney stones
Amitriptyline	N	1	30–150 mg/day	Useful in patients with mixed migraine and tension-type headaches	Frequent side effects	Weight gain, dry mouth, blurred vision, mental clouding, constipation, nausea, urinary retention, reflex tachycardia	Contraindicated in heart arrhythmia, heart block, recent MI, and severe liver disease. Caution advised in cardio-vascular disease, glaucoma, elevated intraocular pressure, impaired liver function, urinary retention, and constipation.

Drug	FDA	Group[a]	Dosage[b]	Advantages	Disadvantages	Side Effects	Contraindications/Comments
Flunarizine	N	4	5–10 mg/day	Wide use outside U.S.	Side effects, Not available in U.S.	Sedation, Weight Gain, Abdominal Pain, Depression, Occasional Extrapyramidal Syndromes	Extrapyramidal symptoms more common in elderly; Depression may be more common in the elderly and in those with a history of depression
Nimodipine	N	2	40 mg tid		Side effects, Uncertain efficacy	Constipation, Fatigue, Peripheral Edema, Postural Hypotension	
Verapamil	N	2	160–640 mg/day	Efficacy in patients with prolonged or atypical aura	Limited data, Frequent side effects	Constipation, Fatigue, Peripheral Edema, Postural Hypotension	Blood levels increased markedly by grapefruit juice
Cyproheptadine	N	3	2 mg bid		Limited data	Fatigue, Weight Gain	Should not be used with MAO inhibitors.
Methysergide	Y	4	2–8 mg/day	Effective for short-term use in episodic cluster headache and menstrual migraine	Risk of severe side effects if used continuously for greater than 6 months	Cardiac, pulmonary, and retroperitoneal fibrosis; nausea, vomiting, abdominal pain, diarrhea, leg pain, restlessness, dizziness, weight gain, peripheral edema, peripheral artery insufficiency, vasospasm	Not for long-term (>6 month) use. Contraindicated in pregnancy, peptic ulcers, peripheral vascular disorders, coronary artery disease, severe hypertension, severe arteriosclerosis, collagen disease, fibrotic disorders, lung diseases, liver or renal impairment, valvular heart disease, leg cellulitis or thrombophlebitis, severe infection or debilitation
Pizotifen	N	4	1.5 mg/day	Wide use in Britain	Side effects, Not available in U.S.	Weight gain, increased appetite, sedation	
Candesartan	N	—	16 mg/day	Few side effects or drug interactions	Little studied for migraine	? dizziness	Contraindicated by renal artery stenosis, diffuse intrarenal vascular stenosis, pregnancy, or breastfeeding.

Notes. FDA: U. S. Food and Drug Administration-approved for preventive treatment of migraine. [a]Group: Efficacy rating in the U. S. Headache Consortium Guidelines (see text for key). [b]Dosage: U.S. Consortium guidelines recommend starting any preventive at the lowest effective dose and gradually increasing until therapeutic benefit is achieved. Some medications require divided doses.

decrease neural excitability (Sándor, Áfra, Ambrosini, & Schoenen, 2000). Moreover, the reduction in migraines correlates positively with improvements in the CNV and in the auditory evoked potential (Sándor, Áfra, Ambrosini, & Schoenen, 2000; Schoenen, 1986).

Note, however, that some beta-blockers, such as pindolol, alprenolol, acebutolol, and oxprenolol, are ineffective or only marginally effective in preventing migraines (e.g., Ekbom, 1975; Ekbom & Zetterman, 1977; Nanda, R. H. Johnson, J. Gray, H. J. Keogh, & Melville, 1978). The reason is uncertain, but it is striking that while these agents block beta-adrenergic sites, they also have sympathomimetic activity (Limmroth & Michel, 2001). Other investigators have focused on the fact that beta-blockers tend to be broad spectrum, and to antagonize serotonin as well as beta adrenergic sites. In fact, as we will see below, other serotonin antagonists, *methysergide* (Sansert), and the antihistamines *cyproheptadine* (Periactin), and *pizotyline* can also prevent migraines.

Now we would not be surprised that a medication that antagonizes serotonin receptors could cause or worsen depression, and indeed this appears to be true of methysergide and the beta-blockers. The prophylactic efficacy of beta-blockers in children appears to be low, although occasional studies have found more positive results. Side effects of propranolol (fatigue, depression, sleep disruption, and reduced exercise tolerance) are so similar to the experience of fibromyalgia, that we might question the medication's usefulness when the conditions co-occur. More certainly, beta-blockers are not recommended when asthma, emphysema, or other diseases involving bronchospasm are present. Because they can reduce cerebral vasodilation, beta-blockers are often avoided in basilar migraine, presumably hemiplegic migraine, and migraine with prolonged aura (Garcia-Monco & Mateo, 2005). The antidepressant fluvoxamine (Luvox) may increase plasma levels of propranolol, and the levels of all beta-blockers may be raised by fluoxetine (Prozac) and paroxetine (Paxil), because these SSRI's inhibit the liver's cytochrome P450–2D6 enzyme system. Lower doses of the beta-blocker, 10–50 percent of normal, may be appropriate (Brøsen, 1998). Among herbal remedies, saw palmetto (serenoa repens) is a strong 2D6 inhibitor (Yale & Glurich, 2005).

Serotonin Antagonists

We have seen that the 5-HT 2B and 2C receptors, perhaps in the dorsal raphe nucleus, near the locus coeruleus, or in dural blood vessels, may contribute to the onset of migraines. So, too, may the 5-HT 2A receptors, on the sensory nerves, spine, and frontal cortex, and the 5-HT 7 receptors on the blood vessel endothelium. If so, then blocking serotonergic activity may help in migraine prophylaxis.

Regardless, there is a broad class of migraine prophylactics that seem to work in proportion to their antagonism of 5-HT 2B and 2C sites (Kalkman, 1994). This class includes *methysergide*, *cyproheptadine*, *pizotifen/pizotyline*, and *mianserin*, of which only the first two are available in the United States.

As with all migraine prophylactics, the exact mechanism remains controversial. For example, even though methysergide unquestionably antagonizes 5-HT$_2$ receptors, it is also, like the triptans, an agonist at 5-HT$_{1B}$ and perhaps 5-HT$_{1D}$ sites (Tfelt-Hansen & Saxena, 2000). Tfelt-Hansen & Saxena suggest that it is the resulting chronic constriction of arteries in the carotid bed that is the real reason methysergide is useful in migraine prophylaxis. This, at least, could explain why methysergide seems to potentiate the therapeutic effect of ergotamine (Silberstein, 1998). Thus as we have seen before, the pendulum sways, from the neurogenic to the vascular, and back again.

Methysergide is particularly notable, because the medication has no known analgesic properties, and in fact seems to block descending pain inhibitory pathways (Kharkevich & Churukanov, 1999) and the analgesic effects of acupuncture (Shimizu, Koja, et al., 1981). Nonetheless, the efficacy of methysergide as a migraine preventive has been well established in eleven double-blind, controlled trials (Silberstein, 1998). Six of the trials involved a placebo group, and generally support the use of methysergide. Seven of the trials involve a comparison drug, either with or without a placebo condition. Unfortunately, small sample sizes and unequal drop-out rates sometimes make the drug-drug comparison trials difficult to interpret. However, two studies seem to have good internal validity. In the first, involving parallel groups ($N = 104$ to 78, over the 6-month investigation), methysergide and flunarizine produced a 66 percent and 68 percent reduction in migraine frequency, respectively (Steardo, Marano, Barone, Denman, Monteleone, & Cardone, 1986). In the second, a cross-over study with 49 evaluable patients, methysergide and pizotifen reduced migraine frequency by 26 percent and 39 percent, respectively (P. G. Andersson, 1973).

A caveat in the placebo-controlled trials is that side effects such as nausea and lightheadedness make the actual extent of blinding uncertain (Gaudet & Kessler, 1987). Still, the rough equivalence to flunarizine and pizotifen, the lack of efficacy for tension-type headache, and the existence of plausible mechanisms, all suggest that methysergide is, truly, a migraine preventive.

Methysergide can also cause a medically dangerous complication, **retroperitoneal** fibrosis (formation of scar tissue in the abdomen), and for this reason it is rarely used (G. Solomon, 1995). In the Consortium guidelines, concerns for its side effects led to a Group 4 designation.

Cyproheptadine (Periactin), an antihistamine with antiserotonergic properties, has been regarded as a migraine prophylactic since the early 1960's, when incidental benefit for migraine was found in people being treated for allergies (J. Miller & Fishman, 1961). Formal studies have been surprisingly rare, however, and cyproheptadine achieves no more than a Group 3 listing in the Consortium Guidelines (Silberstein & Freitag, 2003). Still, a recent investigation was supportive: Rao and colleagues compare propranolol 40 mg bid, cyproheptadine 2 mg bid, propranolol plus cyproheptadine, and placebo, in parallel-group, double-blind design. The sample size is impressive (204 evaluable participants), although the study is limited by the somewhat low propranolol dose, and a retrospective outcome measure. Still, Rao et al. found that cyproheptadine, as a single drug or combined with propranolol, outperformed monotherapy with propranolol. All drugs outperformed placebo. Moreover, after the three month intervention ended, only 15 percent of patients went on to relapse by one-year follow-up (Rao, Das, Taraknath, & Sarma, 2000).

As an antihistamine, cyproheptadine is generally used specifically in children (G. Solomon, 1995). Its main side effects are fatigue, increased appetite, and weight gain.

Pizotifen resembles cyproheptadine structurally, and like cyproheptadine it is an antihistamine and anti-serotonergic (Lance, Anthony, & Somerville, 1970). Modest reductions in migraine frequency have been reported with it (Tfelt-Hansen & Saxena, 2000). It is not available in the United States. Weight gain, sedation, and an often high patient dropout rate in clinical trials led to Consortium Group 4 status for pizotifen.

In contrast to the older anti-serotonergic drugs, which are rather broad spectrum, newer compounds, developed for other purposes, are relatively selective for the various types of $5-HT_2$ receptors. Among these, *nefazodone* (Serzone, an antidepressant) has been studied in migraine and will be discussed below. *Olanzapine* (Zyprexa) blocks the $5-HT_{2A}$ and $5-HT_{2C}$ receptors, exactly the sites most strongly stimulated by the migraine-inducing mCPP. As an atypical antipsychotic with potentially severe side effects, it seems unlikely that olanzapine will become a mainstay migraine prophylactic. However, as we will see below, it has been used clinically with benefit for treatment-refractory chronic daily headache (Silberstein, Peres, Hopkins, Shechter, W. B. Young, & Rozen, 2002). On the other hand, headache is a frequent side effect when olanzapine is used in schizophrenia (e.g., 8.5 percent of patients: Costa e Silva, et al., 2001). Further data should help shed light on this compound, and on the role of $5-HT_2$ receptors.

All of the 5-HT$_{2B/2C}$ antagonists facilitate weight gain, by stimulating appetite, and by reducing the metabolism of brown adipose tissue (Silberstein, 1998). Presumably, this is true of the broad-spectrum anti-serotonergics as well. In one study, for example, 26 of 39 patients gained weight during a 12 week trial of pizotifen. The mean weight gain for these 26 patients was 11 lbs, and only 10 had returned to their original weight 4 months after the trial (Cleland, Barnes, Elrington, Loizou, & Rawes, 1997).

Calcium Channel Blockers

Calcium channel blockers have been studied due to their ability to inhibit smooth muscle contraction. That is, the medications could be useful in migraine prophylaxis in the same way that they are useful for preventing episodes of Raynaud's Disease and angina.

The main example of this effect is flunarizine (Sibellium), a calcium channel blocker with an exceptionally long half-life. In both meta-analyses (K. A. Holroyd, Penzien, Rokicki, & Cordingley, 1992) and head-to-head comparisons (Gawal, Kreeft, Nelson, Simard, & Arnott, 1992; Ludin, 1989; Lücking, Oestreich, R. Schmidt, & Soyka, 1988), flunarizine has been shown to have approximately the same efficacy as propranolol. In controlled trials, migraine frequency is about 42 percent lower on flunarizine than on placbo (Toda & Tfelt-Hansen, 2000). When the drug is discontinued, migraine frequency typically returns to baseline values over 7–9 months (Nuti, Lucetti, Pavese, Dell'Agnello, G. Rossi, & Bonuccelli, 1996).

People who have migraine without aura may, between migraine episodes, show a greater-than-normal increase in blood flow velocity of the middle cerebral artery during high blood carbon dioxide caused by breath-holding. Over three months of treatment, flunarizine reduces both the abnormal cerebrovascular reactivity and the number of migraines (Dora, Balkan, & Tercan, 2003). This is consistent with the vascular theory of migraine, of course, but we do not know if these two effects of flunarizine are causally linked. For flunarizine also possesses antihistamine, anticonvulsant (B. Holmes, Brogden, Heel, Speight, & Avery, 1984), anti-platelet (Steardo, Marano, Barone, Denman, Monteleone, & Cardone, 1986), and anti-dopaminergic properties (Belforte, Magariños-Azcone, Armando, Buño, & Pazo, 2001), any of which could account for its efficacy.

Side effects of flunarizine can include weight gain, sedation, major depression (particularly in those with a history of depression) and, uncommonly, extrapyramidal syndromes (Diener, 2000). Thus, the Consortium guidelines place flunarizine in Group 4 (Silberstein & Freitag, 2003), and the drug is not available in the United States. This assessment does not seem to be shared internationally, however, and in Europe flunarizine, not propranolol, is the front-line migraine prophylactic (Limmroth & Michel, 2001).

Surprisingly, other examples are hard to find. *Verapamil* (Calan) outperformed placebo in two small trials, but the internal validity was compromised by a high drop-out rate (Markley, Cheronis, & Piepho, 1984; Solomon, Steel, & Spaccavento, 1983). Potential side effects include constipation and, less commonly, dizziness, flushing, edema, hypotension, nausea, and headache (Silberstein, Saper, & Freitag, 2001). Depression can also be triggered, presumably by verapamil's broad-spectrum effects. Verapamil falls in Group 2 of the Consortium guidelines, reflecting the limited evidence. Case studies have supported its efficacy in at least some cases of hemiplegic migraine, a rare disorder in which the aura includes weakness or even paralysis on one side of the body. Both familial cases (in which there is an **autosomal dominant** inheritance pattern) and sporadic cases (without family history) have been helped (W. Yu & S. H. Horowitz, 2003).

Trials of *nifedipine* (Procardia) have suffered from low statistical power (Ramadan, Silberstein, Freitag, Gilbert, & Frishberg, nd), but so far it has not demonstrated efficacy (Diener,

Kaube, & Limmroth, 1998). Not surprisingly, then, it falls in Group 5 of the Consortium guidelines (evidence indicating no efficacy over placebo; Silberstein & Freitag, 2003). For *nimodipine* (Nimotop; Consortium Group 2) promising initial results (Gelmers, 1983; Havanka-Kanniainen, Hokkanen, & Myllylä, 1985), gave way to a series of trials in which the drug failed to outperform a placebo (Ansell, et al., 1988; Migraine-Nimodipine European Study Group, 1989a; Migraine-Nimodipine European Study Group, 1989b).

Antidepressants

Amitriptyline (Elavil) is accorded Group 1 status in the Headache Consortium guidelines. A tricyclic antidepressant, it is best known as a serotonin- and norepinephrine-reuptake inhibitor. Both of these neurotransmitters are important in descending pain control, but whether they are behind the preventive effects of amitriptyline is quite unknown. For example, amitriptyline has analgesic effects that are uncorrelated with mood elevation, in non-depressed patients, and at dosages lower than those generally used for depression (Bryson & Wilde, 1996). The medication directly antagonizes muscarinic-type acetylcholine receptors, H_1 histamine receptors, and α_1 adrenoreceptors (Bryson & Wilde, 1996). The resulting sedation might contribute to pain reduction (Onghena & Van Houdenhove, 1992). Activated sodium channels are blocked by amitriptyline (Bryson & Wilde, 1996), much as they are by local anesthetics (Sudoh, Cahoon, Gerner, & G. K. Wang, 2003). And amitriptyline antagonizes the NMDA-type glutamate receptors that are likely to be involved in the development of hyperalgesia (Watanabe, Saito, & Abe, 1993). There is evidence that amitriptyline, given early enough, can prevent post-herpetic neuralgia (a burning pain that develops as a long-term consequence of shingles, particularly in the elderly; Bowsher, 1997). Whether the drug can also prevent transformation of migraine or tension-type headache into chronic daily headache, however, does not seem to have been investigated in prospective trials.

Gomersall and Stuart have reported a small, double-blind crossover study, in which twenty subjects faithfully recorded their migraines for 18 *months*. In all, the number of migraine attacks was 42 percent lower on amitriptyline than it was on placebo (Gomersall & A. Stuart, 1973). Similarly, Couch and Hassanein (1979) found that a 4-week trial of amitriptyline brought at least 50 percent improvement (by retrospective, headache index measure) to 55 percent of patients, versus 34 percent of those receiving a placebo. Conversely, 20 percent of the amitriptyline group, versus 42 percent of the placebo group, reported worsening during the trial. This shift in distribution was statistically significant. And while, as has sometimes been noted, the drop-out rate was high (38 percent), nearly all of the attrition took place during the placebo run-in stage, prior to treatment.

In a head-to-head comparison, amitriptyline was as effective as propranolol in migraine prevention (D. K. Ziegler, Hurwitz, Hassanein, Kodanaz, Preskorn, & J. Mason, 1987). However, the two medications may perhaps be effective for different subsets of patients. Amitriptyline is standard therapy for chronic tension-type headache (Schoenen, 2000). In migraine, there is some evidence that it is effective in migraineurs who also have frequent tension-type headaches, while propranolol may be preferable in patients who have only migraines (N. T. Mathew, 1981).

Because of its broad spectrum of action, amitriptyline carries a raft of side effects, including dry mouth, sedation, nausea, constipation, urinary retention, and weight gain. Naturally, then, it may not be a good choice in patients who already have urinary retention, benign prostatic hyperplasia, or constipation, and caution is also indicated for people who have narrow angle glaucoma, increased intraocular pressure, impaired liver function, or cardiovascular disease. It is contraindicated altogether in patients with heart arrhythmias, heart block, severe liver disease, or who have recently had a heart attack (Bryson & Wilde, 1996).

We might expect that other tricyclics would work just as well as amitriptyline for migraine prophylaxis, but there is relatively little data. We could make a case for nortriptyline (Pamelor; Allegron), which is the primary metabolite of amitriptyline, or for doxepin (Sinequan), which seems to have analgesic properties (Onghena & Van Houdenhove, 1992). Both are in Group 3 (efficacy based on clinical experience only) in the guidelines. On the other hand, imipramine (also Group 3) has not performed as well in animal models of pain (Bryson & Wilde, 1996), and it seems to have little efficacy in migraine (Mylecharane & Tfelt-Hansen, 2000), despite its similar effects on **monoamine** reuptake.

Selective serotonin reuptake inhibitors (SSRI's). After several weeks of treatment, SSRI's may down-regulate the sensitivity of 5-HT$_{2B/2C}$ receptors, providing a possible mechanism for migraine prophylaxis (Kennett, et al., 1994). As a class, however, the drugs have performed inconsistently (Tomkins, Jackson, O'Malley, Balden, & Santoro, 2001). Part of the variance seems to depend on which medication is being considered. Femoxetine has failed (Orholm, Honore, & Zeeberg, 1986; Zeeberg, Orholm, J. D. Nielsen, Honore, & J. J. V. Larsen, 1981), and fluoxetine (Prozac) has passed (Adly, Straumarus, & Chesson, 1992; Saper, Silberstein, Lake, & Winters, 1994), double-blind trials. Fluoxetine (Prozac) has achieved Group 2 status in the Consortium guidelines, while several related drugs—fluvoxamine (Luvox), paroxetine (Paxil), and sertraline (Zoloft)—lacking in controlled studies, have been placed in Group 3 due to favorable clinical experience (Silberstein & Freitag, 2003).

Adding to the variance are occasional case reports of migraines that were initiated or worsened by these same agents: fluoxetine, fluvoxamine, paroxetine, or sertraline (Delva, Horgan, & Hawken, 2000; Larson, 1993; Szabo, 1995). Recall that serontonin seems to play a role in both migraine initiation and inhibition. A sensitization process seems to be involved, as the migraines may not appear until six months after the medication was first prescribed (Delva, et al.). Despite the delay, an association is suggested because the migraines resolve when the medication is withdrawn. And SSRI-induced migraines may be unusual, in that they do not seem to respond to triptans (Delva, et al.; Szabo, 1995). Note that in rebound headaches from ergots, triptans, or analgesics, it is the preventive and not acute treatments that lose efficacy. Thus, if a patient who has been started on an SSRI within the last six months reports that a previously effective triptan is no longer working, we might suspect the SSRI or, of course, other newly emergent process.

Possibly, SSRI-induced migraines may be attenuated by valproate, when depression refractory to other agents requires that we continue the SSRI (Delva, Horgan, & Hawken, 2000).

As another source of variance, fluoxetine, fluvoxamine, and paroxetine inhibit the liver's cytochrome P450–2D6 enzymes, preventing the biotransformation of codeine into morphine. Because codeine creates essentially no analgesia itself—it is simply a "prodrug," or precursor, to morphine—these three SSRI's can completely block its efficacy (Brøsen, 1998; C. M. Thompson, Wojno, Greiner, E. L. May, Rice, & Selley, 2004).

Newer antidepressants. In a small, double-blind cross-over study in children, trazodone (Desyrel[5]) at 1 mg per kg, outperformed placebo in reducing migraine frequency and duration (Battistella, Ruffilli, et al., 1993). However, the differential performance was found only in the second study period; the two interventions, trazodone and placebo, were equivalent during the first treatment period of the crossover study. Now, the first period might be less reliable because of stronger placebo effects or regression to the mean. Then again, we could speculate that tra-

---

[5]Not to be confused with Deseril, the trade name for methysergide overseas.

zodone withdrawal increased migraines, reducing the placebo response in the second period. In any event, the favorable results for trazodone should be regarded as quite preliminary. (Consortium Group 3; efficacy based on clinical experience.)

Unlike amitriptyline, trazodone is of doubtful efficacy as an analgesic (M. E. Lynch, 2001; Onghena & van Houdenhove, 1992). Moreover, there is a single case report of trazodone having initiated migraines (Workman, Tellian, & Short, 1992). A connection would not be surprising, as trazodone's primary metabolite is m-chlorophenylpiperazine (mCPP), which is known to produce migraines and migraine prodromes in certain individuals (Leone, Attanasio, Croci, Filippini, et al., 2000; Silberstein, 1998).

MCPP is also a minor metabolic byproduct of *nefazodone* (Serzone; Rothman & Baumann, 2002), but there is no evidence so far that this is clinically important in migraineurs. In fact nefazodone, in addition to mild serotonin reuptake inhibition, provides potent, selective 5-HT_{2A} receptor antagonism and 5-HT_{2A} down-regulation (DeVane, 1998). We saw above that sensitization of the 5-HT_{2A} receptor may confer a vulnerability to migraines, and thus nefazodone could be a useful prophylactic on rational grounds. So far, we have only an open-label study on chronic daily, primarily migrainous, headaches. The results were promising, and were particularly strong in patients with comorbid depression (Saper, Lake, & Tepper, 2001). However, firm conclusions await controlled investigations.

Venlafaxine (Effexor) inhibits the reuptake of both serotonin and norepinephrine. Perhaps, then, it could turn out to have the same efficacy in headache as amitriptyline, but without the anti-cholinergic and -histaminic side effects (L. C. Adelman, J. U. Adelman, Von Seggern, & Mannix, 2000). Moreover, in theory venlafaxine could reduce pain because of its close structural resemblance to the analgesic tramadol (Ultram; Markowitz & Patrick, 1998). Studies, however, have been sparse. A retrospective, open-label investigation essentially conveys clinical experience, that venlafaxine is sometimes useful in the prophylaxis of migraine and tension-type headache (L. C. Adelman, et al.), and in a small crossover study, similar efficacy to amitriptyline has been reported (Bulut, Berilgen, Baran, Tekatas, Atmaca, & Mungen, 2004; Consortium Group 3).

Duloxetine (Cymbalta), too, inhibits the reuptake of serotonin and norepinephrine, but in roughly equal ratio, unlike venlafaxine, whose effect is stronger at the serotonin transporter (Rabasseda, 2004). Duloxetine has shown some efficacy in fibromyalgia (Arnold, et al., 2004), diabetic **neuropathy** (Wernicke, Y. Lu, D'Souza, Waninger, & Tran, 2004), and global ratings of physical pain in major depressive disorder (D. J. Goldstein, Y. Lu, Detke, C. Wiltse, Mallinckrodt, & Demitrack, 2004), but has not yet been studied in primary headache specifically. Side effects include nausea, dry mouth, fatigue, dizziness, constipation, somnolence, sweating, small increases in blood pressure and, in contrast to amitriptyline, decreased appetite (Rabasseda, 2004).

Milnacipran (Ixel), with a pharmacology reminiscent of duloxetine, may also be promising (e.g., Vitton, M Gendreau, J. Gendreau, Kranzler, & S. G. Rao, 2004), but is early in study and not yet available in the U.S.

Mirtazapine (Remeron) has not been studied in migraine, but its pharmacological portfolio is intriguing. It is a 5-HT2$_{2B/2C}$ antagonist (Kasper, 1996), as are methysergide and propranolol. Mirtazapine resembles mianserin, a migraine preventive that has performed well in European studies (Tomkins, Jackson, O'Malley, Balden, & Santoro, 2001). On the other hand, mirtazapine differs from methysergide in having a low affinity for 5-HT_{1B} receptors, and it differs from mianserin in that it facilitates release of serotonin (de Boer, 1996). Either of these properties could blunt its effectiveness as a migraine prophylactic. All this remains to be sorted out empirically, however.

Antiepileptics

Anti-seizure medication is similarly a logical choice, given indications that neural hyperex-citability underlies migraines. And indeed there is some evidence that *valproic acid* (Depakote) and *gabapentin* (Neurontin) are effective. Other anti-epileptics such as Dilantin and Tegretol do not seem to work in preventing migraines (Ferrari, 1998b).

Valproate (Consortium Group 1) is a simple molecule, an 8-carbon organic acid, that was not even suspected of having a pharmacologic role until Eymard used it as a solvent for administering anticonvulsant compounds. The solvent-only control group showed good protection from seizures, and within five years the medication was in clinical use (Löscher, 1999). Valproate seems to increase levels of the inhibitory neurotransmitter gamma-amino butyric acid (GABA) in the brain, by inhibiting the enzyme that breaks it down, GABA transaminase (N. T. Mathew, 2001). Among the antiepileptics, it has received considerable study for migraine prophylaxis. In various double-blind, placebo-controlled trials, valproic acid has reduced migraine frequency by 27 percent (vs. 14 percent for the control group; Freitag, et al., 2002); 38 percent (vs. 8 percent; Klapper, 1996); and 42 percent (vs. 11 percent; N. T. Mathew, Saper, et al., 1995). In a single-blind, head-to-head comparison, valproate and propranolol had nearly identical efficacy (Kaniecki, 1997).

Despite its efficacy, there is little evidence so far that valproate's effects in migraine are mediated by a reduction in neural excitability. In one study, valproate did indeed raise the threshold for reporting phosphors during transcranial magnetic stimulation of the visual cortex (Mulleners, Chronicle, Vredeveld, & P. J. Koehler, 2002). However, this was true only in migraine with aura, not migraine without aura, yet the clinical benefit was the same in both diagnoses. Moreover, clinical improvement correlated only slightly and nonsignficantly (0.06–0.28) with the increase in visual threshold (Mulleners et al.). Other theories are possible as well. For example, gamma-amino butyric acid seems to inhibit serotonergic neurons in the dorsal raphe nucleus, in the migraine generator region of the brain stem (Kaniecki, 1997; Nishikawa & Scatton, 1985).

Valproate is generally well tolerated but potential side effects include nausea, hair loss, tremor, weight gain, sedation, dizziness, irregular menstrual periods and, possibly, polycystic ovary syndrome (Isojärvi, Laatikainen, Pakarinen, Juntunen, & Myllylä, 1993; P. W. Kaplan, 2004; Steiner & Tfelt-Hansen, 2000). Valproate is thought to be teratogenic (it has been associated with birth defects) and is therefore contraindicated by pregnancy (P. W. Kaplan, 2004). Hepatic disease and thrombocytopenia (low platelet count) are also contraindications, and periodic blood work, including checks of drug levels and liver function, is recommended (Steiner & Tfelt-Hansen, 2000). Even with safeguards in place, however, rare cases of hepatitis or pancreatitis can occur (Silberstein, Saper, & Freitag, 2001).

Gabapentin (Neurontin; Consortium Group 2) may increase the brain's concentration of GABA (N. T. Mathew, 2001). It also may regulate voltage-sensitive P/Q-type calcium channels (which we have seen are implicated in familial hemiplegic migraine), block the release of **monoamines** in the central nervous system, slow the release of glutamate and substance P in the dorsal horn, and increase blood levels of serotonin (D. J. Dooley, et al., 2002; Fehrenbacher, C. P. Taylor, & Vasko, 2003; C. P. Taylor, Gee, Su, et al., 1998). Its usefulness as a migraine prophylactic is just now coming under investigation.

In a 12-week double-blind, parallel group study with 63 participants, gabapentin 1200 mg/day reduced migraine frequency more than did a placebo (Di Trapani, Mei, Marra, Mazza, & Capuano, 2000). Of note, patients who had migraine with aura reported greater benefit (52 percent reduction in frequency) than did patients who had migraine without aura (38 percent reduction), who in turn benefited more than the placebo group (13 percent reduction). All pair-wise differences in outcome were statistically significant. If the finding replicates, it will be a very rare example of pharmacological difference between the two types of migraine.

Reported side effects include sedation and dizziness (Silberstein, Saper, & Freitag, 2001).

Topiramate (Topamax; Consortium Group 3) is a broad-spectrum antiepileptic that may lower neuronal excitability by inhibiting voltage-gated sodium and calcium channels, and perhaps AMPA-type glutamate receptors, and by facilitating the action of GABA receptors (Storey, Calder, Hart, & Potter, 2001). Chart reviews and small double-blind studies have shown efficacy in preventing migraine, and three large multi-center trials have been completed (Brandes, et al., 2004; Diener, Tfelt-Hansen, et al., 2004; Silbersetein, Neto, J. Schmitt, & D. Jacobs, 2004; W. B. Young, Hopkins, Shechter, & Silberstein, 2002). The data so far suggest efficacy comparable to that of other migraine preventives. Thus, Brandes, et al. report a 40 percent reduction in migraine frequency with topiramate 50 mg bid (the optimal dose), compared with a 20 percent reduction in the placebo group (Brandes, et al., 2004). Silberstein et al. report a 39 percent reduction at the same dosage, vs. 18 percent with placebo (Silberstein, et al.). Diener, et al., found a 33 percent reduction at that dose, vs. 15 percent with placebo (Diener, Tfelt-Hansen, et al.). These were large, careful trials and the estimates of therapeutic gain are remarkably stable (18–21 percent). The results from smaller, shorter trials (16 vs. 26 weeks) are not too dissimilar: a 36 percent decrease in the topiramate group, vs. a 14 percent decline in the placebo-treated group (Storey et al.), and a 51 percent decrease vs. 21 percent with placebo (Mei et al., 2004). A head-to-head trial found similar efficacy for topiramate 100 mg and propranolol 160 mg (Diener, Tfelt-Hansen, et al.).

A drawback in the multi-center trials has been a high dropout rate from the topiramate groups: 47 percent (Brandes et al., 2004), 47 percent (Silberstein, Neto, et al., 2004), and 44 percent (Diener, Tfelt-Hansen, et al., 2004). Dosages above 100 mg/day seem to be tolerated especially poorly. Although in Brandes et al. the attrition was no lower in the placebo group, the reasons were different: People given a placebo tended to leave because it lacked efficacy; people given topiramate tended to leave because of side effects (Brandes, et al., 2004). In all, 47–59 percent experience paresthesias at 50 mg bid (Brandes et al.; Diener, Tfelt-Hansen, et al.; Silberstein, Neto, et al.). Aside from the threat to internal validity caused by the attrition itself, the high side effect rate makes a topiramate study difficult to blind (Silberstein, Neto, et al.). Because it decreases sweating, topiramate has been associated with hyperthermia, mostly in young children (≤6 years old) in warm climates, taking high doses for epilepsy (Ziad, Rahi, Hamdan, & Mikati, 2005). In addition, significant impairments in memory, word finding, and problem solving have been reported with topiramate, again at least at relatively high doses. Patients may not always be aware of the extent of their impairment (Salinsky, Storzbach, D. Spencer, Oken, Landry, & Dodrill, 2005).

Still, another key side effect, weight loss, may not be a bad thing in overweight patients. And topiramate has the advantage of maintaining a degree of efficacy among patients thought to be refractory to preventive treatment: those with transformed migraine, migraine complicated by clinical depression, or in whom other preventives have failed. The concurrent use of one or more other migraine prophylactics seems to neither enhance nor impede topiramate (W. B. Young, Hopkins, Shechter, & Silberstein, 2002). Moreover, with the large studies now completed, topiramate's Consortium rating is likely to improve.

Nonsteroidal Anti-inflammatory Medications (NSAIDs)

Acetylsalicylic acid.   That taking an aspirin every other day could help prevent migraines emerged as a byproduct of the Physician's Health Study. The primary purpose of the study was to see if aspirin would reduce the incidence of myocardial infarction, and indeed it did. However,

661 of the men also had migraines, and for them, migraine frequency decreased by 20 percent. This is a minor reduction; however, another nonsteroidal anti-inflammatory, *naproxen* (Naprosyn, Anaprox), may be considerably more effective (Diener, Kaube, & Limmroth, 1998). Moreover, naproxen may be useful in preventing menstrual migraine (Sargent, Solbach, Damasio, et al., 1985). As preventives, both aspirin and naproxen are in Consortium Group 2. The main side effects are gastrointestinal, potentially severe, and a history of peptic ulcer or bleeding is generally taken as a contraindication. The selective COX–2 inhibitors (e.g., celecoxib/Celebrex, rofecoxib/Vioxx) do not seem to have been studied in migraine prophylaxis.

We should add that in the Physician's Health Study, rather low dosages of aspirin were used. Thus, the migraine-prophylactic benefits may have been related to the anticoagulant properties of aspirin rather than to its use as an anti-inflammatory (Wind & Punt, 1989). In a general way, this seems to support the older platelet theory of migraine (Chapter 4).

Anti-Coagulants

So far, however, the platelet theory of migraine has generated no controlled trials of its own. Unblinded studies (Thonnard-Neumann, 1973) and case reports (Fragoso, 1997) suggest improvement in migraine with and without aura during treatment with heparin or warfarin (Coumadin). One patient noted long-term worsening above baseline levels when warfarin was discontinued (Fragoso, 1997). And we could, perhaps, find support for the platelet model in favorable results from another study: A double-blind crossover trial with 47 patients found a greater reduction in days with migraine from **lisinopril** (29 percent) than placebo (9 percent; Schrader, Stovner, Helde, T. Sand, & Bovim, 2001). As one of its effects, lisinopril (Prinivil, Zestril) increases the synthesis of an anti-clotting factor, prostacyclin (Goa, Balfour, & Zuanetti, 1996). First and foremost, however, lisinopril inhibits the production of angiotensin II, a molecule to which we now turn.

Angiotensin II Inhibitors

Angiotensin II is a small 10-unit peptide, produced in the inner lining of blood vessels, that raises blood pressure quickly, through vasoconstriction, and slowly, by suppressing sodium excretion (E. K. Jackson, 2001). This hypertensive effect can be reduced by blocking the enzyme that generates angiotensin II (angiotensin-converting enzyme, ACE) or by antagonizing angiotensin II receptors (AT_1 receptors; E. K. Jackson, 2001). **ACE inhibitors** include captopril (Capoten), enalapril (Vasotec), and lisinopril (Zestril, Prinivil) among others. AT_1 receptor blockers include losartan (Cozaar) and candesartan cilexetil (Atacand). All are used to treat high blood pressure. And because angiotensin II has varied effects, AT_1 blockers may be useful in congestive heart failure and chronic renal failure, as well as hypertension (Burnier & Brunner, 2000). Side effects of ACE inhibitors include cough, angioedema, dizziness, and fatigue (Schrader, Stovner, Helde, T. Sand, & Bovim, 2001). There is some evidence that in hypertensive subjects, aspirin or other nonsteroidals may impair blood pressure control, and/or lead to excess mortality, when given with ACE inhibitors (Dubey, Balani, & Pillai, 2003; W. B. White, Kent, A. Taylor, Verburg, Lefkowith, & Whelton, 2002). Side effects of AT_1 blockers are similar to placebo, with dizziness predominating. Both classes of medications are contraindicated in cases of renal artery stenosis, diffuse intrarenal vascular stenosis, pregnancy, and breastfeeding (Burnier & Brunner, 2000).

Now, headache is a very common side effect of medications. Thus, it is noteworthy that in a meta-analysis of 27 published studies of AT_1 blockers in hypertension, patients receiving the active treatment had, on average, a 31 percent lower risk of headache (Etminan, M. A. H. Levine, Tomlinson, & Rochon, 2002).

So far there has been only one direct clinical trial, but its results are supportive: In a double-blind crossover study of 57 patients who had migraine with or without aura, candesartan 16 mg/day gave a 26 percent reduction in number of headache days, compared with placebo. In all, 32 percent of patients had at least a 50 percent reduction in number of headache days (Tronvik, Stovner, Helde, T. Sand, & Bovim, 2003). Of course a connection between angiotensin and migraines is supported also by the favorable results for the ACE inhibitor, lisinopril, noted above. And it may possibly be relevant that β-blockers act in the kidneys to inhibit the production of angiotensin precursors, and thus downregulate the angiotensin system (E. K. Jackson, 2001).

In Chapter 4 we saw that, historically, both the central nervous system and the cardiovasculature have claimed primacy in causing migraines. In the current chapter we have seen benefit from blood pressure medications (β-blockers and certain calcium channel antagonists), serotonin antagonists with their mixed central nervous system-vascular effects, and from the purely neural impact of antidepressants and anticonvulsants. It seems fitting, then, that we have returned to two new classes of blood pressure medications—inhibitors of a molecule that, left unchecked, acts on blood vessels to produce vasoconstriction. Indeed, angiotensin II may work at sympathetic sites in the spinal cord and the periphery to augment sympathetically induced vasoconstriction (A. M. Allen et al., 1998; E. K. Jackson, 2001). Not surprisingly, AT_1 blockers seem to protect the brain against ischemic damage, and promote cerebrovascular autoregulation, at least in animal studies (Pedersen, Paulson, Nielsen, Strandgaard, 2003).

But history will not stop there. For angiotensin II is found at sites throughout the central nervous system, where it is thought to function as a neurotransmitter or cotransmitter. And one of those sites is the trigeminal nucleus caudalis, where pain signals from the head are first processed (A. M. Allen et al., 1998). It seems we cannot get far into either the neural or the vascular model before encountering the other.

Neuromuscular Blockers

Botulinum toxin type A (Botox, Dysport), as the name suggests, is a toxin produced by the Clostridium Botulinum bacterium. It is used as a local agent to inactivate overly tense muscles, and has thus been utilized in cases of tension-type headache, migraine and, even more experimentally, in cluster headache. Once injected into a muscle, botulinum toxin is taken up by the alpha motor neurons at the neuromuscular junction, where it prevents the release of acetylcholine. This blockade of neurotransmission is permanent, except that new nerve terminals grow, reinnervating the junction over approximately three months (Münchau & Bhatia, 2000). Over time, people can develop antibodies that make them immune to botulinum toxin type A, although this seems to be infrequent with the newer, highly purified form (Jankovic, Vuong, & Ahsan, 2003).

Botulinum toxin is relatively new as a therapeutic agent, and its role in headache prevention is still being evaluated. Silberstein and colleagues report that three months after injection of 25 units of Botox into sites at the forehead and temples, there is a 49 percent reduction in the frequency of migraines, versus a 19 percent reduction with injection of the vehicle only (Silberstein, Mathew, Saper, & Jenkins, 2000). These results appear promising, but do not explain why injection of 75 units did not have a similar effect. Also, I wonder if it might be difficult to conduct a truly double blind test of botulinum toxin because its effects (weakness of the injected muscles) should be apparent to subjects (although sometimes it is not: Freund & Schwartz, 2000).

Botulinum toxin type B (*Myobloc*). The various strains of clostridium botulinum produce, between them, eight variants of botulinum toxin. All eight permanently block the release of acetylcholine at the neuromuscular junction by preventing vesicles containing the neurotrans- mitter from docking and fusing with the cell membrane (Callaway, Arezzo, & Grethlein, 2002). However, the eight variants do not all share the same target molecules, are not prepared com- mercially in the same way, and have different molecular weights, which in theory allow for dif- ferences in clinical efficacy (Callaway et al.). Also, antibodies against one of the forms of botulinum toxin will not work against the other forms. Thus, a person who has become immune to botulinum toxin type A may nonetheless benefit from the B type (Callaway et al.).

At this point, only the A and B forms of the toxin (there are also forms C1, C2, and D through G) have been developed into pharmaceutical products. The B form, Myobloc, is very recent to market and there is little published literature of its application to headaches. The few case stud- ies available have been mildly encouraging, and suggest it may work even when Botox does not (Fadeyi & Q. M. Adams, 2002).

Diuretics

Acetazolamide (Diamox) hastens the excretion of bicarbonate, and along with it, water, sodium, and potassium, leaving the blood more acidic (Physicians' Desk Reference, 2004). Empirically, it has been found to have marked prophylactic benefit in some cases of hemiplegic migraine (Athwal & Lennox, 1996). The reason is unclear, but acetazolamide dilates small arteries in the brain, increasing cerebral blood flow (Okazawa, Yamauchi, Sugimoto, Toyoda, Kishibe, & Taka- hashi, 2001) and may open certain ion channels (Tricarico, Barbieri, & Camerino, 2000). There is no support for its use in typical migraines—it is poorly tolerated and there has been no indica- tion of efficacy (Vahedi et al., 2002). However, there is a little bit of evidence that when the migraine is accompanied by vertigo, or by an aura that includes motor, somatosensory, balance, and/or language problems, acetazolamide may be useful (Ambrosini, Pierelli, & Schoenen, 2003). Acetazolamide in some ways resembles topiramate and the main side effects are similar: paresthesias, and fatigue, somnolence, or difficulty concentrating (Vahedi et al.). Kidney stones are a risk with long-term use. Of note, the medication should not be combined with high dose aspirin. Regular monitoring of blood electrolytes and, in diabetics, blood glucose, is recom- mended (Physicians' Desk Reference, 2004).

CLUSTER HEADACHE

Acute Medications

Attacks of cluster headache last between 15 and 180 minutes. This essentially rules out the use of oral analgesics or triptans, which may take 4 hours to reach full effectiveness. Instead, the treat- ment of choice is subcutaneous *sumatriptan*, 6 mg, which can be repeated once in 24 hours if a second attack occurs (Ekbom & Hardebo, 2002; Zakrzewska, 2001).

For more frequent attacks, the second-line option is inhalation of 100 percent *oxygen*, 7 liters/minute for 15 minutes (Zakrzewska, 2001). Oxygen probably works because it con- stricts cranial arteries. Indeed, the degree of improvement seems to correlate with the amount of cranial artery constriction as measured by reduction in cerebral blood flow (Hardebo, Masseter, & Ryding, 1989). During a cluster period, the cephalic arteries seem unusually responsive to oxy- gen. In general, the treatment does not seem to improve migraines (Hardebo et al.).

Of course the contraindications to sumatriptan, particularly in comorbid cardiovascular or cerebrovascular disease, or hemiplegic aura, apply here as in migraine. Also, there are case reports of sumatriptan causing increased frequency of cluster headache, prolongation of the cluster period, and chronic daily headache, all of which seem to resolve rapidly when the sumatriptan is stopped (Hering-Hanit, 2000). The effect seems to be infrequent, however, as it was not apparent in a long-term, large-scale study (Ekbom, Krabbe, et al., 1995).

Olanzapine (Zyprexa), an atypical antipsychotic, has been studied in a small, open-label trial because of its anti-dopaminergic activity. Of the five patients treated, all consistently achieved 60–100 percent relief of their headaches with 2.5 to 10 mg oral olanzapine. Sedation or sleep, and a somewhat slow onset of action (20 minutes) were the primary drawbacks (Rozen, 2001).

Magnesium. Mauskop and colleagues have found evidence that intravenous magnesium may help interrupt cluster headaches in patients with a low serum magnesium ion concentration (Mauskop, B. T. Altura, Cracco, & B. M. Altura, 1995b). The mechanism of action is not known, but we will see below that a low level of magnesium ions in the serum could, in theory, lead to increased pain sensitivity and/or vasoreactivity.

In small clinical series, intranasal *lidocaine* has had modest benefit in interrupting attacks (Kittrelle, Grouse, & Seybold, 1985; Robbins, 1995). During application, patients are asked to tip their heads back 45° and towards the side of the pain. If nasal congestion interferes, a 0.5 percent phenylephrine spray is sometimes used first (Robbins, 1995). Robbins notes only modest results (16 of 30 patients reported mild or moderate relief), but the convenience and mild side effect profile helped balance this out. Efficacy would be suspected from the probable role of the parasympathetic nervous system in cluster headache, and the potential for intranasal lidocaine to block the parasympathetic sphenopalatine ganglion, located above the nose (Edvinsson, 1991; Yarnitsky, Goor-Aryeh, et al., 2003).

Cluster Headache Preventives

The calcium channel blocker *verapamil*, which has only marginal effectiveness in preventing migraines, seems to perform much better in the prophylaxis of cluster headaches (Gabai & Spierings, 1989). The typical dosage is 240–480 mg/day, although in severe cases dosages have gone as high as 1200 mg/day (Ekbom & Hardebo, 2002). Side effects include constipation, fatigue, water retention, and postural hypotension (Ekbom & Hardebo, 2002). Because cluster headache is uncommon, outcome studies generally have small samples, but the results are encouraging nonetheless. For example, in one trial 80 percent (12/15) of the verapamil group had at least a 50 percent reduction in headache frequency by the second week of treatment. No one in the control group met this criterion (Leone, D'Amico, Frediani, et al., 2000).

Lithium carbonate, typically at 300 mg tid, seems to have similar efficacy as verapamil, but with somewhat slower onset, and at the cost of more frequent side effects. The side effects include constipation or gastrointestinal complaints, increased diuresis, and behavior changes (Bussone, Leone, et al., 1990).

Other preventive medications include daily low-dose *ergotamine* (which does not seem to cause rebound cluster headaches as it does in migraines), *sodium valproate*, a *steroid* taper, *methysergide*, and intravenous *dihydroergotamine* (N. Mathew, 1997b). The preventives are generally used only during the cluster period. The steroid taper and intravenous dihydroergotamine are, of course, of even shorter duration, but are intended to bring the cluster period to a close.

There is some evidence that nighttime *melatonin* levels are suppressed during and between cluster periods (Leone, Lucini, et al., 2000). Not surprisingly, then, melatonin 10 mg qhs has been studied in a double-blind trial as a preventive. The melatonin seems to have brought the cluster period to a close over 3–5 days in 5/10 patients; in contrast, no one in the control group left a cluster period (Leone, D'Amico, Moschiano, Fraschini, & Bussone, 1996). The study was small, but quite encouraging.

TENSION-TYPE HEADACHE

Acute Treatments

Muscle relaxants.   Given the long history in which tension-type headaches were attributed to chronic muscle contraction, it is no surprise that muscle relaxants have played a role in their treatment. However, in most cases this use was based on clinical experience. The few published case series (e.g., Blumenthal & Fuchs, 1961 for favorable data on orphenadrine/Norflex) suffer from the methodological limitations characteristic of their era: poor case definitions, absence of blinding, retrospective outcome criteria, and confounding by other ongoing symptomatic and preventive treatments.

An exception is chlorzoxazone (Parafon), which was subjected to at least two double-blind comparisons with a placebo (Ogden & Schockett, 1960). One study was a double-blind crossover trial in which 101 patients took either chlorzoxazone 250 mg or a placebo for myalgia (muscle pain), generally in the occipital or frontal region, or over one side of the head. Presumably a mix of headache diagnoses was represented in the sample, which was recruited from a hospital emergency room. In any event, 77 percent of the patients preferred the active drug, vs. 9 percent who preferred the placebo. In a second trial, a lower dose of chlorzoxazone (125 mg) combined with acetaminophen, was compared with placebo in a double-blind crossover design (N = 102) with similar patient characteristics and recruitment. The results, too, were similar, with 66 percent of patients preferring the active treatment and 2 percent preferring the placebo (Ogden & Schockett, 1960).

Like other muscle relaxants of its generation, chlorzoxazone was thought from animal experiments to inhibit reflex arcs in the brain stem and spinal cord that underlie spasms (Domino, 1974; Physcians Desk Reference, 2004). In people, however, it has been unclear whether its clinical efficacy traces to anything other than a general sedation (Elenbaas, 1980). More recently, though, chlorzoxazone has been shown to open a type of potassium channel, most likely suppressing firing in the basal ganglia, and breathing new life into the theory that chlorzoxazone does, in fact, relax muscles via subcortical inhibition (Syme, Gerlach, A. Singh, & D. C. Devor, 2000).

Butalbital.   For episodic tension-type headaches, butalbital compounds seem to be more effective than placebo at 2 and 4 hours, with few short-term adverse effects (Silberstein & McCrory, 2001). As with its use in migraine, the risks are worth noting: Acute overdose can cause death, daily use can bring tolerance, sometimes addiction, and abrupt withdrawal can provoke seizures (M. Raja, Altavista, Azzoni, & Albanese, 1996) and delirium tremens (Silberstein & McCrory, 2001). We have seen that with migraines, use of butalbital more than 2–3 times per week is associated with rebound headaches, and transition from episodic to daily headache.

Preventive Treatments

Botulinum toxin.   We have seen preliminary evidence, above, of a role for Botox and perhaps Myobloc in the prevention of migraines. A similar role for tension-type headache seems logical, although double-blind trials have not been supportive (Rollnik, Tanneberger, Schubert,

U. Schneider, & Dengler, 2000; W. J. Schmitt, Slowey, Fravi, S. Weber, & Burgunder, 2001; Schulte-Mattler, Krack, & BoNTTH Study Group, 2004).

It seems possible that, as with EMG biofeedback, targeting the trapezius will prove more effective, at least in tension-type headaches, than treating the forehead and temples. Freund and Schwartz (2000), studying 26 persons with daily cervicogenic headache following whiplash, report a 46 percent reduction in median pain level 4 weeks after botulinum injections to trigger points in the neck. No subject was pain-free after the injections, suggesting that an additional pain mechanism such as central sensitization may have been present. Placebo (saline) injections had no beneficial effects. There was no explicit check on blinding but the authors note that none of the patients reported weakness in the relevant muscles or, indeed, any other side effect. This is a small (total $N = 26$) but promising study that bears replication.

As in EMG biofeedback, there is some evidence that a reduction in muscle tension is not essential for botulinum toxin to be effective. For example, pain reduction can occur prior to muscle relaxation, it can occur in muscle groups that have not been injected, and it can last longer than the muscle blockade (Göbel, Heinze, Heinze-Kuhn, & Austermann, 2001). An alternative theory involves retrograde effects: C-type sensory neurons may transport the medication back into the spinal column, where it may block the release of substance P and other pain neurotransmitters (Göbel, Heinze, et al.). However, there is no evidence so far that Botox prevents release of substance P, or indeed has any direct analgesic effects in people (Blersch, Schulte-Mattler, Przywara, A. May, Bigalke, & Wohlfarth, 2002; Voller, et al., 2003). A third theory, so far untested, is that the key site of action is within **muscle spindles** (Filippi, Errico, Santarelli, Bagolini, & Manni, 1993), sensory ogans in muscle tissue that regulate muscle tone and that may mediate some types of muscle pain.

All of this uncertainty would seem to make placebo-controlled trials essential, but there have been few, and their results unfavorable. Göbel et al. point out a difficulty with them: The controlled studies have generally utilized injection of standardized sites, so that the same sites are injected in all patients. In actual clinical practice, of course, the injection sites are selected individually, for example at trigger points (Göbel, Heinze, Heinze-Kuhn, & Austermann, 2001).

Antidepressants.   From its analgesic properties, it would not be surprising if amitriptyline (Elavil) were of use in chronic tension-type headache. And in fact, in several (Bendtsen, R. Jensen, & J. Olesen, 1996c; H. Göbel, Hamouz, Hansen, et al., 1994), although not all (Pfaffenrath, Diener, et al., 1994), double-blind studies, amitriptyline has had just such an effect. Chronic daily headache, also, may perhaps benefit from treatment with the tricyclic (Redillas & S. Solomon, 2000). Amitriptyline seems to lower total headache burden, by reducing headache duration, and to a lesser extent frequency (Bendtsen, R. Jensen, & J. Olesen, 1996c). On average, headache burden delines about 30 percent more with the medication than with placebo (Bendtsen, 2003). A typical starting dose is 25 mg/day, increasing every two weeks as tolerated, until good therapeutic effect is achieved, or until limited by side effects. Typical maintenance doses are 50–75 mg. Side effects include dry mouth, dizziness, weight gain, and sedation (Bendtsen, R. Jensen, & J. Olesen, 1996c). An 8-week trial is reasonable for establishing efficacy. If the treatment is successful, Bendtsen, et al. suggest tapering the patient off after 6–12 months, reinstituting amitriptyline in case of relapse (Bendtsen, R. Jensen, & J. Olesen, 1996c). As in other chronic pain conditions, the tricyclic appears to work regardless of whether the patient is depressed, and independently of any change in mood (Redillas & S. Solomon, 2000).

Surprisingly, a small but well designed study of mirtazapine (Remeron), 15–30 mg per day, suggests that it, too, reduces chronic tension-type headache activity by about 30 percent over placebo (Bendtsen & R. Jensen, 2004). Side effects included drowsiness, dizziness, and weight gain, and although the medication was well tolerated, we might wonder if subjects guessed the active from placebo phases. The efficacy, for which there is some evidence in other types of chronic pain, requires explanation: Mirtazapine antagonizes alpha–2 adrenergic receptors—precisely those involved in the descending inhibition of pain (Pertovaara, 2000)

The utility of SSRI's is less clear. In a direct comparison with amitriptyline, citalopram (Celexa) failed to significantly reduce pain frequency, duration, or intensity in chronic tension-type headache (Bendtsen, R. Jensen, & J. Olesen, 1996c). This limited utility seems true for other types of pain as well (M. E. Lynch, 2001). Moreover, in a meta-analysis of tricyclics, greater analgesia was produced by mixed norepinephrine-serotonin reuptake inhibitors such as doxepin and amitriptyline, than by clomipramine (Anafranil), which is reasonably selective for serotonin (Onghena & Van Houdenhove, 1992). Meta-analysis results are shown in Table 11–4. Note that the effect size for trazodone is negative, suggesting a possible tendency to worsen pain.

CHRONIC DAILY HEADACHE

Only recently has chronic daily headache come into focus as a target for drug therapy, and uncertainties in diagnostic system and outcome measure continue to impede progress. Still, several groups have reported on their clinical experiences, and a few double-blind trials have emerged.

In a retrospective chart review, *olanzapine* (Zyprexa), an atypical antipsychotic, reduced number of headache days by 23 percent, and remembered headache intensity by 75 percent (Silberstein, Peres, Hopkins, Shechter, W. B. Young, & Rozen, 2002). The patients had, variously, transformed migraine (60 percent), chronic posttraumatic headache (24 percent), new daily persistent headache (8 percent), or chronic tension-type headache (8 percent). Nearly all were overusing symptomatic headache medications. Of course it is difficult to know how much stock to put in unblinded, retrospective data. However, the fact that the headaches had been refractory to a minimum of 4 prior preventives suggests that olanzapine deserves further study. And its antagonism of $5-HT_{2A/2B/2C}$ and dopamine D_{1-4} receptors, and stimulation of α_2 adrenoceptors, could all convey anti-migraine and anti-nociceptive properties (Silberstein, Peres, et al.).

Fluoxetine (Prozac) has also received some empirical support for chronic daily headache. For example, Saper, et al. found in a double-blind trial that 47 percent of a fluoxetine group, but only 24 percent of patients given a placebo, improved by at least 50 percent over a placebo run-in phase (Saper, Silberstein, Lake, & Winters, 1994). A favorable change in headache status was predicted by a prior improvement in mood, even though few patients were clinically

TABLE 11–4
Analgesic Effectiveness of Selected Antidepressants

Antidepressant	Analgesia Effect Size	Number of Studies
Doxepin	0.96	6
Amitriptyline	0.73	15
Imipramine	0.57	6
Zimelidine	0.45	2
Mianserin	0.35	4
Clomipramine	0.29	3
Trazodone	−0.29	2

Note. From "Antidepressant-Induced Analgesia in Chronic Non-Malignant Pain: A Meta-Analysis of 39 Placebo-Controlled Studies," by P. Onghena and B. Van Houdenhove, 1992, *Pain, 49,* p. 205. Copyright 1992 by the International Association for the Study of Pain. Reprinted with permission.

depressed. Moreover, the improvement was seen more clearly in global ratings of headache status than in the diary measures. Thus, the the elevation in mood may mediate the drug's effect on headache (Redillas & S. Solomon, 2000; Saper, Silberstein, et al.), or on appraisal of headache. Nearly all of the patients in Saper, et al.'s experimental group were titrated up to 40 mg fluoxetine per day. Note that fluoxetine, by inhibiting the cytochrome P450–2D6 system, very likely blocks the analgesic effects of codeine (Brøsen, 1998; C. M. Thompson, et al., 2004).

Opiates.   Among the opioids, there has been some recent interest in low dose methadone for chronic daily headaches. From open label (non-blinded) studies by Robbins, it appears that the medication is useful for only a subset of people, but can have quite favorable effects within that subset. For example, in one study 42 of 148 people reported improved quality of life and good-to-excellent reduction in chronic daily headaches. The other 106 subjects, however, left the study due to side effects or because the treatment was ineffective (Robbins, 1997). Of course, without blinding we cannot be sure how much of the efficacy was due to the methadone's pharmacological properties.

Very similar results have been reported by Saper, Lake, and colleagues in 3 to 8 year follow-up from their headache center (Saper, Lake, Hamel, Lutz, Branca, Sims, & Kroll, 2004). Of 160 chronic daily headache patients, refractory to other treatments and started on time-contingent opiates (mostly slow-release morphine, OxyContin, or fentanyl patches), 26 percent had a good clinical response (>50 percent reduction in severe pain index). For this minority, the opiates seem to have been helpful. Still, the translation to an office-based practice is difficult. The patients in Saper's study had frequent follow-ups, were involved in a structured program, learned nonpharmacological techniques, had been screened by a psychologist to rule out personality disorders, and had signed a detailed narcotics contract prohibiting multiple prescribers or pharmacies, early refills, etc. Ominously, patients' perceptions of improvement were not only higher than the improvement calculated from serial reports of headache activity, the perceptions were actually *uncorrelated* with the more objective measure. Not surprisingly, then, patients were sometimes insistent about remaining on the medication, even when there was no actual efficacy, and at least one changed providers rather than taper (Saper, Lake, Hamel, et al.).

Tizanidine (Zanaflex), a centrally acting muscle relaxant, has also shown promise in chronic daily headache. In a 12-site, double-blind trial, overall headache activity was 54 percent lower during the last four weeks of treatment with tizanidine than it had been at baseline. In the placebo group, headache activity had declined by only 35 percent by the last four weeks of treatment (Saper, Lake, Cantrell, Winner, J. White, & V. Cross, 2002). There was no change in disability score using the MIDAS questionnaire, but headache frequency, duration and intensity were all differentially reduced in the tizanidine group. The dose was relatively high (titrated to a median of 20 mg/day), but very few patients dropped out due to side effects, and there were no serious drug-related adverse events.

Although helpful clinically, these results do not lend support to the muscle contraction theory of chronic tension-type headache. Most of the patients in this study had chronic migraine. Moreover, tizanidine is an agonist at α2 adrenoreceptors, which are found in pain inhibitory pathways of the spinal cord (Fairbanks, L. S. Stone, Kitto, Nguyen, Posthumus, & G. L. Wilcox, 2002). In experimental animals, tizanidine seems to have an analgesic effect that can be distinguished from muscle relaxation (Saper, Lake, Cantrell, Winner, J. White, & V. Cross, 2002).

Tizanidine should *not* be combined with the antidepressant fluvoxamine (Granfors, Backman, M. Neuvonen, Ahonen, & P. Neuvonen, 2004).

Histamine.   We have seen that histamine is thought to be the active ingredient in a number of migraine triggers, and may be involved in neurogenic inflammation. Moreover, we have seen that receptor sensitivity is often down-regulated in response to chronic exposure to a drug. Putting these together, we might hypothesize that chronic administration of histamine would lead to desensitization to it, and hence to resistance to migraines. An experiment along these lines has been reported by Nicolodi and coworkers. They administered IV histamine for a 15-day period to 680 patients with transformed migraine. The authors report an approximately 62 percent rate of clinical improvement, generally lasting for 2 to 3 months (Nicolodi, Del Bianco, & Sicuteri, 1998). A placebo control was not used in this initial study.

PAROXYSMAL HEMICRANIA AND HEMICRANIA CONTINUA

Although little is known of the pathophysiology of these disorders, they have in common an absolute responsiveness to indomethacin (Indocin), a nonsteroidal anti-inflammatory. The paroxysmal hemicranias are similar to cluster headaches, but they tend to be briefer and more frequent. As we have seen, hemicrania continua is a type of unilateral chronic daily headache (N. Mathew, 1997b). The response rate of these disorders to indomethacin is thought to be so high that it has become an essential part of their definition. Thus, at this writing it is impossible, by definition, to have a paroxysmal hemicrania that does not respond to indomethacin.

Results are swift and complete; at the right dose, the headache should resolve within 3 days. Typical values are 25–150 mg/day for adults. The doses are sometimes started at 25 mg tid, and adjusted up or down as needed (Pareja, Caminero, Franco, Casado, Pascual, & Sánchez del Rio, 2001). There seems to be no loss of effectiveness over time. Over several years, about 50 percent of patients go into sustained remission or else are able to reduce their dosages; for the other 50 percent, of the dose remains constant (Pareja et al.).

Of course like other nonsteroidals, indomethacin can have significant gastrointestinal side effects. A history of peptic ulcer or bleeding may contraindicate the drug. The form of the cyclooxygenase enzyme that protects the gastric mucosa, however, COX–1, differs slightly from the form, COX–2, involved in pain and inflammation. Older nonsteroidals such as indomethacin inhibit both forms, and thus carry significant risk of gastrointestinal side effects, including even hemorrhage and death (G. Singh & Triadafilopoulos, 1999). Newer nonsteroidals target COX–2 specifically, and these COX–2 selectives have sometimes been used in place of indomethacin. Thus, in a case series of 14 patients with hemicrania continua, 3 of 5 treated with Celebrex (celecoxib) 400–600 mg/day, and 3 of 9 receiving Vioxx (rofecoxib) 50 mg/day had a complete response (Peres & Silberstein, 2002). In all, 80–90 percent of patients with hemicrania continua seem to improve to some degree with the COX–2 inhibitors. Similarly, there are case reports of Vioxx-responsive chronic paroxysmal hemicrania (Lisotto, Maggioni, Mainardi, & Zanchin, 2003).

As is now well known, however, rofecoxib, celecoxib, and another selective COX–2 inhibitor, valdecoxib (Bextra), seem to double or triple the risk of thrombotic (blood clotting) events such as heart attack and ischemic stroke (Bresalier, Sandler, Quan, Bolognese, Oxenius, Horgan, et al., 2005; Nussmeier, Whelton, M. T. Brown, Langford, Hoeft, Parlow, et al., 2005; S. D. Solomon, McMurray, Pfeffer, Wittes, Fowler, Finn, et al., 2005). In platelets and the lining of blood vessels, it seems, COX–2 generates a type of prostaglandin, PGI_2 (prostacyclin) that dilates blood vessels, reduces platelet aggregation, inhibits smooth muscle proliferation (a step in atherosclerosis), and thus helps balance out the effects of a pro-clotting prostaglandin called thromboxane A_2 (McAdam, Catella-Lawson, Mardini, Kapoor, J. A. Lawson, & FitzGerald, 1999). Inhibit COX–2, it seems, and the balance is lost. As of this writing, Vioxx and Bextra have both been withdrawn from the market.[6]

And even aside from the clouded future of COX–2 selectives, indomethacin remains the gold standard by which the hemicranias are defnied. Note that besides inhibiting prostaglandin synthesis, indomethacin seems to lower the pressure of cerebrospinal fluid, decrease cerebral blood flow, strengthen the blood-brain barrier, alter plasma melatonin levels, and antagonize nitric oxide (Peres & Silberstein, 2002). Structurally, it resembles melatonin (Peres, Stiles, Oshinsky, & Rozen, 2001; Rozen, 2003). Of course it may have many other, yet undiscovered, effects on the body as well.

HERBAL, NUTRITIONAL, AND NUTRACEUTICAL PRODUCTS

The disquieting experience with the COX–2 inhibitors has been variously interpreted as a lapse of public trust, and as evidence that a regulatory process—in which postmarketing surveillance leads to further controlled study—is successful in bringing new problems to light (Dieppe, Ebrahim, R. M. Martin, & Jüni, 2004; R. Eisenberg, 2005).

Passions no less strident are evoked by herbal and nutraceutical products. On the one hand, our bodies are surely better equipped to assimilate and utilize food components than molecules that did not exist before 1990. On the other hand, the safety and efficacy of supplements in general has been less well studied than for traditional medications. Some outcome literature is available, however, which we will review here.

Feverfew is an aromatic plant, from which the dried leaves of non-flowering specimens were used to combat fever in Roman and medieval times, and as a migraine prophylactic more recently.[7] In the test tube, **feverfew** extract is a cyclooxygenase inhibitor, like aspirin and other nonsteroidals, but it may not have this action in vivo (Pattrick, Heptinstall, & Doherty, 1989). However, feverfew also contains parthenolide, which inhibits secretion of serotonin, at least from platelets, and which may be the key ingredient for migraine prophylaxis. Murphy et al. have reported the results of a fairly small scale, double-blind, placebo-controlled, crossover study (Murphy, Heptinstall, & Mitchell, 1988). Patients were assigned to a one-month placebo condition, followed by two months of either feverfew or placebo, followed by two months of the other treatment (placebo or feverfew). Overall, there was a 24 percent reduction in the number of migraines on feverfew vs. placebo ($p < .005$), a reduction in nausea and vomiting ($p < .02$), and a trend towards decreased headache intensity ($p < .06$). No harm was found on routine urinalysis, blood work, and pulse and blood pressure measurement, and self-reported side effects were no greater than with the placebo (dried cabbage leaves).

Three caveats should be noted. First, only 60 of the 72 subjects completed the 5-month study. Most of the drop-outs were unrelated to condition, but 3 patients receiving feverfew and 1 on placebo withdrew due to failure to improve. Although this is not enough to explain the study's positive results, it does suggest that the efficacy may be slightly over-estimated in this study. Second, the study involved dried feverfew leaves that had been specially cultivated in a university botany department, standardized for parthenolide content and pre-tested for effects on serotonin

---

[6]As it turns out, several older nonsteroidals are selective, to one extent or another, for COX-2: etodolac (Lodine), meloxicam (Mobic), nabumetone (Relafen), and nimesulide (various trade names, not available in the United States; Hooper et al., 2004). Their effects on prostacyclin may vary (e.g., Belton et al., 2000, vs. Jeremy et al., 1990). Clinically, little is known about the cardiovascular risk with long-term use.

[7]According to Webster's, "few" here derives from the Latin word meaning "to drive away," and is related to "fugitive."

excretion. Thus, we do not know how well the results generalize to the preparations available in health food stores. Third, as is often true for standard pharmaceutical products as well, we have only relatively short-term data on side effects for a medication intended for long-term use.

Positive results have been found in two other double-blind, placebo-controlled studies (E. S. Johnson, Kadam, D. M. Hylands, & P. J. Hylands, 1985; Palevitch, Earon, & Carasso, 1997), but not in a third (de Weerdt, Bootsma, & Hendriks, 1996). The null results study differs from the others in that it used an alcohol extract of feverfew rather than dried leaves. If the difference in preparation is crucial, it would argue against parthenolide being the active ingredient for migraine prophylaxis. For example, chrysanthenyl acetate, a feverfew component with anti-inflammatory properties, largely absent in the extract, may be a key ingredient (de Weerdt, et al.). It turns out, however, that while all four studies have acceptable methodological rigor, the null results study had the strongest methods. Not surprisingly, then, the Cochrane group regards the evidence for feverfew as favorable, but not beyond a reasonable doubt (Pittler, Vogler, & Ernst, 2003). The U.S. Headache Consortium concluded similarly: Group 2 status based on Grade B evidence—some, but not optimal, scientific support.

L–5-Hydroxytryptophan (5-HTP) is a precursor of serotonin (**5-Hydroxytryptamine** or 5-HT). Ribeiro (2000) conducted a double-blind, placebo-controlled study of 65 patients with chronic tension-type headache. The treatment group had a statistically significant reduction in analgesic use during the 8 weeks that they took 5-HTP, although the number of headaches did not show a greater reduction than in the control group. During a two-week follow-up period after the 8 weeks, the group that had been treated had fewer headaches than the group that had been on the placebo. Hence, the results are suggestive, but quite preliminary.

Riboflavin, or Vitamin B_2, is the precursor of two coenzymes used in the **mitochondria** for oxidation. Thus, we could perhaps speculate that high dose riboflavin would help improve mitochondrial energy metabolism. In fact, there are several known mitochondrial defects for which high dose riboflavin has shown efficacy (Antozzi, Garavaglia, Mora, et al., 1994; Penn, Lee, Thuillier, et al., 1992). Moreover, there is preliminary animal data to suggest that riboflavin may have analgesic and anti-inflammatory properties (Granados-Soto, et al., 2004).

I am aware of only one double blind, placebo-controlled trial of riboflavin for prophylaxis of migraines specifically. (Still, this was evidence enough for Consortium Group 2.) Schoenen, Jacquy and Lenaerts (1998) randomized 55 patients with frequent migraines to receive either 400 mg B_2 per day or a placebo. Compared to the placebo group, the patients taking riboflavin had an approximately 50 percent reduction in the frequency of migraines. The effectiveness may build slowly, over perhaps two to three months (Mattimoe & Newton, 1998). Whether the mechanism of action is indeed a normalization of mitochondrial function is not definitely known. Because riboflavin does not appear to normalize interictal auditory evoked potentials its mechanism may be different from that of beta-blockers (Sándor, Áfra, Ambrosini, & Schoenen, 2000). So far, there have been no studies combining high dose riboflavin with beta-blockers, behavioral interventions, or both.

Although only one subject left Schoenen et al.'s study due to a side effect (diarrhea), it should be noted nonetheless that 400 mg is approximately *235 times* the U.S. recommended daily allowance for riboflavin used as a vitamin, and that the study was relatively short-term (3 months). In this context, riboflavin seems more like a drug than a nutrient. I know of no studies to suggest a migraine preventive effect at doses near the U.S. RDA.

Coenzyme Q10, a small molecule, participates in energy production by shuttling electrons along the mitochondrial membrane (Rozen, Oshinsky, et al., 2002). As a supplement, coenzyme

Q10 has shown clinical benefit in disorders of mitochondrial function, such as certain muscular dystrophies (Folkers & Simonsen, 1995). In a small non-blinded study, 150 mg per day was followed by a 55 percent decrease in number of migraine days after 5 to 12 weeks of therapy (Rozen, Oshinsky, et al.). In a second, placebo-controlled trial, coenzyme Q10, 100 mg three times a day, led to a statistically significant 27 percent reduction in migraine frequency, vs. a 2 percent reduction in the placebo group. Nausea declined in the treated patients, increased in the control group, and this difference, too, was statistically significant. In all, 48 percent of treated subjects had at least a 50 percent reduction in migraine frequency, compared with 14 percent of the subjects given placebo (Sándor, Di Clemente, et al., 2005). Although the trials have been small and the response rates limited, low cost and an apparent absence of side effects make coenzyme Q10 a possible candidate for migraine prophylaxis (Rozen, Oshinsky, et al.).

Magnesium is an essential dietary mineral, although taken in high doses it is toxic and even fatal. In the 18th century, magnesia—magnesium oxide—was included in a list of migraine preventives (Fothergill, 1784, p. 111). At the time, migraines were thought to be triggered by gastrointestinal distress; magnesia was assumed to work by preventing indigestion. But the mineral is pertinent to current theories of migraine as well. For magnesium may decrease production of nitric oxide, and limit the release of substance P and serotonin. Moreover, magnesium may act as a kind of poor-man's calcium channel blocker, inhibiting NMDA-type glutamate receptors in pain pathways, and reducing vasoconstriction (Mauskop & B. M. Altura, 1998).

Most magnesium in the body is found in the bones, and inside cells, and in the serum both protein-bound and as free ion. Presumably, only the free ions in the serum are important in headaches (Mauskop & B. M. Altura, 1998). Mauskop and Altura cite evidence that approximately 30 percent of headache patients, and 50 percent of migraineurs during a migraine episode, have serum magnesium ion concentrations that are below the 95 percent confidence interval for the healthy population.

Does all this translate into a clinical role for magnesium? In an intriguing study, Mauskop and coworkers took blood samples from people during migraine attacks, and then administered intravenous magnesium sulfate, observing the response. Much later, the blood samples were analyzed for the pretreatment concentration of free magnesium ion. Of those patients whose magnesium ion concentration had been low, 86 percent had improved with the treatment. Of those whose magnesium levels had been normal, only 16 percent had improved (Mauskop, B. T. Altura, Cracco, & B. M. Altura, 1995a).

These results raise the question of whether oral magnesium supplementation can help prevent migraines.[8] In fact, the evidence appears quite mixed (Consortium Group 2). In one multicenter, double-blind study, 81 migraine patients took either trimagnesium dicitrate or a placebo for 12 weeks. Compared with baseline, the frequency of migraine episodes was lowered by 41.6 percent in the experimental group, versus 15.8 percent in the placebo group. However, there was no correlation between initial serum magnesium levels and subsequent response to treatment (Peikert, Wilimzig, & Köhne-Volland, 1996). In a second multicenter, double-blind study, 69 patients having migraine without aura took either magnesium-u-aspartate-hydrochloride-trihydrate or an indistinguishable placebo for 12 weeks. There was no treatment effect on the frequency, duration or intensity of migraines. In fact, the study was stopped after 69 subjects because it was by then statistically impossible that a reasonable effect could be found with the intended

---

[8]Please note that an overdose of magnesium can be quite dangerous. As always, consulting with a physician is *highly* recommended.

full enrollment of 150 subjects (Pfaffenrath, Wessely, et al., 1996). Hopefully, future work will help clarify the reasons for the discrepant results between these two investigations.

Note that if 50 percent of migraineurs have low serum magnesium levels during attacks, as suggested by Mauskop and Altura, then presumably in the best case scenario no more than half of patients would respond pharmacologically to magnesium supplementation. Here, as with triggers and psychophysiological results, we have evidence that migraine is the common presentation of a number of different underlying disorders. Not surprisingly, then, Mazzotta, et al. suggest that migraineurs should routinely be assessed for the level of magnesium in their red blood cells, to identify the subset of patients most likely to benefit from supplementation (Mazzotta, Sarchielli, Alberti, & Gallai, 1999).

Omega–3 polyunsaturated fatty acids (fish oil supplements).   In theory, fish oil supplements are a logical candidate for migraine prevention. They may have anti-inflammatory properties, reduce platelet aggregation, and inhibit platelets' release of serotonin. But does this mean actual therapeutic efficacy? To my knowledge, there has been only one large-scale study of fish oil supplements in migraines, and its results are complicated (Pradalier et al., 2001).

In all, 196 patients completed the 24-week study. After a 4 week placebo run-in, they were randomized to receive either fish oil or placebo (olive oil + lactose) for 16 weeks in a double-blind format. The study concluded with a 4-week run-out period in which both groups received the placebo. Now, the authors had intended to compare the number of migraine attacks for each group during the last 4 weeks (weeks 13–16) of treatment, versus baseline (the 4-week run-in period). And for this analysis, the results did not even approach significance.

The reason may be that traditional bane of headache outcome research: the placebo group had a 45 percent reduction in the number of headaches. If, however, one looks at the number of headaches for the full 16 weeks of treatment, then the fish oil was indeed superior, with an average of 5.99 attacks, versus 7.19 in the placebo group. The authors point out that a reduction of 1 headache over 16 weeks is not an impressive outcome, and from a clinical standpoint they regard their study as a null result (Pradalier, et al., 2001). However, in the treatment group, 74 percent of patients had at least a 50 percent reduction in headache frequency, while in the control group 55 percent achieved this level. Thus, behind the averages there seem to have been some patients who were significantly improved with the fish oil who would not have been so improved with the placebo, and this is at least a modestly positive outcome.

Melatonin.   We have seen that in a double-blind study, melatonin, 10 mg at bedtime. brought a cluster period to a close after 3–5 days in 5 of 10 patients with cluster headache (Leone, D'Amico, Moschiano, Fraschini, & Bussone, 1996). Melatonin has also been suggested as treatment for indomethacin-responsive headaches (Rozen, 2003) because of a structural resemblance between the two molecules (Peres, Stiles, Oshinsky, & Rozen, 2001). In support, case studies suggest complete prophylaxis of idiopathic stabbing headache with melatonin, 3–12 mg at bedtime (Rozen, 2003). So far, melatonin does not seem to have been studied for hemicrania continua or chronic paroxysmal hemicrania.

Phytoestrogens are plant compounds that act at estrogen receptors (Setchell, 1998). The isoflavones found principally in soy are the best known, but other plant constituents seem to have estrogenic effects as well. And the efficacy of a mix of **phytoestrogens** on migraines occurring between 2 days before and 3 days after the start of menstruation has been studied by Burke et al., using a double-blind, placebo-controlled 28-week trial (B. E. Burke, R. D. Olson, & Cusack, 2002). The mixture contained 75 mg soy extract standardized to 40 percent isoflavones,

50 mg dong quai extract standardized to 1 percent ligustilide, and 25 mg black cohosh extract standardized to 8 percent triterpenes (B. E. Burke et al.). Forty-nine women were randomly assigned, of whom 38 completed the trial and were compliant with the treatment protocol. There was no differential drop-out, non-compliance, or baseline difference between groups. Over the last 16 weeks of the study (i.e., after a 4-week placebo run-in and the first 8 weeks of treatment) women in the phytoestrogen group had on average 4.7 perimenstrual migraines, vs. 10.3 in the control group, a 56 percent difference ($p < .01$). There was no change in headache severity at first, but over the last 5 weeks of treatment pain intensity was actually 75 percent lower in the phytoestrogen group (2.3/10 vs. 7.3/10 on a visual analogue scale, recorded in the headache diary; B. E. Burke, et al.). Thus, this initial foray into the realm of phytoestrogens is highly encouraging.

It should be noted, however, that whether soy isoflavones act as agonists or antagonists at the estrogen receptor depends in part on their concentration (Setchell, 1998). Thus, the effects of isoflavones might, perhaps, depend on dosage. Also, the effects of isoflavones depend on level of endogenous estrogen (Setchell, 1998), and thus isoflavones might affect migraines differently in men, or in post-menopausal women. Indeed, we saw in Chapter 10 a case report of a male physician who seemed to develop migraine with aura after starting high dose isoflavone supplements (P. A. Engel, 2002). We have barely begun to explore how plant compounds influence migraines.

IMPLICATIONS FOR BEHAVIORAL TREATMENT

We have seen, then, that the various classes of migraine preventives typically reduce migraine activity by 25–50 percent. And as we will see in Chapter 14, meta-analyses and head-to-head comparisons suggest that certain behavioral treatments have the same level of efficacy as the best pharmacological migraine preventives. Moreover, the U.S. Headache Consortium has reviewed nonpharmacological as well as drug treatments, and concluded that there is sound evidence to support the use of relaxation training, thermal biofeedback combined with relaxation training, EMG biofeedback, and cognitive-behavioral therapy in migraine prevention (Campbell, Penzien, & E. M. Wall, 2000).

Although the consortium has not yet listed guidelines for tension-type headache, the behavioral outcome literature (reviewed in Chapter 14) suggests similar degrees of efficacy for non-pharmacological and medication-based regimens. And in chronic daily headaches, the high frequency of medication overuse, depression, other psychiatric conditions, poor compliance, and disability, brings psychological treatment into the foreground (Lake, 2001).

In a sense, even the trials of medication preventives contain an indirect homage to the role of psychological factors in headache. For a typical trial begins with a 4-week placebo run-in phase, during which patients monitor their headaches. Those patients whose headache frequency falls below a requisite minimum are dropped from the study prior to randomization to either active treatment or control. The run-in period helps correct for regression to the mean and, for chronic daily headache, confirms the diagnosis. But it also helps ensure that placebo responders are excluded from the study.[9] And some patients, of course, are not even considered for the research, because of behavioral factors: severe psychiatric comorbidity, drug dependence, medication overuse, or changing neurological exam (e.g., Saper, Silberstein, Lake, & Winters, 1994).

It is entirely fitting, then, that we not stop at pharmacology, but return our gaze to self-management.

---

[9] I am indebted to Kenneth A. Holroyd, Ph.D. for calling my attention to this.

CHAPTER 12

Clinical Assessment in Behavioral Medicine

. . . to discover the ways in which life and text inform each other.
                                        —A. G. Zornberg (1995, p. xi)

As discussed in Chapter 1, it is important that the patient first be assessed by their primary care provider and/or neurologist to rule out headaches secondary to another disorder. In our practice, we instruct would-be self-referrals to contact their medical providers or, if they do not have providers, to present to our hospital's walk-in clinic. Still, after these steps have been taken there remains much for the health psychologist to assess.

CLINICAL INTERVIEW

Diagnosis

The interview has several purposes. First, the clinician should collect enough information to verify the specific benign headache diagnosis. Referring physicians will sometimes use diagnostic terminology in idiosyncratic ways (for example using "cluster headache" to mean "mixed migraine and tension-type"). At other times a referral may be accompanied by a vague diagnosis (e.g., "headaches") or be coded for only one of several relevant categories (for example, a patient referred with chronic daily headache may also have an underlying episodic headache disorder). Of course it is important that the psychologist be as clear as possible in his or her own mind about the nature of the headache disorder.

A psychologist, moreover, will generally have a luxury of time that is not available to the referring physician.[1] Occasionally a patient will tell the psychologist more of their headache history, or different aspects, than they told their doctor. And sometimes a psychologist who specializes in headache treatment will know of diagnostic possibilities with which the primary care physician may be unfamiliar. For example, in our town it seems that few general practitioners consider hemicrania continua as a possibility. Thus, within the range of chronic benign headaches, a specialist psychologist can sometimes assist in unraveling a diagnostic conundrum.

What a psychologist cannot do, of course, is rule out an underlying and potentially life-threatening physical disorder. Moreover, such disorders can mimic migraines, temporomandibular

---

[1]Note that by the late 1990s, office visits with a general practitioner in the United States were approximately 7 minutes in duration (Carr-Hill, Jenkins-Clarke, Dixon, et al., 1998), potentially for covering more than one presenting problem (Lipton et al., 2001).

dysfunction, and chronic daily headaches. Thus, it is very important that a physician be on the case, to verify that the headaches are primary.

Diagnostic questions should follow the IHS criteria, and the extensions to chronic daily headache, discussed in Chapters 1 and 7 of this book.

A simple screening question for TMD is "Do you have pain in or around your jaw joint, in the muscles of your face, or in your ear when at rest?" (Drangsholt & LeResche, 1999). Again, actual diagnosis needs to be by a physician or dentist, as a psychologist cannot rule out unusual, dangerous origins for the pain.

Sustaining Factors

Secondly, the interview is an opportunity to assess factors that may be contributing to the headaches, including:

Primary current stressors, how the patient is handling them currently, and how successful the patient is at managing them. One should particularly observe whether the problem solving style is focused, whether the problem is being formulated in way that maximizes its tractability, and whether there are negative, **automatic thoughts** that might detract from the patient's self-efficacy.

Overall level of stress and balance between stressors and coping resources. External stresses are especially problematic when they serve as reminders of the pain (e.g., a worker's compensation or personal injury case), cue schemas for bodily harm (e.g., long-term injuries in a family member), include or follow major life events, overwhelm coping resources, or lead to marked negative affect. Level of caffeine and nicotine intake is sometimes a useful indication of unmanaged stress (e.g., Eysenck, 1991). Also relevant is the amount and kind of buffering resources, including social support, recreation, and physical self-care.

Stresses can be queried informally, or with the aid of checklists for children (D. E. Williamson, Birmaher, et al., 2003), adolescents (Compas, G. E. Davis, Forsythe, & B. M. Wagner, 1987) or adults (T. H. Holmes & Rahe, 1967). Checklists can be useful for people so numb to stresses they have lost track of them, but we must remember that it is how stresses and appraised and handled, and not simply their existence, that is relevant to health. When evaluating stress in children, we should attend also to how their parents handle stress, the level of coping resources in the family, the child's social and cognitive development, and the child's overall level of sensitivity to the environment (Compas, 1987).

Possible ergonomics factors that may have been overlooked by the patient's previous treatment providers. A particularly egregious yet still-common example involves typing at a keyboard and, simultaneously, cradling a phone receiver with one's shoulder. Other possible ergonomics concerns may arise in construction or factory work, or in poorly designed offices. Suspected ergonomics factors can be followed up during the surface EMG assessment, and should be noted in the report back to the medical treatment provider. Definitive statements about ergonomics and specific corrective recommendations should be left to the patient's medical care provider or physical or occupational therapist.

An overview of exposure to major triggers. The interview should not substitute for prospective trigger monitoring but can provide information for explaining and tailoring the subsequent data collection. For example, one would probably not focus too strongly on nutritional triggers for a patient who maintains a strict macrobiotic diet.

Overuse of analgesics and/or migraine abortives, including over-the-counter analgesics. This is primarily of relevance to chronic daily headache. For migraines and tension-type headaches medication use is primarily a reflection of headache frequency and intensity, and of how well the patient feels able to cope with the headaches. Even here, however, symptomatic medications can lose their effectiveness with too-frequent use. Medication use should be tracked prospectively, but one can often gauge from the interview whether this will need to be a significant focus of treatment. In computing intake, one should be aware of hidden sources of acetaminophen, such as the muscle relaxant Parafon Forte. Analgesics should be counted, even if they are taken for a condition other than headaches.

Indications of an underlying substance abuse disorder.   Often the most avid interest in pain medications can be traced to a high pain level combined with poor coping resources. For some people, however, pain report is simply a means to the end of obtaining narcotics. Early in treatment, a history of substance abuse and information from the primary care provider about inappropriate medication seeking can provide clues to an underlying substance abuse disorder. Interpersonal turmoil, an unusual number of motor vehicle accidents and, of course, sedation in-session, indirectly raise concerns for medication misuse. The best indicator, however, is the patient's reaction as treatment unfolds. Patients generally become excited at the prospect that their headaches can be reduced by any means, including nonpharmacological. When a patient repeatedly discounts non-narcotic, non-benzodiazepine therapies at the outset, and gives them only cursory attention during treatment, a medication-seeking agenda should be considered.

Pain Coping

The interview is an opportunity to screen for elements of chronic pain syndrome that could otherwise prevent successful treatment. Important variables include the following:

Catastrophizing.   In laboratory studies, catastrophization predicts lower pain thresholds and tolerance (C. R. France, J. L. France, al' Absi, Ring, & McIntyre, 2002), and a greater tendency for pain to capture one's attention (Crombez, Eccleston, Baeyens, & Eelen, 1998a). People who score high in catastrophizing cope with experimental pain better if they use coping self-statements than if they try to distract themselves (Heyneman, Fremouw, Gano, Kirkland, & Heiden, 1990). In clinical studies, catastrophization correlates with subsequent increases in pain, disability, and depression (Keefe, G. K. Brown, Wallston, & Caldwell, 1989). Thus, assessment for catastrophic thinking about pain is particularly important.

In most studies, catastrophizing is operationalized as a high score on the relevant scale of the Coping Strategies Questionnaire (Rosenstiel & Keefe, 1983) or the Pain Catastrophizing Scale (M. J. L. Sullivan, Bishop, & Pivik, 1995), which we will discuss in the next section. However, catastrophic thinking can also be gauged from the interview, by asking whether, how often, and under what circumstances, the person feels emotionally overwhelmed by pain. This can lead naturally to cognitive therapy emphasizing self-instructional training, and behavioral tools for reducing pain intensity and thus for building self-efficacy. A tendency to ruminate about pain and to overestimate its negative consequences is also characteristic of catastrophizing (Sullivan, Bishop, & Pivik, 1995) and, when identified, can similarly be a lead-in to cognitive therapy. Especially when there is a history of childhood trauma, it is helpful to look for catastrophic reactions specific to pain flare-ups, not necessarily evident or recalled between flare-ups.

Pain-related anxiety.   People sometimes harbor specific fears that, understandably, promote a somatic focus. For example, they may be worried that their headache signifies an episode of dangerously high blood pressure, an aneurysm, or a brain tumor. Of course, patients with these concerns should always be referred back to their medical providers to talk them over. A psychotherapist can help make the discussion with the medical provider as useful as possible by helping the patient clarify their specific concerns, and the evidence and reasoning behind them. Note that global reassurances may not be helpful in cases of persistent health anxiety (Salkovskis & Warwick, 1986); delineating the concerns and addressing the evidence and underlying reasoning may turn out to be more useful.

Functioning.   As we have seen in chapter 3, descending endorphinergic pain control is recruited by activities that have emotional priority over the pain, and particularly activities that are enjoyable and intrinsically motivating. In daily life, such activities are often provided by involvement in a vocation, including homemaking, and in vocational equivalents such as school and volunteering. To be useful for coping, it is helpful that the activities not activate a pain schema. For example, preparing one's worker's compensation case, although perhaps absorbing, probably contains too many reminders of the pain to be helpful for pain coping.

Thus, at the interview we are interested in determining the amount of time spent on non-pain activities, and the degree of enjoyment, absorption, and meaning that they evoke.

Pacing.   Thus, involvement in functional activity is an important component of pain coping. However, overactivity leading to flare-ups tends to have several disadvantages. As we saw in chapter 2, afferent pain pathways in the dorsal horn tend to become sensitized by exposure to pain, and hence repeated unnecessary exacerbations could lead, logically, to a long-term erosion of pain thresholds. Moreover, engaging in tasks to the point of intense pain can punish activity and create a frustrating sense that "the pain always wins."

At the interview, pacing difficulties can be assessed as the frequency of activity-related pain flare-ups—how often a person has a pain exacerbation because they did too much. Once a week seems to be a typical frequency for avoidable flare-ups; a higher level especially is grounds for work on pacing. We are also interested in the intensity and duration of activity-related flare-ups. Persisting in an activity to the point of extreme pain, or flare-ups that last longer than a day, suggest that pacing issues are of particular concern.

Naturalistic pain coping style.   Although little is known about the long-term effects of the various approaches to pain coping, we have seen reasons to eschew dissociation and efforts at suppressing pain during acute exacerbations. Even more, efforts to purposefully intensify pain, so as to experience a sense of relief afterwards, would seem to have the potential to sensitize afferent pain pathways. Thus, asking the patient about how they respond to their usual pain, and to pain flare-ups, can be illuminating.

Family.   Concern and helpfulness from one's spouse is, of course, neither unexpected nor necessarily bad. Rarely, the headaches are the only occasion for positive attention from the spouse, the spouse is unusually focused on the headaches despite a benign medical work-up, or the spouse is unusually invested in seeing the patient as disabled. More commonly, a patient may not pace or otherwise accommodate the headaches, preferring to outrun them with medication. In that case, the spouse may try to influence the patient towards greater self-care, inadvertently serving as a reminder of the headaches. When the patient and spouse both have pain concerns, a flare-up in the spouse's condition can be a powerful reminder of pain for the patient. Thus, it is helpful to know the degree of pain focus within the family. When it is high, including the spouse in treatment sessions, or at least in their educational component, can be helpful.

It is also useful to include the spouse in at least part of the interview. The spouse may be more aware of declines in the patient's mood and functioning than the patient is. Including the spouse is also a chance to observe the level of pain behaviors, and of pain-contingent solicitous attention. However, the delicate question of suicidal thoughts, plans, and intentions should generally be asked without the spouse present.

Relationship to disability.   Few topics arouse so much controversy and keen feelings as the relationship between pain and disability. In my experience, by far the large majority of patients with chronic pain find limitations on work to be a primary source of frustration, and even anguish. The loss of financial independence, activity, socialization, and career success can leave individuals with chronic pain feeling marginalized and subtly worthless. At the same time, they receive no shortage of criticism and pressure from acquaintances and neighbors. In chapter 2 we saw how central sensitization and a decline in descending inhibitory controls can make chronic pain much more difficult to control than acute pain, but such differences are far from obvious to the lay public.

Disability benefits often seem to be the only way for an individual to make ends meet in the context of medical limitations. Nonetheless, for a minority of patients the network of motivations around disability becomes a more complicated web. Depending on the case, relevant factors seem to include (from my clinical experience):

1. Financial need. An injury can produce high medical bills and lost earnings that need to be recouped for an individual to remain financially solvent. The case may require, or the injured person may feel it requires, ongoing disability in order to turn out favorably. Sometimes the debts cannot be recovered, but at least remain in forbearance as long as the disability remains in effect.

2. Matters of principle. People often find the process of litigation surrounding injury cases to be insulting. They feel that their integrity and motives are questioned. There may be sharply felt treatment delays while matters of legal responsibility are haggled out. And the pain problem itself may have arisen from a work environment that the patient found to be stressful or unsafe. After months or years, the only way to right these wrongs, and to receive acknowledgement for past suffering, may seem to be winning the case. It can be too unpalatable, or impractical, to walk away from the case regardless of the cost of pursuing it.

3. Coping skills deficit. Individuals may lack the skills to navigate an injury without marked loss of vocational functioning. Also, there is sometimes a family or cultural history in which disability benefits are a primary coping tool.

4. Need to be disabled. Although it does not seem to be common, some individuals, particularly those with a strong substance abuse history, seem to accept pain as way of attaining a dependent position in the family. The pain may still be intense and a source of significant suffering. However, the combination of avoidance of stresses, access to prescribed medications, and concerned attention from one's spouse can be very powerful reinforcers for some people. At times, the injury occurs (sometimes through poor pacing) shortly after an addiction is ended, or recovery from the pain is followed by the development of a different type of disability.

Of course the presence of a disability application, or of debts, or of a substance abuse history, is not sufficient to indicate a problematic role of disability benefits. Rather, a key additional question is how the person relates to treatment. If they are subtly dismissive of therapy from the outset, or seem to have little personal investment in specific treatment goals, or do not follow through on homework assignments, or request that reports be worded according to their lawyer's suggestions, then we must entertain the possibility that the litigation needs to be settled prior to treatment. What matters most is not the fact of a disability application, but the patient's relationship to the application, and to specific treatment goals.

Expectations

Finally, the interview is a chance to clarify expectations about the treatment and its likely outcome. Note in particular that it is rare for behavioral medicine treatment to cure or completely eliminate a headache disorder. More realistic goals are usually to reduce the frequency of headaches or, in the case of chronic daily headache, to reduce distress and disability and to increase the patient's ability to cope.

PSYCHOMETRICS

Depression

This should be assessed due to the high comorbidity between headaches and depression. A true clinical depression will often need to be treated before behavioral interventions for tension-type headache can be effective. For other types of headache, and for subclinical dysphoria, the increase in self-efficacy, the experience of success, the reduction in symptoms, the improvements in stress coping, and possibly the behavioral mobilization associated with headache treatment may help reduce the depression as well.

The Beck Depression Inventory (BDI; A. T. Beck, Ward, Mendelson, Mock, & Erlbaugh, 1961; A. T. Beck, Rush, B. F. Shaw, & Emery, 1979) appears to have good validity in pain populations (Geisser, Roth, & Robinson, 1997; Holzberg, Robinson, Geisser, & Gremillion, 1996). Because some items tend to receive endorsements simply as a result of pain, the cut-off score should be higher than the 10 used in psychiatric populations. Love (1987) found that correct classification vs. structured interview was maximized with a cut-off score of 12, J. A. Turner and Romano (1984) achieved good results with a cut-off of 13, and Geisser et al. obtained optimal classification with a threshold of 21. It is unfortunate that the cut-off varies over such a large range. Presumably, variations in the sample and in the exact definition of depression account for the differences (Geisser, Roth, & Robinson, 1997). In our own clinic we use a cut-off of 16, because we found that for 6 items (irritability, sleep difficulty, fatigue, difficulty working, not enjoying things as much, and concern about one's health) the 1-point choice is endorsed more frequently than the 0-point choice, suggesting that the six extra points are an artifact of the pain.

The Depression scale of the Center for Epidemiological Studies (CES-D; Radloff, 1977) has similarly been validated for clinical use with individuals who have chronic pain (Geisser, Roth, & Robinson, 1997; D. C. Turk & Okifuji, 1994). As with the Beck, there is considerable range in the optimal cut-off. D. C. Turk and Okifuji recommend using 19 (versus 16 in a non-medical population) while Geisser et al. recommend 27.

Anxiety

The high comorbidity between migraines and panic disorder, and in clinical samples between chronic tension-type headache and generalized anxiety disorder, suggests that screening measures for anxiety should be included for headache patients. There are several choices in wide use. The

Beck Anxiety Inventory (BAI; A. T. Beck, N. Epstein, G. Brown, & Steer, 1988) is comprised of 21 symptoms designed to maximize discrimination between anxiety and depression. An advantage of the BAI is that it captures both cognitive/subjective symptoms and various types of somatic symptoms (autonomic, motoric, panic sensations), giving a sense of how anxiety presents in that individual (A. Osman, Kopper, Barrios, J. R. Osman, & T. Wade, 1997). In general, a score of 20 or greater is considered strongly suggestive of an anxiety disorder, while a score above 14 should be followed up with diagnostic questions at the interview (R. Ferguson, 2000).

The Penn State Worry Questionnaire (PSWQ), naturally, is a measure of worry (T. J. Meyer, M. L. Miller, Metzger, & Borkovec, 1990). A cutoff score of 62–65 seems to provide maximum sensitivity and specificity in distinguishing generalized anxiety from closely related anxiety disorders (Behar, Alcaine, Zuellig, & Borkovec, 2003; Fresco, Mennin, Heimberg, & C. L. Turk, 2003).

The PRIME-MD (an acronym for Primary Care Evaluation of Mental Disorders; R. L. Spitzer, J. B. W. Williams, Kroenke, et al., 1994) consists of a patient screening questionnaire to which positive responses are followed up by a targeted structured interview designed to give DSM-III-R diagnoses. Mood, anxiety, alcohol, eating, and somatoform disorders are covered. As a whole, the instrument appears to have good sensitivity and specificity. However, when the screening questionnaire is used by itself, accuracy for anxiety disorders is modest due to a high false positive rate.

In contrast to depression, anxiety symptoms are not assumed to show confounding with pain, and no adjustment from the standard norms (Gillis, Haaga, & G. T. Ford, 1995) has been made.

Locus of Control

In chronic tension-type headache, improvements in pain tend to be preceded by improvements in self-efficacy, and by shifts to a more internal **locus of control**. That is, a feeling of control over the headaches tends to become a self-fulfilling prophecy, perhaps because it leads to better problem solving and decreases the emotional impact of stressors. Thus, locus of control is relevant as a process measure, for ensuring that treatment is indeed empowering. The construct seems best measured with the Headache Specific Locus of Control Scale (HSLC; N. J. Martin, K. A. Holroyd, & Penzien, 1990; VandeCreek & O'Donnell, 1992), inspired by the Multidimensional Health Locus of Control Scale (K. A. Wallston, B. S. Wallston, & DeVellis, 1978). The HSLC has three subscales, whose meaning is reflected in the highest loading items:

1. Health Care Professionals locus of control: Following the doctor's medication regimen is the best way for me not to be laid-up with a headache.
2. Internal locus of control: When I drive myself too hard I get headaches.
3. Chance locus of control: When I have a headache, there is nothing I can do to affect its course.

The test has 33 items in total, with good **internal consistency** and test-retest reliability, and preliminary evidence of **construct validity** (N. J. Martin, K. A. Holroyd, & Penzien, 1990; Vande-Creek & O'Donnell, 1992). The full HSLC is given at the end of this chapter.

When a person has an internal locus of control, they hold a model of their illness in which their behavior matters (D. J. French, K. A. Holroyd, Pinell, et al., 2000). For patients in chronic pain, this perspective can be freeing and empowering, but it is still on the conceptual plane. To be useful, the person must also have confidence that they possess specific skills that give them control over headaches on an actual, concrete level. This further step is the domain of self-efficacy, best evaluated with the Headache Management Self-Efficacy Scale (HMSE): a 25-item questionnaire with evidence for internal consistency (Cronbach's alpha = 0.90) and construct validity (D. J. French, K. A. Holroyd, Pinell, Malinoski, O'Donnell, & Hill, 2000). Sample items include "When I'm tense, I can prevent headaches by controlling the tension" and, scored in reverse, "Nothing I do reduces the pain of a headache."

There is evidence that having little internal locus of control, having poor self-efficacy, and high total pain ratings, contribute independently to headache disability (D. J. French, K. A. Holroyd, Pinell, Malinoski, O'Donnell, & Hill, 2000).

Catastrophization

Catastrophization, as we have seen, involves rumination, feelings of helplessness, and an exaggerated appraisal of the negative consequences of the pain (M. J. L. Sullivan, Bishop, & Pivik, 1995). In practice, the construct has been defined as a high score on the relevant scale of the Coping Strategies Questionnaire (CSQ; Rosenstiel & Keefe, 1983). In the literature, the scale is not usually used in isolation from the rest of the CSQ. However, the flavor of the construct can be seen by looking at the scale items, scored 0 ("never do that") to 6 ("always do that"), with the middle value, 3, anchored as "sometimes do that":

It's awful and I feel it's never going to get any better.

It's awful and I feel that it overwhelms me.

I feel my life isn't worth living.

I worry all the time about whether it (the pain) will end.

I feel I can't stand it anymore.

I feel like I can't go on.

Alternatively, Sullivan et al. have developed the Pain Catastrophizing Scale, a 13-item instrument with normative data (M. J. L. Sullivan, Bishop, & Pivik, 1995).

Note, however, that the full construct need not be present to have deleterious effects on pain coping. For example, a person may harbor a more specific fear—that the pain will not end, that it will get worse, and that neither self-management nor treatment will be able to bring it under control. The patient may seem to use narcotics as much to treat the fear as the pain. Relevant items on the Pain Catastrophizing Scale may provide an indication of this process.

Note, too, that reports in the interview of feeling overwhelmed by pain need not be synonymous with catastrophization. Some patients, particularly those who do not pace themselves, may use the term matter-of-factly, without much anguish or fear, to mean that the pain has temporarily defeated their efforts to contain it.

Fear of Pain

Fear of pain may be particularly relevant in patients who are highly disabled by headaches, who are overusing headache medications, or whose lifestyles have become very constricted. The primary instrument in this area is the Fear of Pain Questionnaire—III (D. W. McNeil & Rainwater, 1998; A. Osman, Breitenstein, Barrios, Gutierrez, & Kopper, 2002). An earlier version was shown to predict self-ratings of the emotional and functional impact of headaches (Hursey & Jacks, 1992). Surprisingly, there is some evidence that fear of pain is independent of pain catastrophizing, self-efficacy, and internal locus of control (Hursey & Jacks, 1992).

Disability

In a factor analysis of headache-related self-report items and scales, K. A. Holroyd and coworkers found that three questions seemed to best capture the disability factor (K. A. Holroyd, Malinoski, M. K. Davis, & Lipchik, 1999). Each question is answered on a 0–10 scale anchored by "no interference" at 0 and "unable to carry out any activities" at 10.

1. In the past 6 months, how much have your headaches interfered with your daily activities?
2. In the past 6 months, how much have your headaches interfered with your ability to take part in recreational, social and family activities?
3. In the past 6 months, how much have your headaches interfered with your ability to work (including housework)?

Holroyd et al.'s study also included the SF–20, or Medical Outcomes Study Short Form General Health Survey (Ware & Sherbourne, 1992; Ware, Sherbourne, & A. R. Davies, 1992). However, the social and role functioning subscales of the SF–20 had much lower loadings on the disability factor than the above three questions, and the physical functioning subscale loaded instead on an affective distress factor.

An alternative measure is the *Migraine Disability Assessment Scale*, or MIDAS, which was designed to be brief, intuitive, and psychometrically sound (Stewart, Lipton, Whyte, et al., 1999). In fact, the MIDAS scale consists of only seven questions:

Instructions.   Please answer the following questions about ALL the headaches you have had over the last 3 months. Write your answer in the box next to each question. Write zero if you did not do the activity in the last 3 months. (Please refer to the calendar below, if necessary.)

1. On how many days in the last 3 months did you miss work or school because of your headaches?
2. How many days in the last 3 months was your productivity at work or school reduced by half or more because of your headaches (do not include days you counted in question 1 where you missed work or school)?
3. On how many days in the last 3 months did you not do household work because of your headaches?
4. How many days in the last 3 months was your productivity in household work reduced by half or more because of your headaches (do not include days you counted in question 3 where you did not do household work)?
5. On how many days in the last 3 months did you miss family, social, or leisure activities because of your headaches?
A. On how many days in the last 3 months did you have any headache (if a headache lasted more than one day, count each day)?
B. On a scale of 0 to 10, on average how painful were these headaches (0 = no pain at all, and 10 = pain is as bad as it can be)?

A person's score on the MIDAS scale is simply the sum of their answers to questions 1 through 5. The score is then sometimes condensed into a disability grade: I (0–5 on MIDAS;

little disability); II (6–10; mild); III (11–20; moderate); and IV (>20; severe; Lipton, Stewart, A. M. Stone, Láinez, & J. P. C. Sawyer, 2000).

Stewart et al. studied the instrument's reliability in two population-based studies, one in Great Britain and one in the United States. (The samples were not precisely random because not all eligible subjects agreed to participate.) The researchers found a coefficient α of 0.76 in the United States and 0.73 in Britain, suggesting that there is indeed a single domain of content underlying the five items. Three-week test-retest reliability (which is likely to have been suppressed due to some degree of true change in migraine disability over the interval) was low at approximately 0.64 for the individual items, but quite favorable (0.80, United States; 0.83, Britain) for the scale as a whole (Stewart, Lipton, Whyte, et al., 1999).

At first glance, the MIDAS would seem to have muddled measurement properties. People who are unemployed, even if it is because of headaches, skip the first two items and thus have a lower possible maximum score. Days of substantially reduced effectiveness are counted the same as days of complete absenteeism. Moreover, one day can count as three, if employment, housework, and leisure activities are all disrupted. Yet the MIDAS has much to commend it. It is easy to complete and score. Its approximate unit of measurement, lost part-days due to migraine, is intuitively meaningful (Stewart, Lipton, Dowson, & Sawyer, 2001). And it correlates reasonably well with a prospective diary measure of the same variables (Stewart, Lipton, Kolodner, Sawyer, Lee, & Liberman, 2000), is sensitive to treatment effects (D'Amico, et al., 2003), and predicts the intensity of pharmacological treatments needed to effect improvement (Lipton, Stewart, Stone, Láinez, & Sawyer, 2000). Despite its name, items on the MIDAS refer to "headache" in general; thus despite the absence of specific validation, it seems reasonable to use the instrument for other primary headache disorders.

Other instruments are available as well. The *Headache Disability Inventory* (HDI) is relatively short (25 items) and straightforward to score, with excellent **internal consistency** and good 1-week ($r = .95$) and 2-month test-retest stability (G. P. Jacobson, Ramadan, Aggarwal, & Newman, 1994; G. P. Jacobson, Ramadan, Norris, & Newman, 1995). Scores correlate reasonably well with spouse perceptions (G. P. Jacobson, Ramadan, Norris, & Newman, 1995) and improve with treatment (Holroyd, O'Donnell, Stensland, Lipchik, Cordingley, & B. W. Carlson, 2001). Despite its name, however, the HDI assesses the effects of headache on emotional well being as well as functioning, and seems to be a slightly better measure of affective distress than disability (Holroyd, Malinoski, M. K. Davis, & Lipchik, 1999). The items that deal with functioning are rather global (e.g., "Because of my headaches I feel restricted in performing my routine daily activities"), and seem to be sensitive to intensity but not frequency of headache (G. P. Jacobson, Ramadan, Aggarwal, & Newman, 1994). It seems to be similar in spirit, and to give similar results, to the Life Interference scale on the West Haven-Yale Multidimensional Pain Inventory (J. E. Magnusson & Becker, 2003).

The *Migraine-Specific Quality of Life Questionnaire* (MSQ) is a 14-item scale designed to assess three dimensions of perceived migraine-related impairment: interference in activities ("Role Restrictive"), interruption of activities ("Role Preventive"), and emotional reactions to impairment ("Emotional Function"). The instrument has excellent reliability (coefficient α = 0.86–0.96 for the three scales), and evidence of **construct validity** (B. C. Martin, et al., 2000). The MSQ appears to have a strong monotonic relationship to other headache disability measures, and in fact seems to be covering essentially the same range of the same underlying construct (Ware, Bjorner, & Kosinski, 2000).

The *Headache Impact Test* (HIT) differs from the other instruments in two respects. First, it was derived through **item response theory** (Ware, Bjorner, & Kosinski, 2000). This approach allowed each individual item to be calibrated for the range of disability it covers, and the degree of disability at which it is most sensitive (Embretson & Reise, 2000). This, in turn, permits computerized adaptive testing: Broad early questions allow the computer to make a rough estimate of headache impact, and to select subsequent questions to hone in more precisely (Wainer, 2000). As a result, computerized versions of the Headache Impact Test can usually give precise estimates after 5 items have been administered (Ware, Bjorner, & Kosinski, 2000). Alternatively, there is a 6-item pencil-and-paper version (the HIT–6). Both are available on the internet, at www.headachetest.com.

The HIT is distinguished also in covering milder forms of impact, for example, feeling irritable during a migraine (Pryse-Phillips, 2002). Such breadth of coverage seems to make the instrument more sensitive for detecting change (Ware, Bjorner, & Kosinski, 2000), but whether it is clinically useful to measure such subtle forms of disability is unclear.

Oral Habits

As we have seen, parafunctional oral behaviors, such as clenching one's teeth or thrusting one's jaw, appear to play a perpetuating role in temporomandibular disorders and may contribute to migraines and tension-type headache. Moss et al. have presented research, and hence validational data, on a simple questionnaire quantifying parafunctional behaviors (Moss, Ruff, & Sturgis, 1984). In the questionnaire, respondents are asked to estimate the frequency with which they engage in nine oral behaviors:

How often do you

1.   Clench your teeth together?
2.   Bite your lips or tongue?
3.   Chew on pens or pencils?
4.   Bite the side of your mouth?
5.   Cup your chin in your hand?
6.   Rest your head with the hand on the side of your face?
7.   Thrust or jut your jaw forward?
8.   Hold the telephone receiver between your chin and shoulders?
9.   Chew gum?

(Moss, Ruff, & Sturgis, 1984). Responses are given on a 5-point scale, in which 1 = almost never, 2 = occasionally, 3 = often, 4 = very often, and 5 = almost always. Responses to four items (clenching one's teeth, cupping one's chin in one's hand, resting one's hand on the side of the face, and thrusting one's jaw forward) distinguish patients with temporomandibular disorders, migraines, or tension-type headaches from non-pain control subjects. In some cases, these items distinguish the three pain categories from each other (Moss, Ruff, & Sturgis, 1984). The most important item appears to be the first one, clenching one's teeth. At this point, the questionnaire does not appear to have published norms, and it is undoubtedly less accurate than prospective self-monitoring of the behaviors. However, the questionnaire is brief and efficient, and the variables for which it screens appear quite relevant to headache assessments.

Chronic Pain

In our experience, most people with even frequent headaches do not show an overlying chronic pain syndrome. However, because chronic pain syndrome requires a different treatment approach, and generally will not remit with standard headache treatments, it is best to screen for it at the outset. At our clinic we use the West Haven-Yale Multidimensional Pain Inventory (Kerns, D. C. Turk, & Rudy, 1985), the Multidimensional Health Locus of Control Scale (K. A. Wallston, B. S. Wallston, & DeVellis, 1978), and the Survey of Pain Attitudes (M. P. Jensen, J. A. Turner, Romano, & Lawler, 1994).

A Minimal Battery

The headache burden itself (frequency, intensity, duration, and associated features) is best captured through a prospective diary, described later in the chapter. Disability is also important to assess, as a measure of the impact of headaches, and of the efficacy and cost-effectiveness of treatment (K. A. Holroyd, Lipchik, & Penzien, 1998). Disability can be recorded in the diary, or quantified psychometrically. Questionnaires are also useful in screening for depression, Generalized Anxiety Disorder, and other forms of psychiatric comorbidity (e.g., Panic Disorder, Posttraumatic Stress Disorder) that might need to be addressed in or before treatment (Lipchik, K. A. Holroyd, & Nash, 2002). Thus, in episodic headaches, a useful minimal battery might include, for example, the Beck Depression Inventory, the MIDAS, and the PRIME-MD (Lipchik, K. A. Holroyd, & Nash, 2002) or the Beck Anxiety Inventory. I also recommend including the Headache Specific Locus of Control Scale, for its pedagogic use in highlighting a key construct in treatment.

When medication overuse is suspected, a measure of catastrophic thinking can help in gauging readiness for a medication taper. Thus, the Pain Catastrophizing Scale or the Coping Strategies Questionnaire should be included. Patients with high scores may need to work on pain tolerance and coping before or during the detoxification. (However, the psychometrics should not substitute for the interview or headache diary. The scales can give false negatives, it seems, when catastrophization does not emerge until the taper gets underway, or when pain-related thoughts are more depressive than anxious.)

At this point, chronic daily headaches seem best approached as a type of chronic pain syndrome, for which the West Haven-Yale Multidimensional Pain Inventory, the Survey of Pain Attitudes, and a measure of pain catastrophization are appropriate. In clinical work, the oral habits questionnaire seems useful mostly as a form of self-assessment, so that patients can gauge their progress.

PSYCHOPHYSICAL ASSESSMENT (SENSORY TESTING)

We have seen that a decreased threshold for pressure pain (**mechanical allodynia**) is the most consistent physical finding in chronic tension-type headache. Episodic migraines are accompanied by a spread of hyperalgesia from the affected side of the head, to the unaffected side, and ultimately to the ipsilateral forearm. As headaches become more frequent, we might suspect that central sensitization, or impaired descending inhibition, or both, play a progressively greater role (Buchgreitz, Lyngberg, Bendtsen, & R. Jensen, 2006).

Thus, a complete description of a person's headaches would include measures of central sensitization and of the effectiveness of descending pain inhibitory systems. As the basic research develops, sensory testing might allow patient subtyping (Hurtig, Raak, Kendall, Gerdle, & Wahren, 2001), and perhaps more refined treatments. At this point, however, detailed psychophysical assessment has just begun to make the transition from laboratory to clinical application. Much more work is needed in the basic science, and direct sensory testing is not yet part of the traditional repertoire of clinical psychology. However, we can sketch some of the components such testing might include.

Pressure pain thresholds are commonly assessed in the laboratory with von Frey filaments or, to use the original term, "hair esthesiometer" (Boring, 1932; Fruhstorfer, Gross, & Selbmann, 2001; von Frey, 1896). Each of several filaments in turn is pressed perpendicularly into the skin (J. Campbell, Lahuerta, & Bowsher, 1996). The force at which each filament bends is known, and hence a series of filaments of increasing stiffness can be used to measure the limen of punctuate pain. An alternative is the use of **algometers**. As the tip of the algometer is pressed against the skin, the pressure at which the patient reports pain is read from the instrument's strain gauge (Antonaci, Sand, & Lucas, 1998). A third device, of very high ecological validity but so far extant only as a specially built device, consists of a force transducing film held over the fingers. This allows the examiner to palpate muscles as would be done in a physical exam, but to simultaneously obtain measurements of the degree of pressure exerted (Bendtsen, Jensen, & Olesen, 1996b; Tunks, Crook, Norman, & Kalaher, 1988). A reduction in pressure pain threshold can be due to tissue damage, peripheral sensitization, and/or central sensitization. The case for a central process is stronger when abnormal sensitivity is widespread, or is well removed from sites of injury.

Note that the three devices for pressure pain are not strictly comparable. As punctuate stimuli, Von Frey hairs deform the skin, and thus primarily activate receptors in the epidermis. In contrast, pressure algometers, particularly those with large, rubber tips, and manual palpation, deform the skin only minimally, and primarily activate receptors in underlying deep tissues such as muscles and tendons (Treede, Rolke, Andrews, & Magerl, 2002). In tension-type headache, temporomandibular dysfunction and fibromyalgia, it is these deep tissues specifically that appear sensitized (Treede, Rolke, Andrews, & Magerl, 2002). By contrast, in conditions such as reflex sympathetic dystrophy it is the cutaneous afferents that seem to be affected.

Electrical stimuli are, of course, unnatural. There are no dedicated receptors for electricity in the skin; the current seems to directly stimulate the sensory nerves (Gracely, 1999). Nonetheless, as a pain stimulus electricity has several advantages. The precise control of timing allows measurement of temporal summation of pain, which can be an indicator of central sensitization (Curatolo, Petersen-Felix, Arendt-Nielsen, Giani, Zbinden, & Radanov, 2001; Staud, Vierck, Cannon, Mauderli, & D. D. Price, 2001). And different frequencies of stimulation can be used to selectively target a particular type of nerve. Thus, $A\beta$, $A\delta$, and C fibers can be stimulated separately (Radwan, Saito, & Goto, 2001).

Thresholds (or, alternatively, tolerance) for hot and cold pain are usually tested with a thermode, whose surface is heated or cooled electrically at known rate and within safe ranges (Fruhstorfer, Lindblom, & W. G. Schmidt, 1976). The patient indicates pain threshold by pressing a button, which automatically records the temperature and reverses the temperature back to a comfortable value. There is some evidence that in neuralgia, cold allodynia predicts responsiveness of the pain to a sympathetic block (Wahren, Torebjörk, & Nyström, 1991). Thus, it would be intriguing to know whether cold allodynia in other conditions predicts improvement from thermal biofeedback, learned reduction in sympathetic tone, and whether the biofeedback is best focused on the hand or on the site of pain.

In contrast, central sensitization may not extend to heat (Curatolo, Petersen-Felix, Arendt-Nielsen, Giani, Zbinden, & Radanov, 2001; P. Svensson, List, & Hector, 2001), and thus heat-induced pain may be useful as a control condition. Threshold for heat-induced pain can be affected by anxiety (Rhudy & Meagher, 2000).

In the cold pressor test, a person submerges their non-dominant hand in circulating ice water for 5 minutes or until tolerance is reached. Although normed only for immersion time (N. E. Walsh, Schoenfeld, Ramamurthy, & J. Hoffman, 1989), the test allows qualitative assessment of thoughts and feelings in response to pain increase, and sensory experiences (such as the spread of pain to the shoulder or shoulder blade, reminiscent of secondary hyperalgesia). Thus, the cold pressor test provides a way of separating behavioral, cognitive/emotional, and sensory aspects of pain tolerance.[2]

PSYCHOPHYSIOLOGICAL ASSESSMENT

As we have seen, the underlying pathophysiology of migraines, and of the episodic form of tension-type headache, seems to be adversely affected by stress. Thus, the psychophysiological assessment, in which we gauge the level of stress-related physiological responding, can help focus behavioral treatment. The assessment should include a surface EMG component, finger temperature, and heart rate and/or skin conductance level.

If treatment is clinic-based and biofeedback equipment is readily available, the routine inclusion of psychophysiological assessment can be useful. Patients feel validated, the mind-body effect is more vivid, and in a significant minority, signs of very high vigilance, arousal, or muscle tension suggest the specific utility of biofeedback training. This seems especially important in cases of posttraumatic headache and frequent migraines, for which more intensive treatment is often needed. On the other hand, episodic migraine and tension-type headache often respond to briefer intervention, and a biofeedback assessment can generally be omitted without loss of efficacy.

Surface Electromyography (sEMG)

As noted in chapter 6, active muscle contraction requires propagation, along muscle cells, of action potentials, similar to those that propagate along the axons of nerve cells. In surface **electromyography** (sEMG) we record, with electrodes at the skin, the voltage changes that arise from these muscle action potentials (De Luca, 1979; Stern, W. J. Ray, Quigley, 2001). A number of variables can then be extracted from the signal. For example, with an array of microelectrodes and sophisticated signal processing software, we could triangulate and track individual muscle action potentials, and then calculate their rate of travel along single muscle fibers (Zwarts, Drost, & Stegeman, 2000). Or with a simple bipolar electrode we could examine the frequency distribution of the EMG signal, extracting the median and mean frequencies. The possible utililty of these three variables—mean frequency, median frequency, and single fiber conduction velocity— is the object of ongoing research (Zwarts, Drost, & Stegeman, 2000). For now, however, the primary variable extracted from the surface EMG signal is generally its total amplitude. As amplitude is monotonically and in some cases linearly related to force of isometric contraction, amplitude is an index of muscle tension (Stern, W. J. Ray, Quigley, 2001).

The surface EMG assessment should include the major pericranial muscles: frontalis, temporalis, masseter, upper trapezius, cervical paraspinals, splenius cervicis, and sternocleidomastoids. The accuracy of the assessment seems to go up as the number of sites increases, as we generally do not know a priori which sites will be important in a given patient's headaches (Arena, Hannah, Bruno, J. D. Smith, & Meador, 1991; Schoenen, 1991). At our clinic, we generally take readings at rest (initial baseline) and during and after voluntary contraction of the muscle (dynamic assessment).

---

[2]E. H. Weber, the first modern psychophysicist, found that in right-handed subjects, thresholds for temperature and weight (and by extension for pain) were lower on the left side of the body (Weber, 1834/1996). This effect has been verified for punctuate and thermal pain (e.g., Özcan, Tulum, Pinar, & Ba_kurt, 2004; Sarlani, Farooq, & J. Greenspan, 2003), and may relate to specialization of the right cerebral hemisphere (Pauli, Wiedemann, & Nickola, 1999). Whether norms for clinical practice will need to take account of laterality is unclear, however. Side differences are not generally found for deep pressure pain (Rolke et al., 2005).

A number of factors affect the values obtained in surface EMG recordings. Clinicians should be familiar with the characteristics of their equipment, of course, and take into account the characteristics of equipment used in research monographs. Important features include the following:

Filtering.   The EMG signal is not concentrated at a single frequency, but is spread out over the range of approximately 20 to 1000 Hz. The distribution of amplitudes as a function of frequency is highly skewed, having a mode at roughly 60 Hz. Filtering is necessary because unless the room is electrically shielded it will have strong extraneous electrical fields, especially at the oscillation frequency of wall current (60 Hz in North and much of South America, 50 Hz nearly everywhere else).

Three approaches have been taken to filtering. The first, used in most commercial biofeedback machines, is termed "common mode rejection." Machines utilizing this have two active sites on each electrode (bipolar electrodes) and circuitry that filters out signals reaching the two active sites simultaneously. Because electrical interference travels at the speed of light, it will be picked up at the two active sites at the same time and be screened out. Common mode rejection introduces interesting properties into the equipment: (a) The two active sites should be arranged in parallel to the muscle fibers. If the arrangement is perpendicular, then some amount of the muscle signal will reach the two sites simultaneously and be treated as noise. Note that this can allow some monitoring of an underlying muscle if it is perpendicular to a more superficial muscle, as the electrode can be oriented to partially screen out the overlying muscle's activity. We have had some success reading the rhomboids in partial isolation from the lower trapezius in this way. (b) Some of the EMG signal will be deleted by common mode rejection circuitry if the two active sites straddle the neuromuscular junction, as discussed below.

A second technique, which is sometimes used along with common mode rejection, is to place a notch filter at 60 Hz, to focally screen out interference from wall current. This actually does not remove all of the interference, both because the notch filter will inevitably let some noise through, and because wall current can induce "overtones" at multiples of 60 Hz, especially at 120 Hz.

The third technique, implemented differently by different equipment manufacturers, is to truncate the frequency range of the EMG signal. At least 3 versions are in common use. (a) The recorded frequency band can be limited to the 100–200 Hz range, popularized as the J&J narrow filter. Now, as most of the EMG signal is around 60 Hz, this filter removes a great deal of signal as well as noise. It would only be appropriate if the power at 100–200 Hz is a relatively constant proportion of the power in the full EMG signal. It would not be appropriate if the power can shift substantially to lower frequencies, for example with cooling or with muscle fatigue. (b) At the other extreme, the EMG can be measured across the full 20–1000 Hz signal bandwidth (with a notch filter at 60 Hz). There is reasonably good evidence, however, that the skin screens out frequencies above 400 Hz (e.g., A. Van Boxtel, 2001) and hence frequencies above this may contain more noise than signal. (c) In between these two extremes are filters that pass a 30–300 Hz or a 20–400 Hz, or similar bandwidth. These filters are designed to pick up the frequencies having most of the EMG signal.

In general, wider bandwidths give higher readings, due to both increased signal and increased noise. Cram et al. report that shifting from the traditional J&J narrow filter (100–200 Hz.) to a wide filter (25–1000 Hz.) is *approximately* equivalent to multiplying the readings by 1.41 (Cram, Kasman, & Holtz, 1998). Cram and Garber (1986) found that the correlation between readings obtained with the narrow and wide J&J filters was 0.97 at the temporalis, 0.97 at L3 paraspinals, 0.96 at the masseter, and 0.91 at the frontalis. However, the correlation was only 0.89 at the upper trapezius, 0.83 at the sternocleidomastoids, 0.76 at the cervical paraspinals, and 0.71 at the abdomen. Whether these regional differences are due to differences at frequencies greater than

200 or less than 100 Hz is not known, nor is the relative contribution of signal and noise to the discrepancies. Because the correlations are between the same signals, sent through a Y-coupler to the two different bandpass units, simple unreliability of measurement is not playing a role.

On theoretical grounds, however, we would assert that if the surface EMG signal has little power above 400 Hz., then a 20–1000 Hz. bandpass should allow in more noise, and hence give less reliable readings, than a 100–200 Hz. bandpass. There is some evidence to support this. For a Schwartz-Mayo electrode placement (described below) Hudzinski and Lawrence report average test-retest correlations of approximately 0.64 for the J&J wide filter, and approximately 0.77 for the narrow filter (Hudzinski & Lawrence, 1990).

Integration.   The raw EMG signal involves both positive and negative voltage deviations. Thus, total EMG activity cannot be computed as the sum of these deviations because the opposite signs will cancel, partially nullifying the signal. Two alternatives have been adopted in practice. One is to take each deviation's absolute value before adding. After correcting for time and area, this is called the mean rectified value of the EMG signal. The second approach is to square the deviations, average them, and then take the square root. This is analogous to computing the standard deviation and, naturally enough, is called the root mean square (RMS) of the EMG. For the same signal, the results of these two integrating techniques are highly correlated.

Skin preparation.   The top layer of the epidermis, the stratum corneum, is dehydrated, lipophilic and, together with skin oils, an electrical insulator. The amount of electrical artifact that this introduces depends on the ratio of electrical resistance at the electrode-skin junction to the internal resistance, or input impedance, in the biofeedback equipment. In general, the electrode-skin impedance should not exceed 10 percent of the machine's internal impedance. For newer equipment, internal impedance is usually at least 100 mega-ohms, and hence high external resistance can be tolerated. Still, some skin preparation is needed. The most important ingredient is mild abrasion, which can be accomplished by rubbing the area 4 to 6 times with an alcohol pad (Cram & Rommen, 1989). Use of electrically conducting gel is not strictly necessary on newer machines, but it is helpful for preventing movement artifacts. That is, if the electrode pulls away from the skin *slightly*, the gel can act as a bridge, maintaining the electrical contact. When artifact persists despite extensive skin prep, it is helpful to ask the patient whether they have used a rich lotion or soap and, if so, to have them avoid it before future biofeedback sessions.

Careful skin preparation may be particularly important when assessing children. Pritchard noted in passing unusually high skin resistances in the course of an EMG study in children (Pritchard, 1995).

Electrode placement.   The standard electrode placement sites as given in surface EMG chapters and textbooks (e.g., Fridlund & Cacioppo, 1986; Lippold, 1967; see Figure 12–1) are generally useful as ways of coordinating one's work with the larger body of literature. However, especially for older texts, there are exceptions. Significantly for headache treatment, two of these exceptions are the upper trapezius and the frontalis.

For the upper trapezius, one tradition has been to place the sensor at the midpoint of the line joining the C7 spinous process (the big bone at the base of the neck) with the acromion (the bony prominence at the outside of the shoulder). However, at this location the sensor will approximately straddle the motor endplate. Now, motor action potentials spread out symmetrically from the endplate, and thus will reach the two active sites on the electrode at overlapping periods of time. This is a problem because, as noted above, surface EMG equipment generally includes a noise-reducing algorithm, common mode rejection, in which a signal that reaches the two active

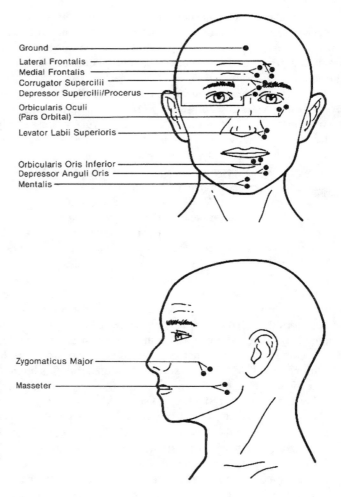

FIGURE 12–1. Standard electrode placements for cranial surface EMG. From "Guidelines for Human Electromyographic Research," by A. J. Fridlund and J. T. Cacioppo, 1986, *Psychophysiology, 38*, p. 571. Copyright 1986 by the Society for Psychophysiological Research, Inc. Reprinted with permission.

sites simultaneously is filtered out. Thus, some portion of the EMG signal is lost if the sensor straddles the motor endplate. Worse, the amount of lost signal will depend on the exact location of the sensor and of the motor endplate. Hence, the readings will be unreliable, and will be affected by arm position (which causes the skin to move over the muscle and thus changes the sensor's position slightly). After studying 16 possible upper trapezius sites, Westgaard and coworkers concluded that an alternative region is preferable, approximately 2 cm (0.8 inches) closer to the acromion than the C7-acromion midpoint (C. Jensen, Vasseljen, & Westgaard, 1993). This site is approximately 70% of the distance from C7 out to the acromion. Readings there have a number of desirable properties including maximum reliability, minimum influence of arm position, little "cross talk" (interference) from neighboring muscles, and a linear relationship to force. That is, during scapular elevation (hunching one's shoulders), the EMG signal expressed as a percent of maximum voluntary contraction is approximately equal to the force generated by the muscle, expressed as a percent of maximum force (C. Jensen, Vasseljen, & Westgaard, 1993). Note that sensor placements far lateral on the shoulder, near the acromion, will miss most of the trapezius signal and read primarily from the underlying supraspinatus (C. Jensen, Vasseljen, & Westgaard, 1993).

For the frontalis, the convention has been to use a bipolar electrode with one active site over each eyebrow, approximately 2 inches from midline. Note, however, that this orients the electrode perpendicularly to the muscle fibers. In theory, this would maximize signal loss due to common mode rejection. More accurate readings should result when one active site is above (closer to the vertex than) the other, in a vertical arrangement (C. M. Davis, Brickett, Stern, & Kimball, 1978). In an experimental study, however, Williamson et al. found that the EMG signal recorded above one eyebrow correlated only 0.13 with the signal from the contralateral side (D. A. Williamson, L. H. Epstein, & Lombardo, 1980). Presumably this is because the left and right frontales are actually two separate muscles, albeit with the same function. Moreover, in the Williamson et al. study, readings from the horizontal placement provide better discrimination between subject-produced high, medium and low levels of muscle tension. Thus, the horizontal placement appears to give a stronger and more reliable signal, perhaps because it is integrating over a larger area (D. A. Williamson, L. H. Epstein, & Lombardo, 1980). Still, two caveats should be noted before recommending the horizontal placement. First, as Davis, et al. point out, it makes more sense to locate each active site above the pupil of one eye, rather than two inches from midline, for in the latter placement the actual anatomic location will depend on the size and shape of the head. Second, in modern bipolar electrodes the active sites are built in at a fixed distance, e.g., 2 cm from center to center. In this case, a horizontal arrangement will read primarily from one of the two frontales, the advantages of a large area of integration will not accrue, and common mode rejection may indeed emerge as a source of signal loss. It appears that the best approach in such a case is to use snap leads to extend the effective size of the electrode. If these are not available, the vertical arrangement appears preferable.

So far, our interest has been in assessing specific muscles with as much accuracy and discrimination as possible. A radical departure from this approach is found in the Schwartz-Mayo placement, apparently first proposed by B. G. Nevins and M. S. Schwartz (1985, cited in Hudzinski & Lawrence, 1988). In this system, the two active posts of a bipolar electrode are separated. One post is placed on the frontalis, above the pupil of, say, the right eye. The second post is attached to the mid-cervical paraspinal muscles on the right side. The resulting readings should be a broad summary of tension in the right-sided pericranial muscles. Now, Hudzinski and Lawrence (1988) reasoned that if this placement were valid, muscle tension readings should be higher in individuals with chronic tension-type headache during a headache state, as compared with outside of a headache state, and as compared with healthy control subjects. In fact, with a standard frontal placement, headache patients did have higher readings than the nonpatients, but only on the left (3.38 microvolts vs. 1.31, $p < .05$). There was no difference on the right (0.52 vs. 0.28, ns). In contrast, the Schwartz-Mayo placement gave strong results on both the left (7.20 vs. 3.32; $p < .01$) and right (6.95 vs. 3.09; $p < .01$). Similar results were found when comparing patients during vs. outside of a headache attack.

Static assessment.   In the static assessment, readings are taken at rest, and interpreted with respect to normative values. The literature for normative values is surprisingly sparse, but there appears to be reasonably good agreement among the available studies.

For pericranial placements, these norms are shown in Tables 12–1 to 12–6. For a given site, the clinician would find the study whose equipment, subjects and posture (e.g., sitting or standing, eyes open or closed) most closely resembles the conditions of assessment. Then, the mean and standard deviation of the study can be used to convert the client's baseline reading into a z-score:

$$z = (\text{baseline reading}-\text{normative mean})/\text{normative standard deviation}.$$

This rough benchmarking can give a sense of the magnitude of elevation, and seems particularly informative in cases of posttraumatic headache and temporomandibular dysfunction arising from a dental injury, when the readings at rest may be as high as 30 standard deviations above the general population mean.

Frontalis.   For static assessment of the frontalis, it seems preferable that the patient be sitting, have their eyes closed, and not be anticipating a laboratory stressor (Wittrock, 1997).

Norms for the frontalis are shown in Table 12–1. The difference between the norms of the Jensen et al. study and those of the other studies probably in part reflects the wider bandpass. In addition, we must remember that "general population" is not equivalent to "pain free population" when it comes to headaches. Nine percent of the Jensen et al. sample had either chronic tension-type headaches or migraines, and another 26% met IHS criteria for episodic tension-type headache.

Anterior temporalis norms are given in Table 12–2. Again, the higher values obtained by Fogle and Glaros (1995) and by Jensen, et. al. (1994) seem explained by the wider bandpass.

Upper trapezius.   Norms for the upper trapezius are given in Table 12–3.

In the literature, the best discrimination for the upper trapezius seems to be when the subject is prone or else sitting without back support (Arena, Hannah, Bruno, J. D. Smith, & Meador, 1991), or during the recovery phase following, say, 5 seconds of scapular elevation (Middaugh & Kee, 1987; Middaugh, Kee, & Nicholson, 1994). In our practice, static readings of the trapezius seem to offer the best discrimination when the patient is standing, arms at their sides. However, this may be an artifact of our patient population, in which headaches are often secondary to

TABLE 12–1
Surface EMG Norms—Frontalis

Source	Population	Position	Equipment	Left Mean	Left Std. Dev.	Right Mean	Right Std. Dev.
Cram & Engstrom, 1986	104 Adult Ed Students, No Pain Problem in Past 2 Years	Sitting	J&J M–501 100–200 Hz. Bandpass	2.0 μVolts	2.1 μVolts	1.8 μVolts	1.9 μVolts
Cram & Engstrom, 1986	104 Adult Ed Students, No Pain Problem in Past 2 Years	Standing	J&J M–501 100–200 Hz. Bandpass	2.0 μVolts	2.0 μVolts	2.1 μVolts	2.0 μVolts
R. Jensen, Fuglsang-Frederiksen, & Olesen, 1994	Random Sample of General Population, $N = 547$	Supine	Dantec Counterpoint 20–1000 Hz. Bandpass, RMS Values	not measured	not measured	4.1 μVolts	2.1 μVolts
Matheson, Toben, & de la Cruz, 1988	73 College Students, No Pain Difficulties	Sitting	J&J M–53 100–200 Hz. Bandpass	2.0 μVolts	1.4 μVolts	1.8 μVolts	1.4 μVolts

TABLE 12–2
Surface EMG Norms—Anterior Temporalis

Source	Population	Position	Equipment	Left		Right	
				Mean	*Std. Dev.*	*Mean*	*Std. Dev.*
Cram & Engstrom, 1986	104 Adult Ed Students, No Pain Problem in Past 2 Years	Sitting	J&J M–501 100–200 Hz. Bandpass	2.4 μVolts	2.0 μVolts	2.4 μVolts	2.2 μVolts
Cram & Engstrom, 1986	104 Adult Ed Students, No Pain Problem in Past 2 Years	Standing	J&J M–501 100–200 Hz. Bandpass	2.5 μVolts	2.1 μVolts	2.1 μVolts	2.0 μVolts
Fogle & Glaros, 1995	96 Student, Staff and Community Volunteers, No Head, Neck or Facial Pain	?Sitting Viewing a Movie	J&J M–501 20–1000 Hz. Bandpass	not measured	not measured	3.3 μVolts	2.4 μVolts
Gervais, Fitzsimmons & Thomas, 1989	24 Student Volunteers, No Signs or Symptoms of TMJ	Sitting Upright, Eyes Closed	Biocomp 2001, 80–400 Hz. Bandpass RMS Values	2.0 μVolts	1.0 μVolts	1.8 μVolts	1.3 μVolts
R. Jensen, Fuglsang-Frederiksen, & Olesen, 1994	Random Sample of General Population, N = 547	Supine	Dantec Counterpoint 20–1000 Hz. Bandpass, RMS Values	3.2 μVolts	1.4 μVolts	3.3 μVolts	1.4 μVolts
Matheson, Toben, & de la Cruz, 1988	73 College Students, No Pain Difficulties	Sitting	J&J M–53 100–200 Hz. Bandpass	2.4 μVolts	1.5 μVolts	2.0 μVolts	1.3 μVolts

work- or motor vehicle accident-related **myofascial pain syndrome** at the neck and/or upper trapezius. The recovery period following shoulder abduction has also seemed informative, although no norms are yet available.

Masseter.   Norms for the masseter are reproduced in Table 12–4. Fogle and Glaros (1995) note no effects of age, gender or facial bony morphology on resting values at the masseter.

Schwartz-Mayo placement.   Recall that in the Schwartz-Mayo placement, one active site of a bipolar electrode is placed at the frontalis, and the other active site is placed on the ipsilateral cervical paraspinals. The Schwartz-Mayo placement is designed to read broadly from the muscles on one side of the head. Norms are given in Table 12–5.

TABLE 12–3
Surface EMG Norms—Upper Trapezius

Source	Population	Position	Equipment	Left Mean	Left Std. Dev.	Right Mean	Right Std. Dev.
Cram & Engstrom, 1986	104 Adult Ed Students, No Pain Problem in Past 2 Years	Sitting	J&J M–501 100–200 Hz. Bandpass	2.2 μVolts	2.5 μVolts	2.3 μVolts	2.8 μVolts
Cram & Engstrom, 1986	104 Adult Ed Students, No Pain Problem in Past 2 Years	Standing	J&J M–501 100–200 Hz. Bandpass	3.1 μVolts	2.7 μVolts	3.3 μVolts	2.9 μVolts
Matheson, Toben, & de la Cruz, 1988	73 College Students, No Pain Difficulties	Sitting	J&J M–53 100–200 Hz. Bandpass	3.1 μVolts	3.2 μVolts	3.0 μVolts	2.9 μVolts
Matheson, Toben, & de la Cruz, 1988	73 College Students, No Pain Difficulties	Standing	J&J M–53 100–200 Hz. Bandpass	4.5 μVolts	4.5 μVolts	4.6 μVolts	4.1 μVolts

TABLE 12–4
Surface EMG Norms—Masseter

Source	Population	Position	Equipment	Left Mean	Left Std. Dev.	Right Mean	Right Std. Dev.
Fogle & Glaros, 1995	96 Student, Staff and Community Volunteers, No Head, Neck or Facial Pain	? Sitting Viewing a Movie	J&J M–501 20–1000 Hz. Bandpass	2.4 μVolts	2.5 μVolts	2.8 μVolts	2.9 μVolts
Gervais, Fitzsimmons & Thomas, 1989	24 Student Volunteers, No Signs or Symptoms of TMJ	Sitting Upright, Eyes Closed	Biocomp 2001 80–400 Hz. Bandpass RMS Values	2.5 μVolts	1.1 μVolts	2.0 μVolts	1.2 μVolts
Matheson, Toben, & de la Cruz, 1988	73 College Students, No Pain Difficulties	Sitting	J&J M–53 100–200 Hz. Bandpass	1.7 μVolts	1.4 μVolts	1.8 μVolts	1.6 μVolts

TABLE 12–5
Surface EMG Norms—Schwartz-Mayo Placement

Source	Population	Position	Equipment	Left Mean	Left Std. Dev.	Right Mean	Right Std. Dev.
Hudzinski & Lawrence, 1990	51 Volunteers, 14–29 yrs. No Pain History	Sitting Upright, No Back Support	J&J I–330 100–200 Hz. Bandpass RMS Values 2-sec Integration	4.0 μVolts	1.1 μVolts	3.9 μVolts	0.9 μVolts
Hudzinski & Lawrence, 1990	39 Volunteers, 30–49 yrs. No Pain History	Sitting Upright, No Back Support	J&J I–330 100–200 Hz. Bandpass RMS Values 2-sec Integration	4.2 μVolts	1.5 μVolts	3.9 μVolts	1.1 μVolts
Hudzinski & Lawrence, 1990	10 Volunteers, 50–74 yrs. No Pain History	Sitting Upright, No Back Support	J&J I–330 100–200 Hz. Bandpass RMS Values 2-sec Integration	5.2 μVolts	2.0 μVolts	4.8 μVolts	1.5 μVolts
Hudzinski & Lawrence, 1990	51 Volunteers, 14–29 yrs. No Pain History	Sitting Upright, No Back Support	J&J I–330 25–1000 Hz. Bandpass RMS Values 2-sec Integration	9.1 μVolts	2.6 μVolts	8.5 μVolts	2.2 μVolts
Hudzinski & Lawrence, 1990	39 Volunteers, 30–49 yrs. No Pain History	Sitting Upright, No Back Support	J&J I–330 25–1000 Hz. Bandpass RMS Values 2-sec Integration	8.7 μVolts	3.6 μVolts	7.7 μVolts	2.8 μVolts
Hudzinski & Lawrence, 1990	10 Volunteers, 50–74 yrs. No Pain History	Sitting Upright, No Back Support	J&J I–330 25–1000 Hz. Bandpass RMS Values 2-sec Integration	12.2 μVolts	5.3 μVolts	10.2 μVolts	3.4 μVolts

Schneider and Wilson's TMD placement.   In this placement, no attempt is made to isolate an individual muscle. Rather, for each bipolar electrode, one active site is placed at the anterior temporalis, one active site is placed at the digastric on the underside of the chin close to the front, and the angle of the mandible is used for the reference site. The goal is to summarize activity from a range of muscles involved in mastication, and to teach clients to relax the entire area. Norms are shown in Table 12–6.

TABLE 12–6
Surface EMG Norms—Schneider and Wilson's TMD Placement

Source	Population	Position	Equipment	Left		Right	
				Mean	Std. Dev.	Mean	Std. Dev.
Hudzinski & Lawrence, 1992	100 Volunteers, No TMD, Headache, or Muscle Pain	Sitting Upright, No Back Support	J&J I–330 100–200 Hz. Bandpass RMS Values 2-sec Integration	3.7 μVolts	1.1 μVolts	3.6 μVolts	1.0 μVolts
Hudzinski & Lawrence, 1992	100 Volunteers, No TMD, Headache, or Muscle Pain	Sitting Upright, No Back Support	J&J I–330 25–1000 Hz. Bandpass RMS Values 2-sec Integration	6.5 μVolts	1.7 μVolts	6.3 μVolts	1.6 μVolts

Corrugator supercilii.   The corrugator muscle is found just above the bridge of the nose. It "knits" the eyebrows, drawing them down towards the bridge of the nose, such as when frowning. Its effects are thus somewhat opposed to the frontalis, which raises the eyebrows. To my knowledge, there are no normative data for the corrugator, and it is rarely used as a site for biofeedback. The corrugator may deserve more attention, however, for it is active during stress and pain (Crombez, Baeyens, & Eelen, 1997), and in proportion to sustained mental effort (Van Boxtel, 2001; Van Boxtel & Jessurun, 1993; Waterink & Van Boxtel, 1994). Moreover, in open label (non-blinded) trials, Botox injections to the corrugator, and even surgical removal of the muscle, have had dramatic effects on migraine frequency and intensity (Guyuron, Tucker, & J. Davis, 2002). A branch of the trigeminal nerve, called the supratrochlear nerve, passes through the corrugator, and thus tension at the corrugator could, perhaps, incite the trigeminovascular system (Guyuron, Tucker, & J. Davis, 2002).

Caveats and confounds.   The validity of normative comparisons is badly compromised by an important confound, the amount of adipose tissue beneath the skin. The amplitude of the electrical signal picked up from the muscles is approximately inversely proportional to the distance between the muscles and the electrode (De Luca, 1979). Of course, adipose tissue increases this distance (Hemingway, Biedermann, & Inglis, 1995). Moreover, subcutaneous tissue acts as a low-pass filter whose bandwidth becomes narrower as the tissue becomes thicker (De Luca, 1979). Thus, Persson and colleagues found that body mass index (a person's weight divided by the square of their height, generally in kg/cm²) correlated -0.6 with EMG amplitude at the upper trapezius during isometric contraction, and -0.5 with amplitude at the deltoid (Persson, Hansson, Kalliomäki, Moritz, & Sjölund, 2000). Similarly, Hemingway, et al., obtained correlations of -0.6 between body mass index and surface EMG readings during isometric contraction at two sites in the low back: the multifidus and the iliocostalis (Hemingway, Biedermann, & Inglis, 1995). Further, Hemingway, et al., suggest that the reason these correlations are not stronger is that body mass index is not an entirely accurate indicator of local adipose tissue thickness. They found that skinfold measures at the recording site correlated -0.65 at the iliocostalis and -0.85 at the multifidus with EMG amplitude. After log-transforming to correct for skew in the skin fold readings, the correlations increase further in magnitude, to -0.7 at the iliocostalis and -0.9 at the multifidus! (Hemingway, Biedermann, & Inglis, 1995). This may be a reason to focus on the frontalis, whose readings are presumably less affected by body fat. Hemingway, et al. present a regression equation for correcting one's data. However, they are for isometric contraction at the low back and not resting baseline at pericranial sites. Moreover, because the equation is based on only 20 subjects, its reliability is uncertain.

Nonetheless, the results of Hemingway, et al. themselves appear to contain a confound. Their sample included both men and women. The women tended to have higher body mass indexes and numerically, if not always significantly, lower EMG readings. Thus, strength differences between the men and women may account for some proportion of the variance ascribed to subcutaneous tissue thickness. It seems doubtful that this would account for all of the variance, however, and further work on eliminating body composition as a confound is clearly needed.

A second, less dramatic caveat pertains to terminology. Although common mode rejection can give electrodes a fair amount of selectivity, the activation picked up in surface EMG is rarely from a single muscle only. Neighboring muscles are particularly likely to contribute to the EMG signal. Therefore, it is appropriate to refer to sites by the area being read, rather than by a specific muscle. For example, while one could refer to an electrode "at the frontalis area" it would not be ideal to refer to "readings from the frontalis muscle" (Fridlund & Cacioppo, 1986). One can gain a sense of the amount of cross-talk between muscles by reading from one muscle area while the patient actively contracts a different muscle. For example, a temporalis placement can be checked informally by recording values when the patient tenses the temporalis (jaw clenching) and then, separately, when patient tenses the frontalis (raising one's eyebrows). Ideally, of course, temporalis site readings will increase much more during the jaw clenching condition.

Thirdly, aside from providing a rough benchmark, interpretation with respect to population mean and standard deviation does not seem to have a strong theoretical rationale. In the ergonomics literature, the most meaningful comparison of EMG readings is not to normative values but to the maximum voluntary contraction for the muscle. Moreover, if pain is due to sustained contraction of a small number of motor units, then the therapeutic goal is not "average readings" but something approaching electrical silence of the relevant muscle. Normative comparisons could be misleading, as even small levels of tension could cause pain in susceptible subjects.

Surface EMG readings tend to increase with age (Hudzinski & Lawrence, 1990). However, the effects appear to be so small that they are without clinical significance. Specifically, Hudzinski and Lawrence (1990) find that the average reading for the Schwartz-Mayo placement in their oldest age group (ages 50–74) was approximately 1 microvolt higher than in their lowest age group (ages 14–29). This apparently refers to microvolts per two-second interval, and hence the difference should be 0.5 microvolts per second. Again using a Schwartz-Mayo placement, in a seated position, Hudzinski and Lawrence (1990) found no significant differences in readings between 80 female and 20 male pain-free volunteers.

Within-subjects design.   The data from Hemingway, et al., and to a much lesser extent the influence of age and gender, suggest that the level of extraneous between-persons variance is rather high in surface EMG. Moreover, the usefulness of an individual's maximum voluntary contraction is a reminder of the comparative power of within subjects analyses. Indeed, van Boxtel and colleagues have suggested that surface EMG readings are more physiologically meaningful when expressed as a proportion of maximum voluntary contraction (Goudswaard, Passchier, & Orlebeke, 1988; van Boxtel, Goudswaard, & Schomaker, 1984).

Still, in our clinic we generally do not encourage maximum contraction of a muscle that may already be sore. And there is some controversy about whether the maximum voluntary contraction is the best approach to normalization. The extent of contraction may be limited, automatically or volitionally, in individuals who are in pain (Marras & K. G. Davis, 2001). And maximum voluntary contraction depends on one's strength as well (Marras & K. G. Davis, 2001). Correcting for strength may be reasonable in ergonomics studies of job tasks, but it seems to introduce a confound when our interest is baseline levels of muscle activation. An alternative is to use a sub-maximal but standardized reference contraction (Mathiassen, Winkel & Hägg, 1995). For the upper trapezius, this could mean asking the patient to hold their arms horizontally out to the side (90° abduction) for ten seconds. When no weights are held in the hands, the abduction corresponds to around one-sixth of the maximum voluntary force, and thus corrects primarily for body composition rather than strength (Mathiassen, Winkel & Hägg, 1995).

Other within-subjects comparisons are possible as well. For patients with unilateral pain, the pain site could be compared with the corresponding location on the other side of the body. For patients whose pain site is bilateral, comparison of the readings under usual vs. stressed vs. relaxed conditions (verified, say, with finger temperature) might be an alternative. I am unaware of norms for these types of comparisons, for example norms of the expected ratio of upper trapezius readings from the dominant vs. nondominant side.[3] This seems to be a useful area for further development. In the meantime, one type of within persons assessment is used somewhat often: dynamic assessment, to which we will turn next.

Dynamic assessment.   For dynamic assessment, voluntary contraction may be elicited by the movements shown in Table 12–7.

The actions of muscles and the specific motions that tense them are given in books of manual muscle testing (e.g., Kendall, McCreary, & Provance, 1993).[4]

For dynamic assessment, motions should be reasonably standardized. For example, Cram (1999) notes that when cervical flexion is produced from the top of the neck, the sternocleidomastoids have to tense strongly to pull the head forward. The subsequent re-righting requires little effort from the cervical paraspinals, however, as the elastic properties of the neck provide most of the force. In contrast, cervical flexion from the base of the neck requires little effort from the sternocleidomastoids because gravity brings the head forward. The cervical paraspinals have to work hard in the subsequent re-righting, however, to oppose gravity. Cram recommends that the two motions be combined in clinical assessment, first asking the patient to tuck their chin down towards their neck, and then rolling the head towards the chest. He recommends that patients be asked to practice the maneuver 3–5 times first, and then be paced through the motion by the clinician during the actual assessment (Cram, 1997).

High readings at baseline, or high readings after voluntary contraction that do not self-correct, raise the possibility that muscle tension is a contributor to the headaches. Donaldson et al. suggest that dynamic assessment can also indicate with reasonable probability that trigger points are present. Specifically, during forward cervical flexion, if one side (i.e., left vs. right sternocleidomastoids) has a maximum reading that is more than 20 percent higher than the maximum reading on the contralateral side, a trigger point is suspected in the side with the higher readings. Similar considerations apply to the cervical paraspinals during re-righting from forward flexion (Donaldson, Skubick, Clasby, & Cram, 1994). Qualitatively, myofascial pain seems

---

[3]Of course Tables 12–1 to 12–6 can tell us the expected ratio of *average* readings from the two sides of the body for various pericranial muscles. However, they do not tell us how much this ratio varies across persons, and hence whether any particular person's ratio is abnormal.

[4]I am grateful to Toni Cavanaugh, PT, for the information on manual muscle testing, and to Jeff Matranga, Ph.D., ABPP, for the idea of using alternative psychophysiological measures to verify stressed vs. relaxed conditions.

TABLE 12–7
Surface EMG—Dynamic Assessment

Muscle	Action to Elicit Contraction
Frontalis	Eyebrows Raised
Corrugator	Eyebrows Knitted
Temporalis	Jaw Clenched
Masseter	Jaw Clenched
Upper Trapezius	Scapular Elevation ("hunching" one's shoulders), Shoulder Flexion (arms out in front), Shoulder Abduction (arms out to the sides)
Cervical Paraspinals	Re-Righting From Neck Flexion
Sternocleidomastoids	Neck Rotation (contralateral: e.g., right rotation activates left SCM), Neck Lateral Flexion (ipsilateral: e.g., right side bend activates right SCM), Neck Forward Flexion (should activate both sides equally)

sometimes to be associated with brief spikes in the electrical signal. This sign of irritability may be the equivalent in surface EMG of the spikes seen on needle EMG when a taut band of muscle is snapped or poked (Rivner, 2001). However, the spikes seem to occur infrequently in surface readings and hence their diagnostic utility is limited by low sensitivity.

Åkesson et al. found that upper trapezius readings during shoulder abduction (90° out to the side, holding a 1 kg dumbbell with the hand facing downwards, for 10 seconds) correlated 0.95 across subjects and occasions with maximum voluntary contraction (Åkesson, Hansson, Balogh, Moritz, & Skerfving, 1997). This is an encouraging result, suggesting that shoulder abduction can serve as a reference contraction, giving some of the same information as maximum voluntary contraction, but presumably without as high a risk of exacerbating the pain.

Kollmitzer et al. report on the test-retest reliability of surface EMG readings taken at three sites at the quadriceps: the rectus femoris, vastus lateralis and the vastus medialis. Subjects were seated in a Cybex knee flexion machine that both standardized the movement and provided subjects with visual feedback about the force of movement, so that they could engage in, for example, a contraction to 50% of maximum. For maximum voluntary contraction, Pearson correlations averaged 0.79 over a 3-minute retest interval, and 0.77 over a 90 minute interval. With a retest interval of 6 weeks, the correlation decreased to 0.35. In contrast, contractions at 50% of maximum had average test-retest reliabilities of 0.98, 0.80, and 0.50 at 3 minutes, 90 minutes, and 6 weeks, respectively (Kollmitzer, Ebenbichler, & Kopf, 1999). Here, then, is another advantage of submaximum reference contractions over maximum voluntary contractions. The poorer reliability at 6 weeks probably reflects at least in part small changes in the positioning of the electrodes across sessions.

Barton and Hayes, meanwhile, studied the time needed for sternocleidomastoid surface EMG readings to return to baseline after maximum voluntary contraction. Subjects were lying supine and contracted the SCMs by flexing their neck forward against resistance. The EMG relaxation times showed modest within-session repeatability, having within-session intraclass correlation coefficients of 0.60 at the right SCM and 0.67 at the left (Barton & Hayes, 1996).

Ideally, a stress condition should be included as well, in which the patient imagines a personally-relevant stressor. Generic stress conditions such as timed mental arithmetic may not be as useful (e.g., Flor, Birbaumer, Schugens, & Lutzenberger, 1992) although the evidence on this is mixed.

Finger Temperature

Finger temperature is generally recorded from the ventral (palmar) surface of the outer most segment of the left index finger. Blanchard, et al., have published norms for their laboratory at SUNY Albany (Blanchard, Morrill, Wittrock, Scharff, & Jaccard, 1989). Readings were taken under the following conditions: (1) The thermistor (a YSI/Yellow Springs Instruments thermistor feeding into a Med Associates ANL–410 temperature unit) was attached with paper tape that did not encircle the finger. (2) The room was dimly lit, the monitor was not visible, and subjects sat in a recliner with their eyes closed. (3) Although subjects had their arms on the arms of the chair, they positioned themselves so that the thermistor was not in contact with the chair arm. (4) There was at least a 10 minute adaptation period, followed by a 10 minute baseline. The published norms are for the average across minutes 8 and 9 of the baseline. (5) Headache diagnostic groups were based on the 1962 criteria.

Median and first and third quartiles (25th and 75th percentiles) for the temperature data are shown in Table 12–8. The original article provides a great deal more data than the brief summary here.

The conditions used by Blanchard et al. illustrate the classic recommendations of Taub and School (1978). Notice in particular the long adaptation period—effectively 17 minutes—prior to measurement. In biofeedback, one wants to train patients in a specific skill, beyond the level of relaxation achieved by simply sitting quietly in the recliner. Taub and School recommend an initial stabilization period of 6 minutes, and more if need be, until the temperature does not fluctuate by more than 0.25 °F during four consecutive minutes (E. Taub & School, 1978, p. 618). They note that in practice, 15 minutes is typically required for adaptation.

In the Blanchard, et al. study, the tape did not encircle the finger so that it would not impede blood circulation. Taub and School further recommend that not just the sensor tip, but 5 cm of wire leading up to the tip, be taped to the skin, to standardize the amount of contact. The reason is that the wires can conduct quite a bit of heat to the tip, where the actual measurement takes place (stem effect).

Note that blood flow to the hands varies for purposes of thermoregulation as well as in response to stress. Thus, ambient temperature should be consistent and comfortable, generally around 72 °F, but sometimes 75 °F for older, slightly built individuals.

Heart Rate and/or Skin Conductance Level

These measures are useful for interpreting the finger temperature readings. Low finger temperature combined with other signs of high sympathetic tone suggests that general stress level may be

TABLE 12–8
Hand Temperature Norms

Statistic	Migraine	Mixed	Tension	Healthy Controls
N	65	70	86	56
% Female	75%	71%	60%	73%
1st Quartile (°F)	93.0–93.9	92.0–92.9	93.0–93.9	94.0–94.9
Median (°F)	88.0–88.9	86.0–86.9	90.0–90.9	92.0–92.9
3rd Quartile (°F)	78.0–78.9	78.0–78.9	82.0–82.9	81.0–81.9

Note. From "Hand Temperature Norms for Headache, Hypertension, and Irritable Bowel Syndrome," by E. B. Blanchard, B. Morrill, D. A. Wittrock, L. Scharff, and J. Jaccard, 1989, *Biofeedback and Self-Regulation, 14,* p. 319. Copyright 1989 by Plenum Publishing Corporation. Reprinted with permission.

the best initial focus of intervention. Low finger temperature in the absence of other signs of psychophysiological arousal points towards vasoreactivity, and suggests thermal biofeedback as an intervention. However, finger temperature will sometimes remain low, not varying even when other autonomic measures indicate a shift towards deep relaxation. If we have ruled out a high dose of beta-blockers (or a low dose interacting with a selective serotonin reuptake inhibitor), the cause may be endothelial dysfunction—an impairment of the lining of the blood vessels—seen mostly in heavy smokers. Regardless, when finger temperature is clearly not varying we must adopt another measure, such as frontalis muscle tension, as our primary focus.

Skin conductance level must be interpreted carefully, for it seems to be more a measure of mental activation than of stress per se. Thus, skin conductance level may be increased by mental effort and exposure to novel stimuli (Dawson, Schell, & Filion, 2000), and even by absorption in pleasant imagery (Alden, Dale, & DeGood, 2001). In our clinic, we sometimes find that early in relaxation training, a patient's finger temperature and skin conductance level will both increase. Later in treatment, skin conductance level declines during relaxation while finger temperature continues to rise. Presumably, early in treatment the patient has indeed achieved a reduction in sympathetic tone, but with considerable effort. Moreover, the relaxation is often quite novel at that point. With practice, the relaxation becomes less novel and effortful, and the degree of relaxation presumably deepens. Some biofeedback applications correct for the novelty effect by basing feedback not on skin conductance level itself, but on its rate of decline (Critchley, Melmed, Featherstone, Mathias, & Dolan, 2001).

HEADACHE DIARY

The gold standard for quantifying the frequency, intensity, and duration of headaches is prospective recording in a headache diary.

The standard scale for home recording of headache pain has been, since the earliest days of biofeedback, Budzynski's 6-point Headache Intensity Scale (Budzynski, Stoyva, & Adler, 1970; Budzynski, Stoyva, Adler, & Mulhaney, 1973).

    0 = no pain or discomfort

    1 = very mild pain or discomfort, not usually noticeable

    2 = noticeable pain, but one from which you can be distracted

    3 = moderate pain, always hurts, but allows normal activity

    4 = strong pain, restricts some but not all activity

    5 = severe pain, totally restricts activity.

We might quibble that the scale, which suggests an effort at absolute scaling of pain, has two primary disadvantages: The presence of descriptors, anchoring each scale point, can disrupt what might otherwise be equal-interval properties, and the wording of the descriptors seems to confound pain intensity with deficits in pain coping (see, e.g., K. A. Holroyd, Malinoski, M. K. Davis, & Lipchik, 1999). The alternative, of course, is a simple visual analogue scale, anchored by the descriptors "no pain" and "worst pain imaginable," which has been well-validated in pain studies. Still, the disadvantages of Budzynski's scale seem more theoretical than actual. The anchor points may, as undoubtedly was intended, make the scale easier to use. Standardizing a scale by convention will often allow it to be treated as if it were giving parametric data (F. M. Lord, 1953; Cliff, 1993). Moreover, the results of a careful scaling study suggest that pain and disability actually are on the same dimension, with disability indicating the more severe levels of chronic pain syndrome (Von Korff, Ormel, Keefe, & Dworkin, 1992). And using the

Budzynski scale allows one's results to be coordinated, at least to a degree, with those of a large set of previous studies.

Once a scale has been selected, how often should pain level be recorded? In the original studies by Budzynski, the ratings were every hour. Study participants were given grids, with hours represented on the x-axis and pain level on the y-axis; the task was to graph one's pain level prospectively. Blanchard, while retaining the 6-point scale, found that good research data could be obtained by asking subjects to record pain level 4 times a day, at meals and at bedtime. This seems like the best format for research. I have not seen any different recommendations for general clinical treatment, but it seems to me that having patients record at bedtime the time of onset, time of offset, and peak intensity of any headaches occurring during the day, would be reasonable when the goal is simply verifying treatment effectiveness.

At several points in treatment, however, the goals for the headache diary are considerably more ambitious. Then, Blanchard's finer grained tracking is preferable. For the diary should do more than simply quantify headache burden—it should help patient and therapist better understand the headache pattern. Thus, during the assessment phase or early in treatment, a more detailed diary is appropriate (as an example, see Worksheet 1 in the chapter appendix). In it, patients record the date and time, pain level if any, associated features such as photophobia (to help in distinguishing type of headache), warning signs or early symptoms, and the situation and any possible triggers. I recommend that patients complete a diary entry at the first onset of a headache, so that subtle cues are not missed. For migraines, warning signs might include the aura, if present. Aura occurs rather late for prevention, however, and preferably the patient will be able to identify earlier, prodromal changes, such as in mood, appetite, physical functioning, or level of consciousness. For tension-type headache, warnings might include tension at the neck or shoulders, tightness at the jaw, physical or mental fatigue, or symptoms of anxiety. When headaches are largely continuous, we would ask instead about how and where pain increases are first manifest. Ideally, triggers can be identified that will allow self-management skills to be used preventively. In the absence of known triggers, however, warning signs and early symptoms allow a similar, proactive response.

A degree of emotional processing of pain can be helpful in session, but I ask patients to avoid affective pain descriptors or emotional journaling in the headache diary. Such ground can be covered more constructively, it seems, as a separate exercise involving a structured thought record (Eimer & A. Freeman, 1998).

Thus, later in treatment, the diary shifts to include one's instantaneous, **automatic thoughts** and consequent emotional responses to trigger situations, and to the pain. This "Dysfunctional Thought Record," shown as Worksheet 2 in the chapter appendix, then provides an opportunity for objectively evaluating the automatic thoughts, and for substituting more precise and accurate appraisals. Catastrophic or depressive responses to pain, stressors, or both, would make this use of the diary particularly important. We will discuss ways of evaluating and correcting automatic thoughts in the next chapter, under "cognitive coping skills."

Patients experiencing the pain in affectively laden terms (pain-distress) may be helped by focusing on the sensory characteristics of the pain—its objective qualities, location, and exact intensity level. An extensive list of sensory descriptors may be found in the sensory and miscellaneous scales of the McGill Pain Questionnaire (Melzack, 1975).

Further in treatment, the recordings are an opportunity for the patient to track the application of pharmacological and self-management skills, their effectiveness, and ways of fine tuning the approach. By tracking the situation or early prodromal signs, the medication or self-management tool employed, and the outcome, patients can identify ways of targeting or changing the tool to have greater efficacy in real life (see Worksheet 3, chapter appendix). Even small reductions in pain, seen clearly in the diary and noted in treatment, can lead to self-efficacy and further gains.

Used actively in this way, as pain and negative emotions unfold in real time, the various phases of the headache diary are perhaps the most demanding aspects of treatment. Nothing, however, seems so empowering to patients as discovering when and how to intervene in their headaches. The detailed knowledge plays a key role in helping patients gain control of their pain.

Thought Sampling

In thought sampling, patients randomly note their thoughts (Hurlburt, 1997) and circumstances (Csikszentmihalyi & Larson, 1987) over the course of the day. Two days of c. hourly self-monitoring seems sufficient to collect a useful amount of data. To be conducted properly, the patients should wear a programmable wristwatch or carry a beeper or notebook computer, to cue the recording at random intervals. However, even a simple alarm watch, set to beep on the hour, can provide data that would not be available otherwise.

Thought sampling, I feel, deserves to make the transition from research to clinical practice. The data might be recorded as a simple checklist: whether the person was thinking of pain, and whether the thoughts were positive or negative. However, I prefer a more open-ended approach, asking the patient simply to record a single sentence that captures the thought they were having just before the alarm sounded. For example, a patient might record at 11 A.M.: "At the keyboard—I wish my shoulders would stop hurting." The data of interest can be coded later: the frequency of pain-related thoughts, the proportion of such thoughts that are positive vs. negative (e.g., coping vs. catastrophizing), and the circumstances in which pain-related thoughts, and especially negative pain-related thoughts, occur.

The disadvantage of thought sampling is that its validation in the laboratory is still in its early stages, at least for pain. We do not know, for example, whether pain-related cognitions measured in this manner are predictive of adjustment the way, say, psychometric measures of catastrophizing are. We do not know if there is a dose-response relationship between frequency of negative pain cognitions and subsequent pain, disability, or distress, or what form such a relationship would take. Certainly there are no norms yet; we cannot tell a patient "your level should be down here."

Yet even in its current, primitive state, thought sampling seems to me to have clinical utility. The data seems intuitively meaningful to patients, and of course it is quite easy to grasp. Like other forms of behavioral self-monitoring, the activity seems inherently therapeutic, as patients begin to reflect on how and how often they think about pain. And the connections between specific stimuli and specific pain-related thoughts are not easily discovered otherwise.

SUMMARY

From the interview we can hone in on the diagnosis, and get a sense of the scope of the problem—the intensity, frequency and duration of pain, the impact on mood and functioning, and the life situation, stresses and coping resources in which the problem is embedded. We also want to understand the person's journey with the headaches, the treatments that have been tried so far and their effects, to avoid repeating past mistakes, and to understand how our own efforts are likely to be viewed. For the interview, too, is a chance to clarify the pateint's goals for treatment, to introduce the idea of self-management, to make note of any barriers, to process the reasons for any skepticism, and to begin coordinating expectations for the therapy and its outcome.

A brief psychometric battery allows us to screen for likely comorbid conditions (especially depression and anxiety) for which a full diagnostic interview would be time consuming. Psychometrics provide the most validated means for assessing factors, such as catastrophic thinking, fear of pain or external locus of control, that can impede recovery if not addressed in the course of treatment. Moreover, as measures of symptom severity, the psychometrics allow us to assess functioning and mood quantitatively, giving useful secondary endpoints for tracking the effectiveness of treatment.

The headache diary, of course, gives us the primary endpoints—headache frequency, duration, and intensity. But as we have seen, the diary is also a means by which patients examine the circumstances, triggers and thoughts antecedent to pain and negative emotions, and the effectiveness of cognitive, behavioral, and medication strategies. By turning patients into scientists, the diary blends assessment and treatment, and can be intrinsically empowering.

When the time and equipment are available, and especially for frequent headaches ($\geq$4 days per month) I recommending including a psychophysiological assessment. Finger temperature and frontalis and upper trapezius surface EMG (temporalis and masseter EMG in the case of temporomandibular dysfunction) comprise a useful minimal battery. The cogency and substantiality these measures give to treatment, and their connection to empirically validated biofeedback therapies (see Chapter 14) can fully repay the additional effort.

We must take care, however, that the vividness of the psychophysiological data not cause us to overlook the cognitive, emotional, behavioral, and systems (family and disability) aspects of pain coping. For if there is any secret to being able to speak intelligently about cases, I am convinced it is this: to always seek to understand the pain on multiple levels. These include physical diagnosis and pathophysiology, sensory characteristics, psychophysiological contributors, behavior (including self-management, functioning, and medication use), cognitive and emotional responses, and the influence of family and workplace—indeed, all of the dimensions we have covered in this chapter. Treatment can then be targeted to the levels at which it will do the most good. In an effort to keep these levels in mind I sometimes use the following mnemonic. It derives from the biopsychosocial, multiaxial system embodied in DSM-IV (American Psychiatric Association, 1994; G. L. Engel, 1977), but elaborated slightly to emphasize variables relevant to pain:

A: Affect and arousal (Axis I)
B: Behavioral reinforcers for pain and non-pain focus.
C: Cognitive coping vs. catastrophizing.
D: Diagnosis of headaches, using the IHS system (Axis III).
E: Ergonomics and surface EMG.
F: Family and individual functioning (Axis II).
G: Goals and expectations for treatment.
H: Hassles and life events stress; coping resources (Axis IV).
I: Impairment—overall level of functioning (Axis V).

P: Psychophysics, sensory testing.
S: Substances, including overuse and addiction issues.

For communicating with other professionals, however, a more compact format is needed. Lake, et al. have proposed a concise multiaxial system, comprising headache diagnosis, frequency, and severity (Axis I), analgesic or abortive use, overuse, and abuse (Axis II), behavioral and stress-related risk factors (triggers, aggravators; Axis III), comorbid psychiatric disorders (Axis IV), and functional impact and disability (Axis V; Lake, Saper, Hamel, & Kreeger, 1995). It seems reasonable that Lake et al.'s system become standard in headache work, as the DSM-IV has in psychiatric diagnosis.

HSLC: Headache Specific Locus of Control Scale

© Kenneth A. Holroyd, Ph.D. (reprinted with permission)

Instructions. This is a questionnaire designed to determine the way in which people view certain important headache-related issues. Each item is a belief statement with which you may agree or disagree. Below are numbers which correspond to a scale on which you may rate the extent to which you agree or disagree with each item. The values range from "Strongly Disagree" = 1 to "Strongly Agree" = 5. Write the number that represents the extent to which you disagree or agree with the statement. Please make sure that you answer every item and that you write only one number per item. This is a measure of your personal beliefs; there are no right or wrong answers.

> **1 = Strongly Disagree**
> **2 = Moderately Disagree**
> **3 = Neutral**
> **4 = Moderately Agree**
> **5 = Strongly Agree**

1. When I have a headache, there is nothing I can do to affect its course. _____
2. I can prevent some of my headaches by avoiding certain stressful situations. _____
3. I am completely at the mercy of my headaches. _____
4. I can prevent some of my headaches by not getting emotionally upset. _____
5. If I remember to relax, I can avoid some of my headaches. _____
6. Only my doctor can give me ways to prevent my headaches. _____
7. My headaches are sometimes worse because I am overactive. _____
8. My headaches can be less severe if medical professionals (doctors, nurses, etc.) take proper care of me. _____
9. My headaches are beyond all control. _____
10. My doctor's treatment can help my headaches. _____
11. When I worry or ruminate about things, I am more likely to get headaches. _____
12. Just seeing my doctor helps my headaches. _____
13. No matter what I do, if I am going to get a headache, I will get a headache. _____
14. Having regular contact with my physician is the best way for me to control my headaches. _____
15. When I have headaches, I should consult a medically trained professional. _____
16. Following the doctor's medication regimen is the best way for me not to be laid-up with a headache. _____
17. When I drive myself too hard, I get headaches. _____
18. Luck plays a big part in determining how soon I will recover from a headache. _____
19. By not becoming agitated or overactive, I can prevent many headaches. _____
20. My not getting headaches is largely a matter of good fortune. _____
21. My actions influence whether I have headaches. _____
22. I usually recover from a headache when I get proper medical help. _____
23. I'm likely to get headaches no matter what I do. _____
24. If I don't have the right medication, my headaches will be a problem. _____
25. Often I feel that no matter what I do, I will still have headaches. _____
26. I am directly responsible for getting some of my headaches. _____
27. When my doctor makes a mistake, I am the one to suffer with headaches. _____
28. My headaches are worse when I'm coping with stress. _____
29. When I get headaches, I just have to let nature run its course. _____
30. Health professionals keep me from getting headaches. _____
31. I'm just plain lucky for a month when I don't get headaches. _____
32. When I have not been taking proper care of myself, I am likely to experience headaches. _____
33. It's a matter of fate whether I have a headache. _____

Internal Subscale: Items 2, 4, 5, 7, 11, 17, 19, 21, 26, 28, 32
Health Care Professionals Subscale: Items 6, 8, 10, 12, 14, 15, 16, 22, 24, 27, 30
Chance Subscale: Items 1, 3, 9, 13, 18, 20, 23, 25, 29, 31, 33

Chapter Appendix—Headache Worksheets for Successive Stages of Treatment

1. Discovering Patterns

Please complete when a headache first begins, or as soon as possible afterwards. Please record the situation in which the headache began, any possible triggers in the situation, and early warnings—the first indications, however subtle, that a headache was beginning. These will all be useful later in treatment, for knowing when to use self-management tools.

Date and Time	Pain Level[1]	Associated Symptoms (if any)[2]	Early Warnings, Symptoms	Situation	Possible Triggers

[1]0 to 10, where 0 is "no pain" and 10 is the "worst pain imaginable."
[2]For example, nausea, runny nose, lights are painful, sounds are painful, walking makes the pain worse.

2. Record of Automatic Thoughts (Dysfunctional Thought Record)

Please complete if the pain or negative emotion intrudes as a problem, or as soon as possible afterwards. The goal is to characterize the effects of automatic thoughts on mood or pain, and to examine how changing the thoughts changes the associated feelings.

Date and Time	Situation	Pain Level and Emotions Before[1]	Automatic Thought[2]	Pain Level and Accurate Reappraisal	Emotions After

[1]Depending on the patient's needs and stage of treatment, this column may focus on degree of belief in maladaptive thought, level of pain sensation, level of pain distress, stress level, or catastrophic or depressive reactions (see P. R. Martin, 1993, pp. 175–198).
[2]In response to situational stressor or to the pain itself, depending on patient's needs and stage of treatment.

3. Fine Tuning Treatment Effectiveness

Please complete if the pain intrudes as a problem.

Date and Time	Pain Level Before[1]	Warning Signs (Situation or Symptom)	Intervention	Pain Level After

[1]0 to 10, where 0 is "no pain" and 10 is the "worst pain imaginable."

CHAPTER 13

Elements of Behavioral Medicine Treatment

> *The separation of physical pain from displeasure . . . though it may seem at first sight*
> *"a bold assumption" will, I think, be found both a necessary and a fruitful one.*
> —Strong, 1896, cited in Kugelmann, 2001

We have drawn heavily on the published literature on chronic pain and headaches. Of course this literature can be quite useful, and therapeutic avenues it illuminates will be our focus in this chapter. We must not overlook, however, what the literature fails to show: the effort, energy, and courage that coping with chronic pain involves. Like other forms of illness, pain requires energy when energy is lowest, and a sense of hope precisely when one is most isolated. For no matter how much other people sympathize, their lives are going on. In this chapter, we will discuss ways of managing this burden that have the support, to a greater or lesser degree, of the outcome literature. Then, in the four chapters that follow, we will examine that literature more closely.

TREATMENT RATIONALE

As is often true in counseling, the initial evaluation can be therapeutic. It is an opportunity for the client to examine the pain and its impact in a supportive environment, to review and let go of past, strenuous efforts to find a cure, and to look for the parts of the pain problem that admit of a solution. In essence, it is a time for making the transition from trauma to mature self-management. Of course the transition is by no means completed with the evaluation, or with the compassionate, precise, and realistically positive feedback that should follow it. Acknowledgement and support for this transition may be appropriate throughout the course of treatment. But after the evaluation is done, it is often helpful to shift focus to the sequential mastery of a set of pain management skills. For these skills, more than any other aspect of treatment, are a path to recovery.

Parts of the bridge from evaluation to treatment are often apparent from the interview. The person may have noticed a connection between stress and at least some of their headaches. Or bright lights may bother her mostly when she is tired, or a tension-type headache may follow mental fatigue. Perhaps the neck becomes tense and knotted, the jaw hurts from clenching, the superficial temporal artery distends, or the scalp is too tender to comb one's hair. The person's symptoms allow us to synthesize, from the material in parts I and II of this book, a heuristic, rational, individualized model of the headaches. The model will draw in various proportions from findings and theories for the specific headache diagnosis, and the information on pain in chapters 2 and 3.

A key step in treatment is to explain this model, first in its physical aspects, and then in the influence of stress and other psychological factors on it. In most cases, the main elements of treatment will follow from the symptoms, and not need elaborate explanation. But the model is important anyway, for after years or decades of seemingly random suffering, of failed medications and vertiginous side effects, of procedures and consults awaited and regretted, the idea that the headaches have an underlying order is intrinsically empowering. Here, the potential to control the headaches first emerges. And here treatments become orderly experiments, so that even a failed attempt helps inform the patient, and sets the stage for the next rational intervention.

Although the focus here is primarily on behavioral tools, a severe disorder such as a continuous, high intensity, disabling headache seems to respond best to the total momentum of treatment arrayed against it. For these headaches, combining behavioral therapy with preventive medications and physical interventions (e.g., physical therapy, physiatry, or anesthesiological procedures as appropriate), discussed in Chapter 16, is usually the best approach.

PATIENT EDUCATION

Thus, the first step in treatment is education, to minimize pain-related anxiety that could cause vigilance to physical sensations, and to promote an internal locus of control. For if a patient is to successfully learn how to prevent and manage headaches, it helps if they first have a model of the disorder in which what they do matters (D. J. French, K. A. Holroyd, Pinell, Malinoski, O'Donnell, & K. R. Hill, 2000). This educational process continues throughout treatment, both didactically and through the patient's careful observations. Sometimes, well into treatment, a patient will accidentally discover that vivid imagery of a trigger is enough to elicit pain, or that imagining warmth or medication helps alleviate it, to their pleasure, for it opens up a new realm of tools. From this perspective, identifying psychological contributors that can be brought under the patient's control can be empowering.

In a classic article, Russell Packard asked 50 physicians of various specialties what headache patients want from a consult. Logically enough, 66 percent nominated pain relief as the primary goal. In second place, at 22 percent, was an explanation for the pain (Packard, 1979). But when Packard gave the same survey to 100 neurology outpatients with headache, the priorities were reversed: The most frequent top goal (46 percent) was an explanation for the pain; relief (31 percent) came in second (Packard, 1979). Twenty years later, this divergence still held true. Patients rated a "willingness to answer questions" as a more important physician attribute than "medical expertise in diagnosis and treatment." When physicians answered, the priority ordering was reversed (Lipton & Stewart, 1999). First and foremost, the patients want an understanding of their pain.

Ideally, of course, patients are well-informed and their questions answered by their medical providers before the psychologist is consulted. However, in reality a medical care provider may not have enough time, or may have difficulty translating information into terms that the patient finds useful. The provider may have a purely physiological model in which patient behavior plays no important role. And a general practitioner simply may not know as much about headaches as a psychologist who devotes his or her life's work to the area. Therefore, much of what the patient learns about migraines, tension-type headaches or chronic daily headaches may need to come from the psychologist.

Nonetheless, there are certain questions that the psychologist should not answer, and for which the patient should be referred back to their medical provider. These are questions about physical or medical treatment, about new symptoms, or about whether the patient's headaches are in fact benign. Obvious examples that have arisen in practice include "My sister died from an aneurysm—could my headaches be from an aneurysm?," "I stopped taking my medication; is that all right?," and "I've started seeing gray dots before a headache; is that normal?." The last symptom might indeed be normal for a patient with migraines, but new symptoms should always be evaluated by the medical provider.

IDENTIFYING HEADACHE PATTERNS

Instinctively, people tend to avoid becoming aware of a headache until it overtakes them. As a result, the headaches may seem more sudden, random, and uncontrollable than need be. Conversely, there is often nothing more empowering than identifying the earliest possible prodromal signs (e.g., a change in mood or arousal, in mental clarity or sensory acuity, in muscle tension, in yawning, in thirst or urination, in bowels) as an opportunity to prevent or blunt a migraine (Lipchik, K. A. Holroyd, & Nash, 2002). And even when true prevention is not effective, the chance to prepare, to plan, and to have acute medications on hand, can be invaluable (Lipchik, K. A. Holroyd, & Nash, 2002). The headache diary, with space for recording the earliest warnings, is a useful way of raising awareness (see Chapter 12). Then, the patient knows when to bring to bear the skills that work for them, such as deep relaxation, biofeedback, and cognitive coping.

RELAXATION TRAINING

Deep relaxation is comprised of several related techniques that may help reduce pain through such mechanisms as (1) A reduction in sympathetic tone (psychophysiological relaxation); (2) Absorption in external, pleasant imagery, inducing appetitive motivational states that are relatively incompatible with pain; (3) A focus on internal, non-pain sensations, to capitalize on the competition between submodalities of somatosensory perception; (4) Redirection of attention to other parts of the body; and (5) A reduction in pain-related distress through the induction of positive affect.

Before teaching relaxation, it is good to set the tone. Even chronically stressed people can often remember an environment in which they saw the world differently because they felt safe. Especially valuable are times spent in activities that feel more important than the stressors: worship, nurturing a child, caring for a pet, or creating a work of scholarship or art. Formal training in relaxation can bring a physiological depth and a mental quiescence not readily available in the course of other pursuits. But remembering core values and naturalistic relaxation can be a good starting point.

Three forms of relaxation training are in common use (McGrath, 1999). We will describe them here. A relaxation script based loosely on one of these techniques, autogenics, is given at the end of the chapter.

Progressive muscle relaxation is based on the work of Edmund Jacobson (1924, 1929), and involves tensing and then relaxing successive muscle groups. Traditionally, it has been used primarily for tension-type headache (e.g., Blanchard, Andrasik, Ahles, Teders, & O'Keefe, 1980), on the belief that muscle contraction plays a key role in the pain (Budzynski, Stoyva, & C. S. Adler, 1970). However, as a vivid, concrete, and easily learned skill, it is a useful starting point for all types of relaxation training.

In the classic Jacobsonian approach, progressive relaxation is simply a learned muscle skill. Patients begin by lying on their backs and focusing on a single muscle group, for example the wrist extensors. They tense the muscle lightly, extending the wrist, just enough to become aware of the feeling of muscle tension. Note that this feeling is different from the sense of strain in the joints or of the stretch of nearby tissues. Then the patient stops tensing the muscle and focuses on relaxing it as deeply as possible. The relaxation is not an active process but an absence of muscle tension. Much more time is spent on the relaxing than on the tensing. As the person's skills in discrimination improve, less and less tension, and ultimately none at all, are needed at the start of the exercise. Skills are learned for each muscle group in turn. Once the patient has learned the skills while supine, he or she would practice engaging in activities while tensing only those muscles necessary for the activity. The time required depended on the patient, but Jacobson's standard course involved 44 hours of training. (E. Jacobson, 1964; Lehrer, 1982, 1996).[1]

Of course, 44 hours is quite lengthy by current standards of therapy, although it is not long when compared with learning other skilled behaviors such as driving, dancing, or playing a musical instrument (see J. Holroyd, 1996, for a similar point regarding hypnosis). In any event, therapists nowadays generally use an abbreviated technique, first proposed by Wolpe and Lazarus (1966) and described in detail in D. A. Bernstein, Borkovec, and Hazlett-Stevens (2000). In the abbreviated approach, the muscles are combined into larger groups. For example, the patient may begin by making a hard fist, thus tightening numerous muscles in the hand and forearm. The tension is implemented as a strong isometric contraction, to heighten the contrast, and so that muscle fatigue can contribute to the subsequent relaxation. The relaxation is treated not simply as the absence of tension, but as a vivid, comfortable, enjoyable experience in its own right. Thus, suggestions for attending to relaxed sensations are included. Early on, cycles of tensing and relaxing help facilitate discrimination between the two states. Then, patients gradually learn to reproduce the relaxed sensation directly from memory, and to self-cue the relaxation response. For example, a person may learn to breathe in deeply, and then to say the word "relax" as they exhale (Lipchik, K. A. Holroyd, & Nash, 2002). Thus, the traditional and abbreviated techniques of progressive muscle relaxation differ somewhat in assumptions and implementation (Lehrer, 1982). We will consider this further in Chapter 15, when discussing research on the components of behavioral treatment for headaches.

The techniques of progressive muscle relaxation may be familiar and intuitive, and are well described in Bernstein, Borkovec, and Hazlett-Stevens (2000) and in Blanchard and Andrasik (1985). Briefly, patients are asked to tense each of 16 muscle groups in turn, using the actions shown in Table 13–1. In general, patients should hold the tension for 5–7 seconds, and then release, attending to the change in sensation, and maintaining the relaxation for at least 30–40 seconds. The pace should be slow, of course, c. 15–20 minutes in total. It helps for the patient to be comfortably dressed, without watch or glasses, and well supported (including the head and neck) in a soft recliner (Blanchard & Andrasik, 1985). In early sessions, the room should be quiet, dim, and relatively free of distractions, although later practice may be in progressively more challenging circumstances. Most important, of course, is that the therapist be comfortable with relax-

---

[1]Although Jacobson is known as the founder of scientifically based relaxation training, we learn from Gessel (1989) that his career ran much deeper than this. Jacobson's graduate studies in psychology were at Harvard University, where he published in symbolic logic under the guidance of Josiah Royce, and then completed his Ph.D. dissertation under William James. James is considered the father of American psychology, but Jacobson didn't really respect him because, as a person, James was very nervous. Jacobson then pursued postdoctoral studies in introspection with Titchener at Cornell University, and in physiology with A. J. Carlson at the University of Chicago. After taking time out to obtain his MD from Rush College of Medicine, Jacobson returned to his studies of tension and relaxation, first at the University of Chicago, and then at a private laboratory, basically inventing electromyography in the process. His last book was published in 1983, when he was 95 years old, and he died that same year. Gessel points out that in Jacobson's work we can see the influence of his background. His skeletal muscle theory of tension is concordant with his dissertation advisor's belief in the peripheral origins of emotion, the James-Lange theory: "Can one fancy the state of rage and picture . . . limp muscles, calm breathing, and a placid face? The present writer, for one, certainly cannot" (W. James, 1884, p. 194). And even though progressive muscle relaxation is the core technique of behavioral therapy, we can see in Jacobson's emphasis on the *awareness* of muscle tension, his training in the earlier paradigm, introspectionism (Gessel, 1989).

TABLE 13–1
Tensing Procedures for Progressive Muscle Relaxation

Area	Tensing Procedure
Dominant hand and forearm	Clenching one's hand into a fist
Dominant upper arm	Pressing one's elbow down into padded chair arm
Nondominant hand and forearm	Clenching one's hand into a fist
Nondominant upper arm	Pressing one's elbow down into padded chair arm
Forehead	Raising one's eyebrows
Upper face	Squinting one's eyes while wrinkling the nose
Jaw and mouth	Clenching one's jaw while smiling
Neck	Simultaneous forward flexion and (backward) extension
Chest, shoulder and upper back	Holding a deep breath while engaging in scapular retraction
Abdomen	Tightening the abdominal wall muscles
Right upper leg	Simultaneously tensing one's hamstrings and quadriceps
Right lower leg	Dorsiflexion of one's right foot (flexing foot upward at the ankle)
Right foot	Curling one's toes, turning one's foot lightly inward, and plantar flexion (pointing the toes forward)
Left upper leg	Simultaneously tensing one's hamstrings and quadriceps
Left lower leg	Dorsiflexion of one's left foot (flexing foot upward at the ankle)
Left foot	Curling one's toes, turning one's foot lightly inward, and plantar flexion (pointing the toes forward)

ation, in no great hurry, and enjoy the process. Of course supervised training in the procedure, and familiarity with the full technique and manual, are quite important.

Depending on the pain sensitivity of the head, neck, or other muscles, a patient may need to tense the area more briefly, or only minimally, or skip it altogether. Sometimes, the exertion of tensing any muscles will worsen a headache. In these cases, autogenics training (described below) may be more useful. With autogenics, the forehead may relax on its own with the general relaxation, or as the person imagines feelings of coolness there. Surface EMG biofeedback may also be useful, for teaching deep levels of muscle relaxation without prior tensing. Generally, though, except in rare cases of medical contraindication (e.g., severe osteoporosis for neck rotation) I encourage patients to experiment with lightly tensing the muscles as a way of gaining a deeper relaxation. The goal is to teach a flexible, empirical approach, learning from the pain how best to manage it, in place of fearful avoidance (Philips & Rachman, 1996).

Details are especially important—how a patient individualizes the skills. Thus, in mastering muscle relaxation, patients may give extra attention to a few "trouble spots." For example, if the suboccipital muscles are a site of chronic discomfort, a person may explore the effects of jaw movements, or of lifting their head slightly while supine, learning to substitute a feeling of relaxation for the tension. This type of self-examination is best done in a globally relaxed state.

Patients should also be coached to notice subtle behaviors that can produce static muscle tension under stress. A person may clench their fist, hunch their shoulders, brace themselves against the chair, or adopt an uncomfortable position for their neck, to name a few. Progressive relaxation of the involved muscles is a natural substitute.

Once the capacity to relax deeply has been mastered, it is developed through a series of steps into a tool that can be used for handling daily stresses. First, the 16 tense-and-release cycles are grouped into 7 (dominant arm, nondominant arm, head, neck, trunk, dominant leg, nondominant leg), and then 4 (both arms, head and neck, trunk, both legs), so that the relaxation response can be invoked more readily. Ultimately, no muscles are tensed; they are relaxed directly from memory. Then, the client learns to deepen the relaxation further by counting to ten, timing each count to an exhalation.

With two further steps the skills are then brought into daily life. To deal with uncomfortable physical tension, the client attends to their muscles when sitting upright, and then in progressively more complex and distracting activities. The goal is to relax all muscles except those needed for the task, and to not tense the needed muscles to the point of discomfort ("differential relaxation"). To deal with specific psychosocial stresses, the client pairs relaxation with a cue, such as lowering the shoulders and thinking the word "relax" while exhaling. In time, the behavior itself elicits a relaxed feeling ("cue-controlled relaxation") and can be used to optimize one's approach to stressful situations.

Autogenics training (Schultz & Luthe, 1959) involves focusing on sensations of relaxation in one's body. In the classic autogenics script, a person imagines first that each arm and leg in turn is feeling warm and heavy. Later steps include imagining a calm and regular heartbeat, effortless, passive breathing ("it breathes me"), and feelings of warmth at the abdomen, and of coolness at the forehead. Other types of relaxation involving somatosensory imagery, for example feeling that each part of the body in turn is enveloped in a comfortable, warm, peaceful sense of relaxation, are sometimes described as extensions of the autogenics paradigm. Nowadays, passive attention to the sensations remains the cornerstone of autogenics, but self-statements (e.g., "my right arm is heavy"), visualization (e.g., of increased blood flow to the extremity, or of heat radiating from it), and direct suggestion by the therapist, are included as well (e.g., J. Harvey, 1998, which includes a particularly appealing rendition of the classic script).

Autogenics has been used primarily for migraines (Blanchard & Andrasik, 1982), because of its focus on autonomic relaxation, and so that the imagery of warmth can facilitate success in thermal biofeedback. I have found it to be a useful technique for chronic pain in general. Still, autogenics requires access to memories of relaxed sensations, which may not be available to some chronically tense people, or which may be achieved only with great mental effort. For these individuals, progressive muscle relaxation may be a more vivid starting place. Also, as a teaching device for the seemingly obscure image of warmth at the abdomen I sometimes encourage patients to place a warm "hot pack" on their abdomen early in the autogenics training. Not only does this seem to facilitate a sense of deep relaxation, but patients will often sense a lowering of pain intensity. Presumably the novelty of the task, and the focus on a different part of the body and on a competing somatosensory experience, add to the relaxation in producing the improvement in pain. Learning to reproduce this effect without the hot pack is then a goal for further practice.

Even at its first development by Johannes Schultz in the 1920's, autogenics was remarkably modern. The emphasis was on self-management; patients learn to produce the relaxed, hypnosis-like state on their own. Indeed, Schultz's term "autogenics" emphasizes the "self-created" or self-induced nature of the state. Also, it treats the disorder at the level of the symptoms. Schultz regarded the full psychoanalytic armamentarium as overkill for psychosomatic disorders. And autogenics was programmatic: Schultz's first book was an attempt to present autogenics in a skills-acquisition protocol (Linden, 1993).

In ***meditative relaxation***, the third technique, one's attention is focused on deep, slow abdominal breathing. Generally, a rate of 6 breaths per minute is adopted spontaneously, vs. 12 breaths per minute outside of a meditative state (Guyton & J. E. Hall, 2000). The therapist demonstrates and coaches patients on the slow pace, on the expansion of the abdomen during inspiration, and on the quietness of the accessory muscles in the neck, shoulders, and chest. Patients may appreciate knowing that deep, slow breathing raises the efficiency of oxygen uptake in the lungs (Giardino, Glenny, Borson, & L. Chan, 2003), and reduces the vasoconstrictive response to stress (M. T.

Allen, & Crowell, 1990; McCaul, S. Solomon, & D. S. Holmes, 1979). Gradually one's skills increase. Successive improvements in subjective relaxation and in the mechanics of breathing seem to interleave each other. A surface EMG sensor on the abdomen, for training very low levels of muscle tension at the abdominal wall (c. 0.4 μV) can be quite helpful.

This approach to relaxation derives from Yoga and certain Zen meditative practices, and was popularized in America by Herbert Benson (e.g., 1984). More generally, Benson suggests that the essence of all relaxation techniques is a focus on a repetitive stimulus and a passive disregard of distracting thoughts. Thus, a mindful awareness of slow, steady walking can sometimes take the place of abdominal breathing. For pain control, patients sometimes find a surprising degree of benefit from imagery that they are breathing into the painful area, and that their breath has a light, soothing, healing quality (Eimer & A. Freeman, 1998).

Barriers.   From the outset, it is helpful to discuss with patients when, where and how they will be able to practice with a minimum of distraction (Bernstein, Borkovec, & Hazlett-Stevens, 2000). Still, patients initially may be frustrated by outside noises, and thus it is important to remember that it is the defensive response to noises, and not the noises themselves, that is distracting. In time, acceptance and passive disregard of routine distractions should become part of the relaxation practice. Similarly, early in clinic training, patients may be distracted by anxious thoughts, or they may approach the relaxation in a too tense and effortful way (Lipchik, K. A. Holroyd, & Nash, 2002). With reassurance, and with instruction in acceptance and passive intention, both problems tend to resolve easily, as facility with relaxation is acquired. Breath counting may help focus attention (Blanchard & Andrasik, 1985). Still, difficulties will sometimes persist and should be explored with the patient. Some people fear losing control of their emotions and becoming overwhelmed, or losing control of their environment causing inadequacy, failure or rejection. Some may feel that they look unattractive when relaxed, or they may feel weak, or they may think of relaxation as an unwelcome compromise with the pain. Often, processing these feelings will make relaxation possible, but sometimes they are a sign that cognitive behavioral work for Generalized Anxiety Disorder, or depth-oriented psychotherapy, needs to take place before headache treatment. Of course successful psychotherapy is a crucial first step for patients prone to emotional decompensation.

Generalization.   Typically, patients are instructed in the relaxation technique, or in a combination of techniques, and are then given an audiocassette for daily home practice. Generalization training may be explicit: After a solid foundation of relaxation skills has been acquired, the patient is then encouraged to take brief relaxation breaks, for perhaps a minute each, as often as every hour. In one technique, the patient affixes a red dot, say, to the face of their watch, as a cue to relax whenever they check the time (Ahles, A. King, & J. E. Martin, 1984). The goal is to connect relaxation skills, via classical conditioning, to as many settings in the patient's life as possible, and to make tension a more abnormal or infrequent state. Crucially, the relaxation is then used as an active coping skill for dealing with stressors.

BIOFEEDBACK

Biofeedback involves taking accurate, real-time measurements of some aspect of the patient's physiology, and displaying the measurements back to the patient. The basic paradigm is that a person can bring even autonomic functioning under volitional control if the right information is available. Even when the focus is purely on relaxation skills, biofeedback can be helpful for verifying the amount and type of physiological relaxation, selecting a relaxation technique, demonstrating the mind-body effect to patients, achieving a criterion level of relaxation, and documenting the results of treatment (Andreassi, 1995). For while the absorption, pleasant affect, and competing somatosensory experience of subjective relaxation are all important, they are not a guarantee that physiological relaxation is taking place.

For headaches, biofeedback may be brought into treatment when the psychophysiological assessment shows marked tension in the relevant physical measure. Alternatively, biofeedback may be included in a **stepped care** approach, (e.g., if the patient does not improve significantly with relaxation training; Blanchard & Andrasik, 1985), or as **stratified care** (e.g., for chronic daily headache, when it is helpful for treatment to have as much momentum as possible).

For headaches, two forms of biofeedback are in common use. In *thermal biofeedback*, a thermistor is attached to the (usually ventral) surface of a patient's index finger, and temperature readings are collected and displayed (Sargent, Walters, & Green, 1973). A baseline finger temperature of approximately 89 degrees has been reported in the literature, although at our own clinic we find a norm of around 87 degrees. The goal is for the patient to volitionally warm their hands. Techniques include autogenics phrases, imagery of warmth at the hands (for example, lying on the beach with the hot sun warming them), attempting to feel the pulse in one's hands, and simply learning from the biofeedback display. There is some evidence of a threshold-type response, in which achieving a finger temperature of 95–96 °F predicts a greater probability of improvement in migraines (Libo & Arnold, 1983; Morrill & Blanchard, 1989). (Note, however, that for individuals with poor circulation from reflex sympathetic dystrophy or diabetes, we should avoid very high finger temperatures. In these disorders, extraction of oxygen by the tissues may be impaired. Thus, we would not want too much blood bypassing the capillaries, and shunting directly from arterioles to venules, as happens at the higher hand temperatures; Baldi, Aoina, Oxenham, Bagg, & Doughty, 2003; Koban, Leis, Schultze-Mosgau & Birklein, 2003; Tayefeh, Kurz, D. I. Sessler, C. A. Lawson, T. Ikeda, & Marder, 1997; Veves, & Sarnow, 1995).

Generally, initial hand-warming skills are seen by the second or third session. Early on, an inverted U-shaped function is common, with finger temperature declining after a 7–12 minute rise (Kluger, Jamner, & Tursky, 1985). Later in training, more sustained increases may be achieved. Note that there is no evidence that warming the hands externally, for example with a heating pad, has any efficacy for headaches.

It helps for the patient to already have a solid grounding in relaxation skills. The primary challenges in biofeedback are then to introduce the machinery as a way of deepening these skills, to suggest passive intentionality in place of trying too hard, early on to encourage the patient, and to solve the occasional technical problems as they arise. Beyond this, biofeedback is self-learning. Later in treatment, the therapist—a potential distraction—need not, and perhaps should not, be present.

The classic recommendations for thermal biofeedback are due to Taub and School. In their studies, the variable that had the greatest impact on whether a person acquired hand-warming skills was the attitude and manner of the therapist. When the therapist was not interpersonally warm, essentially no skills acquisition took place (E. Taub & School, 1978). A pleasant physical environment is helpful as well, and of course room temperature should neither be cool nor fluctuate. For most people, an ambient temperature of 70–72 °F is sufficient but for older people, slightly built, 75° or even 76 °F may be necessary. Other factors pertain to the mechanics. On older equipment, Taub and coworkers found that sensitive feedback (0.02 °F resolution) delivered at a slow rate (display updated two times per second) enhanced satisfaction and learning (E. Taub & Emurian, 1976; E. Taub & School, 1978). Most biofeedback equipment nowadays interfaces with computers. On them, we have found that a line graph display seems to work well, with sensitivity adjusted to clearly show the effects of the patient's efforts.

Why is the manner of the therapist so important? The greatest barrier to successful hand warming skills seems to be performance anxiety. An initial phase of relaxation training or surface

EMG biofeedback (skills that may be easier to acquire; Middaugh, Haythornthwaite, at al., 2001) can further help patients to succeed at thermal biofeedback (Tibbetts, Charbonneau, & Peper, 1987). Digital indoor-outdoor thermometers make for inexpensive home trainers (the "outdoor" probe is taped to the finger). Practice is often harder in the mornings, at least at first, because of the diurnal surge of cortisol,[2] but can also set a relaxed tone to the day that makes coping with stresses easier.

In *surface EMG biofeedback*, the electrical power output of the muscles is measured at the surface of the skin, and displayed for the patient (Budzynski, Stoyva, & C. S. Adler, 1973). There is a direct relationship between electrical power and force of muscle contraction, and hence the surface EMG readings indicate muscle tension. The readings may be used to teach the patient to relax the muscles, to teach the patient how posture and ergonomics affect muscle tension (Middaugh, Kee, & Nicholson, 1994), and in cotreatment with physical therapy, to verify the effects of the patient's stretching exercises.

I generally introduce the muscle tension readings by describing briefly the voltage changes in muscles as they contract, and how these changes can be read at the surface of the skin. For patients who have had painful experiences with diagnostic needle EMG, it helps to emphasize the surface nature of the sensors, and the fact that biofeedback is a way of facilitating relaxation skills. Patients should also be made aware that no electricity will be entering their bodies; rather, the sensor is designed to read the electricity emanating from them. I then generally demonstrate the skin prep, and readings before, during and after muscle contraction, on myself, using the opponens pollicis muscle at the base of the thumb as a convenient site.

Once the person has adapted to the sensors, and practiced their general relaxation skills without feedback, they can begin using the biofeedback display to deepen the relaxataion. The tense and release cycles of progressive muscle relaxation,[3] imagery of breathing into the area, imagining an alternative sensation (e.g., a pleasant coolness), and directly experimenting with the biofeedback display can all be helpful. As in thermal biofeedback, passive intention, "not trying too hard," is a key skill that comes with practice.

Some patients, even those whose muscle tension readings are not elevated beyond general population norms, report a temporary, complete resolution of pain when they reduce muscle tension readings to near zero. I generally encourage patients to aim for 0.3 μV (the level of machine noise on our equipment), although the effect seems to appear between 0.7 and 0.5 μV. The approach has seemed quite useful for imparting a sense of control over pain in tension-type and cervicogenic headaches.

Much rarer is a third approach: In *cephalic blood volume pulse* biofeedback, the diameter of an extracranial cephalic artery, usually the superficial temporal artery, is measured indirectly by the reflectance of infrared light (photoplethysmography) from the skin surface over the artery. Participants are taught to constrict the artery, for use in interrupting migraine episodes. It has very high face validity, so to speak, for people whose migraines include a flushed, visible pulsing. The equipment is not as readily available as for thermal or EMG biofeedback (Speckenbach & Gerber, 1999). However, reflectance plethysmographs for finger pulse are commercially available, and can be attached over the temporal artery with a dark headband. The readings seem to be more reliable if ambient lighting is kept low. Relatively few research studies have been conducted on

---

[2] I am indebted to Jeff Matranga, Ph.D., ABPP, for information on the home trainer, and to Richard J. Corbett, MD (1934–2000) for the information on cortisol.

[3] And I am indebted to Laura E. Holcomb, Ph.D., for pointing out to me the power of this approach, especially for the paraspinals in the neck and low back.

this method (e.g., Kropp, Gerber, Keinath-Specht, Kopal, & Niederberger, 1997). The preliminary data have been encouraging (Blanchard, 1992). However, more research is needed to be sure that the superior results are not simply due to the expectancies for improvement raised by new, plausible types of treatment.

Logically, cephalic pulse volume biofeedback would be primarily useful for patients with "extracranial migraines," in which dilation of the superficial temporal artery, often visibly distended on the headache side, is a key contributor to the pain (see Chapter 5). For these patients, when plethysmographic measurement is unavailable, it is often helpful to read the temperature at the affected vs. unaffected temple. In extracranial migraines, the temperature is generally higher on the affected side (Drummond & Lance, 1983). I have not known patients to be able to alter cephalic temperature directly, but it generally declines during autogenics training, giving extra intuitive validity to the skills.

On cluster headaches.   In the next chapter, we will review the scant research on behavioral treatment for cluster headaches. The literature is too sparse to suggest any behavioral modality as empirically supported. Logically, however, it makes sense to inquire about triggers, as discussed in Chapter 10. Of course if stress or letdown is a trigger, relaxation or stress management training is implied directly. In addition, temperature or pulse volume at the temples may show side-to-side differences and/or lower variability on the symptomatic side interictally. It remains for future research whether trying to change these differences with biofeedback training will be worthwhile, for example when aura or altered sensory experience gives a warning period in which self-regulatory skills can be applied.

Although measures of electrodermal responding such as *skin conductance level* are rarely mentioned in the headache literature, they respond much faster than finger temperature, and hence can be a wonderful way of introducing biofeedback, for example to older children. Children love seeing how the machine responds when they talk about how their younger sister bugs them, or when they say things about themselves that are not true. Once the general idea of biofeedback is learned, transition to the slower measure, finger temperature, can be made.

Moreover, the sensitivity of skin conductance to degree of mental activation may be a particular advantage. For some migraineurs describe continuous vigilance, and the feeling that they never allow their brains to rest. People with chronic tension-type or posttraumatic headaches may report mental fatigue as an antecedent to pain. Although direct attempts to lower skin conductance seem especially prone to backfire, the measure can be useful as a secondary index. By keeping it in the corner of one's eye, a patient can use it as a guide to a more mentally quiescent, passive, and restful approach to relaxation. The respiration artifact—increases in skin conductance with laughter, coughing, or deep breathing, should be pointed out, so that patients do not mistake it for a sign of stress.

Regardless of the specific form of biofeedback, three steps are typically taken in the later stages of treatment to generalize the self-regulatory skills to the patient's daily life:

- Practice in self-regulation without feedback. For example, a person may continue decreasing muscle tension with the biofeedback signal turned off. The machine's recordings during this interval can help show when a patient is ready to practice independently.
- Rehearsal of the skills at home, typically for twenty minutes a day.
- Application of the skills as a coping tool for handling personally relevant stressors. This last step may be implemented as a homework assignment, or as an in-session goal of maintaining relaxed readings while discussing stressful issues (e.g., C. S. Adler, S. M. Adler, & Packard, 1987).

We have seen in Chapter 6, and will explore more deeply in Chapter 15, that recovery in tension-type headache (and in chronic pain more generally) seems to be preceded by the expectation of control over pain. This seems reasonable, for as long as the pain is regarded as an overbearing problem, the mind will remain vividly engaged with it. Thus, all signs of progress, however meager in themselves, should be celebrated as steps to recovery, and as pointers to what the person is capable of achieving.

TRIGGER IDENTIFICATION AND MANAGEMENT

Patients often enter treatment with an intuitive sense of their headaches' precipitating factors. However, because the effect of triggers is probabilistic, and may depend on the number of triggers present, both illusory correlations and overlooked connections can occur. Even as salient a trigger as stress can go unnoticed—recall Wolff's classic results in Chapter 5 suggesting a 4-day delayed effect between a major stressor and a migraine. Some patients find that this association holds like clockwork, and gives them ample time for prevention, but only after they know to look for such a distant cause.

Thus, triggers are generally tracked prospectively using a daily headache diary and a candidate list, such as that given at the end of Chapter 10. The prospective measurements of pain level and headache frequency also help in quantifying the effectiveness of treatment (Lake, 2001). Triggers can be determined from the diary by inspection, or by computing lagged correlations between exposure to a given trigger and the subsequent occurrence of a headache.

Once triggers have been identified, attempts are made to eliminate them. For dietary triggers this may be relatively easy. For other triggers, such as caffeine, stress or missed sleep, patients may benefit from behavioral tools in habit control, to help bring about the needed lifestyle changes.

We saw in Chapter 10 that there is theoretical reason, and a little bit of data, to believe that desensitizing to triggers is a better strategy than avoidance. At this point the evidence seems too scant to recommend desensitization/purposeful exposure as a general strategy. However, when triggers are frequent and truly unavoidable (for example, certain ambient smells), and elicit strong arousal, muscle tension (e.g., grimacing), and/or expectation of a headache, desensitization may be the best approach. In that case, **imaginal desensitization**, with much attention to maintaining a relaxed state (Philips & Jahanshahi, 1985), is a good starting point. Desensitization might be useful to consider also for patients whose lives have or would become highly constricted by trigger avoidance.

Of course when there is a large number of environmental triggers, avoiding them becomes impractical. In that case it makes sense to focus more on reducing pain sensitivity than on changing the environment. Chronic migraines in particular, especially with comorbid fibromyalgia, seem best treated by analogy to other types of chronic pain.

COGNITIVE COPING SKILLS

As we have seen, chronic headaches can be a source of stress that in turn contributes to further headaches. And outside stresses may take on added significance when they are known triggers. The person may fear the stressor, and dread the headache to follow. A deficit in effective coping is even more problematic in medication overuse headaches, in which the patient may not see an alternative to the medication, even though it is contributing to their pain. The targeted use of relaxation skills as a part of one's response to the stressor is thus very helpful, for clearer and more flexible thinking, and to prevent a subsequent headache. In addition, it may be helpful to go beyond this and address more directly the patient's manner of thinking about and responding to stresses.

A particularly well-validated approach begins by helping the patient to identify stressors that are contributing to headaches, and for which behavior change is feasible. The stressors may include the headaches themselves. If the patient is avoiding stressors that should be dealt with, or is dealing with them in an unfocused and ineffective manner, then the therapist helps promote effective problem-solving. If the patient is engaging in sound problem-solving but is also thinking in anxious ways about the stressors, then the therapist teaches skills for redirecting one's thoughts in directions that promote greater self-efficacy. The treatment approach is quite similar to **Problem Solving Therapy**, which was originally developed for depression (D'Zurilla & Nezu, 1999; Nezu, 1986). As we will see in the next chapter, there is evidence that cognitive coping skills, combined with relaxation, are particularly effective for tension-type headache (Tobin, K. A. Holroyd, Baker, Reynolds, & Holm, 1988).

As forms of treatment, cognitive and problem solving therapy deserve and have manuals of their own (e.g., J. S. Beck, 1995; D'Zurilla & Nezu, 1999). Here, we will simply outline a few salient principles.

We are all capable of reasoning that is precise, clear, and accurate. We do not grade roads, wire houses, conduct research, or balance our checkbooks based on vague, emotional generalizations. But we also tend to be "cognitive misers" (S. E. Taylor, 1981): We expend such thought only when we have to, typically at work or school. And the more personal and emotionally laden a topic is for us, the more likely we are to apply biased, overgeneralized, poor quality thought. Thus, in chronic pain, problem solving may be supplanted under stress with the thought "If only the doctors would find out what's wrong." When this is part of a constructive attempt to collect more information it can be quite helpful, but often it is vague, inchoate and wishful, disempowering the patient by formulating the problem in essentially unsolvable terms.

Moreover, we may attend to only the part of the data that fits our beliefs (selective abstraction), overgeneralize, exaggerate the importance of single events (arbitrary inference), oversimplify into all-or-none categories, and take things far more personally than would be warranted (A. T. Beck, 1976). This results in ideas that are neither accurate nor useful. Indeed, **cognitive distortions** are typically so vague, stereotyped and saturated with emotion that they could not possibly be true; they are virtually a disengagement from problem solving.

Note that the source of distress need not be our conscious thoughts, but can be the automatic, moment-to-moment appraisal and encoding of stresses as they arise. A person may not notice these appraisals until attending carefully to them, filling out a thought record (see Chapter 12) immediately after stressors. Sometimes behavior is the first clue. A patient may report no pain-related distress, yet have an expression of exquisite suffering during brief paroxysms of pain.

To correct automatic thoughts, the client should first question and test them, rationally and with simple behavioral experiments. The client should satisfy himself in the accuracy of a more sophisticated, nuanced, well thought out appraisal of key stress situations. The more accurate thoughts should then be kept readily accessible in one's mind and rehearsed when stressors arise. It can also help to review stresses in clear visual detail while maintaining the more accurate perspective in consciousness.

Thus, we can go far in managing stresses if we treat reactions of depression, anxiety, or distress as markers of a problem for which we need a more effective solution. It helps to then pause, disengage from our current way of responding to the problem, and drop back into a more objective, accurate, and dispassionate mode of thought. Moreover, we should restate the underlying problem in terms that are as precise, detailed, and unbiased as possible. We should then approach the problem systematically, generating as many possible paths to a solution as we can. And we should then test these solutions by careful trial and error, expecting surprises, and being as prepared to learn when our predictions are wrong as when they are right. In short, we proceed as "naïve scientists" studying the problem (Fiske & S. E. Taylor, 1991).

Because problem solving skills are procedural rather than intellectual (declarative) knowledge, acquisition and fluency can take months. We should expect to slowly get better at them, recognizing that mistakes along the way are both inevitable and useful.

Some problems, such as the death of a loved one, are unsolvable in concrete terms. Then our task is emotional coping, treating our feelings as the problem to be worked on. Except in cases of death, however, I tend to be very cautious about shifting from problem- to emotion-focused coping. We can conclude too readily that a problem is objectively insurmountable. And unless we know for sure that a problem is unsolvable, there is something to be said for the patient, dispassionate, careful pursuit in its own right. We are meant to solve problems.

Williams and coworkers have suggested that the effectiveness of coping skills training is enhanced if patients have specific behavioral goals for the amount of daily practice, say, for 20 minutes once a day and for three 10 minute breaks. At this point, the evidence for the efficacy of time goals seems stronger for laboratory than for clinical pain, but a degree of support has been found (L. D. James, Thorn, & D. A. Williams, 1993).

TREATMENT FOR TEMPOROMANDIBULAR DISORDERS

The main ingredients of biobehavioral treatment of headaches are useful in treating temporomandibular disorders (TMD) as well. After assessment, education about the role of parafunctional behaviors, stress-induced muscle tension, and trigger points, is often a key first step, which surface EMG monitoring can make more vivid. Biofeedback to reduce tension at the masticatory muscles (especially the masseter and anterior temporalis) to low values, relaxation and stress management skills, and generalization of this new self-regulatory capacity to stressful situations, are often useful in turn (Gevirtz, Glaros, Hopper, & M. S. Schwartz, 1995; J. J. Sherman & D. C. Turk, 2001). For muscle relaxation, jaw stretching exercises, taught by a physical therapist, can be a helpful adjunct, and may substitute for a tense-and-release approach (C. R. Carlson, F. L. Collins, Nitz, Sturgis, & J. L. Rogers, 1990; C. R. Carlson, Okeson, Falace, Nitz, & D. Anderson, 1991). When trigger points are present, the global relaxation should be trained to a high finger temperature criterion. If needed, elements of chronic pain treatment, described later in this chapter, also may be included. There are, however, two emphases in treating TMD not often applied in headaches: The treatment team generally includes a dentist, of course, and if bruxism is present, considerable focus is given to oral habit change (Gevirtz, et al.).

Oral habit change.   Eliminating parafunctional behaviors such as daytime jaw clenching can be difficult even when a person knows that they may be contributing to pain. Gramling and associates report benefit from a behavioral habit reversal protocol (Gramling, Neblett, Grayson, & Townsend, 1996). In this approach, patients first engage in self-monitoring parafunctional oral behaviors. Relevant behaviors from the Oral Habits Questionnaire (Moss, Ruff, & Sturgis, 1984), discussed in the previous chapter, are reasonable targets. The purpose of self-monitoring, of course, is to bring the behavior into awareness, so that it is more susceptible to change. The next step is to teach breathing relaxation and facial exercises as alternative, incompatible responses. Patients learn to substitute the breathing relaxation and facial exercises for the oral habits. Other components of the program are progressive muscle relaxation, to be practiced at least four times a week, and skills for eliminating irrational beliefs about stressors. Sometimes, self-monitoring will show that the parafunctional behaviors are consistently occurring in certain types of situations, for which assertiveness, problem-solving, or stress-management skills may be useful (Gevirtz et al., 1995).

For nocturnal bruxism, deep relaxation at bedtime is a reasonable starting point, combined with self-statements (e.g., "lips together, teeth apart"), and the somatosensory imagery of a relaxed jaw (Foster, 2004). Surface EMG trainers can be adapted as an alarm to awaken a patient when they brux. Sensitivity should be low enough that swallowing will not trigger the unit. Volume is set high enough to awaken the patient, and the pitch is changed every 2–3 nights to prevent habituation (Foster, 2004). Help with lifestyle change, or referral for appropriate resources, are also logical (Foster, 2004), given correlational data suggesting that tobacco use, and excessive intake of alcohol and coffee are risk factors for nocturnal bruxism (Lavigne, Lobbezoo, Rompre, T. A. Nielsen, & Montplaisir, 1997; Ohayon, K. K. Li, & Guilleminault, 2001).

MEDICATION TAPER

We have seen that overuse of symptomatic headache medications is thought to be a common cause of chronic daily headache, and should be considered as well in chronic posttraumatic headache. For patients with rebound headache, discontinuing the medications is usually a crucial part of recovery. For other patients, a taper may be mandated by side effects such as sedation, dizziness, impaired concentration, or flattened affect. When the overused substance is a benzodiazepine, narcotic (e.g., codeine) or barbiturate (e.g., butalbital, Fiorinal), a slow tapering is in order, to prevent severe withdrawal symptoms, such as seizures (N.T. Mathew, 1993). When the rebound headache is due to a simple analgesic, ergotamine, or triptan, the usual course is abrupt withdrawal (Hering & Steiner, 1991). In either case, the change in medication requires a collaboration between the patient, psychologist, and prescribing physician. The psychologist will sometimes be the first person on a case to discover the frequent use of symptomatic medication. At times, a psychologist who specializes in headache treatment will know more about medication rebound than the physician, and be in a consulting role to physician and patient about this. Sometimes the problematic medication may nearly escape notice, such as the acetaminophen in Parafon Forte. And some patients will be strongly and understandably resistant to a taper until they have good pain coping skills in place.

As we have seen, vigilance to headaches and medication intake can sometimes become quite ingrained. Moreover, the transition from primary to daily headache is subtle; there is usually little intuitive evidence that the medications have become a cause of the headaches (Henry, Daubech, Lucas, & Gagnon, 1988). All of this makes the taper a leap of faith. Several behavioral steps can make the recovery easier. First, education about rebound headaches, and about some of the possible underlying mechanisms (see Chapter 7), can make the taper more plausible. It can also help to sketch the likely course of a taper as realistically as possible. Second, in theory it can be helpful behaviorally for the physician to first switch medications to long-acting varieties and time contingent intake, so that the medications are no longer reinforcing attention to pain (Gerber, Miltner, & Niederberger, 1988). I have not always found this to be useful, however. It seems to prolong the anxious period before getting through the taper. Note, too, that this step would be self-defeating if it substitutes for the taper. Third, because the patents are likely to be afraid and relying on the reassurance of the treating professional, confidence, structure, and close coordination with the physician are important.

Seeing health as deriving mostly from medical care ("powerful others" locus of control; N. J. Martin, K. A. Holroyd, & Penzien, 1990) may be a risk factor for high medication intake (Reynaert et al., 1995). When an opiate reduces pain, for example, an individual with a variety of self-management tools may conclude, "the pain is tractable; I can gain control of it." But the lesson for a person with an external locus of control may be, "I need narcotics to control the pain."

A tendency to interpret anxiety symptoms as dangerous (anxiety sensitivity; Asmundson, K. D. Wright, P. J. Norton, & Veloso, 2001) may also be a risk factor. Indeed, we should look closely at anxiety, and its possible confounding with pain, whenever there is overuse of pain medications (Reynaert et al., 1995). For example, a person who immediately reaches for their narcotics upon learning that their son was severely injured may not be treating pain then, given the strong distraction and possible stress-induced analgesia. Logically, catastrophization is also a risk factor, for a patient with rebound headache may be afraid of being overwhelmed by pain, and of being unable to function, without symptomatic medication. Thus, acquisition of pain coping skills is a very useful part of treatment for medication overuse.

Education about psychological factors in headache, and training in pain management techniques, can help balance out a "powerful others" locus of control. For anxiety sensitivity, the key treatment ingredients are similar to those for treating panic disorder: giving information on the stress response and its advantages for survival, and ultimately conducting desensitization to the physical experience of arousal. As always, it is important to proceed slowly to, and through, the desensitization, and to maintain exposure until distress has subsided, so that self-efficacy is bolstered by the process. Because pain-management skills do not seem to be as effective during high medication use, it is best not to wait for good pain control before beginning the taper. However, skills for reducing anxiety should ideally be well established.

Still, in my own experience, the majority of patients with rebound headaches simply have no idea that medications can have this effect. For them, the challenge is to be sure that they are discussing a reduction in medications with their physician, and not abruptly discontinuing use of a barbiturate, benzodiazepine, or narcotic.

Several detoxification regimens have been reported useful in easing the pain and autonomic symptoms that frequently (but not invariably) follow withdrawal. Traditionally, detoxification was performed in an inpatient setting, to help ensure compliance and control of withdrawal symptoms. More recent protocols cover outpatient withdrawal, although presumably medical concerns (such as poorly controlled hypertension) or difficulty with compliance would call for an inpatient setting.

Generally, the protocols include medications that have been found useful in status migrainosus: corticosteroids, and long-acting nonsteroidals or anti-migraine agents. Simultaneously, migraine prophylactics are instituted.

The classic inpatient protocol consists of intravenous dihydroergotamine (0.25–1.0 mg) and metoclopramide (Reglan, 10–20 mg) per eight hours (Raskin, 1986; Silberstein, Schulman, & M. M. Hopkins, 1990). For outpatients, Bonuccelli, et al. recommend 4 mg dexamethasone IM and prn oral antacid daily for 2 weeks, amitriptyline 25 mg po for 1 week, followed by amitriptyline 50 mg for 6 months (Bonuccelli, Nuti, Lucetti, Pavese, Dell'Agnello, & Muratorio, 1996). Alternatively, Krymchantowski and Barbosa (2000) use a 6-day burst of oral prednisone (60 mg for 2 days, 40 for 2 days, and then 20 mg for the last 2 days) plus 300 mg of daily ranitidine (Zantac). Hering and Steiner (1991) used amitriptyline 10 mg and prn naproxen. Naproxen is preferred to other nonsteroidals because it is long-acting. N. T. Mathew (1987) reported good results with naproxen, 500 mg bid, beginning one day before withdrawal and continuing until the withdrawal was complete. Behaviorally, time-contingent medication is generally more appropriate than prn for reducing psychological dependency.

Some clinicians also allow use of sumatriptan, 6 mg subcutaneous, for acute exacerbations during and after withdrawal (Bonuccelli et al., 1996). The practice was started before triptan overuse headaches were identified (Diener, Haab, Peters, Ried, Dichgans, & Pilgrim, 1991), and logically would seem problematic in patients already dependent on symptomatic medications (Krymchantowski & Barbosa, 2000).

So far there have been no controlled studies, and hence the evidence is in the form of clinical series at single treatment centers. The data from Krymchantowski and Barbosa may have an advantage, in that it is based on a sample size of 400. However, no comparative trials are available.

SELF-APPLIED MODALITIES

Cooling.   Perhaps the classic home remedy for migraines is a cool washcloth placed across the forehead. In a variant, some patients place the washcloth at the back of their neck instead, to reduce nausea rather than pain. There may be several reasons that this method would help. If the forehead has not become sensitized, the cool stimulus may compete with pain for access to central processing resources. Also, cold is the quintessential stimulus for constricting superficial blood vessels via alpha-adrenergic, heat-conserving mechanisms. Superficial vasoconstriction would be particularly useful for people with "extracranial migraines"—migraines in which distension of the extracranial blood vessels contributes significantly to the pain. Moreover, coolness applied to the forehead or face elicits a "**diving reflex**"—a set of physiological changes aimed at reducing oxygen consumption (Gooden, 1994; Reyners, Tio, Vlutters, van der Woude, Reitsma, & Smit, 2000). In essence, the body assumes that if your forehead is cool, you are probably underwater. Not surprisingly, the diving reflex overlaps to a degree with the relaxation response, particularly in a reduction in heart rate (M. T. Allen, Shelley, & Boquet, 1992; Heath & J. A. Downey, 1990; recall the inclusion of images of forehead coolness in autogenics).

For a headache that is present continuously, it is theoretically plausible that consistent, time-contingent application of heat or cold could help reduce central sensitization, particularly if the patient focuses their attention on the competing stimulus. The goal is to strengthen their sensitivity to heat or cold at the expense of pain sensitivity. The warm or cool stimulus itself should be very weak; the practice is in imagining the temperature sensation as clearly as possible, and then retaining it in memory. This approach capitalizes on intracortical inhibition and diffuse noxious inhibitory controls, as discussed in Chapter 2. Nonetheless, I know of no research that verifies the utility of such a "psychophysical therapy." Its benefits, although rational, are uncertain.

On similarly rational grounds we may suspect that the effects of a modality could vary considerably depending on how the stimulus is applied. Some patients, for example, use a cold stimulus to intensify pain to the highest tolerable level, holding this for as long as possible, and then removing the stimulus. The relief is reinforcing, and gives them a brief sense of control over the pain. Presumably, the pain reduction is mediated by an increase in blood pressure, the cognitive sense of control, and/or a large scale recruitment of endorphinergic pathways. (Cold water swim is used to elicit an endorphin response in laboratory animals; Lapo, Konarzewski, & Sadowski, 2003). But such an extreme approach seems likely to have the opposite effect of the sensory reeducation discussed in the previous paragraph. By maintaining pain at a very high intensity, one gives the pain system ample opportunity to acquire further sensitization. Here too, however, the psychophysical hypothesis requires testing. The long-term effects of various types of counter-stimulation have not yet been explored.

TENS.   A **TENS** unit, or transcutaneous electrical nerve stimulator, is a portable device that supplies a mild electric current to the skin. The sensation from the electricity masks or blocks the pain. TENS units were originally inspired by the gate control model (D. M. Walsh & McAdams, 1997): Stimulating large diameter nerve fibers, which encode non-noxious touch or pressure, should block the input from small-diameter "pain" nerves (Melzack & P. D. Wall, 1965). However, the devices are often set to deliver a stimulus that is itself mildly painful, producing some of the relief via pain-on-pain inhibition (diffuse noxious inhibitory controls; Chesterton, Barlas, Foster, Lundeberg, C. C. Wright, & Baxter, 2002). A fatiguing of peripheral nerves, "electrogenic blockade," is a third possible mechanism (Pertovaara & Hämäläinen, 1982).

TENS units are prescribed medically and dispensed by a physical therapist, who instructs the patient in their use and helps find the optimal placement of the stimulation pads. In practice, the electrodes are often applied at or near the site of pain. However, when a region has been sensitized by prolonged pain, the additional input can be noxious, and in that case it seems more logical to place the electrodes at a related site: an adjacent dermatome, the same dermatome on the opposite side of the body, or the same dermatome but proximal to the pain. Different frequencies of stimulation seem to work through different spinal mechanisms. In particular, the effects of low (but not high) frequency TENS seem to be mediated by serotonin ($5-HT_{2A}$ and $5-HT_3$) and μ-opioid receptors (Radhakrishnan et al., 2003). Thus, in animal studies low frequency TENS shows **cross-tolerance** with narcotic analgesics (Chandran & Sluka, 2003). This may not be a concern clinically, however, as units are generally set to alternate between frequencies (e.g., "burst" mode; Chesterton, et al., 2002). A single study on mice suggests that **5-hydroxytryptophan** (5-HTP), a serotonin precursor, may increase the efficacy of TENS (Shimizu, Koja, Fujisaki, & Fukuda, 1981). It is unknown whether this is true in people as well, or whether serotonergic antidepressants would likewise show a synergy with TENS (Radhakrishnan et al.).

Very few adverse effects have been reported for TENS units, but a number of theoretical concerns have been noted (Geddes, 1998; Hansson & Lundeberg, 1999). Implanted on-demand cardiac pacemakers or automatic defibrillators could malfunction. TENS electrodes on the anterior-lateral neck could cause the laryngeal muscles to spasm, or affect blood pressure or heart rhythm via stimulation of the vagus nerve or receptors in the carotid sinus. And the use of TENS for labor pain could involve possible risks if the electrodes are placed near the uterus or fetus (Geddes, 1998; Hansson & Lundeberg, 1999).

Of course, TENS electrodes applied to the head, unlike those on the back or shoulder, are highly visible, and the advantages for pain control must be balanced against the behavioral and social effects of so visibly calling attention to one's pain. For this reason, I tend to be very cautious about raising the idea of medical consideration for a TENS unit in the case of headaches. However, when the stimulation is applied intermittently and in private, the benefits can sometimes predominate.

Scents. We saw in Chapter 2 that pleasant smells can reduce pain, especially in women. Some patients report that by carrying a light spray of lavender or lilac with them they can prevent such odors as diesel, fresh asphalt, or even the strong perfumes of others from triggering migraines. Of course, as with all forms of trigger management, we must weigh the averted migraines against the risk that avoidance will perpetuate the stimulus sensitivity.

GENERAL PAIN COPING SKILLS

As we will discuss further in the next chapter, various combinations of biofeedback, relaxation training, and cognitive stress management therapy have been empirically supported for migraines and tension-type headache. However, they may not be sufficient for continuous headache, refractory chronic daily headache, or for many cases of posttraumatic headache. For patients with these disorders, skills for managing pain, and for minimizing the impact of pain on one's functioning and emotional well being, are important.

Note that the application involves a leap of faith. Behavioral chronic pain treatment has been validated primarily for chronic low back pain, with a smaller amount of literature for other conditions such as rheumatoid arthritis, fibromyalgia, and sickle cell disease. The theories underlying cognitive-behavioral therapy are not pain-site specific, however. And given the paucity in general of empirical treatment data for continuous headache and posttraumatic headache, chronic pain treatment seems a reasonable, if inferential step.

From Chapter 3, we know the variables to address in chronic pain treatment. These variables are summarized in Table 13–2, below.

We have already encountered several of the primary treatment modalities, including problem solving therapy and training in a variety of pain management tools. In addition, two further approaches are taken in behaviorally oriented chronic pain programs: operant conditioning, and cognitive-behavioral skills training.

Operant conditioning.   The pain sensation is sometimes surrounded by a penumbra of behavior: rest and withdrawal, foregoing activities, talking about pain, and accelerating medication use. The pain behaviors can be a source of unhappiness in their own right, and can increase pain through deconditioning, perhaps distress, and frequent attention to the sensation. Operant approaches focus on decreasing the pain behaviors, within safe and reasonable medical limits set by the patient's physician (Sanders, 1996).

Like all behaviors, the pain-related behaviors are thought to be maintained by their consequences, two in particular. The first is reduction in pain, and in the anxiety that the pain may cause. This reduction can reinforce inactivity, even when activity would give a better long-term outcome, avoidance of activities, even beyond what may be medically necessary, and dependence

TABLE 13–2
Primary Goals in Chronic Pain Treatment

Treatment Goal	*Means of Assessing*	*Primary Treatment Modalities*
Promote Internal Locus of Control	Headache Specific Locus of Control Scale	Patient Education
Increase Self-Efficacy	Headache Management Self-Efficacy Scale	Skills Training
Decrease Catastrophizing	Pain Catastrophizing Scale or Coping Strategies Questionnaire	Skills Training, Cognitive Therapy, Problem Solving Therapy
Decrease Fear of Pain	Fear of Pain Questionnaire	Skills Training, Graded Exposure to Avoided Situations
Increase Involvement in Non-Pain Activities of High Emotional Priority	Interview	Problem Solving Therapy and In-Session Reinforcement
Increase Positive Affect	Beck Depression Inventory	Behavioral Mobilization, Cognitive Therapy, Problem Solving Therapy, Assertiveness Training
Decrease Exposure to Reminders of Pain and Injury	Interview	Behavioral Mobilization, Pacing, In-Session Reinforcement of Functioning, Education of Patient and Spouse
Reduce Anxiety Sensitivity	Interview	Patient Education, Desensitization to Symptoms of Arousal
Decrease Overt Pain Behaviors and any Reinforcements that Support Them	Interview, West Haven-Yale Multidimensional Pain Inventory	Education of Patient and Spouse

on medications and procedures, even when these have a long track record of failure. Occasionally, a patient for whom several surgeries have provided no lasting benefit, whose pain in fact is worse than ever, presents as almost desperate for one more operation to fix the problem. The second major source of reinforcement is thought to be the patient's spouse or significant other, whose efforts to protect the patient from pain and overactivity may have developed in time into a pattern in which only pain is reinforced.

In pain, as in other applications, the operant approach involves identifying key behaviors, and developing realistic and medically appropriate targets for these behaviors. The goal, of course, is to work with the patient in arranging things to promote greater involvement in meaningful non-pain activities. In part, this implies problem-solving, so that barriers to the activities are removed. In part, it may imply working with the spouse to be sure that the natural reinforcements are encouraging recovery. And in part, direct reinforcement by the therapist has a role to play. In therapy, patients may learn to coach others not to ask about the pain, or they may learn to answer such questions briefly and confidently, gently steering the conversation to other topics. Such intervention by the patient can be especially powerful, and by educating others the patient reinforces their own sense of knowledge and mastery over the pain. And patients are often relieved when others stop asking about the pain. It's bad enough to have pain without having to think about it all the time.

For patients receiving worker's compensation, it is helpful for the larger system to be reinforcing wellness. Of course, a treating psychologist's impact on the system is likely to be limited. However, a team meeting, in which all sides in a case agree on a realistic plan for increased functioning, can implicitly create incentives for recovery.[4]

Cognitive-behavioral skills training. Cognitive-behavioral interventions are designed to counter the feelings of helplessness and depression that can undermine chronic pain coping. Individuals first learn skills for producing a favorable impact on their situation. They learn relaxation and biofeedback as ways of controlling psychophysiological processes that may be relevant to the pain, and to the tension and distress caused by pain. Similarly, they learn skills in mental imagery. Note that although imagery is often described as a relaxation technique, there is little evidence that by itself it produces a decrease in sympathetic tone. However, imagery is a particularly effective way of decreasing the subjective experience of pain, presumably through absorption-mediated activation of descending pain modulatory circuits. Third, participants learn skills in assertiveness and effective problem-solving. Thus, specific coping skills are taught, relevant to physiological tension, subjective pain experience, and external stressors. Then, individuals examine their habitual thoughts when encountering a stressor. They identify catastrophic thoughts, maladaptive beliefs, and **cognitive distortions** that may underlie depression or low self-efficacy in reaction to the pain. Finally, individuals are given considerable practice in integrating and implementing the skills: setting goals, developing strategies, self-reinforcing, and engaging in constructive, solution-focused internal dialogue (Bradley, 1996).

Hypnosis may be defined simply as "a procedure wherein changes in sensations, perceptions, thoughts, feelings, or behavior are suggested" (Kirsch & Lynn, 1995, p. 846; after the American Psychological Association's Division of Psychological Hypnosis). In clinical practice, hypnosis usually involves an induction process including deep relaxation, focused attention on the clinician's voice, and a suspension of critical judgment. In the research literature, however, it seems that none of these ingredients are necessary, and that their effect in increasing suggestibility is small (Kirsch & Lynn, 1995).

---

[4]I am indebted to Melvin Attfield, Ph.D, for pointing this out to us in a long-ago talk.

A number of suggestions have been used for pain control, including dissociation from one's body, transforming the pain into a different type of physical sensation, and deep absorption in pleasant imagery. We saw in Chapter 2 that vibration and pain may compete for activation in primary somatosensory cortex. Thus, not all sensory modalities need work through the same mechanism, or be equally effective. In hypnosis, the prototypical suggestion is of numbness and anesthesia in the affected body part, and there is a little evidence that this may be a particularly useful type of imagery (H. J. Crawford, Knebel, L. Kaplan, et al., 1998; Zachariae & Bjerring, 1994).

The effects of hypnosis are usually short-term. For example, in studies of laboratory pain, the suggestions are generally repeated throughout the pain exposure. With practice, however, a patient may become progressively more skilled at self-inducing the hypnotic experience. Then they can use the experience as needed as an active coping tool. We will examine hypnosis at some length in Chapter 15.

Somatic awareness has been proposed as a pain management skill (Bakal, Demjen, & Duckro, 1994). Individuals with somatic awareness are cognizant of the moment-by-moment fluctuations in their pain, but this awareness differs from an anxious pain focus. In somatic awareness, the perceptiveness goes beyond the pain itself, to include: (1) a sense of the internal (thoughts, feelings, behaviors) and environmental factors that are affecting pain level; (2) an almost automatic sense of when to use relaxation, a change in activity, or other coping skills to reduce the pain before it escalates too far; and (3) a sense of confidence in one's ability to manage the pain. Note that as pain becomes more severe and disruptive, seeking an awareness of its nuances is quite counter-intuitive. It is far more natural to try to ignore the pain as a coping strategy. Bakal and his coauthors argue, however, that ignoring chronic pain simply allows the pain to escalate to the point that it becomes much harder to reduce.

As we have seen, the headache diary can be a useful tool for building somatic awareness. As the individual tracks his or her pain, and its antecedents and consequences, they begin to notice that its fluctuations have a certain amount of predictability. This in turn gives a sense of which coping skills to use, and when to use them.

Somatic awareness is a component of a very well designed and popular self-help guide, *Managing Pain Before It Manages You* (Caudill, 1995), and of a very useful book we will discuss further below, *Taking Control of Your Headaches* (Duckro, W. Richardson, J. E. Marshall, Cassabaum, & G. Marshall, 1999).

Acceptance vs. pain suppression.   As we saw in Chapter 3, effortful attempts to exclude pain from consciousness can make pain more noxious and intrusive, delay recovery from flare-ups, disrupt concentration, and can undermine one's confidence in pain management skills. Pain suppression seems to be too tiring, difficult, and paradoxical in its effects to be useful. Of course, if the approach is working for a patient there is no need to change it. And we must distinguish sustained, effortful pain blocking from brief use of suppression while a patient refocuses on an absorbing, enjoyable task. Still, a shift from sustained suppression to acceptance of the pain is often the single most useful change that an otherwise well functioning person can make (McCracken & Eccleston, 2003), and sometimes leads to dramatic drops in pain intensity.

In acceptance, we relinquish strategies that have not worked, such as attempts to eliminate or find a cure for the pain. We are willing to continue in pain, and seek a renewed engagement in life (McCracken & Eccleston, 2003). Paradoxically, by shifting attention from control over the pain to control over our thoughts, feelings, and life, acceptance can be associated with more rather than less pain control (Viane, et al., 2003).

For patients angry about an injury, acceptance may mean acknowledging the anger and examining its sources, including on a cognitive level. It also means looking at the personal costs of the anger, and the degree to which it is precluding a fuller life. For some people, this processing will need to be in the realm of depth-oriented, but not necessarily long-term, psychotherapy. Depending on the patient's readiness to take responsibility for their lives, and the relevance of the injury to their sense of self, the course of therapy may be long or short.

A similar process is to mourn and ultimately move beyond activities that are no longer feasible. All-or-none thinking should be avoided, however, for there is often some part of the former activity that can be retained, or there is an alternative route to the same rewards.

Functioning.   As my boss, Jeff Matranga Ph.D., ABPP has patiently pointed out over many years, considerable gains in pain coping can often be made simply by promoting increased functioning, that is, involvement in absorbing non-pain activities. Often, this can be accomplished through a combination of problem-solving and encouragement. Note, however, that pain is sometimes a source of anxiety, as when a person feels unable to cope with it. Then they may anxiously self-monitor for early signs of a pain flare-up, and limit their activities. The patient may describe this process explicitly, or we may suspect it from the combination of a very low activity level, poor perceived control over the pain, avoidance (e.g., in an almost desperate-sounding use of pain-contingent analgesics) and catastrophic thinking (Philips, 1987). When present, such anxious expectancies can block attempts to increase functional activity.

Sometimes it is possible to correct the anxiety through **graded exposure**, such as in an exercise-to-quota program in physical therapy for low back pain. Headaches, however, seem particularly susceptible to top-down influence. For them, anxious vigilance to pain may be enough to trigger a self-fulfilling prophecy. In this case, it is important to counteract the expectancies. Ways of doing so include combining the functional activity with relaxation or other tools that build confidence in one's ability to control the pain; combining the activity with outside distraction from pain monitoring; and removing external cues, such as clocks, that could be used to gauge amount of effort.

Pacing.   Often, it is the impediments to productivity—work, housecleaning, and playing with children and grandchildren—that people find most frustrating about their pain. Not surprisingly, they try to make up for lost time whenever their pain is at a tolerable level, discontinuing activity only when the pain again becomes unbearable. Although this is a highly intuitive strategy, it has a number of disadvantages. It can turn every activity into a contest that the pain ultimately wins, adding still further to frustration. Although pain-related frustration is not as harmful as pain-related anxiety in promoting a somatic focus, the frustration still can work against emotionally "de-prioritizing" the pain. Also, the contingency in which activity is regularly followed by increased pain would, at least in theory, punish involvement in nonpain endeavors. Conversely, pain-contingent rest may reinforce the body for heightened pain sensitivity. And repeated intense flare-ups can presumably contribute to central sensitization, causing a long-term reduction in pain thresholds and increased susceptibility to future flare-ups.

The alternative, of course, is to treat pain like a stressor, i.e., as something to be managed proactively, before it reaches a crisis stage. On the level of skills, pacing means prioritizing activities, focusing on those of high priority, and discovering the duration of involvement, roughly, that triggers a flare-up. The goal is then to engage in planned rest breaks before the threshold for an exacerbation is reached. Note that the rest breaks should be time-contingent, prompted perhaps by an alarm wristwatch, a stopwatch, or a small timer, so that the person does not have to monitor their pain level.

It is important, too, that the patient break the cycle of anger with the pain. Addressing all-or-none thinking, responding assertively to criticism by others who may be concerned by the patient's seeming lack of motivation, and learning to notice and enjoy the numerous intermediate steps to a goal may all be important. Before the pain, it may have been possible to please others with frenetic activity, but now setting boundaries, requesting assistance, and negotiating expectations are crucial.

So, too, is education. Patients are aware that short-term flare-ups are the price of poor pacing. They may not know that deconditioning and, potentially, a subtle decrease in pain thresholds may linger long after the flare-up has passed. On a deeper level, pacing often requires therapeutic work on accepting the pain as a matter of current reality. Sometimes finding a productive "downtime" activity during rest breaks, or combining them with an enjoyable activity such as relaxation practice, can make them more palatable and lessen the need for accepting the pain (Caudill, 1995). Relapses into overactivity should be explored carefully for the eliciting circumstance and emotion, for example guilt at seeing one's spouse working, so that a more constructive response, compatible with pacing, can be developed.

IMPROVING ACCESS TO SERVICES

The majority of headache sufferers have never encountered the techniques discussed in this chapter, for the nearest biofeedback therapist may be fifty miles away, or have a long waiting list. From a public health perspective, then, it is reasonable that the behavioral skills of headache self-management be communicated as broadly and as cost-effectively as possible. Efforts to realize this goal include home-based treatment, group therapy, educational programs in the workplace, books for the lay reader, internet sites, and even television and radio programs (de Bruijn-Kofman, van de Wiel, Groenman, Sorbi, & Klip, 1997).

Home-based treatment.   Many of the treatment components for episodic headache—identification of triggers and prodromal signs, acquisition of deep relaxation skills, developing expertise in problem solving—rely heavily on home practice. It is thus a small and logical step for the skills themselves to be taught partially through workbooks and audiotapes, with the therapist serving to introduce, model, and suggest refinements (Lipchik, K. A. Holroyd, & Nash, 2002). Treatment may then require only 3 or 4 sessions of therapist time, with 3 scheduled, interspersed, 15-minute phone consultations (Lipchik, K. A. Holroyd, & Nash, 2002). Provided the patient is able to follow the written materials, is prepared to work independently, and is not overly burdened by psychiatric comorbidity, there is no loss of efficacy in taking such an approach (see Chapter 14). Indeed, a particularly large outcome study of behavioral treatment for tension-type headache has used a home-based format (K. A. Holroyd, O'Donnell, Stensland, Lipchik, Cordingley, & B. W. Carlson, 2001).Medication overuse and other forms of chronic daily headache, however, are thought to require more intensive therapist contact (Lipchik, K. A. Holroyd, & Nash, 2002).

To my knowledge, no standard set of materials is yet available for home-based treatment. Each center produces its own workbooks and tapes. However, relaxation instructions, headache record sheets, lists of potential triggers and prodromal symptoms, and materials on cognitive therapy are the raw ingredients, and are all widely published. For migraines, log sheets may include a headache diary, checklists of warning signs (prodromal symptoms, aura, and early migraine symptoms) and potential triggers, records of home relaxation practice and thermal biofeedback, and sheets for problem solving barriers to skills acquisition and for systematizing a self-management plan (Lipchik, K. A. Holroyd, & Nash, 2002). For tension-type headache, there is usually little or no emphasis on thermal biofeedback, and greater focus on problem solving skills, including a record of stressful situations, especially those in which a headache occurs, identifying dysfunctional thoughts, objectively appraising these thoughts and substituting more effective alternatives. Thus, the "dysfunctional thought record" of cognitive therapy is often a useful component of treatment (J. S. Beck, 1995; P. R. Martin, 1993). A fuller description of home-based treatment is given in Lipchik et al. (Lipchik, K. A. Holroyd, & Nash, 2002).

Groups.   Relaxation training (Janssen & Neutgens, 1986), cognitive therapy (P. R. Johnson & Thorn, 1989), and perhaps even biofeedback (Gauthier, G. Cote, A. Cote, & Drolet, cited in K. A. Holroyd, Lipchik, & Penzien, 1998) can be administered to groups rather than individually (Napier, C. M. Miller, & Andrasik, 1997). There, the support, sense of community, and opportunity to learn from each other may become a natural part of the treatment. For tension-type headache, there is enough data to suggest that group therapy can be as effective as the individual form (Rains, Penzien, & K. A. Holroyd, 1993).

As in home-based treatment, significant psychiatric comorbidity may require a more intensive, individual approach. However, for refractory headaches, intensive group treatment might be effective. In this approach, home exercises, postural correction, dietary and other lifestyle changes, relaxation and stress management skills, and proper use of medication, are all covered in a small, interactive group conducted in turn by people from various disciplines (Scharff & Marcus, 1994). It is very important that any group discussion be structured to maintain a positive focus.

Note that in a single study testing the hypothesis, groups run by a more experienced therapist had better results (K. A. Holroyd & Andrasik, 1978). Of course group therapy, like headache management, is its own area of expertise, and the therapist should have grounding in both.

Internet.   Instructional materials that might be sent as workbooks and audiotapes can of course now also be sent as web pages, streaming video, and file attachments—an on-demand self-help program. If we also allow the therapist to respond to emails, the treatment approximates a (very) minimal-therapist-contact format. The advantages are a remarkable level of accessibility, convenience and cost-effectiveness (Ström, Pettersson, & G. Andersson, 2000). On-line psychometrics and headache diaries could allow a degree of treatment matching and documentation of efficacy. And people are already using the internet extensively for health-related information (Peroutka, 2001). On the other hand, the intervention seems constrained to a relatively low level of intensity, and there seems no opportunity to truly diagnose or assess the participants. Serious illness could be missed. Security and confidentiality concerns must also be addressed in the website design (Ström, Pettersson, & G. Andersson, 2000).

So far, empirical results have been sparse and inconsistent, although at least mild benefit is suggested (G. Andersson, Lundström, & Ström, 2003; Ström, Pettersson, & G. Andersson, 2000). The treatment populations have been poorly specified, and a sometimes high dropout rate (Ström, Pettersson, & G. Andersson, 2000) does not seem prevented by telephone contact with the therapist (G. Andersson, Lundström, & Ström, 2003). Still, in the mix of treatment delivery models, sheer ease and efficiency will surely give the internet a place.

Books.   In addition to direct outreach to headache sufferers who may not be involved in formal treatment, a book intended for the lay public can provide useful homework assignments to reinforce in-session material. The variety available allows some tailoring to the individual patient.

In *Taking Control of Your Headaches* (Duckro, W. Richardson, J. E. Marshall, Cassabaum, & G. Marshall, 1999), patients learn to identify patterns in their pain and the subtle factors (medication overuse, muscle tension, environmental exposures, unhealthful lifestyles, psychological strain, and stressful ways of thinking and acting) that may be contributing. Through recognizing the early beginnings of a headache and learning skills to eliminate or counteract the triggers, the reader is helped to regain a sense of control over the headaches. This book was written as a guide for patients in a multidisciplinary headache center. It is not intended as stand-alone treatment, but it can go a long way in explaining and deepening behavioral and multimodal therapy. I have found it particularly helpful for instilling a sense of openness and optimism in patients who have been disappointed by numerous medication trials.

In *The Headache and Neck Pain Workbook* (DeGood, Manning, & Middaugh, 1997), the emphasis is on instruction in mental and physical relaxation skills, posture, a home exercise program, and the judicious use of modalities and medication, to build self-regulatory capacity. Consistent with this focus, the presentation is of the skills themselves, and on immediately relevant concepts such as stress and the fight-or-flight response. A chapter is devoted to medication options, appropriate use, and contraindications, but predates the newer triptans. This workbook may be particularly useful for people whose headaches have a significant myofascial component.

In the first third of *What Your Doctor May Not Tell You About Migraines*, the authors, Mauskop and Fox (2001), advocate for the combined use of magnesium, high dose riboflavin, and feverfew. The remainder of the book discusses self-management tools: an elimination diet with an emphasis on whole, unprocessed foods; avoidance of environmental triggers, especially allergens and pollutants; exercise; sleep hygiene; and rudimentary stress management techniques. Migraine medications are also reviewed, although the focus is clearly on self-management and supplements.

Migraine: The Complete Guide (American Council for Headache Education, 1994) is a comprehensive migraine treatise written for the lay public. Prevalence, genetics, and pathophysiology, for example, are covered in much greater depth than in other popular works. The book is not focused on self-management, so much as on helping patients become knowledgeable, active participants in their healthcare. Self-advocacy tips for communicating with doctors, family members, employers and health insurers are also included.

Even more than the Council's book, Lance's (1998) *Migraine and Other Headaches* is like a medical textbook written for an intelligent and motivated lay audience. Reading it is like having the luxury of a long consult with a very experienced physician-researcher. Detailed neurophysiology of nearly all forms of headache, clinical anecdote, advice on treatment, reassurance, and avuncular counsel for a more relaxed lifestyle are blended into a highly informative mix. However, this is not a treatment manual, and techniques for changing one's behavior are touched on only lightly.

In contrast, *Conquering Your Migraine* (S. Diamond & Franklin, 2001) distills Seymour Diamond, M.D.'s extensive clinical experience into an informal, easy-to-read, non-technical guide. Academic knowledge is included sparingly and only to help in understanding practical headache management. Although it is not a stand-alone manual, and refers frequently to professional consultation, Diamond's book has a particularly vivid description of biofeedback, relaxation therapies, and lifestyle triggers that can be a helpful introduction to behavioral treatment.

CHILDREN

Most treatment components for adults can be adapted also to pediatric headaches. Thus, children can often benefit from tracking antecedents and looking for triggers (usually with help from their parents), learning to problem-solving stressful situations, and applying tools in relaxation and physiological self-regulation to change their ways of responding to stress (P. A. McGrath, D. Stewart, & Koster, 2001). It is generally beneficial to involve the parents throughout, for prompting and coaching the child and to support the legitimacy of the intervention (P. A. McGrath, et al.). Parental involvement is especially important when pain is leading to excessive social withdrawal and school absence, suggesting that support for increased functioning should be an explicit part of treatment. Of course when parents are worried about the pain, either for its medical implications or its impact on their children's lives, then providing precise information, and referring back to the physician for answers to medical questions, is crucial.

Generally, biofeedback and relaxation training are taught to children in the same way as for adults, with a few modifications. The sessions may be a half-hour, or they may be punctuated by play periods for coloring or playing a game with the therapist. Even a short ball game might be included, for children who need activity (Kröner-Herwig, Mohn, & Pothmann, 1998). Reinforcement is used much more frequently, for example during biofeedback. For each day's entry in a headache log or home practice record, the child may be allowed to select a colorful sticker to place next to it (K. D. Allen & Shriver, 1998; Kröner-Herwig, Mohn, & Pothmann, 1998). Verbal reinforcement during relaxation practice may be gradually faded across sessions (Bussone, Grazzi, D'Amico, Leone, & Andrasik, 1998).

For relaxation skills, children are often taught slow, paced breathing (P. A. McGrath, et al., 2001) and a progressive muscle approach (Bussone, Grazzi, D'Amico, Leone, & Andrasik, 1998). The muscle relaxation is like play, for example wrinkling the forehead to shoo off an imaginary fly, or reaching far overhead to tense the arms before letting them drop back down (Forman, 1993; Koeppen, 1974). For young children, imagery may be preferred to the progressive muscle component, with the child selecting pleasant scenes such as "going skiing," "koala bear," or "a unicorn" (Olness, H. Hall, Rozniecki, W. Schmidt, & Theoharides, 1999). The key step is absorption in an enjoyable scene, after which attention to relaxed sensations, especially at the head, neck, and shoulders, can be included (P. A. McGrath, et al.). Children's openness to imagination often allows them to learn relaxation and mental hand warming in just a few sessions. From clinical experience, Whiteside reports that hypnosis seems to work wonderfully with children: "They do not have the built-in resistance that many adults have and can easily be hypnotized in quite large groups. Not only that, but to them it is great fun and certainly something to boast about to their mates at school. It is a simple progression to teach them self-hypnosis which they can use at the onset of an attack" (Whiteside, 1990, p. 109). Related techniques such as analgesic imagery ("magic glove") can then be taught as well (Olness, H. Hall, Rozniecki, W. Schmidt, & Theoharides, 1999).

* * *

RELAXATION EXERCISE[5]

This script can be taught to patients in session, or recorded for home practice. It should be spoken slowly, with frequent pauses. If the patient is having pain in any area during the session, it may be helpful to skip that body part, at least early in training, to avoid calling attention to the pain.

Begin by sitting in a comfortable chair, or lying on a soft surface, so that your entire body is supported. Adopt a comfortable position. Allow all the muscles in your body to let go and relax. Allow feelings of relaxation to replace any tension in your body.

---

[5]In writing this exercise, I have been influenced by a similar script created by Natalie Morse, director of Community Health at MaineGeneral Medical Center. Natalie's adaptation of autogenics is the first exercise on her Journey to Relaxation tape.

If there are any outside sounds, any distracting thoughts, let them drift through on their own. Don't try to block them. Don't try to hold onto them. Let them come and go while you simply relax deeply.

Now, take a deep breath and, with your chest filled, bring your shoulders back slightly. Notice the tension in your chest and upper back. Hold the tension for a few seconds . . . and then exhale. Sink back into a comfortable position. Notice the feeling of relaxation in your chest and upper back.

Now, take a deep, slow breath, without the tension. Let your abdomen expand as your lungs fill with air. As you exhale, lower your shoulders, and allow yourself to sink more deeply into relaxation. Let your breathing become slow and regular, with each breath feeling more deeply relaxed.

As you relax, you may notice a feeling of comfortable, pleasant heaviness at your right arm. Allow your right arm to feel comfortable, warm and heavy, letting go of any tension. A pleasant, relaxed, warm feeling. Let the feeling spread, from your fingers to your wrist . . . your forearm, too, becoming warm and relaxed . . . the feeling now at your upper arm, your shoulder . . . your entire arm feeling warm, relaxed, and comfortably heavy.

And as you continue breathing deeply and slowly, breathing out tension, breathing in relaxation, notice the comfortable relaxed feelings also in your left arm. Your left arm feels warm and pleasantly heavy, as the feeling of relaxation spreads from your fingertips to your wrist . . . from your wrist to your forearm . . . and then to your upper arm . . . so that your left arm, like your right arm, feels very comfortable, warm, and heavy.

As your breath continues, slowly and deeply, you may notice that the feeling of relaxation is spreading also to your shoulders and neck, the muscles letting go of tension, releasing, resting, feeling comfortable and relaxed. Your face, too, relaxes, your jaw slightly open, your face smooth and expressionless . . . feeling peaceful . . . as your muscles relax completely . . . as you breathe deeply and effortlessly, simply enjoying the relaxation.

Notice, too, a feeling of warmth and heaviness in your right leg, a peaceful, comfortable feeling. Allow that feeling of relaxation to deepen, so that your right leg feels warm and comfortably heavy. Your feet, calves, thighs, all feel warm and heavy. . . . And notice, too, the feelings of relaxation in your left leg, a warm and pleasant feeling, the muscles relaxing deeply, so that your left leg, like your right, feels comfortably warm and heavy.

As you continue breathing deeply and effortlessly, allow the relaxation to spread also to your abdomen, your abdomen feeling warm and relaxed, comfortably warm and relaxed. And allow the feeling of relaxation to spread also to your chest, the muscles in your chest relaxing as you breathe easily and effortlessly. With each breath, the relaxation deepening, so that your upper back, too, feels warm, relaxed, and comfortable, the muscles peaceful and relaxed. And allow that feeling to spread to your midback, and then your lower back, so that your entire body feels warm, peaceful, and relaxed . . . (pause)

Continue breathing slowly and deeply, allowing the feeling of relaxation to deepen with each breath . . . (pause)

Now, slowly open your eyes . . . noticing your surroundings . . . moving and stretching . . . and coming back into the present. Notice that you can feel alert, aware, and relaxed at the same time. Notice that by breathing deeply you can create relaxed feelings in your body.

* * *

For Eliza, there were many small turning points. Learning about the physiology of migraine was an unexpected relief, for until then the attacks had been her personal hell, and frighteningly unpredictable. The idea that there was an objective mechanism, a dependent variable for which she could conceivably identify the independent variables, seemed remarkable.

In fact, she had been tracking pain, but moment-by-moment, to gauge whether its trajectory required rest, ice, heat, TENS, Axert, Percocet, or whether she could chance a small foray into housework. The moment-by-moment tracking was too fine to show patterns. She needed to control the tempo of the game (she had played basketball in college), for which recording her pain level four times a day was satisfactory. Gradually, she noticed earlier warnings—incoordination, subtle numbness at her hand, and before all of these, a premonitory uptick in energy. Particularly striking, though, were the results of tracking her hand temperature. Over eight weeks of tracking, a decline in temperature over a 12-hour period was almost always followed by a migraine. Conversely, no migraine ever followed a 12-hour increase in hand temperature. Of course, this suggested mental hand warming directly.

Attempting to learn the skills, however, made clear to her that she would need to take on her constant worry and her perfectionism. She was continuously vigilant, remembering her children's and her husband's appointments, attempting to keep a spotless home, and multitasking at her job. As it turned out, she did not need treatment for Generalized Anxiety Disorder (although another patient might have). Rather, when she saw the connection to her migraines, perfectionism lost its lure; it just wasn't worth it. At the first hint of vigilance she would remind herself of this, and substitute mental hand warming. As she gained skills in prevention, she gave up the public accoutrements of migraine, especially her dark glasses. She still has chronic migraines, but her total headache burden has declined by 60 percent, to which a reduction in duration, frequency, and for some attacks, intensity have all contributed.

* * *

When Sam began treatment, work stresses activated a "helplessness schema," a conviction of the insurmountability of the problems, the futility of effort, and the inevitability of pain, with such strength that even mention of the stresses made him morose, angry, and achy. At first, simply noticing this process intellectually and the thoroughness with which it took control of his feelings was a step forward. Only gradually could he observe it with enough distance to entertain that there could be other options. Once he had taken that step, though, a host of possibilities tumbled forward. He analyzed the stresses in precise detail, in terms of his relationship with his boss and his coworkers, the work tasks, and his vocational skills. With much encouragement at first, he was able to generate solutions along every dimension. He also became able to put the schema into words, identifying the rapid automatic thoughts by which it dominated his mood. This allowed him to catch himself and substitute more considered, accurate thoughts, much as he had taught himself, when his children got old enough to talk, to stop using curse words. In this context, thinking of the pain as like a behavior over which he could have control did not seem so far-fetched. Progressive muscle relaxation was a pleasant contrast to his chronic sense of tension, and he applied it avidly, especially at stress-times: after lunch, when he ordinarily felt depleted and painful, and when his boss first arrived at work. He still gets headaches, but they no longer seem so disruptive or formidable.

* * *

The muscle tension readings from his forehead startled Brian. Even before the first assessment had ended, he was experimenting with the display, to see if he could reduce them. Developing the skill in-session proved to be straightforward enough; remembering to practice at home, and especially at work, were the real challenges. Then, when he caught a flare-up at its earliest stages, and eliminated it, and felt palpably for the first time that the headaches could be under his control, the momentum shifted. From then on, it was simply a matter of finding the right techniques at the right times, and enjoying the sense of progress.

* * *

When Marion learned to manage her posttraumatic headache, now in its third year, the change was so gradual it was nearly imperceptible. First, the diagnosis was clarified, that it was not a chronic tension-type headache and was unlikely to remit with yet another medication trial. This medical endpoint was surprisingly liberating, for it freed her from a constant cycle of wondering, disappointment and frustration with each new consult. She then began thinking about other things—household chores, outdoor work, and activities with her children—that she wanted to regain. At first, each new project was like a duel, to see how much she could accomplish before succumbing to a flare-up. Tracking her pain and resting preventively were maddening, and then strange, but they worked, and gradually brought her life more under her control. She began thinking of projects that she had always wanted to do, which did not require the prolonged exertion that triggered exacerbations. The pain seemed changed from a disease needing a cure, to an object that she needed to work around in order to regain her connection to life. As the pain became more of a "given," it became less relevant to her.

PART V

Behavioral Medicine Treatment Outcome Literature

CHAPTER 14

Outcome: Meta-Analyses and Representative Studies

Well, my dear fellow, that is the most astonishing thing I have ever heard. Here you have spent a lifetime trying to discover the North Pole, that nobody in the world cares tuppence about, and you have never even tried to discover a cure for headache, which the whole world is crying for.

—George Bernard Shaw, on meeting Nansen,
an arctic explorer (Henderson, 1911, p. 504)

In Chapter 11, we discussed the effectiveness of medications for benign headaches. Not surprisingly, behavioral treatment has generated a large outcome literature of its own. Here, and in the chapters to follow, we will examine the main elements of that literature. First, we will look at how well treatment works, for adults and children, through the lens of meta-analysis and a few of the largest controlled studies. Then in Chapter 15, we will examine relaxation, biofeedback, hypnosis, and other behavioral tools in greater detail, to understand their mechanisms of action, and to fine-tune their clinical application. The next Chapter, 16, deals with patient selection and treatment matching, for choosing which behavioral treatment to use, and for choosing between medication, self-management, and their combination. Finally, we will turn in the last chapter to long-term outcome, and the prospects for our ultimate goal: a cure for chronic headaches.

But first, how well do behavioral interventions work? There are a few relatively large-scale studies on the behavioral treatment of chronic headaches. We will examine these studies, and then survey the rest of the literature—a fair number of small-scale investigations—from the vantage point of meta-analysis. In the process, we will seek out information on three types of efficacy: overall (is the treatment better than no treatment?), substantial (is it better than a placebo?), and relative (is it better than alternative behavioral and/or pharmacological treatments?).

MIGRAINES

The largest study to date on the behavioral treatment of migraines seems to be that of J. D. Sargent and coworkers at the Menninger Foundation (Sargent, Solbach, Coyne, Spohn, & Segerson, 1986). Although 136 migraineurs completed the study, the authors note that the power to detect a moderate effect size was only 0.68, apparently in part because of the nonparametric multivariate analysis that was employed. But the study has many strengths. Participants were randomly assigned to conditions, and, heroically, kept daily headache records for 9 months. Of course subjects were not informed of the study hypotheses during their involvement. The technicians who trained the participants also did not know the hypotheses and did not have access to the headache data.

In the study, four conditions were contrasted: autogenics, frontalis EMG biofeedback plus autogenics, thermal biofeedback plus autogenics, and a no-treatment control. Actually, the no-treatment condition was perhaps more of a placebo, as the participants in it attended the same number of sessions as the other patients, sitting quietly in a recliner while psychophysiological data were collected without feedback. Thus, the "no treatment" subjects had 22 sessions of "time out" from daily stresses, and indeed their readings became more relaxed over the course of the study. On the other hand, sitting quietly was not a very credible treatment, as 47 percent of subjects in the no treatment group felt that in fact they had obtained no benefit.

They were probably wrong, however; on average, subjects in all groups showed a decline in headache frequency and intensity. However, the improvement was greater for subjects in the active treatments versus those in the no treatment group (frequency, $p < .05$; intensity, $p < .005$). Moreover, there was a trend for patients receiving thermal biofeedback to show more improvement than those receiving frontalis biofeedback or autogenics without biofeedback (frequency, $p < .09$; intensity, $p < .08$).

Although a superb study, it has two limitations. First, 23 percent of the initial sample dropped out of the research. These people did not differ in treatment group membership or headache variables, but they were more likely to be young, single, non-white, and receiving public assistance. Thus, the generalizability of the results across demographic groups may be impaired.

Secondly, and more seriously, subjects were not restricted in amount of medication. On average, medication use did not change. However, it appears that for patients in the thermal biofeedback group, medication use increased over the study.[1] This confound, although serious, presumably affects only the intensity variable, and not frequency, as any occurrence of a headache on a given day, no matter how brief or successfully treated, would increment "frequency" by the same amount.

Sargent et al.'s study, then, suggests that various forms of relaxation training are more effective than what is most likely a weak placebo treatment. The study also gives a faint, equivocal hint that thermal biofeedback might be better than autogenics or frontalis EMG biofeedback. It would be preferable, however, to compare behavioral treatments to a strong placebo, that is, a placebo identified as being equally credible, and as inspiring the same expectations for recovery as the active treatment.

This test was undertaken in a methodologically crisp study by Blanchard and associates (Blanchard, Appelbaum, Radnitz, Morrill, et al., 1990). The placebo was "pseudomeditation" and it had two parts. The first part was "body awareness" training, in which subjects learned to become aware of each part of their body in turn, focusing on any sensations arising from it. The second part was "mental control," in which subjects worked on imagining routine daily activities as clearly as possible. In both parts, the participants were asked not to relax, lest it interfere with the "meditation." This placebo was indeed rated as equally credible and was felt to be as likely to help as the two actual treatments: A combined progressive muscle relaxation—autogenics—thermal biofeedback condition, and a condition in which cognitive stress management training was added to the combination of relaxation and biofeedback.

The outcome, statistically, was that the active treatments and placebo outperformed a waiting list control, and were not different from each other. The data also contained two hints that the relaxation-biofeedback training (with or without cognitive therapy) might be better than the placebo. First, 52 percent of the treated patients, but only 38 percent of the placebo group, showed a 50 percent or greater reduction in headache activity. However, this difference was not statistically significant ($p = .24$). Second, at three-month follow-up, the placebo group had relapsed to

---

[1]The amount of increase is not clear. However, the F-ratio for the Group (thermal biofeedback vs. the 2 other active treatments) X Time interaction contrast is small enough ($F = 2.04$) that a large increase in medication use does not seem likely.

their baseline level of headache activity, while the gains of the treated groups were unabated. However, this conclusion is based on only 40 percent of the study participants, in part because patients who did not improve with the study intervention were referred on for clinical treatment.

Now, if we assume that relaxation-biofeedback and the pseudomeditation are equivalent, how could this be? With 116 subjects in total, the study's statistical power was more than adequate. It appears, however, that the "pseudomeditation" was more "meditation" than "pseudo." It has some similarities to mindfulness meditation, which has a degree of empirical support for managing chronic pain (Kabat-Zinn, Lipworth, & Burney, 1985). Taking time away from stresses, noticing non-pain bodily sensations, and refocusing one's thoughts on neutral topics are not inappropriate for pain coping. Indeed, the members of the placebo group showed an increase in hand temperature, and some described actively using their skills for stress management.

Clearly it would be nice to have more data. One source is a clinical series of 156 patients (72 with migraine and 84 with migraine plus tension-type headache) who had participated in studies in Blanchard et al.'s laboratory (Blanchard, Andrasik, Evans, Neff, Appelbaum, & Rodichok, 1985). Although they did not all participate in the same study, they received nearly identical treatments, and hence combining the samples seemed justified. In this series, Blanchard et al. found that 24 percent of the patients who received relaxation training had at least a 50 percent reduction in headache activity, pre- to post-treatment, as measured prospectively with a headache diary. In contrast, 52 percent of those who received relaxation training plus thermal biofeedback showed at least a 50 percent improvement. The difference in proportions was significant by chi square testing, $p < .01$. Now, the samples were not independent, in the sense that the 132 patients who received thermal biofeedback included 39 who had previously received, and failed, relaxation training. Thus, the assumptions behind the statistical test were violated. Substantively, however, what are the likely effects? As Blanchard, et al. always incorporated relaxation training into the thermal biofeedback, the 39 do not seem to have received an "extra dose" of behavioral treatment. Moreover, as Blanchard, et al. suggest, the 39 patients had shown themselves to be relatively unresponsive to a behavioral treatment, and hence their inclusion would have biased the study against thermal biofeedback. Even so, thermal biofeedback had more than twice the success rate of relaxation training by itself.

Note that a differential effectiveness does not necessarily imply that thermal biofeedback works through some mechanism other than relaxation. It might be, for example, that thermal biofeedback is simply a good pedagogic tool for teaching relaxation. We will examine this question further in Chapter 15, when we look at the components of behavioral treatment in greater detail.

Meta-analyses.   There have been many other studies of behavioral treatments for migraines, but the sample sizes are often between 10 and 30 subjects per group.[2] Thus, the best way to draw conclusions from this literature is through meta-analysis. In meta-analysis, information on the strength and direction of treatment effects is extracted from a large and representative sample of studies. These estimates of treatment effects are then examined statistically. Behavioral treatment of chronic headaches was among the first areas to be subjected to meta-analysis, and hence some of the earlier reports lack contemporary rigor. However, even fairly primitive meta-analyses are a marked improvement over qualitative literature reviews.

---

[2]In psychological research, large scale studies are sometimes looked upon with suspicion, due to their capacity to detect small and therefore clinically meaningless effects. On the other hand, large scale studies are the standard in medical research, presumably because they can hint at the generality of an effect (in the absence of true random sampling), accurately estimate effect size (D. H. Barlow, 1983) and increase the probability of detecting unusual side effects.

An important distinction among studies centers on the type of outcome measure they use. In more recent studies, the key variables have generally been derived from headache diaries. In the diaries, pain intensity is recorded hourly or 4 times per day. Overall pain level is usually operationalized as the sum of pain ratings over a given period of time. Information on headache frequency, intensity and duration can also be extracted from the diaries. Importantly, as a prospective measure it is relatively resistant to bias. The alternative outcome measure in use is of global ratings of improvement, either by the patient, the treating physician, or both. Global ratings generally show large biases when compared directly with diary measures (Blanchard et al., 1981; Cahn & Cram, 1980).

K. A. Holroyd and Penzien have published a meta-analytic comparison of propranolol with the combination of autogenics and thermal biofeedback. Their analysis, shown in Table 14–1, distills 60 studies comprised of 2445 patients in total (K. A. Holroyd & Penzien, 1990). As can be seen, propranolol and the behavioral intervention have identical efficacy (43 percent reduction in headache activity), and out-perform placebo (14 percent reduction) and no-treatment controls. Post-hoc testing found no effect on outcome of client gender, dropout rate, age, diagnosis (with vs. without aura), or (for the medication studies) dose or single vs. double vs. not blind conditions.

Note that no attempt was made in the meta-analysis to contrast behavioral treatments with each other. That question was addressed in an earlier meta-analysis. Blanchard and Andrasik (1982) reviewed 23 prospective studies contrasting various behavioral treatments with each other, and with psychological placebos and/or headache monitoring. For comparison, the response rate to placebos in the pharmacological literature was also included.

Results are shown in Table 14–2. In this early meta-analysis, the treatments sort themselves into three overlapping groups. The first group, to which only the combination of autogenics and thermal biofeedback belongs, had significantly better outcomes than all other treatments except for relaxation training by itself. The second group consists of relaxation training, cephalic biofeedback, and thermal biofeedback, each offered as a single modality. They are superior to headache monitoring and to pharmacological placebos, but not to psychological placebos, which are also in the second group. The third group consists of the two types of placebo and the headache monitoring (no treatment) condition.

An updated meta-analysis has since been reported (McCrory, Penzien, Rains, & Hasselblad, 1996) and is shown in Table 14–3. Only controlled trials were included.

TABLE 14–1
Propranolol vs. Behavioral Treatment in Migraine Prevention

Type of Treatment	Any Outcome Measure		Headache Diary Outcome	
	Mean Effect Size[a]	N[b]	Mean Effect Size	N
Propranolol	55*	25	44*	12
Thermal Biofeedback + Relaxation	56*	35	43*	22
Placebo	14	20	14	15
No-treatment Control	3	17	2	15

Note. From "Pharmacological versus Non-Pharmacological Prophylaxis of Recurrent Migraine Headache: A Meta-Analytic Review of Clinical Trials," by K. A. Holroyd and D. B. Penzien, 1990, *Pain, 42,* p. 11. Copyright 1990 by the International Association for the Study of Pain. Reprinted with permission.
[a]Mean Effect Size = Mean % improvement in ratings from baseline
[b]N = number of studies on which the analysis is based.
*= Significantly different from placebo.

TABLE 14–2
Behavioral Interventions for Migraine Prevention: Relative Efficacy (Blanchard & Andrasik, 1982)

Type of Treatment	Prospective Outcome Measure	
	Mean Effect Size	N
Autogenics + Thermal Biofeedback[a]	64.9	10
Relaxation[a,b]	47.9	7
Cephalic Vasomotor Biofeedback[b]	42.3	4
Thermal Biofeedback[b]	34.6	7
Psychological Placebo[b,c]	27.6	5
Headache Monitoring (No treatment)[c]	17.2	6
Medication Placebo[c]	16.5	6

Note. Adapted from "Psychological Assessment and Treatment of Headache: Recent Developments and Emerging Issues," by E. B. Blanchard and F. Andrasik, 1982, *Journal of Consulting and Clinical Psychology, 50,* pp. 866–867. Copyright 1982 by the American Psychological Association. Adapted with permission.

[a,b,c]Treatments with no superscripts in common are significantly different on *t*-test

Mean Effect Size = Mean % improvement. Depending on the study, these are % improvement in headache ratings from baseline, when these are available, or else the % of subjects whose headaches improved.

N = number of studies on which the analysis is based.

TABLE 14–3
Behavioral Interventions for Migraine Prevention: Relative Efficacy (McCrory, et al., 1996)

Type of Treatment	Effect Size	N	Mean % Improvement[a]	N
Thermal Biof. + Relaxation[b]	0.60	11	37.6	21
Relaxation[b]	1.30	6	35.0	17
Cognitive-Behavioral Therapy[b]	0.87	3	38.9	10
Placebo	0.13	4	14.8	4
Waiting-List Control	—	—	1.7	12

Note. Data from "Efficacy of Behavioral Treatments for Migraine and Tension-Type Headache: Meta-Analysis of Controlled Trials," by D. C. McCrory, D. B. Penzien, J. C. Rains, and V. Hasselblad, 1996, *Headache, 36,* p. 272. Copyright 1996 by the American Headache Society. Adapted with permission.

[a]For the mean % improvement, the outcome for each treatment arm of each study was weighted by the sample size.
[b]Significantly different from waiting-list control.

Here, relaxation training, alone and in combination with thermal biofeedback, and cognitive-behavioral therapy, were superior to the waiting list controls, while the placebo conditions were not (McCrory, Penzien, Rains, & Hasselblad, 1996).

Effect size, here used in a restricted sense, was almost certainly computed as a *z*-score:

$$\frac{\text{(mean improvement in treatment group} - \text{mean improvement in control group)}}{\text{control group standard deviation}}$$

and was significantly *larger* for relaxation training alone than for the combination of relaxation training with thermal biofeedback. However, not all studies provided enough data for the computation. The mean percent improvement is based on a greater number of studies, and should be more stable. (Percent improvement is a perfectly good measure of effect size in the broad sense of the term; Lipsey & D. B. Wilson, 2001.) With this measure, thermal biofeedback plus relaxation shows a slight numerical advantage over relaxation training by itself.

U. S. Headache Consortium.   In Chapter 11 we discussed the evidence-based guidelines for migraine medication developed by the U.S. Headache Consortium, a group comprised of the American Academy of Neurology, American Academy of Family Physicians, American College of Physicians, American Headache Society, American College of Emergency Physicians, American Osteopathic Association, and the National Headache Foundation. The consortium reviewed behavioral treatments as well, determining that there is consistent evidence from multiple, well-designed clinical trials ("Grade A evidence") to support the use of relaxation training, thermal biofeedback combined with relaxation training, EMG biofeedback, and cognitive-behavior therapy as treatment options for migraine prevention (J. K. Campbell, Penzien, & E. M. Wall, 2000).

TENSION-TYPE HEADACHE

In the last section, we reviewed a key study from Blanchard's research group, in which behavioral treatment for migraines was compared to a highly credible psychological placebo. A similar study on tension-type headaches has been published by the same group (Blanchard, Appelbaum, Radnitz, Michultka, Morrill, Kirsch, Hillhouse, Evans, Guarnieri, Attanasio, Andrasik, Jaccard, & Dentinger, 1990). Sixty-six patients participated. As before, the placebo was pseudomeditation, involving practice in body awareness and neutral mental imagery, without relaxation. The active treatments were progressive muscle relaxation, and the relaxation plus cognitive stress management training. A headache monitoring group served as an additional control. In this study, prospectively-monitored headache activity declined significantly, pre- to post-treatment, with the relaxation training ($p < .001$) and the relaxation plus cognitive therapy ($p < .001$) but not in the pseudomeditation or headache monitoring groups. Similar results were found for medication intake, with only the two active treatments showing a statistically significant decline.

A somewhat murkier picture is given by the proportion of subjects showing a clinically significant (>50 percent) reduction in headache activity. Among the patients receiving relaxation plus cognitive therapy, 62 percent were clinically improved, and this was nearly a higher proportion ($p = .065$) than for the patients receiving relaxation without cognitive therapy (32 percent). Pseudomeditation came out in the middle (45 percent) and headache monitoring was relatively ineffective (20 percent).

Of course it is always helpful to have more data, and for this we may turn to a meta-analytic review of 78 studies, comprising 2866 patients in total, presented in Table 14–4 (Bogaards & ter Kuile, 1994). Relaxation, EMG biofeedback, cognitive therapy, and the combination of relaxation training and biofeedback, all gave better outcomes than the placebo conditions.

Psychological placebos used in the studies included headache discussion, pseudomeditation, client-centered therapy, and false biofeedback. No effects were found on treatment efficacy of patient gender, quality of the study design, number of patients in the study, diagnostic system in use, or method of patient recruitment.

Across all treatments, greater chronicity of headaches implied poorer prognosis ($r = .31, p < .012$). On the other hand, short-term therapy was supported: No correlation was found between outcome and number of hours of therapy ($r = .06$, *ns*). This is consistent with results, given below, that home-based treatment is as effective as its clinic-based counterpart (e.g., Blanchard, Appelbaum, Guarnieri, Neff, Andrasik, Jaccard, & Barron, 1988).

The medications whose trials were entered into the meta-analysis include diazepam, amitriptyline, clomipramine, doxepin, naproxen, ibuprofen, aspirin, acetaminophen, acetaminophen plus codeine, and butalbital compound. When these trials are considered together, the medications outperformed placebos only when global improvement ratings were used. Of course such a broad grouping is pharmacologically meaningless. It can be useful as a benchmark, however, to give

TABLE 14–4
Behavioral Interventions for Tension-Type Headache (Bogaards & ter Kuile, 1994)

Type of Treatment	Any Outcome Measure		Headache Diary Outcome (Prospective Measure)	
	Mean Effect Size[a]	N[b]	Mean Effect Size	N
Biofeedback + Relaxation	56*	11	59*	9
Cognitive Therapy	53*	15	53*	15
EMG Biofeedback	47*	29	48*	28
Relaxation	36	38	36*	37
Pharmacological	39	17	17	5
Placebo	20	28	16	21
No-treatment Control	−5	17	1	16

Note. From "Treatment of Recurrent Tension Headache: A Meta-Analytic Review," by M. C. Bogaards and M. M. ter Kuile, 1994, *Clinical Journal of Pain, 10.* p. 174. Copyright 1994 by Raven Press. Reprinted with permission.

[a]Mean Effect Size = Mean % improvement in ratings from baseline

[b]N = number of trials on which the analysis is based.

*= Significantly different from placebo.

TABLE 14–5
Behavioral Interventions for Tension-Type Headache (McCrory, et al., 1996)

Type of Treatment	Effect Size	N	Mean % Improvement	N
EMG Biofeedback	1.10*	9	49.1*	24
Relaxation	0.71*	13	31.7*	25
Cognitive-Behavioral	0.70*	3	53.0*	7
Hypnosis	0.64*	3	18.7*	4
Placebo	0.29	5	21.2	8
No-treatment Control	—	—	2.8	15

Note. Data from "Efficacy of Behavioral Treatments for Migraine and Tension-Type Headache: Meta-Analysis of Controlled Trials, by D. C. McCrory, D. B. Penzien, J. C. Rains, and V. Hasselblad, 1996, *Headache, 36,* p. 272. Copyright 1996 by the American Headache Society. Adapted with permission.

*Significantly different from control condition.

us a sense of where behavioral treatments fall in the spectrum of effectiveness. Nonetheless, we cannot directly compare behavioral treatments with medications in this analysis because the studies are drawn from different literatures that may have different policies about publishing null results.

A similar meta-analysis was published shortly after the Bogaards and ter Kuile review by a different group of researchers, as shown in Table 14–5 (McCrory, Penzien, Rains, & Hasselblad, 1996). Not surprisingly, the results are broadly consistent with those of the earlier meta-analysis. Relaxation (32 percent reduction in headache activity), EMG biofeedback (49 percent reduction) and cognitive-behavioral treatment (53 percent reduction) each outperformed the waiting list control condition. The meta-analysis also included hypnosis, whose effects were statistically significant but modest (19 percent reduction) and not numerically superior to the placebo conditions (21 percent reduction).

Finally, in the largest and most recent meta-analysis, shown in Table 14–6, the main behavioral treatments (EMG biofeedback, relaxation training, cognitive-behavioral stress management skills, and EMG biofeedback combined with relaxation) outperform placebo, with roughly the same

TABLE 14–6
Behavioral Interventions for Tension-Type Headache (McCrory, et al., 2001)

Type of Treatment	Effect Size	N	Mean % Improvement	N
EMG Biofeedback with relaxation	0.84*	5	50*	7
EMG Biofeedback without relaxation	0.70*	8	48*	14
Cognitive-Behavioral	0.64*	10	39*	13
Relaxation	0.64*	15	37*	19
Amitriptyline	0.51*	3	33*	3
Placebo	0.15	8	17	11
No-treatment Control	0	9	1.6	13

Note. Adapted from *Evidence Report: Behavioral and Physical Treatments for Tension-Type and Cervicogenic Headache* (pp. 43 and 44), by D. C. McCrory, D. B. Penzien, V. Hasselblad, and R. N. Gray, 2001, Des Moines, Iowa: Foundation for Chiropractic Education and Research. Copyright 2001 by Duke University. Adapted with permission.

*Significantly different from no-treatment control.

efficacy as the best pharmacological treatment, amitriptyline. In this meta-analysis, no significant differences emerge between active treatments (McCrory, Penzien, Hasselblad, & R. N. Gray, 2001).

Now, these analyses lead naturally to three closely-related follow-up questions (Blanchard, Andrasik, Ahles, Teders, & O'Keefe, 1980): (1) Can we predict whether a patient is likely to benefit from a given treatment? (2) Are the patients who respond to one treatment the same as those who respond to another, or are the different treatments benefiting different subsets of patients? And: (3) Can we identify predictors that would allow patients to be matched to the treatment to which they would be most likely to respond? We will take these questions up later, in Chapter 16.

HOME-BASED TREATMENT

Haddock et al. conducted a meta-analytic review of 13 studies that directly compared largely home-based with largely clinic-based behavioral treatment (Haddock, Rowan, Andrasik, Wilson, Talcott, & R. J. Stein, 1997). Home-based treatment involved an average of 2.7 visits (or 162 minutes) with a therapist and two telephone contacts, while clinic-based treatment involved 8.6 visits (484 minutes) on average, and no phone calls. The two forms of treatment were essentially equal in efficacy when compared with control groups or with each other, in both immediate outcome and subsequent (4–20 week) follow-up. On some measures, home-based treatment may have performed slightly better. Needless to say, home-based treatment was far more cost-effective.

The authors point out three caveats, however. First, patients in the studies had been screened for an absence of comorbid conditions, and for an ability to adhere to treatment with minimal supervision. It seems reasonable that the cost of the screening be included in the total cost of home-based treatment. Second, the studies have so far been conducted in research settings by investigators who are likely to be proponents of home-based treatment. Third, studies to empirically develop patient selection and treatment matching criteria have not yet been conducted (Haddock, Rowan, Andrasik, Wilson, Talcott, & R. J. Stein, 1997). And to these we may add a fourth caveat: Studies of home-based treatment generally involve monitoring treatment effectiveness with a headache diary. The diary is to be turned in to the investigators, and this in itself may augment compliance beyond what would be found in an applied setting. Of course this caveat would not obtain if a headache diary were incorporated into the actual treatment.

Despite these qualifications, the home-based format clearly seems to be a promising way of getting the benefits of behavioral treatment to large numbers of headache sufferers who otherwise could not afford it.

Now, in Haddock, et al.'s meta-analysis, the average number of clinic visits was 2.7. We may ask, can the visits be reduced still further without losing efficacy? Powers, et al. provide some preliminary evidence on this (Powers, Mitchell, Byars, Bentti, LeCates, & Hershey, 2001). As part of multidisciplinary treatment of pediatric migraine, children were seen for a single session of relaxation training (involving deep breathing, progressive muscle relaxation, and guided imagery) and thermal biofeedback. Before the session, the children were not able to increase their finger temperature appreciably. With the training, they increased finger temperature by an average of 3.3 °F. They were then encouraged to practice at home. At 5-month follow-up they were able to raise finger temperature by an average of 3.7 °F. Now, the children showed a modest decrease in headache intensity (-10 percent) and frequency (-25 percent) that in theory could have been due to any of the interventions in the multidisciplinary treatment. However, finger temperature change and change in headache frequency were negatively correlated ($r = -.45; p < .05$), providing some suggestion that the thermal biofeedback skills were playing a role. Needless to say, it would be premature to conclude too much from this uncontrolled pilot study. Moreover, it is not clear whether the rather limited nature of the improvements is due to the tertiary care sample or the brevity of the treatment. Still, more research is clearly warranted on this highly cost-effective intervention.

TEMPOROMANDIBULAR DISORDERS

There is much less data available for behavioral treatments of temporomandibular disorders than for tension-type and migraine headaches. However, Crider and Glaros (1999) have summarized the results to date, for studies involving surface EMG biofeedback, with or without additional stress management or relaxation training. Nearly all of the biofeedback focused on the masseter. In total, the literature consisted of three trials comparing biofeedback to a credible placebo, three trials in which the comparison was to a no-treatment control, four trials in which active treatments were compared with each other, and three uncontrolled trials. Fortunately, this sparse literature is also fairly consistent, showing a moderately large effect of biofeedback in improving the clinical exam (see Table 14–7).

The difference in percent of subjects rated as improved is significant ($p < .05$). However, this appears to be a retrospective measure of uncertain validity. The effect size for pain ratings is based on a prospective measure and approaches significance ($p < .10$). Clinical exam is also prospective and the effect size is significant ($p < .01$).

Additional training in stress management or relaxation skills did not add measurably to the outcome in these studies. The meta-analysis does not address the mechanisms by which biofeedback had an effect, a topic to which we will return shortly.

TABLE 14–7
Biofeedback for Temporomandibular Disorders

Treatment	N	Pain Effect Size	N	Exam Effect Size	N	% Improved
Biofeedback	4	1.04	6	1.33	7	68.6%
Control	3	0.47	3	0.26	4	34.7%
Follow-Up[a]	2	1.33	3	1.84	6	69.3%

Note. From "A Meta-Analysis of EMG biofeedback treatment of temporomandibular disorders," by A. B. Crider and A. G. Glaros, 1999, *Journal of Orofacial Pain, 13,* pp. 34–35. Copyright 1999 Quintessence Publishing. Adapted with permission.

[a] The studies in which follow-up data (3–24 months) are reported are a subset of the biofeedback studies in the first line of the table.

Several outcome studies have directly compared biofeedback and cognitive-behavioral skills training. Flor and Birbaumer (1993) report that while both treatments produced increases in active coping, only the biofeedback treatment produced long-term (2 year) reductions in pain, distress, and health care utilization. Mishra and coworkers randomly assigned 94 patients with chronic temporomandibular dysfunction to receive biofeedback, cognitive behavioral skills treatment for managing stress, combined biofeedback and cognitive behavioral treatment, or conservative dental care as a control. All three of the active treatment groups, but not the control group, showed a statistically significant reduction in pain scores pre- to posttreatment. Tests comparing groups with each other showed that the biofeedback group improved to a greater extent than the control group, with no other significant pairwise comparisons (Mishra, Gatchel, & Gardea, 2000). Thus, this study too provides at least faint evidence that biofeedback by itself is the best approach, when assessed immediately posttreatment. The reason is not clear. Mishra et al. suggest that the biofeedback, as a physically-oriented intervention, may have inspired more effort and adherence. When it was combined with a more psychologically-oriented intervention, some of this intuitive applicability may have been lost (Mishra, Gatchel, & Gardea, 2000). However, fine-grained studies to shed empirical light on this question do not seem to have been conducted yet. We will consider this question further in Chapter 15.

And in fact, the results look different at one year (Gardea, Gatchel, & Mishra, 2001). Then, both the biofeedback and combined treatment produced a greater reduction in pain than the no-treatment control. For a pain-disability measure, only the combined therapy showed greater efficacy than the control. For self-reported mandibular functioning, the combined treatment and cognitive-behavioral therapy by itself were more effective than no treatment. Thus, at one-year follow-up, the combined treatment appears to have had broader results than the biofeedback. It is not unusual for the benefits of cognitive therapy to increase during the first year after treatment.

The results of Gardea et al.'s study differ from those of Flor and Birbaumer. The two studies diverge on a number of particulars, including diagnostic criteria for temporomandibular dysfunction, type of cognitive intervention, and placement of the biofeedback sensors (masseter in Flor and Birbaumer, frontalis in Gardea et al.) The frontalis is not a muscle of mastication, and thus in Gardea et al.'s study, the biofeedback was primarily a way of teaching relaxation and illustrating psychophysiological effects.

At least two studies suggest that adding a cognitive-behavioral intervention can improve outcomes, when compared with conservative dental treatment alone (D. C. Turk, Zaki, & Rudy, 1993). Generally, conservative dental treatment involves medication, physical therapy, and/or an oral appliance to correct malocclusion (Mishra, Gatchel, & Gardea, 2000).

Dworkin et al. have suggested that brief cognitive behavioral treatment in a group format is unlikely to be intensive enough to benefit patients who somaticize or who are depressed (S. F. Dworkin, J. A. Turner, et al., 1994). On the other hand, Turk et al. have examined whether cognitive therapy for depression could improve outcomes for people scoring in the "dysfunctional" cluster of the West Haven-Yale Multidimensional Pain Inventory (high levels of pain, negative mood, and life interference/dissatisfaction due to pain, and low levels of perceived control over one's life; D. C. Turk & Rudy, 1987). All 48 research participants received an intraoral appliance, biofeedback, relaxation training, and instruction in cognitive pain coping tools such as distraction. Twenty four of the participants also received standard cognitive therapy, targeting maladaptive thoughts and beliefs, for specific concerns in the person's life. As a control, the other twenty four participants received supportive counseling. The outcomes for the two groups differed in a specific way: While both groups showed reductions pre- to posttreatment in ambient pain, depression, and muscle pain with palpation, only the cognitive therapy group went on to show further gains between the end of treatment and 6-month follow-up (D. C. Turk, Rudy,

Kubinski, Zaki, & Greco, 1996). We will see this phenomenon again, of behavioral therapy reaching full effectiveness 6 or 12 months after the conclusion of treatment, again in Chapter 17 when we consider long-term outcome studies.

MENSTRUAL MIGRAINES

Menstrual migraines are, as the name implies, those reliably triggered by menstruation. An exact definition of a menstrual migraine has not been universally accepted, and the term is used variously to mean any migraine occurring perimenstrually, or migraines occurring perimenstrually with predictable regularity, or migraines in women whose headaches occur exclusively perimenstrually. Because of the presumed strong endogenous, hormonal component, there has been some effort to determine whether biofeedback is useful in menstrual migraine.

Gauthier and coworkers selected 39 female patients who had both menstrual and nonmenstrual migraines by self-report. Menstrual migraines were defined broadly as those occurring during or within three days of menstruation. Participants were treated with either thermal or cephalic pulse amplitude biofeedback. Within subjects, there were significant reductions in headache frequency, duration, and intensity, and in medication intake, both for those migraines that occurred perimenstrually, and those that did not. There were no significant differences between the two treatment groups. Moreover, an analysis of effect size suggested that if such a difference were detected it would account for at most 1 percent of the variance in headaches. When participants were divided into those whose migraines were chiefly perimenstrual (based on prospective monitoring) and those whose headaches occurred chiefly at other times, there was again no significant difference in treatment outcome (Gauthier, Fournier, & Roberge, 1991).

Kim and Blanchard compared 38 migraineurs who reported that their headaches were associated with menstruation, with 60 female migraineurs who reported that their headaches were not associated with menstruation. There was a strong treatment effect for both groups. The two groups did not differ in their treatment responses (M. Kim & Blanchard, 1992).

A potential weakness in these studies is the division into groups based on a single self-report item. The reliability of the menstrual-nonmenstrual distinction is uncertain, and the failure to find significant differences in treatment response may reflect this. On the other hand, some of the overlap between groups is most likely characteristic of migraines themselves, as perimenstrual phase (and perhaps mid-cycle as well; M. Kim & Blanchard, 1992) is, after stress, the most common trigger of migraines in general.

Kim and Blanchard attempted to circumvent these difficulties by selecting a group of female migraineurs for whom menstrually-related migraines were verified prospectively over three menstrual cycles (M. Kim & Blanchard, 1992). The phase of the menstrual cycle involved in the migraines was allowed to vary between, although not within, subjects. Kim and Blanchard found that for these women, menstrual and nonmenstrual migraines decreased by the same amount with behavioral treatment. The menstrual migraines were as readily treated as the nonmenstrual migraines. However, the conclusion is blunted by the fact that the two types of migraine showed only a trend ($p = .085$) towards statistically significant improvement. This may be due to the small sample size ($N = 15$) and hence under-powering, or it may indicate that the migraines in this group of people were harder to treat behaviorally.

M. Kim (1995, cited in Blanchard, 1998) applied the term "menstrual migraine" to migraines occurring during declining estrogen levels: the interval immediately preceding ovulation, and the interval from 3 days before menstruation through day 8 of the next cycle. She found a significantly better response of nonmenstrual migraines (60.7 percent decrease) vs. menstrual migraines (43.7 percent decrease) to thermal biofeedback plus relaxation.

Note that in no behavioral study to date, to my knowledge, have women been isolated who have pure menstrual migraines—that is, for whom hormonal cycle invariably triggers a migraine and whose migraines occur at no other times. Thus, menstrual migraine remains an area in which further behavioral research is needed.

POSTTRAUMATIC HEADACHES

Outcome data on behavioral treatment for posttraumatic headaches are almost completely lacking. Hickling, et al., however, report on a clinical series of 12 patients who had been in a motor vehicle accident, and who were treated in the first author's private practice (Hickling, Blanchard, S. P. Schwarz, & Silverman, 1992). Of the 12 patients, 9 had some level of Posttraumatic Stress Disorder (8 diagnosable, 1 subsyndromal), 8 were depressed (6 with a Major Depressive Episode, 1 with Dysthymia, and 1 with Adjustment Disorder with Depressed Mood), and 5 had a phobia of driving. Treatment was individual cognitive-behavioral psychotherapy for coping with anxiety- and depression-inducing situations, desensitization, supportive therapy, relaxation training and, if needed, thermal or EMG biofeedback. In essence, they were being treated for all of their disorders, and not simply the headaches. Patients received between 8 and 50 sessions (mean = 20), and two thirds showed at least a 50 percent reduction in headaches as measured prospectively with a headache diary. Hickling et al. suggest that the relatively long treatment course was required by the high prevalence of comorbid emotional disorders (Hickling, Blanchard, S. P. Schwarz, & Silverman, 1992). These results are quite helpful for those of us in clinical practice, but as the authors note they are merely suggestive, and await replication in controlled studies.

Similar uncontrolled data is available for multidisciplinary treatment of chronic posttraumatic syndrome (Medina, 1992). This syndrome involves posttraumatic headache and the constellation of comorbidities that surround it: irritability, dizziness, reduced endurance, and difficulty with memory and concentration. Medina reports that over an average of 18.8 treatment days, taking place over an average of 7 weeks, 14 of 20 patients were markedly improved, and 17 out of 20 returned to work. This was a small study, and of course without suitable controls we do not know what the active ingredient was that led to the improvements. However, the research seems quite promising as a starting point.

More recently, Packard and Ham (1997b) have proposed that EEG biofeedback, with training to decrease theta activity (4–7 Hz., associated with low arousal) and increase 15–18 Hz beta activity (associated with high arousal) would help reduce post-concussion symptoms, including headache. So far, however, the available data are too preliminary to permit conclusions.

CLUSTER HEADACHES

To my knowledge, there have been only five studies of the effects of behavioral treatment on cluster headaches.

The first was a study by Benson and coworkers of the effects of Transcendental Meditation. Of their 21 participants, 4 had cluster headaches. All were taught to meditate for 20 minutes, twice a day, and all provided daily headache records beginning 1–3 months before the meditation and continuing for 4–14 months afterwards. Of the patients with cluster headache, 1 had no change in symptoms, 2 improved for several months but relapsed thereafter, and the last subject, who had had severe daily cluster headaches, experienced a complete remission that was still ongoing at one-year follow-up (Benson, Klemchuk, & Graham, 1974). The participants were trained at the Students International Meditation Society at a cost of $75, which, along with the extended practice, perhaps added a cognitive dissonance motivation for expecting a reduction in headaches. Note, too, that improving for several months and then relapsing is also characteristic of *untreated* cluster headaches, as people move in and out of cluster periods.

The second study, by C. S. Adler and S. M. Adler (1976), involved 58 patients, of whom 5 had cluster headaches. Treatment was combined psychodynamic therapy and biofeedback, in which the machines were used both for teaching relaxation skills and for fostering insight into which topics were anxiety provoking. Of the 5 patients, 3 (60 percent) had at least a 75 percent reduction in headache frequency, at $3\frac{1}{2}$ to 5 year follow-up. A weakness of the study, noted by the authors, is that it was retrospective.

The third study, by Blanchard and coworkers, was a trial of progressive muscle relaxation training and thermal biofeedback (Blanchard, Andrasik, Jurish, & Teders, 1982). The subjects had presented during a study on migraines and tension-type headaches. For ethical reasons, they were informed in advance that the treatment was purely experimental, given the paucity of empirical literature. Of the 11 patients, all of whom had the episodic form of the disorder, 4 declined treatment. For two other patients there were no outcome data, as they were not yet scheduled to enter a new cluster period by the time follow-up ended. Thus, the effective sample size was 5. Assessment was prospective and follow-up periods ranged from 15 to 22 months.

Of the 5 patients, 4 showed some degree of improvement. That is, two of the 5 patients experienced a reduction in the duration, frequency, and intensity of headaches, and were able to prevent some cluster headaches at their earliest stages. One of the 5 patients experienced only a reduction in headache frequency, and one had a reduction in intensity and duration only. For these patients, there was no consistent change in the timing or duration of cluster periods. The fifth patient was definitely worse, having apparently changed from the episodic to the chronic form during the follow-up period. Thus, the results are inconclusive.

Since the study by Blanchard, et al., there have been two reports of successful treatment, but both are in the form of case studies. Hoelscher and Lichstein (1983) report that cephalic pulse amplitude biofeedback, used to treat a 61 year old man with chronic cluster headaches, produced a 70 percent reduction in headache frequency and a 45 percent decrease in pain severity that was maintained at 1-, 3-, 6-, 12-, and 21-month follow-ups. King and Arena (1984) report that in a 69 year old man with chronic cluster headache, thermal biofeedback and elimination of pain-contingent responding by the spouse produced a decrease in pain reports that was maintained at 1-, 4-, and 15-month follow-ups. In both cases, the improvements were accompanied by marked reductions in medication use. Of course case study data cannot be regarded as compelling.

Thus, the literature contains, in effect, 3 very favorable case studies suggesting particular effectiveness for the chronic form of the disorder. Given the graveness of the diagnosis, a trial of behavioral treatment for chronic cluster headache does not seem unreasonable. The literature is quite sparse, however, and the trial could not be regarded as evidence-based.

Before leaving the topic of cluster headache, recall that alcohol, exertion, a hot environment, and other causes of vasodilation have been implicated as triggers. Recall, too, the epidemiological link to smoking. To my knowledge, studies of systematic trigger-elimination, and of smoking and alcohol cessation, have not been conducted in the context of cluster headache.

CHRONIC DAILY HEADACHE

Medication overuse.   We saw in Chapter 7 that overuse of symptomatic headache medications can drastically lower the effectiveness of preventive drug treatment. Does high medication use also impair the effectiveness of behavioral treatment? There is some evidence that it does. Blanchard and coworkers reviewed the outcome data for over 400 individuals who had participated in behavioral treatment studies, culling out 51 patients who consumed high amounts of symptomatic medications and 51 matched controls (Michultka, Blanchard, Appelbaum, Jaccard, & Dentinger, 1989). The treatments that had been studied were biofeedback, relaxation training, and/or cognitive therapy. Blanchard et al. found that the high medication users had the same *absolute* reduction in headache activity as the matched controls. However, because baseline headache activity was more intense among the high medication patients, their relative improvement was lower—a 23 percent reduction, versus 43 percent for the low medicators. Not surprisingly, then, only 29 percent of the high medicators were clinically improved by conventional standards, compared with 55 percent of the low medicators (Michultka, Blanchard, Appelbaum, Jaccard, & Dentinger, 1989).

In this analysis, however, we are presuming that cognitive-behavioral treatments will be applied with no special attention to the high medication use. Clinically, it appears that a medication taper is a key component in recovery from rebound headaches.

Moreover, we saw in Chapter 7 that patients who feel dependent on symptomatic medications might have an external locus of control in regard to headaches. Thus, self-management training could perhaps be particularly important for promoting self-efficacy in patients who are being tapered from medications. There is a little bit of evidence to support this supposition. Specifically, Grazzi, et al. followed 61 patients for 3 years after treatment. All of the patients had transformed migraine with high medication use, and for all of the patients the acute medications were stopped and replaced by appropriate prophylactic drugs (Grazzi, Andrasik, D'Amico, Leone, Usai, Kass, & Bussone, 2002). Nineteen of the patients, however, also received 8 weekly sessions of progressive muscle relaxation, enhanced with frontalis muscle tension biofeedback. During the first year after treatment, 10 percent of the subjects who were taught relaxation skills, and 20 percent of those who were not, relapsed back into high medication use. After three years post-treatment, 13 percent of the cognitive-behavioral group, and 42 percent of the preventive-medication-only group, had relapsed into overuse. The difference at year 3 was statistically significant (χ^2 [1] = 4.41, $p < .04$; Grazzi, Andrasik, D'Amico, Leone, Usai, Kass, & Bussone, 2002). This result seems reasonable, and consistent with the evidence that self-management skills increase self-efficacy. However, subjects were allowed to opt out of the relaxation training if they lived too far from the hospital. Now, "too far" can be a subjective judgment, and hence we might wonder whether the relaxation group was, on average, more committed to their treatment (Grazzi, Andrasik, D'Amico, Leone, Usai, Kass, & Bussone, 2002). More research, of course, will be helpful.

Continuous headache. Thus, we usually cannot simply apply short-term biofeedback, relaxation, and cognitive therapy to medication-overuse headache and achieve good results. In fact, the same appears to be true for another type of chronic daily headache. Blanchard et al. found that among patients who were experiencing headaches almost continuously, only 13 percent were clinically improved after short-term treatment, versus 52 percent of patients with almost-daily headache, and 70 percent whose headaches were frequent but episodic (Blanchard, Appelbaum, Radnitz, Jaccard, & Dentinger, 1989). Note, however, that the near-daily headaches, which nominally would meet the criteria for chronic daily headache, did respond to short-term behavioral treatment. The dividing line seems to be between headaches 5–6 days per week on average, which generally do respond, and continuous headaches, which generally do not respond.

Now, these negative results are for the standard relaxation, biofeedback, and cognitive therapies, applied at their usual level of intensity. In the study, Blanchard et al. simply culled out data from patients with daily headache from a large data set of treatment trials previously conducted at their clinic. In a subsequent study, Barton and Blanchard made an intensive effort to get daily headaches to yield, by applying the treatments for a total of 20 sessions (Barton & Blanchard, 2001). On process measures, the treatments had a degree of efficacy. Despite literally daily headaches, patients reported a subjective sense of relaxation and appeared reasonably relaxed by a checklist of behavioral signs. The patients were able to increase finger temperature, and they rated themselves at the end of treatment as somewhat more able to prevent, control and cope with their headaches (Barton & Blanchard, 2001). However, actual headache activity essentially did not change, prospectively measured. That is, 2 of 20 patients (10 percent; or 2 of 16 treatment completers; 12.5 percent) achieved at least a 50 percent reduction in headache activity at post-treatment follow-up. This, of course, is about the same proportion as were successful in the data-mining study noted above.

Barton and Blanchard's study has attracted respectful, cogent criticism. Holroyd, for example, drawing on the Treatment of Chronic Tension-Type Headache Trial, suggested that the post-treatment measure (12 weeks after baseline) may have been too soon to see clear results (K. A. Holroyd, 2001). Moreover, although the patients were fairly low on average medication intake (the equivalent of 3 over-the-counter pills per day) they were still a bit over the threshold of 14 pills per week for potential rebound headache (Baskin, 2001). Also, the heterogeneity of diagnosis (e.g., chronic tension-type headache, transformed migraine), small sample size, and the lack of control groups and predefined end-points have similarly been questioned (Ramadan, 2001). Still, all the data so far available seems to point to the same, minimal, 10 percent success rate for headaches that occur literally daily.

Where does this leave us? Some investigators have suggested that future research should focus on identifying risk factors for daily headache, and then on prevention (e.g., Loder & Biondi, 2003). The potential efficacy of combined medication and behavioral treatment has also been suggested (K. A. Holroyd, J. L. France, Cordingley, Rokicki, Kvaal, Lipchik, & McCool, 1995). While these issues are being worked out in studies, the best approach clinically may be to treat daily headaches by analogy to other types of chronic pain syndrome, for which well-established pain coping skills are available. Behavioral treatment for pain has acquired a degree of supporting data in its own right, as we will see in the next section.

Hospitalization.   In a few studies, the focus has been on intensive inpatient treatment for chronic migraine, in which the primary intervention was intravenous dihydroergotamine or hydrocortisone, oral preventives, individual and family therapy, and educational groups on relaxation and pain management. Other modalities, such as biofeedback or physical therapy, were included as needed (Lake, Saper, Madden, & Kreeger, 1993). Thus, the data do not allow us to tease out the effects of the behavioral components specifically. Still, the few results available have been impressive.

Thus, Lake et al. found that shortly after an average of 8.5 days of inpatient treatment, the number of pain-free days per 2-week interval had increased from 1.03 to 4.78, with further improvement over the next 8 months. Depression, sleep disruption, use of acute medications, functional impairment, pain-distress, and pain behavior (discussion of headache) all improved significantly as well (Lake, Saper, Madden, & Kreeger, 1993), replicating the results of a prior, short-term study (Lake & Saper, 1988).

The response rate in Lake, et al. (1993), 66 percent, was high for a mailed questionnaire, but low for an outcome study, and there was no control group. Still, given the refractoriness of chronic daily headache, a strong treatment effect seems likely.

CHRONIC PAIN

Beyond this, there is little empirical literature on the behavioral treatment of chronic daily headache or of posttraumatic headache. However, we might be able to anticipate the likely degree of efficacy by examining the behavioral treatment literature for other chronic pain conditions, such as rheumatoid arthritis, osteoarthritis, and chronic low back pain. This general chronic pain literature has been examined in a meta-analysis by Morley, Eccleston and A. Williams (1999), and is given in Table 14–8. We should note that in the meta-analysis, studies of headaches were specifically excluded. This is because the vast majority of behavioral studies of headaches focus on migraines and tension-type headaches, which are presumed to be easier to treat behaviorally than is the pain of, say, arthritis or failed back surgery.

In the meta-analysis, behavioral treatment included studies of relaxation training, biofeedback, behavior modification, cognitive therapy, and coping skills training.

The patients in the waiting list control condition most likely continued to receive treatment, for example medications or physical therapy, from their regular treatment providers. Thus, in this meta-analysis "waiting list control" is not synonymous with "no-treatment control." However, the regular treatments were presumably ineffective for the patients given that they had been referred to a behavioral chronic pain program. Note that these patients tended to benefit from behavioral treatment on every dimension of outcome, including pain, activity, mood, catastrophic thinking, and social role functioning. On each of these measures, the effect size of behavioral treatment was approximately 0.50. By comparison, amitriptyline appears to have an effect size of c. 0.73 as an analgesic in chronic pain (Onghena & Van Houdenhove, 1992). However, because amitriptyline is such a standard intervention, we might speculate that the patients were already taking it, or had failed it.

The alternative treatments are those against which behavioral treatment was explicitly compared in the studies entered into the meta-analysis. They vary from study to study and include physical therapy, occupational therapy, arthritis education, and even non-behavioral pain clinic treatment. Here, the advantages of behavioral treatment are more modest, but it still outperforms alternatives on three of the outcome dimensions: pain, pain behaviors, and coping thoughts, with an effect size of 0.27 to 0.40. Moreover, this is likely to be an underestimate, as physical therapy, occupational therapy, work hardening, and rehabilitative medical care for chronic pain now often include behavioral components, such as time-contingent (vs. pain-contingent) medication, gradual increase of activity, and reinforcement for gains in functioning (Keefe & Lefebvre, 1999).

TABLE 14–8
Efficacy of Behavioral Treatment for Chronic Pain

Outcome Measure	Behavioral vs. Waiting List		Behavioral vs. Alternative Treatment	
	Effect Size	N	Effect Size[a]	N
Pain Experience	0.40	28	0.29	22
Depression	0.36	24	—	15
Mood-Other	0.52	16	—	16
Catastrophizing	0.50	16	—	14
Coping Thoughts	0.53	11	0.40	15
Pain Behaviors	0.50	12	0.27	11
Activity	0.46	14	—	0
Social Role Functioning	0.60	25	—	14

Note. Adapted from "Systematic Review and Meta-Analysis of Randomized Controlled Trials of Cognitive Behaviour Therapy and Behaviour Therapy for Chronic Pain in Adults, Excluding Headache," by S. Morley, C. Eccleston, and A. Williams, 1999, *Pain, 80,* pp. 9 and 10. Copyright 1999 by the International Association for the Study of Pain. Adapted with permission.

[a]Only effect sizes significantly different from zero on at least the $p < .05$ level are shown.

Operant methods seem to have their strongest support for increasing activity and exercise tolerance, and reducing medication use, in chronic low back pain (Compas, Haaga, Keefe, et al., 1998; Keefe & Lefebvre, 1999; Keefe, Gil, & S. C. Rose, 1986). Keefe and Lefebvre suggest that in practice, a pain reduction of 20–30 percent is typically achieved. This is not unimpressive, given the simultaneous reduction or elimination of pain medications, and the refractoriness of the pain to other treatments. Note, however, that the effect sizes for chronic pain treatment are considerably smaller than those for migraines and tension-type headache, confirming the impression that chronic pain is harder to treat successfully.

The source of the pain reduction is not certain. It could be a response artifact: Patients might report their pain as lower, without any change in sensation, as a generalization of decreased pain-related conversation. Alternatively, the improvement in quality of life may lower pain along its affective dimension (reduced pain-distress). As a third possibility, the resumption of activities may provide a continuous diversion of attention from the pain, thus decreasing the pain's sensation intensity. A fourth possible mechanism, for which we found a degree of evidence in chapters 2 and 3, is that the sensitivity of the pain system may respond to operant and classical conditioning.

Several studies have examined whether cognitive-behavioral therapy leads to improved outcomes. For example, Gil, et al. used prospective pain diaries to study the effects of pain coping skills (relaxation, imagery, distraction, etc.) in adults with sickle cell disease. Use of coping skills was associated with a decrease in hospital and doctor's office visits and a lowered intake of narcotics, and with an increase in phone calls to doctors, time off from school or work, and intake of non-narcotic analgesics (Gil, Carson, Sedway, Porter, Schaeffer, & Orringer, 2000). The coping skills apparently allowed individuals to manage the pain with less intensive external support.

There is some evidence that when the patient's spouse helps provide training in pain coping skills, outcomes are better than when the spouse is simply present for support (Keefe, Caldwell, et al., 1996; Radojevic, Nicassio, & Weisman, 1992). Presumably, the spouse is more likely to reinforce pain coping when his or her participation is actively elicited. There is also a little bit of evidence that patients' pain and mood are better on time-contingent than pain-contingent schedules of analgesics (e.g., Berntzen & Götestam, 1987).

We will examine operant and cognitive chronic pain treatment, and other components of behavioral therapy, in greater detail in Chapter 15.

TREATMENT OUTCOMES FOR CHILDREN WITH HEADACHES

The outcome literature for children, although still sparse, is beginning to accumulate to the point that tentative conclusions can be drawn. And there is reason for optimism. From a structured review of 57 published trials, Sarafino and Goehring conclude that biofeedback brings about a greater reduction in headache activity, from baseline to the end of treatment, in children than it does in adults. Further, from the end of treatment to post-treatment follow-up, children show greater additional gains than do adults (Sarafino & Goehring, 2000).

Migraines

A thorough meta-analysis of controlled comparisons of two or more treatments for pediatric migraine, 1970–1992, was presented by Hermann, M. Kim and Blanchard (1995), and is shown in Table 14–9. To be included in the analysis, studies had to include 3 or more subjects in each treatment condition, provide sufficient detail that effect size could be computed or inferred, and

TABLE 14–9
Efficacy of Behavioral and Pharmacological Interventions for Pediatric Migraine

Treatment	Effect Size	N
Behavioral		
Thermal Biofeedback + Autogenics[a]	3.33 (2.57)[1]	4 (5)
Biofeedback + Progressive Muscle Relax.[a]	2.84 (3.09)	3 (4)
Progressive Muscle Relaxation[b]	1.43 (0.95)	4 (5)
Multicomponent Treatment[b]	1.41	3
Psychological Placebo[c]	0.56	4
Waiting List Control[c]	0.56	5
Medication		
Propranolol[a]	2.84	2
Ergotamine[2]	1.55	2
Clonidine	1.46	2
Dopaminergic Drugs	1.42	2
Serotonergic Drugs[b]	1.18 (1.30)	9 (10)
Calcium Channel Blockers[b]	1.06 (1.15)	10 (11)
Placebo Medication[c]	0.71	13

Notes. Adapted from "Behavioral and Prophylactic Pharmacological Intervention Studies of Pediatric Migraine: An Exploratory Meta-Analysis," by C. Hermann, M, Kim, and E. B. Blanchard, 1995, *Pain, 60*, p. 246. Copyright 1995 by Elsevier Science BV. Adapted with permission.

[1]Effect size and number of studies are given with the outliers excluded. The corresponding figures with the outliers included are given in parentheses.

[2]Ergotamine, clonidine, and dopaminergic drugs (domperidone, metoclopramide) were not included in the statistical comparisons due to the small number of studies. Numerically, however, their effect sizes are equivalent to those of progressive muscle relaxation and multicomponent behavioral treatment, and thus to the "b" group of treatments.

Calcium-channel blockers: flunarizine, nimodipine

Serotonergic medications: amitriptyline, trazodone, cyproheptadine, pizotifen, 5-HTP

Dopaminergic medications: domperidone, metoclopramide

[a,b,c]Treatments that do not share a superscript are significantly different in terms of estimated efficacy. Significance is at the $p < .01$ level except for calcium channel blockers, which are superior to medication placebo at the .05 level.

not have severe methodological flaws (for example, comparing two drugs in a cross-over design without sufficient washout period between them). The inclusion of behavioral and pharmacological treatments in the same meta-analysis allows for tentative, but intriguing, cross-modality comparisons.

The treatments coalesce into three categories. The highest efficacy, with rather extraordinary effect sizes of 2.8–3.3, were achieved with thermal biofeedback plus autogenics, with biofeedback (thermal or EMG) plus progressive muscle relaxation and, among the medications, with propranolol. The second group, with effects sizes of 1.1–1.4, includes progressive muscle relaxation, multicomponent behavioral treatment, serotonergic drugs, and calcium channel blockers. These, in turn, were superior to psychological and pharmacological placebos, and to time itself (waiting list controls) with still respectable effect sizes of 0.6–0.7. Hermann, M. Kim and Blanchard stress the preliminary nature of their results owing to the relative sparseness of well-controlled studies.

Note that the category of serotonergic drugs is so pharmacologically diverse, including a serotonin precursor (5-HTP), antagonists (cyproheptadine, pizotifen), and reuptake inhibitors (amitriptyline, trazodone) that one could argue that it is meaningless. In terms of effect size, however, the subcategories do not differ significantly.

Five conditions (thermal biofeedback, biofeedback plus progressive muscle relaxation, progressive muscle relaxation by itself, calcium channel blockers, and serotonergic drugs) had statistically significant within-groups heterogeneity of variance. In each case, this could be corrected by eliminating a single study whose results were an outlier. In most cases, there was a plausible reason for the aberrant results. For example, a study by Guarnieri and Blanchard used home-based vs. clinic-based treatment, did not check for compliance, and achieved notably poorer results than other studies of the same treatment. In Table 14–9, effect size and number of studies are given with the outliers excluded. The corresponding figures with the outliers included are given in parentheses.

Methodological adequacy differed considerably across studies. It did not correlate with effect size for the behavioral studies ($r = -.06$, ns). However, for the medication studies it accounted for approximately 16 percent of the variance in effect sizes, with the poorer studies showing greater reduction in headaches ($r = -.4$, $p < .01$). This is of some concern. However, Hermann et al. suggest that it is a relatively minor factor in the variation of effect sizes in their study. Also the assumption, implicit in the use of the Pearson r, that the quality-effect size relationship is linear, has been criticized (Goodkin & McGrath, 1996).

An updated review, performed according to the criteria of the Cochrane Collaboration, found broadly similar results: evidence in favor of autogenics training, alone or in combination with biofeedback or cognitive-behavioral therapy, when compared with waiting-list controls. Again, methodology was found suboptimal, particularly in the areas of sample size, blinding, and method of randomization (Damen, Bruijn, Koes, M. Berger, Passchier, & Verhagen, 2006). Thus, there is definite need for larger and more definitive studies in pediatric migraine.

Hermann, et al.'s meta-analysis suggests that, for children, biofeedback leads to better outcomes than relaxation training by itself. In a direct comparison, Labbe (1995) found that autogenics plus finger temperature biofeedback had greater efficacy (80 percent of children symptom-free) than autogenics-only (50 percent of children symptom-free), or waiting-list controls (0 percent symptom-free). This seems to lend itself to a psychophysiological explanation, but the matter has not been settled. Allen and Shriver (1997) present data from a small study ($N = 6$) suggesting that belief in efficacy, rather than true physiological control, is the primary determinant of success for children. On the other hand, Scharff and colleagues found that for 36 children and adolescents with migraine, hand warming biofeedback and stress management led to greater clinical improvement than an equally credible hand cooling condition (Scharff, Marcus, & Masek, 2002).

In the meta-analysis, it is tempting to make post-hoc comparisons between behavioral and pharmacological treatment. As with the meta-analyses for adults, however, data on the two forms of treatment may appear in different journals with differing policies about publishing null results. We are on safest grounds if we simply conclude that the best behavioral and medication treatments are of roughly similar effectiveness. To go further, it would be preferable to have head-to-head comparisons, and there have been only two so far.

Olness and colleagues conducted a double-blind, placebo-controlled, single crossover study of propranolol 3 mg/kg/day, to which self-hypnosis was added as a final treatment stage (Olness, MacDonald, & Uden, 1987). That is, children received either placebo or propranolol for 11 weeks, followed by a 1 week washout period, an 11 week treatment with propranolol or placebo, and another 1-week washout period. After the second washout period, the children received 3 sessions of self-hypnosis training, followed by 2 monthly review sessions, and were followed for another 12 weeks. All of the 28 children, ages 6–12, had migraine with aura. There was no effect of any treatment on headache intensity or duration. The number of headaches per 12-week study period was 13.3 during the placebo condition, 14.9 on propranolol, and 5.8 following self-hypnosis. The self-hypnosis outperformed propranolol ($p = .01$) and the placebo ($p < .05$). The reason for the inefficacy of propranolol was unclear, and might perhaps have been related to insufficient study duration (Olness, MacDonald, & Uden, 1987). Also, only 19 of the children received propranolol. By design, the other 9 children received placebo during both arms of the cross-over study.

In a similar study, Sartory et al. randomized 43 people with migraine, ages 8–16, to receive progressive muscle relaxation, temporal pulse amplitude biofeedback, or metoprolol (50 or 100 mg/day, depending on body weight). Each of the two psychological treatments was combined with stress- and pain-management training to increase its efficacy, and headache activity was monitored prospectively. Now, at the end of treatment (6 weeks for the psychological treatments, 10 weeks for the metoprolol) the relaxation group had a significant reduction in headache frequency and intensity, and a trend towards reduction in duration. The pulse amplitude biofeedback group had significant reductions in headache frequency and duration. In contrast, improvements in the metoprolol group were small and statistically nonsignificant for all measures (Sartory, Müller, Metsch, & Pothmann, 1998). As in Olness' study, the failure of a **beta-blocker** to show efficacy is surprising. The trial length, however, ten weeks, was a bit shorter than the twelve weeks generally recommended for the medication. Also, the post-treatment measures were derived from headache diaries kept over the four weeks following treatment. Thus, the effects of metoprolol, like those of the behavioral interventions, were assessed after the treatment phase had ended. More commonly, response to a medication is assessed while the medication is still being taken.

Predictors of outcome.   Hermann, Blanchard, & Flor (1997) obtained excellent results in treating 36 migraine patients, ages 8–16, with biofeedback. This is consistent with meta-analyses showing that youth is a predictor of good outcome. Indeed youth may be a predictor even within the pediatric age range. In Hermann, et al.'s study, pre-teens showed more improvement than teenagers. Despite the reliance of treatment on home practice, family organization and structure did not predict treatment outcome. Overall results, for the 32/36 treatment completers, included a 60 percent reduction in the headache index, a 50 percent reduction in headache frequency, a 65 percent drop in medication use, and a 55 percent improvement in school absenteeism (see Table 14–10).

On the other hand, Olness, et al. found that the effectiveness of self-hypnosis for migraines with aura was unrelated to age, sex, baseline headache frequency or severity, child's IQ on the Wechsler Intelligence Scale for Children—Revised, presence of EEG abnormalities, or degree of hand warming achieved during self-hypnosis (Olness, MacDonald, & Uden, 1987). (Note that children with abnormal EEG's received a CT or brain scan, and were excluded from the study if the imaging was positive. Children with an IQ below 85 were also excluded from the study.)

TABLE 14–10
Treatment Results for Pediatric Migraine (Hermann, Blanchard, & Flor, 1997)

Outcome Measure	Pre-Treatment	Post-Treatment
Headache Intensity X Duration	168.9 ± 133	68.2 ± 84
Headache Frequency	8.0 ± 4.9	4.0 ± 4.4
Medication Frequency X Strength	12.7 ± 13	4.4 ± 7.5
Days of School Absence	1.1 ± 1.8	0.5 ± 1.1

Note. Adapted from "Biofeedback Treatment for Pediatric Migraine: Prediction of Treatment Outcome," by C. Hermann, E. B. Blanchard, and H. Flor, 1997, *Journal of Consulting and Clinical Psychology, 65,* p. 613. Copyright 1997 by the American Psychological Association. Adapted with permission.

Tension-Type Headache

There have been fewer studies of behavioral treatment of tension-type headache in children and adolescents, and hence no meta-analyses are available. Therefore, we will simply discuss salient examples from the literature.

B. Larsson and Melin (1988) treated 16–18 year old students with therapist-assisted or home-based progressive muscle relaxation. No significant effects were obtained for the 23 migraineurs in the study. However, for the 85 subjects with tension headache, 59 percent showed at least a 50 percent reduction in headache intensity X duration, vs.11 percent in a placebo condition and 0 percent in a self-monitoring control condition (χ^2 [4] = 30.35, $p < .01$).

The primary predictors of headache improvement in the relaxation group were baseline headache intensity ($r = .46$, $p < .01$) and satisfaction with home life ($r = .42$, $p < .01$). Greater satisfaction and greater initial headache activity were associated with greater improvement. These correlations, although potentially of theoretical import, are not high enough to be useful clinically for selecting patients.

Kröner-Herwig and coworkers compared the effects of waiting-list control, progressive muscle relaxation and frontalis EMG biofeedback in 50 children, ages 8–14, with tension-type or both tension-type and migraine headaches (Kröner-Herwig, Mohn, & Pothmann, 1998). Also studied was the effect of combining child treatment with instruction to the parents to model and reinforce good pain coping behaviors. Outcome measures were derived from 4-week headache diaries, completed before treatment, immediately after treatment, and again at 6-month follow-up.

The analyses of variance in this study showed only a main effect for time. Each group improved, although for the control group the numerical change was rather meager. If, however, we categorize the children on each variable as improved by greater than 50 percent, versus a 50 percent improvement or less, a more nuanced picture emerges. Calculating chi-squares from the published data (and correcting for small expected frequencies in some cells), we find that post-treatment, the biofeedback group had a better outcome than the control group on headache frequency, intensity, and duration. The remaining comparisons (progressive muscle relaxation vs. control, progressive muscle relaxation vs. biofeedback) were not significant for any of the variables. At the 6-month follow-up, biofeedback outperformed progressive muscle relaxation on headache frequency, duration, and intensity.

Of note, neither treatment led to a reduction in functional impairment, that is, in the frequency with which activities were interrupted or prevented by a headache. Parental involvement seemed to have weak effects. It improved results for one outcome measure, headache intensity, immediately post-treatment, but this effect was no longer apparent at the follow-up (Kröner-Herwig, Mohn, & Pothmann, 1998). We will consider the effects of parental involvement further in the next section.

A third controlled study of biofeedback, this one of pediatric episodic tension-type headache, has been reported by Bussone, et al. Their treatment consisted of 10 twice-weekly sessions of frontalis biofeedback. The control condition consisted of 10 sessions of sitting quietly in the biofeedback room while frontalis EMG was measured but not used therapeutically. The control condition was thus intended to replicate the attention, expectation, and quiet rest of the biofeedback condition, but not the active psychophysiological control. Participants receiving biofeedback were asked *not* to practice between sessions. Headaches were measured prospectively using 4-week headache diaries completed hourly at baseline, and 1 month, 3 months, 6 months, and 12 months after treatment. A booster session was offered at each of the 4 follow-up periods.

Compared with baseline, the placebo group achieved a respectable c. 60 percent reduction in total headache activity at 1 month, and maintained this level of improvement through the

12-month follow-up. The biofeedback group achieved approximately the same level of improvement at 1 month, but then continued to improve at later follow-ups, so that at one year they had an 86 percent reduction in total headache activity. Although conceptually the result is thus a group X time interaction, in the ANCOVA only the group main effect is significant, with biofeedback outperforming the placebo. Follow-up contrasts showed that the biofeedback was superior specifically at the two later periods, 6 months and 12 months post-treatment (Bussone, Grazzi, D'Amico, Leone, & Andrasik, 1998).

The reason for the delayed effect of biofeedback is not clear. The authors speculate that the instructions to eschew home practice, which were intended to provide a "cleaner" test of biofeedback and to minimize demands on the subjects, may have been responsible. On the other hand, gradual improvement over the first year post-treatment is not uncommon in cognitive-behavioral interventions.

Now, two qualifiers must be added. First, the degree of improvement in headaches was unrelated to surface EMG values, and in fact the surface EMG changed very little over the study for either group. Thus, the true active ingredient of treatment is unknown. Second, 5 of 15 patients in the control group, and 0 of 20 in the biofeedback group, dropped out of treatment. We could suggest that the difference between groups was thus underestimated, as the 5 dropouts, had they not been excluded from all data analysis, would most likely have suppressed the average improvement in the control group. On the other hand, we may suspect that the placebo was not fully credible, and possibly, this is the true difference between the two interventions.

Parental Involvement in Treatment

The weak effect of parental involvement, and the absence of an effect on functioning in the study by Kröner-Herwig et al., is in contrast to a study by Allen and Shriver, who focused on the effects of parent training, and who obtained clear improvements in functioning (K. D. Allen & Shriver, 1998). The 27 children in Allen and Shriver's study all had migraines and were slightly older (average age 12 years vs. 11 years). However, it seems likely that the key difference is in the nature of the intervention. For Kröner-Herwig, et al., the intervention with parents was primarily educational, and lying down and resting was, reasonably enough, considered an appropriate coping strategy for severe headaches (Kröner-Herwig, Mohn, & Pothmann, 1998). In the intervention by Allen and Shriver, parents periodically self-rated their responses to their children's headaches, and no discontinuation of normal activities was to be encouraged. Although the intervention sounds rather draconian, Allen and Shriver found that the parental involvement indeed gave better functional outcomes than biofeedback without parental involvement. Moreover, in the parental involvement condition there was also a greater number of children whose headache frequency was clinically improved, post-treatment, and at 1-month and 3-month follow-ups. This effect had disappeared at one-year follow-up, but a change to a potentially less reliable outcome measure at 1 year (single telephone report vs. prospective diary), and a small amount of subject attrition may be the reason.

On the other hand, Whiteside describes an intervention in which parents were, it seems, encouraged to help their children use self-hypnosis/relaxation skills. There was no formal outcome study, but the project seems to have been successful, and a very positive experience for the participants (Whiteside, 1990). Recall that Aromaa et al. had found that it was the father's poor tolerance for pain (modeling), rather than reinforcement for pain, that was the main parental factor in children's severe headaches (Aromaa, Sillanpää, Rautava, & Helenius, 2000). Implicitly, Whiteside's approach reduces *parents'* anxiety about pain.

But Whiteside's approach does not seem to have arisen from theory; more, it was inspired by a school essay, written by his 8-year-old daughter. Now, we have seen that for the best behavioral and pharmacological treatments, the clinical outcome literature, although preliminary, is quite favorable. Yet perhaps in our efforts to apply scientific methodology to the problem, we are in danger of becoming too clinical, too dispassionate. We will close this chapter, therefore, with a portion of the essay by Michael Whiteside's daughter (from Whiteside, 1990, p. 106):

"I wished my dad would come home cause he's a doctor and would make my terrible headache better. All day at school my head had been hurting and now I was in bed waiting for my dad. I was gazing round my room when I thought one of my posters had fallen off the wall and then it jumped back on again. I got out of bed to go and look and then I was sick. I got back into bed and thought the television was on. I began to shiver violently and knew I was going to be sick again because I always shiver and shake when I have these headaches. Oh why won't my dad come home and make this awful pain in my head go away. I went to sleep and when I woke up my dad was there and said it was my migraine again. He had brought some pills in a tiny glass but I hate pills and pleaded with my dad but it didn't work. Then I said I was a bit hungry so he went downstairs and I poured the pills down the sink and don't think he knows even now. I cried because all I really wanted was my dad to put his arms round me and hug me till I was better."

CHAPTER 15

Process: Studies of the Components
of Behavioral Treatment

(1) Walking about gently for a considerable time. The movement softens or relaxes the tissues. (2) Fats of thin consistence, and the oils already named. (3) Agreeable music—especially if it inclines one to sleep. (4) Being occupied with something very engrossing removes the severity of pain.
        —Avicenna (1930/11th century, p. 529) on "other means of allaying pain"[1]

While meta-analyses and outcome reviews can tell us whether and how well a treatment works, they shed little light on the underlying mechanism, or on how the therapies can be improved. For this we need more in-depth study of the individual treatment components. It is to this study that we will turn next.

RELAXATION TRAINING

Progressive muscle relaxation. We have seen that progressive muscle relaxation as it was taught by Jacobson differs from the abbreviated procedures in common use currently. Lehrer argues on rational grounds that the abbreviated procedures may be equivalent or even superior when the relaxation is a subsidiary component of a cognitive or cognitive-behavioral treatment such as systematic desensitization. However, Lehrer suggests that when the primary goal is to produce a deep relaxation response, such as when treating a psychophysiological disorder, the traditional approach may be preferable (Lehrer, 1982). Why? First, it is considerably more intensive. Second, there is much greater focus on relaxation as a physical skill, as opposed to a subjective experience. Third, Lehrer notes that the strong, repeated, isometric contractions of the abbreviated approach could increase tension due to slow recovery, and impede discrimination of low levels of muscle tension.

There appears to be little empirical literature addressing this point. Lehrer and coworkers, however, used surface EMG and magnitude estimations of subjective muscle tension to test the underlying assumptions of the abbreviated approach. They found that the repeated cycles of tension and relaxation in fact did appear to reduce tension, although slowly and only at the frontalis, and not the wrist extensors. Discrimination among low levels of muscle tension was poor among

---

[1]The lead for this quote is from C. S. Adler, S. M. Adler, & A. P. Friedman (1987). It is a sad irony that Avicenna ultimately died from an overdose of self-administered opium.

the subjects (all of whom were healthy) and did not improve with training (Lehrer, Batey, Wool-folk, Remde, & Garlick, 1988). The authors suggest that the perceived relaxation may be pri-marily a cognitive phenomenon, due to expectancy effects, contrast with the very high levels of tension during the isometric contraction, and/or the subjects' interpretation of the muscle's increased blood flow after the contraction (Lehrer, Batey, Woolfolk, Remde, & Garlick, 1988).

In Chapter 2 we saw that certain types of pain might derive from a distortion of the homuncu-lus in somatosensory cortex. In that case, a slow and detailed course of discrimination training, whether involving proprioception and tension, as in progressive muscle relaxation, or light touch, or both, would presumably be a key step in recovery. In theory, an abbreviated approach would not be useful: Contracting multiple muscles of the hand and arm simultaneously, for example, most likely would not restore ordered representations of the individual digits. When used as a form of discrimination training, Jacobsonian relaxation would presumably be enhanced by focus-ing visually on the tensing and release, because visual feedback facilitates proprioceptive (Ramachandran & Rogers-Ramachandran, 1996) and somatosensory (McCabe, Haigh, Shenker, J. Lewis, & Blake, 2004; Rock & J. Victor, 1964) awareness. For areas such as the forehead, a mir-ror would be necessary. However, additional research is needed to verify these hypotheses.

Abdominal breathing.   It appears that long-term practitioners of meditative techniques, such as Transcendental Meditation, show a decrease in sympathetic tone during the meditation (e.g., Barnes, Treiber, J. R. Turner, H. Davis, & Strong, 1999). This may be due partially to the cogni-tive shift of focusing on a repetitive stimulus rather than on stressors. Nonetheless, the physical effects of slow abdominal breathing are more subtle than a simple reduction in autonomic tone.

Short-term training in slowed respiration does not seem to change other psychophysiological variables such as heart rate, skin conductance or, importantly for headaches, hand temperature or frontalis EMG (G. T. Montgomery, 1994). Emotionally, however, deep slow breathing may induce a feeling of relaxation, perhaps by activating the relevant cognitive schema or **neural network** (Philippot, Chapelle, & Blairy, 2002). Moreover, slow, paced breathing, even when it does not produce physical relaxation, seems to reduce the physical effects of stress, especially the α-adren-ergic, vasoconstrictive effects relevant in migraine (M. T. Allen & Crowell, 1990). This stress-buffering property seems to arise from slow breathing itself, rather than from the involvement in the task or the expectation that it will be relaxing (McCaul, S. Solomon, & D. S. Holmes, 1979).

The clearest effect of abdominal breathing, however, is on heart rate. More specifically, note that heart rate speeds up briefly when one inhales, and momentarily slows down during exhalation. Because the average respiration rate is c. 9 breaths per minute, heart rate changes about once every 6.67 seconds, or 0.15 times per second (0.15 Hz). This is the "respiratory sinus arrhythmia" (RSA): the change in heart rhythm due to respiration (Berntson, Bigger, et al., 1997). In part it is due to the effects of the respiratory centers in the medulla on the cardiac center, and in part it reflects the influence on heart rate of stretch receptors in the chest (Berntson, Cacioppo, & Quigley, 1993). Biologically, the RSA may increase the efficiency of gas exchange in the lungs, by coupling the pulse of blood in the alveoli to the timing of inhalation (Giardino, Glenny, Borson, & L. Chan, 2003).

If this 0.15 Hz variability is removed statistically, heart rate is still not exactly constant. The variability is spread over many frequencies, which may reflect both a multiplicity of influences on heart rate, and the fact that synapses conveying rhythmic information from the medulla do not transmit the signal perfectly, but tend to smooth it over nearby, and especially lower, fre-quencies (Berntson, Cacioppo, & Quigley, 1993).

Now, if a person slows their breathing to 6 times a minute, then of course the respiratory sinus arrhythmia will shift downward in frequency to 0.10 Hz, corresponding to one breath every ten seconds. But additionally, the amplitude of the RSA increases markedly, in fact so much so that there is an increase in total heart rate variability (Lehrer, Sasaki, & Saito, 1999). What accounts for this increase? Lehrer, et al. argue that 0.10 Hz. is also the frequency at which baroreceptors (which detect blood pressure changes in the aorta) influence heart rate. When breathing slows to 0.10 Hz., the RSA and baroreceptor rhythms coincide, and the resulting resonance increases heart rate variability (Lehrer, Sasaki, & Saito, 1999). There are other explanations as well, however (Berntson, Cacioppo, & Quigley, 1993): First, the synapses between the cardiac rhythm generator in the medulla and the heart muscle do not respond very rapidly. Thus, the synapses act like low-pass filters: A lower frequency signal will be conveyed more completely than a high frequency signal, producing a stronger effect. Secondly, sympathetic activation attenuates the RSA. If a person relaxes because, cognitively, they are focusing on their breathing, the magnitude of the RSA may increase. Thirdly, when people are breathing slowly, they are also breathing deeply. The result is greater activation of stretch receptors in the chest, which then exert a greater influence on heart rate, raising the amplitude of the RSA.

Now, the respiratory sinus arrhythmia is useful to psychophysiologists as a relatively pure measure of vagal (parasympathetic) control of heart rate, relatively unaffected by sympathetic tone. It is not clear, however, whether the changes in RSA produced by slow abdominal breathing imply a general influence on the body, or are simply a behavioral artifact. Lehrer et al. argue for the former interpretation. Drawing on the theory that at 0.10 Hz. the RSA and baroreceptor influences are in resonance, they suggest that breathing at 6 times a minute augments baroreceptor effects. As the baroreceptors send afferent signals to the limbic system, there is room for slow breathing to have emotional effects. Note, however, that the nature of these effects, and indeed their existence, is quite open to speculation. While it is relatively easy to measure a physiological effect of slow breathing on heart rate, the implications for relaxation skills or headache management are unknown. For example, in a true relaxation effect, heart rate would decrease globally, which does not appear to be the case with slow abdominal breathing alone.

General effects.   With the exception of abdominal breathing, there is no consistent evidence that the various approaches to relaxation training have different effects. All of the approaches seem to lower autonomic tone (for example, heart rate and skin conductance) and levels of urinary catecholamines (Lehrer & Woolfolk, 1993). A few studies suggest that Transcendental Meditation produces more of a cognitive relaxation (for example, greater EEG alpha rhythm) accompanied by somatic arousal (such as increased heart rate) but the majority of studies find lower somatic arousal with meditation (Lehrer & Woolfolk, 1993). Possibly, the same protocol may produce different effects in different subjects. Given the discrepant findings among studies, it seems safest clinically to use psychophysiological (biofeedback) monitoring to verify a physiological relaxation response in the patient. This would be particularly true for migraines, in which a decrease in autonomic tone is presumably a core ingredient in treatment efficacy.

Just as one should not assume that adherence to a given protocol is producing physiological relaxation, so too should one avoid treating self-report estimates of stress as the equivalent of a physical measure. In fact, self-report and physiological indicators of stress may be relatively independent dimensions. For example, Cohen and associates have published findings on the degree to which cardiovascular (heart rate, systolic blood pressure, diastolic blood pressure), immunological (number of CD8 cells, number of CD56 cells, natural killer cell activity) and endocrinological (plasma norepinephrine, salivary cortisol) measures of stress reactivity intercorrelate. With the exception of those involving cortisol, all of the entries in the correlation matrix were statistically significant, and at least 0.34. Self-rated anxiety, however, which had shown a level of test-retest reliability equivalent to that of the other measures, correlated with *none* of the physiological variables. Now there are a number of possible explanations, some specific to the study's particular methodology. Moreover, a different self-report scale, assessing degree of interest and energy for the task, did correlate with the physiological measures (S. Cohen, Hamrick, Rodriguez, Feldman, Rabin, & Manuck, 2000). Still, the results clearly caution against the use of self-report as a substitute for psychophysiological recording. On the other hand, as indicated elsewhere in the discussions of cognitive variables in tension-type headaches and in chronic pain syndrome, self-report variables are certainly valuable in their own right.

BIOFEEDBACK

Surface EMG biofeedback. The mechanism by which EMG biofeedback brings improvement in tension-type headaches is not fully known. In general, the degree of reduction in muscle tension with EMG biofeedback does not appear to correlate with the degree of improvement in symptoms (Rokicki et al., 1997), although some authors have found evidence to the contrary (C. Philips, 1977b; Schoenen, 1991). Schoenen et al. (1991) found that the primary effect of EMG biofeedback was an increase in pressure pain thresholds at a number of sites, including the Achilles' tendon, which implies a central process. There are at least three theories of what this process is. Flor, et al. note that, compared with control subjects, patients with tension-type headache were less able to discriminate levels of muscle tension. At low muscle tension levels, perceived tension and aversiveness were higher among the patients (Flor, Fuerst, & Birbaumer, 1999). We may speculate, then, that EMG biofeedback helps patients to better discriminate level of muscle tension, and perhaps to distinguish it from pain. Thus, patients with TMD or chronic back pain show a degree of clinical improvement when taught to better discriminate EMG levels (Flor & Birbaumer, 1991).

A second theory is that frontalis EMG reflects general sympathetic arousal, so that reducing the EMG signal is a way of learning physiological relaxation. Thus, McGrady and coworkers found that behavioral treatment, emphasizing autogenics relaxation and frontalis EMG biofeedback, was successful for some patients as a treatment for essential hypertension. The patients most likely to show a significant improvement in blood pressure were those whose baseline stress was high, as reflected in particular by low finger temperature and high heart rate and frontalis EMG (Weaver & McGrady, 1995). Moreover, there was a trend ($p = .08$) for higher post-treatment frontalis EMG to predict relapse in blood pressure at one year follow-up (McGrady, Nadsady, & Schumann-Brzezinski, 1991). The meta-analytic finding of Gauthier et al., that relaxation training adds relatively little to the efficacy of EMG biofeedback (Gauthier, Ivers, & Carrier, 1996) similarly suggests that the two techniques may have considerable overlap.

A third possibility, with quite a bit of evidence, is that EMG biofeedback works by increasing the patient's sense of self-efficacy. In support of this are deductions from placebo-controlled studies.

Two general types of biofeedback control conditions have been used: noncontingent feedback, in which the signal displayed to the patient is unrelated to actual muscle tension, and feedback with altered contingency, in which the signal has a different biological source than what the subject has been told. The key example is a study by Andrasik and Holroyd. All subjects were told that by controlling the feedback signal they were learning to lower frontalis EMG readings. For some subjects, however, the signal had been inverted: They were actually learning to increase frontalis muscle tension. For other subjects, meanwhile, the display was reading from their wrist extensors; tension at the forehead was not being changed at all (Andrasik & K. A. Holroyd, 1980).

Now, from its inception in the treatment of tension-type headaches, veridical surface EMG has tended to outperform random, noncontingent "feedback" (e.g., Budzynski, Stoyva, C. S. Adler, & Mullaney, 1973; Kondo & A. Canter, 1977). Actual muscle tension feedback, however, even when it is inverted or from an irrelevant site, tends to produce lasting reductions in headache activity, of the same extent as veridical feedback. For example, in Andrasik and Holroyd's study, participants changed muscle tension in the direction of training (decrease, increase, or no change). However, subjects in all three groups achieved similar improvement in their headaches (Andrasik & K. A. Holroyd, 1980). Moreover, at 3-year follow-up patients in all three groups still had a greater than 50 percent reduction in total headache activity (Andrasik & K. A. Holroyd, 1983). There was no advantage for the group that had actually lowered frontalis muscle tension. In contrast, a group that simply recorded headache activity showed a 7 percent increase in headaches over the three years, suggesting that there was no spontaneous remission (Andrasik & K. A. Holroyd, 1983).

Now, why would an irrelevant or even inverse contingency have therapeutic efficacy when random feedback does not? Holroyd et al. suggest that the key is the subject's perception of control (K. A. Holroyd, Penzien, Hursey, Tobin, L. Rogers, Holm, & Marcille, 1984). Random feedback, no matter how favorable, might "feel" random. In effect, the subject would be thinking "I seem to have done well, but I can't figure out what I did and I doubt I'd be able to do it again." When the contingency is merely altered, subjects feel internally that they have achieved physiological control. Holroyd, et al. propose that the resulting increase in self-efficacy leads to better problem-solving, and hence resistance to stress (K. A. Holroyd, Penzien, Hursey, Tobin, L. Rogers, Holm, & Marcille, 1984). The sense of control changes how subjects think about headaches and stressors, and how they respond to them.

To test this more directly, Holroyd et al. manipulated frontalis muscle tension (veridical vs. inverse feedback) and perception of success (high- vs. low-success feedback) independently. In this study, improvements in headache activity were generated by the high success feedback, but not by actual reductions in muscle tension. Moreover, while improvement was uncorrelated with changes in muscle tension, it was indeed correlated with increases in self-efficacy ($r = .49$, $p < .01$) and internal locus of control ($r = .43$, $p < .01$; K. A. Holroyd, Penzien, Hursey, Tobin, L. Rogers, Holm, & Marcille, 1984). Similar results come from a fine-grained analysis by Rokicki, et al. Rokicki's group found that in tension-type headache, changes in self-efficacy correlate with future rather than with current improvement in pain (Rokicki, K. A. Holroyd, C. R. France, Lipchik, J. L. France, & Kvaal, 1997). It appears that the perception of success precedes the success itself.

Thus, we see that surface EMG biofeedback is quite effective as a treatment for tension-type headache, but that its effects may be mediated by cognitive rather than psychophysiological changes. There are three catches, however. First, the subjects in the studies by Andrasik, Holroyd and coworkers were having at least three headache days per week prior to treatment. Thus, most would probably now be diagnosed with chronic tension-type headache, a form of chronic daily headache, for which central pain sensitization may be particularly important.

Second, nearly every study ever conducted of surface EMG biofeedback has used a frontalis electrode placement (Arena & Blanchard, 1996), yet we have seen that muscle pain is thought more likely to be referred to the frontalis than generated there. Thus, surface EMG biofeedback from other sites, such as the sternocleidomastoids or upper trapezius, might have greater efficacy and show a more direct role for muscle relaxation.

To date, two studies have compared EMG placement sites. Hart and Cichanski (1981) did not find a greater reduction in tension headache activity with placement at the posterior cervical muscles than with placement at the frontalis. However, use of analgesics declined more in the group receiving biofeedback from the neck muscles. Moreover, the "neck" group had a better numerical reduction in headache activity (57 percent vs. 45 percent) and at 10 subjects per condition the study may simply have been under-powered.

In a second study, Arena and coworkers compared EMG biofeedback from the upper trapezius to frontalis biofeedback and progressive muscle relaxation. The participants had tension-type headaches that usually began at the occipital, suboccipital, or posterior cervical (back of the neck) region. The percentage of subjects showing a prospectively measured, clinically significant (>50 percent) reduction in headache activity was higher with the trapezius placement (100 percent) than with frontalis placement (50 percent) or progressive muscle relaxation (37.5 percent). The difference was statistically significant with chi-square testing (Arena, Bruno, Hannah, & Meador, 1995). Averaging across subjects, the degree of improvement in headache diary scores was highest in the trapezius group (74 percent improvement), lowest in the relaxation group (34 percent) and intermediate for the frontalis biofeedback (44 percent). The difference between the trapezius and relaxation groups was statistically significant.

Although these results are intriguing, they do not necessarily rescue the psychophysiological hypothesis. Degree of improvement in headaches did not correlate in any obvious way with the amount of reduction in the EMG. Moreover, the authors note anecdotally that participants seemed to find the trapezius placement more credible than the frontalis. Still, it seems appropriate that research on EMG biofeedback be expanded to include at least the upper trapezius and sternocleidomastoid areas.

Indeed, there may be advantages to including multiple sites in the same study. Schoenen (1991) found that reductions in EMG and headache were correlated in his treatment study. However, he measured EMG at three sites (frontalis, temporalis and trapezius) during three conditions (supine, standing, and while doing mental arithmetic). The correlation was between degree of headache improvement and the amount of EMG change at whichever combination of site and condition showed the greatest reduction for that patient. This would make sense if different muscles and conditions were pain generators for different patients. Even so, the correlation between EMG reduction and outcome was modest (Spearman's $\rho = .53$, $p < .005$).

The third catch is that, even within a chronic tension-type headache group, there may be a subset of subjects for whom muscle tension is important. Thus, Rokicki et al. found that women whose pain improved with biofeedback could be distinguished from a group that did not improve, based on the EMG signal. However, it was not mean EMG amplitude that was predictive, but the coefficient of variation (the standard deviation as a percent of the mean). The coefficient of variation in the EMG signal was higher at all sessions in the treatment successes (Rokicki, T. Houle, Dhingra, Weinland, Urban, & Bhalla, 2003). The reason for the association is unclear. Perhaps a higher coefficient of variation implies that muscle fatigue is playing a role in the pain (Enoka, Rankin, Joyner, & Stuart, 1988; Ng, Parnianpour, C. Richardson, & Kippers, 2003). Perhaps a lower coefficient of variation indicates a different type of muscle tension, driven more by the steady, intrinsic firing of spinal motor neurons in the relative absence of control from higher brain centers (Gorassini, Knash, P. J. Harvey, D. J. Bennett, & J. Yang, 2004; Mattei, Schmied, Mazzocchio, Decchi, A. Rossi, & Vedel, 2003). Perhaps high-variability feedback is simply easier for subjects to use, or gives a heightened sense of control over muscle tension (higher self-efficacy; Rokicki et al.) Still, Rokicki et al.'s results need replicating and the explanations are speculative. The area waits promisingly for further research.

Thermal biofeedback: Mechanisms of efficacy.   Much of the literature on thermal biofeedback has focused on two questions: Does thermal biofeedback have specific efficacy, beyond that of relaxation training and, if so, is the hand warming itself the active ingredient?

We have seen that in the meta-analyses and larger outcome studies, there seems to be a consistent, but statistically nonsignificant, tendency for thermal biofeedback plus relaxation to show a greater percent improvement than relaxation training by itself. To truly answer the question, however, we need more direct comparisons. If the numerical advantage turns out to be real (and it is not clear that it does), then the question arises of whether thermal biofeedback has a specific efficacy, or is simply a way of improving relaxation skills.

Thus, it would be particularly useful theoretically to have data about whether thermal biofeedback by itself, in the absence of a general relaxation response, can bring about improvement in migraines. Blanchard and Andrasik (1982) report that thermal biofeedback in isolation may not be effective for migraines, despite its possible usefulness as a single modality in Raynaud's (Freedman, 1987). In a meta-analysis, Gauthier, Ivers and Carrier (1996) note that relaxation training seems to improve success with thermal biofeedback. On the other hand, Ellertsen, et al. report an approximately 65 percent reduction in headache frequency following thermal biofeedback as a single modality (Ellertsen, Nordby, Hammerborg, & Thorlacius, 1987). The improvements were maintained at two-year follow-up. The investigators had been careful not to encourage relaxation or even to mention the word during the biofeedback training. They found that migraineurs showed a significant decrease, relative to control subjects, in the pulse wave amplitude (PWA) at the superficial temporal artery, probably indicating vasoconstriction, c. 10 seconds after a tone was sounded. This response normalized in those subjects whose headaches improved with biofeedback (Ellertsen, Nordby, Hammerborg, & Thorlacius, 1987). Weaknesses in the study are, first, that there was no control group and hence in theory (although unlikely in practice) the clinical improvements could have been due to the passage of time. Second, general arousal was not reported, and thus we do not know whether successful clients intuited the relaxation response as a way of producing the hand warming.

Arguing against a specific efficacy is the fact that no treatment study to date has shown thermal biofeedback to be superior to relaxation training. (Sargent, Solbach, Coyne, Spohn, & Sergerson, 1986, report a statistical near-miss.) However, sample sizes have generally been small and hence the comparative studies may simply have lacked the statistical power needed to detect a difference. Arguing in favor of specificity are the facts that: (1) Thermal biofeedback for Raynaud's does not appear to involve a relaxation effect. (2) The above-noted *possibility* that relaxation training and thermal biofeedback may have greater combined effects than either treatment separately (K. A. Holroyd, Lipchik, & Penzien, 1998). And (3) thermal biofeedback may benefit some patients who do not show benefit from relaxation training (Blanchard, Andrasik, Neff, Teders, Pallmeyer, Arena, Jurish, Saunders, Ahles, & Rodichok, 1982).

If thermal biofeedback indeed has a specific efficacy, we must then clarify the nature of this efficacy. Three hypotheses are current: a specific psychophysiological hypothesis, in which learned control of vasoreactivity is central, a general psychophysiological hypothesis, in which an overall relaxation effect is the active ingredient, and a cognitive hypothesis, in which the key element is an increase in self-efficacy.

Lisspers, Öst, and Skagerberg (1992) examined a large number of demographic, psychometric and pretreatment psychophysiological variables, in looking for predictors of success at 6-month follow-up. The patients had either received thermal biofeedback ($N = 29$) or pulse volume biofeedback of the superficial temporal artery ($N = 28$). Of the 17 predictors, the only one to emerge as significant was whether or not the patient had learned, at least minimally, to produce the criterion response. Patients who acquired the response had, on average, a 68 percent reduction in total headache activity (intensity X duration X frequency, measured prospectively) vs. a 35 percent reduction for those who had not acquired the response. Treatment credibility was not a significant predictor. This seems to favor the psychophysiological hypothesis. Note, however, that by the very nature of biofeedback, patients knew whether they had been successful. Thus, self-efficacy is also a viable explanation for Lisspers, et al.'s results.

A similar study was conducted by Morrill and Blanchard (1989), looking at whether degree of finger temperature increase could distinguish those migraineurs who achieved at least a 50 percent reduction in headaches with thermal biofeedback and relaxation, from those migraineurs who were comparatively unimproved. Overall, finger temperature did not distinguish the two groups, but heart rate did. That is, migraineurs whose headaches were improved by at least 50 percent showed a statistically significant reduction in heart rate with treatment, while migraineurs who were not clinically improved showed, on average, an increase in heart rate over treatment.[2] Of course this suggests that a general relaxation effect is the mechanism of action of thermal biofeedback plus relaxation training. It also raises the question of whether heart rate monitoring should be included in treatment, as a biofeedback modality, or simply as a check for the clinician that the relaxation and biofeedback are progressing properly.

The evidence about whether cognitive changes mediate the effects of thermal biofeedback in migraine is mixed. French, et al. used false temperature feedback to create perceptions of either high or low success in regulating peripheral blood flow (French, Gauthier, Roberge, Bouchard, & Nouwen, 1997). Subjects in the high success condition reported considerably greater self-efficacy, as expected, but they did not show a reduction in headache symptoms or in medication use. Blanchard and coworkers followed veridical thermal biofeedback training with either high-success or low-success feedback. Both groups showed improvement in their headaches, with somewhat greater effects for the subjects given high-success feedback (Blanchard, M. Kim, Hermann, Steffek, et al., 1994). Allen and Shriver (1997) report data from a small sample of children suggesting that self-efficacy may be a particularly strong mediator of success for pediatric headaches.

Another approach to determining whether physiological or cognitive factors are primary is to conduct blinded, placebo-controlled trials of thermal biofeedback. In essence, the biofeedback signal is inverted for some subjects, who then believe they are warming their hand when they are actually cooling it down. A small study of this type was conducted by Largen et al. (Largen, R. J. Mathew, Dobbins, & Claghorn, 1981). Subjects in both the hand warming and the hand cooling groups showed a significant decrease in headache duration. This suggests a common mechanism and, as all subjects had been taught progressive relaxation, autogenics, and frontalis EMG biofeedback, we might suspect a general relaxation response. Alternatively, cognitive distraction during a migraine, or perhaps an expectation of success might be the key variables. Of note, however, only the hand warming group showed a decrease in headache frequency on prospective monitoring. Indeed, while 83 percent of subjects in the hand warming group showed a decrease in headache frequency, 80 percent in the hand cooling group had an *increase* in headache frequency (Largen, R. J. Mathew, Dobbins, & Claghorn, 1981).

A second example is a study by Kewman and Roberts which, additionally, was double-blind: Neither the study participants, nor the research assistants who interacted with them, were told the study hypothesis, or that the signal was sometimes inverted (Kewman & Roberts, 1980). Moreover, no relaxation training was taught; all of the skills acquisition focused on the biofeedback itself. Now, the hand warming and the hand cooling groups achieved similar reductions in migraine frequency (13 percent and 21 percent decreases, respectively). A caveat, however, is that the hand cooling group did not really succeed at their task. Only 3 of the 12 subjects were consistently able to lower finger temperature. Another 3 subjects consistently raised it, while the

---

[2]The increase in heart rate does not necessarily imply that unimproved migraineurs became more anxious. Hand warming might decrease total peripheral resistance and hence lower blood pressure, which in turn would tend to produce a compensatory increase in heart rate.

remaining 6 performed inconsistently. In the hand warming group, 8 of 11 subjects were consistent hand warmers, 2 more achieved the opposite response consistently, and the eleventh subject was inconsistent (Kewman & Roberts, 1980). Of note, the greater success of the handwarming group on the biofeedback display did not seem to translate into greater treatment efficacy.

A different picture emerges from the Kewman and Roberts study if we reclassify subjects according to which response they learned, rather than which response they were supposed to learn. The consistent hand warmers had a 39 percent reduction in number of migraines, measured prospectively, pre- vs. post-treatment. The inconsistent learners, who on average increased finger temperature slightly, had a similar, 32 percent, reduction in migraine frequency. Subjects in a control condition, who merely self-monitored their headaches, had a 16 percent reduction in frequency. In contrast, those subjects whose hands grew consistently colder had a 57 percent *increase* in migraine frequency (Kewman & Roberts, 1980). This is reminiscent of Largen et al.'s results, above. Of course, in reclassifying subjects we run the risk of confounding psychophysiological change with perceived efficacy on the biofeedback task. But recall that the original hand warming group had performed much better at their task than the hand cooling group, and yet had about the same improvement in migraines. A second concern is that only the contrast between hand cooling and the other three groups was statistically significant (Kewman & Roberts, 1980). Thus, we have better evidence that hand cooling is detrimental than that hand warming is helpful. However, we must suspect the study's small sample size (34 subjects spread over 3 groups) for the paucity of statistical findings.

An alternative approach to blinded studies is to present hand cooling to research participants as a credible treatment in its own right. Thus, in a study by Blanchard and others, hand warming was compared to three highly credible placebo biofeedback conditions: hand cooling, hand temperature stabilization, and EEG biofeedback to suppress alpha waves. (Note that alpha wave suppression would not be expected to involve a relaxation response.) The authors report that post-treatment, all four groups showed significant and equivalent reductions in migraines/mixed headaches and in medication use, with no specific efficacy for the hand warming condition (Blanchard, Peters, et al., 1997).

This is an exceptionally well controlled and well documented study. Nonetheless, its interpretation must be qualified by two limitations in particular. First, the comparison among treatment conditions is restricted to pre- versus post-treatment; there is no subsequent follow-up. Blanchard et al. explain that for ethical reasons, subjects in all conditions (who had, after all, presented for the research in order to receive treatment) were offered veridical hand warming biofeedback and autogenics training after the study. The other, and more serious concern, is that only 21 percent of subjects in the hand-warming (active treatment) condition achieved a 50 percent or greater reduction in headache activity. Blanchard et al. note that in their own lab, approximately 50 percent usually achieve this level. Indeed, focusing on just the migraineurs (v. mixed headache), we see improvements in the headache diary index of 19 percent (hand warming condition), 19 percent (hand cooling), 17 percent (temperature stabilization), and 23 percent (alpha suppression). Now, the improvements associated with psychological placebos in meta-analyses are 14 percent (K. A. Holroyd & Penzien, 1990), 28 percent (Blanchard & Andrasik, 1982), and 15 percent (McCrory, Penzien, Rains, & Hasselblad, 1996). If we average these three figures from the meta-analyses we get 19 percent, which is just the level of improvement seen in the Blanchard, et al. study. Thus, the study is noteworthy not for a high efficacy in the placebo conditions but for the unexplained and unusually low efficacy of the active treatment.

Similar designs have been used by others. Marcus, Scharff, and Turk, for example, compared a control condition (hand cooling biofeedback and education about triggers) with an active treatment (hand warming biofeedback, education about triggers, progressive muscle relaxation, and a program of neck exercises) in a group of 25 women who had migraines during pregnancy (Marcus, Scharff, & D. C. Turk, 1995). Subjects rated the two forms of treatment as equally credible, with one exception: At post-treatment the control subjects did not feel that the intervention had been terribly successful. And indeed it had not; the control group experienced a 33 percent reduction in headache activity, versus a 73 percent reduction for the active treatment group. Moreover, subjects who received the active treatment showed little of the expected resurgence in migraine activity during the year after giving birth (Marcus, Scharff, & D. C. Turk, 1995). The caveat, of course, is that we do not know how much of the treatment success was due to hand warming specifically, versus, say, the relaxation or the neck exercises.

A similar study by Scharff et al. was conducted with 36 children, ages 7 to 17, with migraine (Scharff, Marcus, & Masek, 2002). The active treatment involved hand warming biofeedback, progressive muscle relaxation, imagery, and training in cognitive-behavioral stress management techniques. The control condition was comprised of hand cooling biofeedback and general discussion about the child's life and headaches over the preceding week. The children rated the two approaches as equally credible and equally beneficial, at the start of treatment and again at the end. The two approaches, however, were not equally beneficial. At post-treatment, 10 percent of the subjects in the hand cooling group, 54 percent in the active treatment group, and 0 percent in a waiting list control condition, achieved at least a 50 percent reduction in headache activity (χ^2 [2] = 12.65, $p < .002$). Again, we do not know whether thermal biofeedback by itself contributed to the outcome (Scharff, Marcus, & Masek, 2002).

Overall, then, the literature seems to suggest that cognitive factors add to, but do not fully account for, the efficacy of thermal biofeedback. The question of whether thermal biofeedback is simply a particularly effective way of teaching relaxation, versus having a more specific mechanism of action, is unresolved.

Thermal biofeedback: Home practice.   The usefulness of home practice in thermal biofeedback has also been debated. The initial foray into this area was by Blanchard's group, in which migraineurs were either issued small thermometers and instructed to practice daily, or were gently discouraged from trying to rehearse outside of the sessions. In this study, there were small numerical effects of home practice on reducing medication intake and headache activity, but despite an adequate sample size (59 in total) the results do not even begin to approach statistical significance. Indeed, Blanchard et al. note that the effect size, $d = .01$, is clinically trivial (Blanchard, Nicholson, Radnitz, Steffek, Appelbaum, & Dentinger, 1991).

The topic was revisited three years later by a team headed by Gauthier. Gauthier's group noted two weaknesses in Blanchard et al.'s study. First, because home pratice was never explicitly prohibited, 30 percent of the control group had admitted afterwards to engaging in some amount of intentional relaxation practice over the course of the study. Second, a significant minority of the subjects in both arms of the study had mixed tension-migraine headaches. Because the mixed disorder (what would now be called chronic daily headache) did not respond well to the thermal biofeedback, treatment efficacy in the home practice group (and of course the control group as well) may have been suppressed. Gauthier and coworkers addressed these concerns by including only migraineurs, by enjoining the control group against home practice, and by instructing the experimental group to rehearse daily and at the first sign of a migraine. Gauthier, et al.'s results were very different from those of Blanchard's clinic: Despite a smaller sample size, only the home practice group showed significant improvements. In fact, the control group showed a nonsignificant worsening of headache activity (Gauthier, Côté, & D. French, 1994).

Now, Gauthier et al.'s study is not entirely beyond methodological dispute. At mid-treatment (although not pre- or post-treatment, when headaches were assessed) the prohibition against home practice seems to have made the control treatment less credible. Gauthier et al., however, suggest that a key difference was their experimental group's application of biofeedback skills at a time of stress, the threatened onset of a migraine. In Chapter 17, we will see additional evidence that the effects of home practice may vary a great deal depending on when it is applied.[3]

Blood volume pulse (BVP) biofeedback has not been included in meta-analyses, most likely because relatively few studies have been conducted on it to date.

Kropp et al. report the results of a cross-over study: Half of their 38 subjects received BVP biofeedback followed by cognitive-behavioral therapy, while the other 19 received the same treatments in the reverse order (Kropp, Gerber, Keinath-Specht, Kopal, & Niederberger, 1997). Migraines were assessed prospectively pretreatment, post-treatment, and at 2-year follow-up. In this study, the group receiving biofeedback first appeared to have better outcomes, perhaps because the illustration of mind-body effects made the subsequent psychotherapy more persuasive. The biofeedback-first group attained better BVP control, achieving an approximately 19 percent reduction in the pulse volume. Moreover, the degree of pulse volume reduction correlated almost perfectly ($r = .91$) with the degree of clinical improvement. This last result would be expected if the psychophysiological rationale for BVP biofeedback is in fact the mechanism of action. However, it is also possible that greater physiological control elicited greater self-efficacy (Kropp et al., 1997) in this highly face-valid, non-blinded treatment. On the other hand, recall that Ellertsen and colleagues found that efficacy of *thermal* biofeedback could be predicted from a normalization of pulse wave amplitude at the superficial temporal artery (Ellertsen, Nordby, Hammerborg, & Thorlacius, 1987). Because pulse wave amplitude was simply an incidental part of data collection, and not an object of feedback, Ellertsen et al.'s results suggest that it is indeed intrinsically relevant to migraines.

EEG biofeedback for migraines is still in its infancy. Gannon and Sternbach (1971) describe a case study in which a patient with migraines was trained to increase the proportion of alpha waves at an occipital recording site. At three month follow-up the patient reported no change in pain during an episode, but was sometimes able to prevent a migraine. Andreychuk and Schriver (1975) reported that alpha biofeedback, self-hypnosis, and autogenics plus thermal biofeedback were all equally effective in a group study of migraine treatments. More recently, Siniatchkin et al. taught children with migraines to reduce the mean amplitude of contingent negative variation (CNV). Recall that the CNV is an event-related potential that follows the warning signal in a reaction time test. The CNV may correspond to the mobilization of attentional resources. Compared with a waiting list control and with their own baseline values, the children had a reduction in migraine frequency and total migraine activity, but the clinical improvement did not correlate with the improvements in the CNV (Siniatchkin, Hierundar, Kropp, Kuhnert, Gerber, & Stephani, 2000). The results seem worthy of further research follow-up, but are too preliminary to serve as a basis for clinical treatment.

Instructions in biofeedback.   It is widely accepted that patients should have some sort of introduction to the biofeedback equipment and process at the start of training, but there are few studies to guide us in optimizing these instructions. LaCroix and coworkers contrast two theories of biofeedback process. In the first, termed the "feedback" model, patients use the equip-

---

[3]We should add that the results from Blanchard's and Gauthier's clinics have one definite point of correspondence: In neither study did home practice improve the acquisition of hand warming skills.

ment to enhance their sensory discrimination of tense vs. relaxed states. Once their proprioceptive abilities are thus strengthened, patients can then go about bringing their physiology under voluntary control, as a new, learned ability. In the second theory, termed "feedforward," patients do not learn new abilities so much as fine-tune existing strategies. For example, patients may adjust their frontalis muscle tension using the abilities they have now to control their muscles. The biofeedback signal does not lead to improved proprioceptive perception, but simply improved motor performance, as patients use the signal to increase the target behavior (Dunn, Ponsor, Weil, & Utz, 1986; LaCroix & Gowen, 1981).

Now, Dunn et al. and Utz (1994) present evidence that the feedforward model is correct, at least in the early stages of biofeedback training, and that instructions to use more of a feedback strategy do not alter this. Hence, Utz recommends feedforward type instructions at the first stages of treatment, with instructions for more proprioceptive learning later on. She gives as an example of feedforward instructions:

> In order to learn this biofeedback task of decreasing your forehead muscle tension, you can simply use the abilities that you already possess. Studies have shown that most people actually know how to decrease forehead muscle tension, but may have never paid attention enough to use this skill. You may use any technique that you possess in order to lower your forehead muscle tension. You will receive feedback through a sound in the earphones. A decrease in the pitch and frequency of the sound indicates a lowering of muscle tension" (Utz, 1994, p. 297).

Of course instructions are not the only factor relevant to learning autonomic control. Guglielmi and Roberts provide evidence that people whose finger temperature is more labile will acquire thermal biofeedback skills to a much higher level (Guglielmi & A. H. Roberts, 1994). As migraineurs often show vasomotor instability, Guglielmi and Roberts' results seem to bode well for treatment.

COGNITIVE PROBLEM SOLVING THERAPY

Cognitive problem solving therapy appears to be quite effective for tension-type headaches, and its combination with relaxation training may be more effective than relaxation training by itself. Indeed, we have seen that the benefits of EMG biofeedback and autogenics in tension-type headache may be mediated by cognitive changes. However, there is so far no indication that cognitive therapy contributes to the treatment response in migraines (Blanchard, 1998; Blanchard, Appelbaum, Radnitz, Michultka, Morrill, Kirsch, et al., 1990).

ORAL HABIT CHANGE

Oral habit change has received some empirical scrutiny from its developers (Gramling, Neblett, Grayson, & Townsend, 1996). They found that, compared to a no-treatment control group, habit-reversal patients showed a trend towards lower average pain diary scores post-treatment ($p = .08$), and had significantly lower scores at 4-month follow-up. As it turns out, the treatment group did not show a greater decrease in parafunctional behaviors, raising questions about whether the pain reduction was due to nonspecific effects, habit change, or other components of the treatment such as progressive muscle relaxation. However, the authors note that the treatment group may have been more aware of their behaviors due to the self-monitoring component, and that as a result, greater reporting of the behaviors might have masked a true decline in their frequency.

Unfortunately, the study has several limitations, including a high dropout rate. Of 24 subjects who completed the assessment phase, 17 elected to continue into treatment, and 9 attended at least 5 of 7 treatment sessions. Thus, only 37.5 percent of the eligible sample completed the treatment (allowing a somewhat lenient definition of "completed"). The authors attribute the dropout to subjects' difficulties working the group sessions into their schedules, and suggest that individual sessions would largely eliminate this problem. Other limitations include the small sample size and the fact that the control group was self-selected due to the scheduling conflicts rather than randomly assigned. Thus, the initial data is supportive of the habit reversal protocol, but a great deal more research is needed.

CHRONIC PAIN TREATMENT

Conditioning techniques. Note that the graded activity increase in operant therapy may or may not result in an exposure treatment of pain-related fear. The reason for the uncertainty is that, in the operant model, no attempt is made to select activities that are feared, much less to obtain a hierarchy of such activities. Vlaeyen and associates provide evidence that graded exposure is effective (and that a graded increase in *non*-feared activities in *not* effective) in reducing catastrophization, perceived disability, and pain-related fear (Vlaeyen, de Jong, Geilen, Heuts, & van Breukelen, 2001). Of course in practice, achieving the treatment goals of an operant intervention, for example, progressing through physical therapy and on to re-employment, will often implicitly contain an informal exposure therapy component. However, the active ingredient in the improved functioning is likely to be the exposure and not the positive reinforcement.

Cognitive pain coping skills training. Therapy to teach pain coping skills, such as pleasant imagery or distraction, has been subjected to a few very well constructed studies, but most of these have been of chronic low back pain. Thus, there is a leap of faith in assuming the results apply to other conditions, such as chronic daily headache or chronic facial pain. At least in theory, however, pain management principles should have general applicability, and hence we will briefly review the literature.

In fact, at least one study is directly applicable: Turner and colleagues examined the degree to which treatment outcome for temporomandibular disorder could be predicted from changes in beliefs and coping strategies (J. A. Turner, Whitney, S. F. Dworkin, Massoth, & L. Wilson, 1995). Specifically, they examined the change from initial assessment to three months after treatment in self-reported passive coping, active coping, sense of control over the pain, and conviction that one suffers from a physical disease. It turned out that all of these, except for passive coping, indeed predicted outcome at three month follow-up. Note, however, that this is prediction in a statistical sense: Because the outcome and the change in beliefs were measured concurrently, we do not know whether the change in belief produced the outcome, or merely reflects the patients' improved condition. A more incisive question is whether the change in beliefs at 3 month follow-up can predict whether additional improvement will occur by 12 month follow-up. And when we turn to this prospective question, the results are much more circumscribed. Specifically, greater use of passive coping at 3 months predicted greater interference from pain in daily activities, but the odds ratio was only 1.10. Patients who felt that they could control their pain at 3 months reported less pain interference at 12 months, with an odds ratio of 0.70. On the other hand, usual pain level, perceived disability, depression, and amount of unassisted jaw opening could not be predicted from a change in beliefs. Thus, we can infer a little bit of support for the idea that changes in beliefs and coping skills are the mechanism by which treatment works, but the results are not strong.

At this point, we might argue on theoretical grounds that beliefs and coping strategies *should* mediate improvement in symptoms, but there are theories to the contrary as well. Notice that in the research by Vlaeyen et al. mentioned above (Vlaeyen, de Jong, Geilen, Heuts, & van Breukelen, 2001), graded exposure (a behavioral therapy) reduced catastrophization (a cognitive variable). The implications of this have been studied explicitly: Kole-Snijders and coworkers randomly assigned 148 patients with low back pain to behavioral (operant) treatment or a waiting list control condition (Kole-Snijders et al., 1999). The operant program was quite structured, inpatient, and included treatment contracts, activity-to-quota, time-contingent rest, and training of the spouses to differentially reinforce behaviors that did not involve expression of pain. Not surprisingly, the treated patients fared better than those on the waiting list. Of greater importance is the fact that half of the treated patients ($N = 59$) received explicit training in pain coping skills along with the operant treatment, while the other half ($N = 58$) participated in a (placebo) discussion group about pain. The coping and discussion groups were equally credible. The question, of course, is whether the training in pain coping skills improved the outcome.

The short answer is "no." That is, people who received the coping skills training had a small advantage in perceived coping immediately after treatment, but this was no longer evident at the 6 and 12 month follow-ups. Now, this result can be debated. For example, in the coping skills group, the amount of home practice during treatment correlated with the amount of improvement at 12 month follow-up ($r = .35; p < .05$). Hence, perhaps the coping skills would have fared better if there had been more compliance with home practice. Moreover, the discussion group was rather elaborate. Patients read passages about pain at home and presented them to the group, they listened to musical passages and discussed them, and they viewed but did not use surface EMG biofeedback. So convincing was the group that other staff members in the program were apparently unaware that it was designed to be a placebo. Certainly the coping skills training was not being compared to "nothing."

However, the authors point out that there is a sound theoretical reason why coping skills would not add to a well-structured operant program. They suggest that the key cognitive variable, catastrophization, exerts its effects through fear of pain and avoidance of activities that could increase (low back) pain. In operant treatment, patients confront and work through the avoidance and fear, simultaneously decreasing catastrophization and the effects of catastrophization. The behaviors change the cognitions.

There is another perspective, however, that might allow us to rescue the concept of coping skills training. It might be that a given coping skill only works for certain individuals, and only when applied in a particular way. There is a bit of evidence for this assertion from laboratory studies of pain coping.

Recall from Chapter 3 that when volunteers try to solve a maze at the same time their hands are immersed in ice-cold water, brain activation for pain all but disappears from their PET scans. When absorbed in solving the maze, the brain does not register the pain. From this result, it seems natural to conclude that patients will cope with pain better if they purposefully distract themselves from it. It seems, however, that the situation is much more complex.

One factor to take into account is the patient's level of anxiety about their pain. Patients high in anxiety who try to distract themselves indeed find themselves able to decrease pain, but they also become more globally anxious, more worried about injury from the task at hand (they were tested during a physical therapy session), and they experience the pain as more intense in its affective component (H. D. Hadjistavropoulos, T. Hadjistavropoulos, & Quine, 2000). What happened? First, the patients who were high in health anxiety had considerable difficulty ignoring the pain, so the strategy was not easy to implement. Secondly, while suppressing awareness may or may not be an effective strategy for reducing pain, it is certainly not a good strategy for reducing anxiety. Harvey and Bryant (1998) report that attempts to suppress trauma-related thought in Acute Stress Disorder actually increase the thoughts and their intrusiveness. In the study by Hadjistavropoulos, et al., the pain patients with a greater amount of health anxiety seemed to cope better when they purposefully attended to the pain during physical therapy.

For low-anxious participants, the results were the opposite: They were more worried about injury when asked to attend to their pain (H. D. Hadjistavropoulos, T. Hadjistavropoulos, & Quine, 2000).

A second moderating variable may be gender. Keogh et al. asked healthy university student volunteers to either attend to the sensations produced by a cold pressor task, or else to avoid, suppress and block out the sensation and associated thoughts and feelings. The authors report that for male volunteers, the pain's sensory intensity was lower in the attention than in the suppression condition, while the female volunteers showed no differential efficacy for one strategy or the other (Keogh, Hatton, & Ellery, 2000). The applicability of this result to clinical samples is unknown.

It may seem surprising that attending to pain would actually decrease its intensity. In most cases, however, the participants are asked to consider the pain sensation as objectively, concretely, and neutrally as possible (H. D. Hadjistavropoulos, T. Hadjistavropoulos, & Quine, 2000). Thus, they might notice the coldness or tingling quality of the pain. This approach would tend to block anxious cognitive elaboration. Moreover, "coldness" and "tingling" are not exactly pain itself, and by deconstructing the pain into component sensations that are not themselves pain, the participants may have actually been attending to competing sensations.

There is at least one example in which attending to an alternative sensation produces a rather strong decrease in pain. In studies of hypnosis, suggestions of local anesthesia seem to be more effective than suggestions of global relaxation, or of whole body dissociation from the pain (De Pascalis, Magurano, & Bellusci, 1999). Now, suggestions of numbness in an area may not seem very comparable to attending to sensations from an area, even if the sensations are tingling or cold. Imagine, however, that after the suggestion of glove anesthesia—of numbness over the hand and wrist—we ask subjects to detect electric shocks given to the area. De Pascalis et al. found that highly hypnotizable subjects were more likely to miss some of the shocks altogether. This is not surprising because the highly hypnotizable subjects also had higher sensory detection thresholds and higher pain thresholds under glove anesthesia than less hypnotizable subjects. However, for those shocks that they detected, the highly hypnotizable subjects had a faster reaction time than less hypnotizable subjects (De Pascalis, Magurano, & Bellusci, 1999). It seems that the perceived anesthesia was associated with increased attention to the area.

HYPNOSIS AND THE REVERSAL OF CHRONIC PAIN

To my knowledge, hypnosis is the only type of psychological intervention, indeed only type of intervention of any form, that has been purported to permanently undo chronic pain. However, the evidence that it can do so is of the weakest type: a handful of case studies. Thus, Daly and Wulff describe treatment of a middle-aged man beginning 17 months after the onset of posttraumatic headaches. He was taught to achieve very deep relaxation, through verbal instruction and through thermal and muscle tension (cervical paraspinal) biofeedback. Essentially, the patient appeared to be entering a trance state through the relaxation alone. Thereafter, he was guided through a series of seven sessions of imagery while in a trance, in which the headache was pictured as a ball that was then destroyed, with the pieces exiting through his hands. In the early sessions his headache improved but the patient had re-onset of his arm pain. In later sessions, both were gone, and he remained pain-free at 1-year follow-up (Daly & Wulff, 1987).

Against these rather remarkable results we must balance the spontaneous remission rate for posttraumatic headaches, the fact that the patient tapered from his daily use of analgesics (which presumably helped to eliminate any rebound component), and the plethora of uncontrolled variables that are a part of case study research.

A similar technique, with similarly positive results, is described by Crawford and coworkers (H. J. Crawford, Knebel, L. Kaplan, et al., 1998). They taught 15 adults with chronic low back pain to use focused analgesia, learned via hypnosis, to increase their tolerance for immersing their hands in ice water (cold pressor task). The patients practiced this over three sessions, and transferred their skills to tolerance for electric shocks. By the end of the third session, they were spontaneously applying their skills to their back pain as well. (Note the elements of shaping and increased self-efficacy implicit in this intervention.) Crawford et al. report that of the 15 adults in their sample, 3 were without pain at 1-month follow-up. Now, the spontaneous remission rate for low back pain of greater than 6 months duration is quite low. However, the conclusions must be qualified by the short-term nature of the follow-up and, as in the Daly and Wulff study, the idiosyncrasies of case studies.

Still, if repeated hypnotic sessions have the potential to eliminate chronic pain in some people, it would be of tremendous importance. Leaving aside, then, the treacherous world of case studies, what can we say about hypnosis and pain?

Certainly there is evidence that hypnosis has some degree of efficacy for pain control. Meier and coworkers studied hypnotic suggestions of analgesia on pain from electric shocks. Because they had previously used the same experimental arrangement to study the analgesic effects of drugs, they could state that for highly hypnotizable subjects, the hypnosis had the same effect on pain ratings as 100 mg of IV Demerol (Meier, Klucken, Soyka, & Bromm, 1993). These were subjects selected for their responsiveness to hypnosis, however. More broadly, Montgomery et al. conducted a meta-analysis of hypnotic analgesia, using 18 research reports involving 933 subjects. Montgomery et al. found that the average effect size was moderately strong, 0.67. However, the average obscured the effects of hypnotizability. For people high on this dimension, the average effect size was 1.22; for people low in hypnotizability the average effect size was essentially nil. There were no significant differences in efficacy between the studies of healthy volunteers undergoing a laboratory pain task, and patients experiencing clinical pain (G. H. Montgomery, DuHamel, & Redd, 2000).

Mechanisms.   How does hypnosis bring about this effect? E. R. Hilgard has suggested that the analgesia is a result of dissociation: The part of consciousness that is registering the pain is segregated from the rest of conscious awareness (E. R. Hilgard, 1986; Kihlstrom, 1998; cref. Kirsch & Lynn, 1998). The evidence supporting this, however, is by no means definite. For example, E. R. Hilgard pointed out that hypnosis does not prevent autonomic responses to pain, such as electrodermal or cardiovascular changes (Sears, 1932; E. R. Hilgard & J. R. Hilgard, 1983). However, increased autonomic activity may also be a byproduct of antinociceptive activity in the brain stem (Bathien & Hugelin, 1969), in which the pain is, presumably, blocked far below the level of consciousness. E. R. Hilgard also pointed out that during hypnotic analgesia, a dissociated part of consciousness could still report pain, through automatic writing or key pressing. However, social-cognitive theorists of hypnosis have cast doubt on the idea that automatic communication is from a deeper level of awareness. They have demonstrated that a person can report either more pain or less pain through automatic responding than they do through standard communication, depending on what is suggested (Spanos, Gwynn, & Stam, 1983).

In an alternative theory of hypnosis, participants are responding to the social role and expectations associated with being subject to a hypnotic procedure (Kirsch & Lynn, 1995; Spanos,

1991). Of course this more mundane explanation would in no way negate the reality or extent of hypnotic analgesia.

More concretely, what is happening neurophysiologically during hypnotic analgesia? The answer is still sketchy, but some early evidence has been turned up. For example, several investigators have found that hypnosis reduces the late components of the somatosensory event-related potential (e.g., H. J. Crawford, Knebel, L. Kaplan, et al., 1998; Spiegel, Bierre, & Rootenberg, 1989; Zachariae & Bjerring, 1994). However, null results have also been reported (Friederich, Trippe, Özcan, Weiss, Hecht, & Miltner, 2001; Meier, Klucken, Soyka, & Bromm, 1993). Moreover, Friederich, et al. suggest that the apparent reduction in ERP amplitude in some studies was actually due to habituation, as the conditions were not counterbalanced. Meanwhile, Rainville, et al. found that when hypnosis was used to alter the degree of unpleasantness of a painful stimulus, without altering the perceived intensity, activation in the anterior cingulate cortex, measured by PET scan, changed accordingly. There were no corresponding changes in primary somatosensory cortex (S1), presumably because S1 encodes the sensory and not the affective characteristics of pain (Rainville, Duncan, D. Price, Carrier, & Bushnell, 1997).

Now, factors such as distraction, habituation, and changes in arousal also affect neurophysiological measures (Meier, Klucken, Soyka, & Bromm, 1993). Thus, it might be that the mechanism by which hypnosis works is one already familiar to us. That is, hypnosis may simply be one way among many of producing relaxation, distraction, and/or placebo/expectancy effects. Just recently, studies have begun appearing in which hypnotic suggestions for focused analgesia are compared with neutral hypnosis, hypnosis with suggestions for relaxation, hypnosis with suggestions of dissociation from the body part to which the pain stimulus will be applied, and placebo. The placebo condition might involve, for example, an alcohol spray that the subject is told is a topical fast-acting anesthetic. In general, focused analgesia seems to be more effective than dissociation and relaxation, which in turn are more effective than a placebo (H. J. Crawford, Knebel, L. Kaplan, et al., 1998; Zachariae & Bjerring, 1994). Insofar as focused analgesia involves turning attention towards and not away from the site of pain, distraction and relaxation do not seem to gain support as explanations for hypnotic effects. However, in the experiments by Crawford et al. and Zachariae and Bjerring, the subjects but not the hypnotist were blind to the study's hypotheses. Thus, there is room for expectancies on the part of the experimenter to have influenced the results. This may account for the inefficacy of the placebo condition in these studies.

Cortical or subcortical? Returning to the event-related potential and PET studies, note that they are of high-level structures. However, in Chapter 2 we saw that there are inhibitory pathways from the cortex down to the dorsal horn. Not surprisingly, then, there is some evidence that hypnosis can reduce a spinal nociceptive reflex, termed **R-III**,[4] suggesting that some of the analgesia involves descending inhibitory pathways (Kiernan, Dane, Phillips, & D. Price, 1995; Sandrini, Milanov, Malaguti, Nigrelli, Moglia, & Nappi, 2000). However, in the study by Kiernan, et al., R-III showed only 2/3 as much reduction from baseline as pain reports did. In contrast, the reductions in R-III and pain reports are in an approximately one-to-one ratio following morphine analgesia (Willer, 1985). Thus, while hypnosis seems to be working at a spinal level, some portion of the analgesia is presumably supraspinal (Kiernan, Dane, Phillips, & D. Price, 1995).

---

[4]The R-III reflex involves contraction of the biceps fermoris (part of the quadriceps muscle in the thigh) in response to an electric shock delivered to the sural nerve at the ankle. The contraction is a withdrawal response, and the strength of the reflex can be measured as the magnitude of muscle contraction on surface EMG. Of course withdrawing can also be voluntary, or involuntary and due to startle. However, the immediate response, from 85–120 milliseconds after stimulation, is a spinal reflex (Kiernan et al., 1995).

Sandrini et al. provide a second type of data about whether hypnotic analgesia involves sub-cortical pathways. Recall from Chapter 2 that pain from one stimulus (the target) can be attenuated by another painful stimulus applied somewhere else on the body (the "heterotopic nociceptive stimulus"). Thus, immersing one's hand in ice water will decrease the pain ratings and the strength of nociceptive reflexes evoked at the ankle by an electric shock. The neural processes mediating this effect are referred to as Diffuse Noxious Inhibitory Controls. They involve an inhibitory loop at the level of the medulla, and can be distinguished from distraction in careful psychophysical studies. Now, what would happen if we applied the ice water bath and hypnosis at the same time? Presumably, if hypnosis is purely a cortical phenomenon, the two sources of analgesia will have stronger combined effects than either one separately, because different processes are being invoked. On the other hand, if hypnosis primarily works through the same medullary and spinal structures as the Diffuse Noxious Inhibitory Controls then presumably the combined effects would be no greater than either one separately. In fact, when we conduct the experiment, something else altogether happens: The effect of Diffuse Noxious Inhibitory Controls and that of hypnosis cancel out, leaving little or no analgesia (Sandrini, Milanov, Malaguti, Nigrelli, Moglia, & Nappi, 2000). The reasons for this result are unclear, but it does imply that hypnosis is exerting a substantial degree of its effect on medullary and/or spinal levels.

So far, we have been assuming that the mechanism by which hypnotic analgesia takes place is the same for everyone. In fact, there may be substantial differences among subjects. Thus, Danziger et al. studied eighteen highly suggestible subjects and found, not surprisingly, strong hypnotic analgesia in all of them. That is, all eighteen participants reported an increase in pain threshold, and had similar decreases in the late components of the somatosensory evoked potential. However, in eleven of the subjects, hypnotic analgesia was associated with a strong decrease in the R-III reflex, while for the other seven subjects hypnosis strongly *increased* the R-III reflex (Danziger et al., 1998). Clearly, there is more work to be done in developing a neurophysiological understanding of hypnosis.

Or of whether hypnosis is always a unique process. For distraction, too, is likely to have subcortical effects—the R-III reflex, for example, is partially inhibited when a person is involved in a competing task (Bathien, 1971; Willer, Boureau, & Albe-Fessard, 1979). The involvement has be significant, however; mere momentary inattentiveness is not sufficient (Dowman, 2001). Thus, it has not yet been established that the effects of hypnosis necessarily go beyond other examples of absorption in a non-pain activity (Farthing, Venturino, & S. W. Brown, 1984).

Moreover, in some approaches hypnosis is used to elicit imagery of movement, such as involvement in a sport (Gay, Philippot, & Luminet, 2002). In that case, the analgesic effects may arise from activation of motor cortex (Moseley, 2004), and be predicted better by capacity for visualization than by hypnotic susceptibility (Gay et al.). Motor imagery may reduce pain through a different physiological mechanism than suggestions of analgesia.

Nonetheless, the results of Danziger et al. may be of great practical significance. In Chapter 2 we saw evidence that a portion of central sensitization takes place at the dorsal horn. Patients whose nociceptive reflexes are enhanced under hypnosis could perhaps be acquiring sensitization at the spinal level, even though they are not consciously experiencing pain. Conversely, patients with reduced nociceptive reflexes might, possibly, be "unlearning" central sensitization. If so, then sustained use of hypnotic analgesia might have beneficial or harmful long-term consequences depending on how, neurophysiologically, the analgesia was produced.

Alternatively, increased self-efficacy and decreased catastrophization from effective pain self-management might render all approaches beneficial in the long run. In truth, we know relatively little about the long-term effects of any of the specific behavioral or naturalistic strategies for coping with pain. This would be an exceptionally useful area for further research. We saw evidence in Chapter 2 that chronic pain leads to atrophy of dorsolateral frontal cortex, and it would be useful to know whether behavioral skills can alter this natural history. In the meantime, we can take comfort in the fact that for headaches specifically, there are a number of long-term follow-up studies, some as far as 8 to 10 years after treatment has ended. We will examine this literature in detail in Chapter 17.

CLINICAL IMPLICATIONS

In the meantime, from the process studies to date we can draw several inferences about therapies for headache patients.

The literature, taken broadly, suggests that episodic migraines should be approached as a psychophysiological disorder, with primary emphasis on acquiring relaxation and mental hand warming skills, and on integrating these skills with daily life. Our goal is relaxation to a specific physiological criterion, the hand warming response. Cognitive factors such as catastrophizing appear subsidiary, relevant mostly when they are barriers to the effective use of physical relaxation.

Although equipment for measuring temporal pulse amplitude is not in wide use, we have seen hints, here and in Chapter 5, that it is closely related to migraine, and possibly may be a mechanism by which relaxation-type therapies work. There are similar hints, in the work of Paul Martin and colleagues, that temporal pulse amplitude may be equally important in tension-type headache (P. R. Martin & Seneviratne, 1997; P. R. Martin, J. Todd, & Reece, 2005). Hence, this variable should see greater inclusion in headache treatment studies. In the meantime, its tentative, qualified use as an intermediate endpoint in the clinic, at least in episodic migraine, does not seem unreasonable.

There is little specific literature yet on slow, paced breathing as a single-modality treatment for migraine. However, evidence that the practice blocks stress-related vasoconstriction without changing related measures such as oveall heart rate, supports its inclusion in migraine therapies.

Schoenen's evidence, that we should examine multiple sites in our surface EMG assessments, and seek to ameliorate tension at those sites at which it appears, is well taken. Moreover, in this chapter we have encountered two reasons for conducting a psychophysiological assessment: its results are not interchangeable, or even correlated, with self-report, and the assessment may be valuable as an orientation to treatment, vividly showing the mind-body effect.

Nonetheless, the weight of evidence suggests that tension-type headaches, especially their chronic form, have a very strong cognitive component. Thus, the development of self-efficacy and an internal locus of control is central, whether approached explicitly through cognitive therapy, or implicitly in the course of EMG biofeedback. It follows, of course, that we should encourage self-efficacy by pointing out, whenever practical, the self-directed nature of the person's gains in psychophysiological monitoring. (No deception is needed; that the discovery of control pays a high dividend in making pain less distressing, more ignorable, and then less intense makes sense to patients, who can then notice and enjoy the process.)

Cognitive factors seem equally important in other forms of chronic pain and hence, by extension, in chronic daily headaches. When headaches are extremely frequent or continuous, assessing catastrophic thinking, fear of pain, and high levels of disability is especially useful. For therapy, however, the active ingredient seems to be the reduction in fear that follows for a patient when they successfully navigate a prolonged graded exposure. When pain is very frequent or continuous, our goal may need to shift from prevention to facing the pain with clarity, equanimity, confidence, and a minimum of disability, until the pain loses its capacity to provoke distress.

Of course, catastrophic thinking or fear of pain need not be present. Some patients with frequent pain need only encouragement to apply skills they already possess, such as capacity for absorption, or for relaxation, or for managing the ergonomics of tasks and the timing of rest breaks.

For in the process literature we have seen hints that a single treatment approach will not benefit everyone with the same disorder. We must be able to match patients to the appropriate therapy. Fortunately, there is an empirical literature to guide us in this project, which we will review in the next chapter.

CHAPTER 16

Patient Selection and Treatment Matching

We know from Babylonic and Egyptian inscriptions that opening up the head was not always indicated; driving out demons with different spells and invocations also came into the picture.

—Isler (1993, p. 9)

In the behavioral realm, some degree of treatment matching seems implicit in the diagnosis and case formulation. We have seen evidence that EMG biofeedback and cognitive therapy are particularly useful for tension-type headache, and that autogenics combined with thermal biofeedback has particular efficacy for migraines. On rational grounds, it may be useful to further subdivide diagnostic categories by the key physiological or psychological process, although such fine-grained treatment matching does not yet have empirical support.

For example, both pericranial pain sensitivity and myofascial neck pain can lead to a diagnosis of chronic tension-type headache. From the interview, a heightened pain sensitivity might in turn seem traceable to pacing issues that cause frequent flare-ups at the neck, shoulders and head; catastrophization or other sources of anxious vigilance to pain; and/or medication overuse. We might approach the myofascial pain with combined muscle relaxation and physical therapy, catastrophization and pacing difficulties with cognitive-behavioral therapy, and of course medication overuse with a concomitant supervised taper.

For migraines, the relevant categories are less clear. Logically, however, we might treat signs of vasoconstriction under stress with deep relaxation and thermal biofeedback. When there are indications that the pain has an extracranial component (e.g., a visibly distended superficial temporal artery) we might include cephalic blood volume pulse biofeedback, or track forehead temperature as a measure of efficacy. When the key trigger is mental overactivity, skin conductance biofeedback, or cognitive therapy for Generalized Anxiety Disorder (e.g., worry exposure; T. A. Brown, T. A. O'Leary, & D. H. Barlow, 2001) seem relevant. Other patients may be reacting to life stresses that call for problem solving therapy, overusing medications that should be tapered, or dealing with muscle tension as a trigger or as an early and perhaps correctable manifestation of migraine. Pain sensitization or a large number of seemingly classically conditioned triggers may call for chronic pain treatment and desensitization, respectively. Again, all of this requires empirical validation in future research.

Similar questions can be asked of medications. We have seen that propranolol helps normalize the build-up in contingent negative variation that precedes a migraine. Does this mean that patients whose migraines seem to have an endogenous quasi-periodicity, even after a careful search for triggers, would benefit from propranolol specifically? If there is comorbid fibromyalgia, is a tricyclic the best choice? If instead the comorbidity is with allergies, asthma, and eczema, should an antiserotonergic with antihistaminic properties—say, cyproheptadine or azatadine—be the starting point? Or if the migraines are preceded by mental fatigue, is a supplement such as riboflavin or coenzyme Q10 indicated, to boost energy production in the mitochondria? We can guess, but empirically the answers to these questions are unknown.

More broadly, treatment matching comprises the question of when patients should be referred for acute or preventive medications, physical therapy, chiropractic adjustments, or other treatment modalities. For although behavioral therapy has, on average, good efficacy for chronic benign headaches, not everyone will benefit or complete treatment. Thus, we must first ask which patients are likely to benefit from behavioral therapies, that is, how should patients be selected?

PREDICTING TREATMENT RESPONSE

Response to behavioral interventions has been predicted from patients' headache characteristics, patterns of psychophysiological response, and scores on psychometric instruments. Most of the correlations have been too low for clinical application and are presented here only for their use in future research. Five results, however, seem reliable and strong enough to suggest clinical guidelines.

IN CLINICAL PRACTICE

First, patients with frequent and severe tension-type headaches, who report high levels of daily stress, are likely to require more intensive treatment than simple relaxation training. In fact, Tobin et al. found that a full 81 percent of the variance in relaxation training efficacy could be predicted from pretreatment stress and headache activity. Work on cognitive coping skills seems particularly useful for these patients (Tobin, K. A. Holroyd, Baker, Reynolds, & Holm, 1988).

Second, depression seems to lower treatment efficacy for tension-type headache (Blanchard, 1992). Thus, treatment for depression may need to precede work on tension-type headaches for patients having both conditions.

Third, continuous, high intensity headaches do not seem to respond well to short-term behavioral treatment (Blanchard, Appelbaum, Radnitz, Jaccard, & Dentinger, 1989). The right behavioral treatment for these headaches is not known. It might involve a longer course with emphasis on cognitive stress management skills (Blanchard, Appelbaum, Radnitz, Jaccard, & Dentinger, 1989), but preliminary results have not been encouraging (Barton & Blanchard, 2001). Alternatively, more general training in chronic pain coping might be indicated. Note that headaches occurring 5 or 6 days a week do seem to respond adequately to standard behavioral intervention, although even here, a longer term treatment course might be considered.

Fourth, individuals who are using enough symptomatic headache medications to be at risk for rebound are likely to fare poorly in behavioral treatment (Michultka, Blanchard, Appelbaum, Jaccard, & Dentinger, 1989). A medication tapering, in conjunction with the patient's physician, is generally necessary as a first step.

Fifth, high scores on scales 1 and 3 of the MMPI seem to lower treatment efficacy for migraines (Blanchard, 1992). High scores on these MMPI scales predict poor responses in other types of pain as well. For example, Wiltse and Rocchio (1975) were able to correctly predict the results of chemonucleolysis for low back pain in 77 percent of patients by using a cutoff of $T = 65$ on these scales. Elevations on MMPI scales 1 and 3 presumably indicate the presence of chronic pain syndrome. Because successful behavioral chronic pain treatment lowers scores on these scales by 5–15 T-score points (Naliboff, McCreary, McArthur, M. J. Cohen, & Gottlieb, 1988), it may be a useful prelude to standard migraine treatments for these patients.

IN RESEARCH

Psychophysiological Reactivity.   Recall two results from Chapter 5. Olness et al. found that children who were successful at reducing migraine frequency through self-hypnosis tended to have higher tryptase levels starting out (Olness, Hall, Rozniecki, W. Schmidt, & Theoharides, 1999). Tryptase is presumably an index of mast cell activity. The prediction of treatment success suggests that tryptase levels are influenced by a psychological variable such as stress. Also, Wauquier and coworkers found that successful biofeedback for migraines was associated with reducing interictal vasoconstriction of the middle cerebral artery. People who did not show the interictal vasoconstriction were less likely to benefit (Wauquier, McGrady, Aloe, Klausner, & B. Collins, 1995). Both of these were single studies, and used measures that are not generally available in clinical practice. From the results, however, we might suspect that other measures of baseline stress would predict treatment response. This question has been addressed in an intensive study in Blanchard's laboratory.

Specifically, Blanchard et al. examined the extent to which a subject's pattern of autonomic responding predicts subsequent treatment efficacy (Blanchard, Andrasik, Arena, Neff, Saunders, Jurish, Teders, & Rodichok, 1983). In the study, four psychophysiological measures—frontalis EMG, finger temperature, skin resistance level, and heart rate—were measured under 1 baseline, 3 relaxation and 3 stress conditions. Results are given in the form of multiple regression-derived prediction equations and classification formulas from discriminant function analysis. For relaxation training, two zero-order correlations are given which would be significant at the (two-tailed, uncorrected) $p < .01$ level: (1) For migraines, treatment outcome from relaxation training is predicted by the decrease in hand temperature during a mental arithmetic stressor ($r = .509$). Thus, an indication of vasoreactivity under stress predicts outcome from relaxation training for migraines. And (2) among all patients, an increase in frontalis EMG during the mental arithmetic stressor predicts a good result from relaxation skills ($r = .290$).

Thus, relaxation training seems to have greater efficacy for individuals who show high physiological reactivity under stress. Vasomotor reactivity is noted for migraines, and frontalis muscle tension for the combined sample of tension-type, migraine, and mixed headaches. These results seem quite sensible and bear further study.

In Blanchard et al.'s treatment protocol, biofeedback was administered only to subjects who failed to show clinically significant improvement with relaxation skills. For this somewhat select group, a single zero-order correlation was significant at the two-tailed, uncorrected, $p < .01$ level. The correlation pertains specifically to a category ("vascular headache") comprised of migraineurs, and of people with both migraines and tension-type headache. For people in this category, the ability to lower frontalis muscle tension by relaxing, prior to learning biofeedback, predicts poorer treatment responsiveness. The interpretation of this correlation seems less clear than the two correlations above. Perhaps people whose muscle tension is already responding to relaxation, but whose headaches are not responding, are unlikely to benefit from further work at reducing arousal. Alternatively, it may be relevant that Blanchard et al. treated vascular headache with thermal biofeedback. Perhaps people who respond to stress with muscle tension are less likely to benefit from non-muscle-tension biofeedback. These interpretations are quite speculative however.

Moreover, we must be careful not to rely too much on a single investigation. The study included 40 predictors (autonomic measures, measurement conditions, and comparisons between conditions). And with as few as 21 subjects in some groups, there is plenty of room for the multivariate results to capitalize on chance. From the published results, it does not appear that any of the predictors are significant at a Bonferroni-corrected .05 level. Thus, pending replication we cannot be sure that they are reliable or have clinical utility.

Psychometrics. Psychometric instruments have similarly been used to predict treatment outcome (Blanchard, Andrasik, Neff, Arena, Ahles, Jurish, Pallmeyer, Saunders, Teders, Barron, & Rodichok, 1982; Blanchard, Andrasik, Evans, Neff, Appelbaum, & Rodichok, 1985). We have already encountered the most robust results: that depression in tension-type headache, and elevations on MMPI scales 1 and 3 in migraine, seem to suppress the efficacy of standard treatments (Blanchard, 1992).

Beliefs and self-management. Ter Kuile, Spinhoven, & Linssen (1995b) treated 130 headache patients, most of whom had tension-type headache, with either autogenics or a self-hypnosis technique that incorporated content from cognitive therapy. Ter Kuile et al. were unable to predict outcome from either pretreatment psychopathology or personality traits, possibly because their sample was relatively homogeneous and rather free of psychopathology. Similarly, demographic and medical variables, and pretreatment pain coping strategies, were not useful in prediction. Patients who expected treatment to work had greater pain reduction immediately post-treatment ($r = .35, p < .0001$). However, this correlation had dissipated by 6-month follow-up. A more durable effect was that people who had clinically significant reductions in headache activity at 6-month follow-up had better control of pain through self-management techniques *before* treatment.

Headache characteristics. Blanchard et al. were able to predict treatment response using linear discriminant functions of headache history variables. The predictors of good outcome are given in Table 16–1 (Blanchard, Andrasik, Arena, Neff, Jurish, Teders, Barron, & Rodichok, 1983).

In the Blanchard et al. study, headache characteristics correctly classified between 87 percent and 95 percent of patients as improved vs. not improved. Depending on headache and treatment type, the headache history information was either as good a predictor or better than psychometric and psychophysiological variables. Note, however, that the multivariate techniques used in data analysis are likely to capitalize on chance, and hence the results would benefit from replication (Blanchard, Andrasik, Arena, Neff, Jurish, Teders, Barron, & Rodichok, 1983).

It appears that the more nearly a patient's headache approaches a chronic daily headache, that is, the more intense, continuous and unvarying the pain is, the less it yields to standard biofeedback plus relaxation training (Blanchard et al., 1982). Again, these headaches may more nearly resemble a general chronic pain syndrome, and require more intensive treatment, directly addressing environmental factors.

Learning Biofeedback

To my knowledge, the most ambitious effort to determine which patients are likely to acquire biofeedback skills has been the multi-site Raynaud's Treatment Study. In this study, 81 persons with Primary Raynaud's Disease and 46 healthy control subjects received thermal biofeedback, 74 persons with Raynaud's received frontalis EMG biofeedback as a behavioral control condition, and another 158 subjects received either a medication or a medication placebo (Middaugh, Haythornthwaite et al., 2001).

For thermal biofeedback, by far the most important predictor of success at learning hand warming skills was the specific clinic at which the skills were taught (odds ratio $\approx$ 9). Skills

TABLE 16–1
Headache Characteristics That May Be Predictive of Treatment Outcome

Headache Type	Treatment	Predictors of Good Outcome
Tension[a]	Relaxation	Shorter duration of headache problem Few or no first-degree relatives with headaches No prior psychological treatment for headaches Pain occurs in temples Pain is *not* throbbing or sometimes one-sided Number of positive items on mental status exam
Tension	EMG Biofeedback[b]	Pain occurs in area behind eye Headache is accompanied by vomiting Low income (?)
Migraine	Relaxation	Shorter duration of headache problem (as % of life) Burning, sharp, or other pain Pain does *not* occur in area behind eye Job problems No change in headache phenomenology during headache
Mixed Tension and Migraine	Relaxation	Pain occurs in back of neck No photophobia Pain is *not* a dull ache Presence of physical precursor to headache Greater number of first-degree relatives with headache problem
Vascular (Migraine or Mixed)	Thermal Biofeedback[b]	Pain occurs in forehead area Pain is sometimes one-sided No photophobia Prior psychological treatment for headaches Greater number of first-degree relatives with headache problem

Notes. Adapted from "Nonpharmacologic Treatment of Chronic Headache: Prediction of Outcome," by E. B. Blanchard, F. Andrasik, J. G. Arena, D. F. Neff, S. E. Jurish, S. J. Teders et al., 1983, *Neurology, 33,* p. 1599. Copyright 1983 by the American Academy of Neurology. Adapted with permission.
[a]Blanchard et al.'s study preceded the 1988 IHS system and terminology.
[b]Biofeedback was administered only to patients who had not improved with relaxation.

acquisition ranged from 12.5 percent of participants at one center to 75 percent at another. Needless to say, the instrumentation and training protocol were the same across sites, and it turns out that ambient outdoor temperature and severity of disease (for those with Raynaud's) had no effect. Hence, it appears that either cultural differences among the clinic cohorts, or differences in the personal characteristics of the therapists, were the key variables (Middaugh, Haythornthwaite et al., 2001). As this was a study of biofeedback in its purest form, no relaxation skills were taught, which may have made the learning particularly vulnerable to therapist personality (Middaugh, Haythornthwaite et al.).

Compared with clinic site, patient characteristics were much less important as predictors of successful learning. However, two dispositional coping strategies, measured with the COPE self-report instrument (Carver, Scheier, & Weintraub, 1989), were correlated with successful learning: a tendency to deal with stress by seeing its positive aspects (odds ratio = 2.0), and a tendency not to simply deny that a stressor took place (odds ratio = 0.76; Middaugh, Haythornthwaite et al., 2001). Perhaps these coping strategies are reflecting the personality characteristic of openness to new experiences.

Psychophysiologically, frontalis EMG biofeedback was an easier task to learn, and in the Raynaud's study clinic site did not matter. Female gender was a moderately strong predictor of successful learning (odds ratio = 5.6) and tendency to use humor as a coping strategy was a weak predictor (odds ratio = 1.3; Middaugh, Haythornthwaite et al., 2001). However, neither was strong enough for making treatment decisions.

Pain Coping Strategies

We saw evidence in Chapter 3 that distraction by a competing activity can activate endorphin-ergic pathways, and thus reduce pain and presumably lower firing rates in the dorsal horn. Yet there were studies that showed no effect of distraction. Moreover, a case can be made theoretically that distraction could harm pain coping. That is, distraction could be a form of cognitive avoidance, inadvertently perpetuating pain-related anxiety (H. D. Hadjistavropoulos, T. Hadjistavropoulos, & Quine, 2000).

In fact, whether or not distraction is beneficial may depend on a person's anxiety level. H. D. Hadjistavropoulos and coworkers found that patients who were anxious about their chronic pain, gave higher pain affect ratings on the McGill when instructed to use distraction during physical therapy, versus when they monitored pain sensations. In contrast, patients who were not anxious about their pain gave lower pain affect ratings when they used distraction (H. D. Hadjistavropoulos, T. Hadjistavropoulos, & Quine, 2000; recall that the effects of sensory self-monitoring may be specific to men; Keogh, Hatton, & Ellery, 2000). Thus, it seems reasonable to assess for pain-related anxiety before instructing patients in distraction techniques. Moreover, there may be benefit in looking for activities that are emotionally absorbing, as the resulting "appetitive motivational state" presumably enhances the effect of distraction.

A similar intervening effect has been found for catastrophizing (Heyneman, Fremouw, Gano, Kirkland, & Heiden, 1990). Recall that patients who catastrophize focus on the negative qualities or reactions to the pain, and feel unable to cope with it. It appears that for people high in catastrophizing, distraction does not increase tolerance for laboratory pain. Rather, benefit accrues from self-instructional training, in which people notice the negative self-statements, and generate problem-solving, coping self-statements in their place (Meichenbaum, 1977). For these individuals, the self-instructional training seems to counteract the effects of catastrophization, and to increase pain tolerance to the baseline level of people who do not catastrophize (Heyneman, Fremouw, Gano, Kirkland, & Heiden, 1990). Meanwhile, people who are not prone to catastrophizing derive little benefit from self-instruction, but benefit greatly from distraction (Heyneman, Fremouw, Gano, Kirkland, & Heiden, 1990).

Distraction techniques, narrowly defined, may be disadvantageous to another group of patients as well. There is a little bit of evidence that people who obtain high scores on the Dissociative Experiences Scale (E. Bernstein & F. Putnam, 1986) are better able to decrease pain-distress and increase pain tolerance by imagining that the affected body part is "numb and insensitive" (Giolas & Sanders, 1992). In contrast, cognitive distraction (focusing on one's breathing) seems to be considerably less effective for people prone to dissociation. Conversely, for low scorers on the Dissociative Experiences Scale, distraction appears to be more effective than the imagined analgesia. Thus, for very imaginative people the optimal coping strategy is presumably to use one's imagination (Giolas & Sanders, 1992). Nonetheless, this finding does not abrogate the cautions in Chapter 3. Dissociation seems best restricted to short-term pain flare-ups, or to use as a temporary strategy for building self-efficacy.

Of course, cognitive-behavioral treatment goes beyond focusing on one's breathing, and includes deep relaxation, imagery, and coping self-statements. In the last chapter, we saw that hypnotic analgesia is more effective for people who are highly hypnotizable than for people who score low in hypnotizability (Montgomery, DuHamel, & Redd, 2000). There is some evidence that hypnotizability also predicts responsiveness to non-hypnotic cognitive-behavioral treatment (Farthing, Venturino, S. W. Brown, & Lazar, 1997; Milling, Kirsch, Meunier, & M. R. Levine, 2002). The reason is unknown; perhaps a contiguous variable, such as capacity for absorption (Tellegen & G. Atkinson, 1974), is the true underlying predictor.

The goal of matching people to treatments implies an additional topic as well: predicting whether a given patient will benefit from pharmacological vs. behavioral therapy. I am not aware of any studies that bear directly on this question. However, we may draw insights from the literature and from clinical practice, as discussed in the next section.

COMBINING BEHAVIORAL THERAPY WITH OTHER TYPES OF TREATMENT

Behavioral treatments are primarily designed to prevent headaches, and thus are relevant when prophylaxis is indicated. By convention these conditions include: frequent migraines (at least 2 per month), tension-type headaches occurring often enough that symptomatic treatment would risk medication overuse (e.g., greater than 3 days per week), headaches affecting functioning or quality of life, complicated migraine (in which the risk of stroke mandates preventive efforts), and patients in whom acute treatments have been ineffective or are contraindicated (S. Diamond, 1999). Given these conditions, however, we must decide among behavioral and pharmacologic options, and their combination with each other, and with other treatment modalities such as physical therapy. Here, there are no hard and fast rules. Let us first examine the empirical evidence, and then discuss possible guidelines.

COMBINATION OF BEHAVIORAL AND PHARMACOTHERAPY

We have seen that propranolol and behavioral therapy give nearly identical improvement rates for migraine (K. A. Holroyd & Penzien, 1990). Thus, a natural question is whether combining the two forms of treatment will yield superior outcomes. Two studies have examined this, and both answer in the affirmative.

Ninan T. Mathew compared propranolol, amitriptyline, and biofeedback, as single modalities and in various combinations, in 340 people with migraines, in a between-subjects design (N. T. Mathew, 1981). A key strength of the study was that headache frequency and severity were assessed prospectively using a headache diary. Improvement was determined by comparing headache activity during months 3–6 with the activity during a 1-month pretreatment baseline. An apparent weakness of the study was an unusually high dropout rate from the biofeedback-only condition: 35 percent, as compared with 17 percent attrition from the remaining seven groups combined.

The results are given in Table 16–2. Certainly biofeedback added numerically to the response to propranolol, to amitriptyline, and to the two drugs in combination. For propranolol, the added benefit of biofeedback was statistically significant. For amitriptyline and amitriptyline plus propranolol, it is unclear from the article whether the addition of biofeedback achieves significance.

Holroyd et al. compared the combination of behavioral treatment and low-dose, long-acting propranolol to behavioral treatment by itself (K. A. Holroyd, J. L. France, Cordingley, Rokicki, Kvaal, Lipchik, & McCool, 1995). They found that the combination therapy brought at least a

TABLE 16–2
Biofeedback and Pharmacological Migraine Prevention, Separately and in Combination

Treatment	Improvement in Headache Index
Propranolol + Biofeedback	74%
Propranolol	62%
Propranolol + Amitriptyline + Biofeedback	73%
Propranolol + Amitriptyline	64%
Amitriptyline + Biofeedback	48%
Amitriptyline	42%
Biofeedback	35%
Control (Abortive Treatment Only)	20%

Note. Adapted from "Prophylaxis of Migraine and Mixed Headache. A Randomized Controlled Study," by N. T. Mathew, 1981, *Headache*, *21*, p. 107. Copyright 1981 by the American Headache Society. Adapted with permission.

50 percent reduction in headache activity (intensity X frequency) for 92 percent of patients. Across all patients in the combination-therapy group, the average reduction in headache activity was 79 percent. This is very close to the 74 percent improvement noted by N. T. Mathew (1981). Holroyd et al.'s patients were judged by a neurologist, who was blind to treatment group, to have had a 90 percent reduction in headache activity. (Global judgments are often about 20–30 percentage points higher than measures from prospective headache diaries.)

The authors note that the modal propranolol dose used in the study was only 60 mg/day, and the average dose was 106 mg/day. This compares with a typical dose of 160 mg/day in clinical trials of propranolol. Thus, behavioral treatment may permit improvement with lower doses of the medication, and hence lower exposure to side effects. Interestingly, there was informal feedback from patients at 6 month follow-up that they had discontinued the propranolol but that their headaches remained well-controlled. Thus, the combination of propranolol and behavioral therapy appears more effective in migraine prevention than either treatment alone.

Is the same true for tension-type headaches? This seems to have been examined only for the "chronic" category, in which the headaches have occurred for at least fifteen days a month, for at least the last six months. Specifically, Holroyd and colleagues randomized 203 patients to receive either a tricyclic antidepressant or a placebo, alone or in combination with stress management training (K. A. Holroyd, O'Donnell, Stensland, Lipchik, Cordingley, & B. W. Carlson, 2001). The antidepressant was nearly always amitriptyline, but substitution with nortriptyline was permitted if the patient was not responding or found the side effects to be unacceptable. The stress management training combined progressive muscle relaxation with cognitive skills in areas such as problem solving, recognizing and correcting cognitive distortions, and use of coping self-statements. The training was provided in a minimal-contact format, with three 1-hour sessions, two telephone contacts, and the rest of the skills acquisition left for home practice with workbook and audiotapes. The results are given in Table 16–3.

By convention, "clinically improved" means at least a 50 percent reduction in total headache activity, as measured prospectively by a headache diary. Thus, it appears that the combination of behavioral and antidepressant medication is more effective than either intervention by itself. To some extent, however, this depends on how one looks at the data. If the dependent variable is total reduction in headache activity, rather than percent of subjects clinically improved, then the results are simply that stress management, antidepressant, and their combination, are all equivalent to each other and better than a placebo. Also, it appears that it takes some time for the stress management intervention to consolidate and begin reducing headaches. The advantage of stress

TABLE 16–3
Stress Management Training and Tricyclic Medication for Chronic Tension-Type Headache

Treatment	% of Subjects Clinically Improved at 6 Months
Antidepressant + Stress Management	64%
Antidepressant	38%
Placebo + Stress Management	35%
Placebo	29%

Note. Data from "Management of Chronic Tension-Type Headache with Tricyclic Antidepressant Medication, Stress Management Therapy, and Their Combination: A Randomized Controlled Trial," by K. A. Holroyd, F. J. O'Donnell, M. Stensland, G. L. Lipchik, G. E. Cordingley, and B. W. Carlson, 2001, *JAMA, 285,* p. 2212. Copyright 2001 by the American Medical Association. Used with permission.

management training over placebo was apparent numerically at 1-month follow-up, but did not become statistically significant until the next follow-up, at 6-months (K. A. Holroyd, O'Donnell, Stensland, Lipchik, Cordingley, & B. W. Carlson, 2001).

Needless to say, this is an impressive and welcome study. Still, we must be mindful that any single study will necessarily have limitations. In this case, the main limitation seems to be the blinding. Subjects, of course, were aware of whether they received stress management training, and there was no "placebo" of an equally credible but inert behavioral intervention. In theory, subjects were blinded to medication, but we may wonder how well this held up in practice, as 80 percent of those who received antidepressants, but only 30 percent of those on placebo, reported adverse effects (K. A. Holroyd, O'Donnell, Stensland, Lipchik, Cordingley, & B. W. Carlson, 2001). It is hard to imagine how the study could be done differently, however, as any sedating or energizing properties of an "active placebo" would hardly be neutral with respect to tension-type headache.

COMBINATION OF BEHAVIORAL AND PHYSICAL THERAPY

Both physical therapy (Hammill, Cook, & Rosecrance, 1996) and chiropractic (Vernon, 1995) have positive outcome studies in tension-type headache. Hence, their combination with behavioral therapy is of interest.

For migraines, Marcus, Scharff, Mercer and Turk (1998) found that physical therapy (including postural correction, cervical range of motion exercises, isometric strengthening of the neck, use of modalities, whole body stretching and reconditioning, and treatment of trigger points) was relatively ineffective. This was despite a very high frequency of muscle problems, including trigger points and mechanical problems, in the migraineurs. However, among subjects for whom prior relaxation training and biofeedback had been unsuccessful, the response rate to physical therapy was much greater. This suggests either that there are subsets of migraineurs for whom different treatments are effective, or that the combination of physical therapy and prior behavioral treatment has greater benefit than either treatment alone.

Broadly speaking, manual therapists attempt to treat hypomobility or stiffness in spinal joints by manipulating, that is, mobilizing, the joints. Chiropractors pursue the same end through high-velocity thrusts (Hurwitz, Aker, A. H. Adams, Meeker, & Shekelle, 1996). The literature for these therapies in headache treatment is sparse and short-term, but reasonably encouraging. For example, Boline et al. compared the combination of amitriptyline, chiropractic adjustment, moist heat and massage, to amitriptyline alone, for chronic tension-type headache. At 4-week follow-up the patients in the multimodality chiropractic group had more improvement from baseline on headache frequency and intensity, and functional status, and were using less amitriptyline (Boline, Kassak, Bronfort, Nelson, & Anderson, 1995). On the other hand, Jensen and coworkers found that for patients with chronic posttraumatic headaches, manipulation outperformed cold packs for only the first 2–5 weeks after the end of treatment (O. K. Jensen, Nielsen, & Vosmar, 1990). For migraines, Parker and colleagues found a greater reduction in pain intensity at 2 month follow-up for patients who received manipulation from a chiropractor versus from a medical doctor or a physical therapist (Parker, Pryor, & Tupling, 1980; Parker, Tupling, & Pryor, 1978).

Due to the paucity of studies, reviewers have hesitated to draw conclusions about the efficacy of manual therapy for headaches (Hurwitz, Aker, A. H. Adams, Meeker, & Shekelle, 1996). For migraines, the U.S. Headache Consortium determined that the evidence for cervical manipulation, acupuncture, TENS, and other physical treatments was too limited and mixed to permit evidence-based recommendations (J. K. Campbell, Penzien, & E. M. Wall, 2000). Similar conclusions were drawn by Lenssinck et al. for tension-type headache (Lenssinck, Damen, Verhagen, M. Y. Berger, Passchier, & Koes, 2004). Still, the early results are intriguing, and further research will undoubtedly shed light on whether, when and how manual therapy is effective.

To my knowledge, there have been no studies on the combination of chiropractic and behavioral treatment. The question of whether the two therapies have additive effects, however, is of theoretical as well as practical interest. For one might assume that physical interventions would work primarily on peripheral sources of pain, while psychological interventions would mostly target descending pain modulatory pathways. In fact, the line is not so clearly drawn. We saw in Chapter 2 that TENS units may work by increasing endorphinergic activity. Hence the same may be true, at least in part, of electrical stimulation in physical therapy. Moreover, Sterling and coworkers found in a double-blind, placebo-controlled study that mobilization of the cervical spine did more than lower resting pain level. The mobilization also raised pain thresholds on the same side as the mobilization, and raised skin conductance level and lowered skin temperature, suggesting an increase in sympathetic nervous system activity (Sterling, Jull, & Wright, 2001). Thus, the authors speculate that manual therapy may have raised the level of descending pain inhibition.

BEHAVIORAL THERAPY AND REGIONAL ANESTHESIA

As regional anesthesia—the use of nerve blocks—becomes more popular, the procedures are finding their way into headache treatment. For headache that follows whiplash, the rationale is clear and the practice supported by a small, controlled literature: It appears that the C2–3 zygapophyseal joint in the neck refers pain to the head. When blocking the afferents from the joint completely removes the headache, then lesioning these same nerves is likely to give longer term relief, c. 6 months (Govind, W. King, B. Bailey, & Bogduk, 2003; S. Lord, Barnsley, Wallis, & Bogduk, 1994). Usually, however, neither the rationale nor the empirical support is well developed. A migraine that begins above the eye may be dulled by numbing the skin and muscles in the area. Yet, there is no theory that the skin or muscles above the eye are a major source of pain in migraine. A steroid may be used for a longer term result, but steroids are anti-inflammatories and there is no evidence that the skin or muscles are inflamed (Bogduk, 2004).

That the procedures may hold promise all the same is suggested by a well-controlled trial comparing occipital nerve blockade with steroids plus local anesthetic, vs. local anesthetic alone, in the treatment of cluster headache. In the experimental group, 8 of 13 patients went on to achieve at least a month of remission, including 3 of 4 patients with chronic cluster headache (Ambrosini, Vandenheede et al., 2005). Again, the explanation is unknown. We saw in Chapter 2 that pain afferents from the head and neck converge, and perhaps this is the basis of the analgesic response. Even more surprising, a block of the sympathetic stellate ganglion in the neck can also reduce cluster headache, even though cluster headaches are *parasympathetic* and should be exacerbated by reduction in sympathetic outflow (Albertyn, Barry, & Odendaal, 2004).

On a practical level, nerve blocks sometimes seem useful as a "transitional preventive" (Peres, Stiles, Siow, T. D. Rozen, W. B. Young, & Silberstein, 2002) for medication overuse headache. By giving partial relief for a few weeks, the block gives the patient time to taper from acute medications, learn self-management skills, and undertake preventive pharmacotherapy. The block works within three days, and complements behavioral treatment, which has a slower onset but a far more durable effect.

CLINICAL GUIDELINES

In the realm of psychological treatment, it seems reasonable to parse patients into those whose concerns call for a cognitive-behavioral approach (for depression, chronic pain syndrome, or for handling a high level of life stresses) vs. those with less complicated presentations who are likely to benefit from simpler, psychophysiological therapy. The interview and psychometrics can help in making this distinction.

For those patients learning pain-management skills, assessment of catastrophization and fear of pain, psychometrically or through the interview, can clarify whether imagery, involvement in non-pain activities, and other distraction-type techniques will be useful, or whether learning to reduce catastrophic thoughts and fear (through self-instructional training, graded exposure, and dispassionate monitoring of the sensory characteristics of pain) will be needed first.

More generally, the interview and psychometrics are a chance to learn the deficits and strengths of an individual's approach to pain coping. This knowledge allows us to remediate unhelpful components, such as catastrophic thoughts, while incorporating the strengths—such as capacity for absorption, sources of meaning, and naturalistic forms of relaxation—into the treatment.

Of course, all this assumes that we are drawing on psychological therapies rather than, or in addition to, medication, but should we do so? That preventive behavioral and pharmacotherapies are equally matched in treatment efficacy (see Chapter 14) highlights the question of when to use one vs. the other. There is as yet no data to guide us in this aspect of treatment matching (K. A. Holroyd, Lipchik, & Penzien, 1998). We do not know which migraine patients will respond best to a beta-blocker vs. an antiepileptic, for example, to relaxation training vs. biofeedback, or more generally to self-management vs. pharmacotherapy. In practice, neurologists in office-based treatment often begin with medications. Migraine texts may recommend behavioral and lifestyle changes as the starting point (e.g., Lance, 1998, pp. 119–120), or as one component of multimodal therapy (e.g., Silberstein, Saper, & Freitag, 2001, p. 136). Behind this diversity, certain clinical considerations appear reasonable, and seem to work in practice (K. A. Holroyd, Lipchik, & Penzien, 1998):

Medications may be contraindicated by concurrent disease (e.g., propranolol by asthma), potential drug interactions, or condition (e.g., pregnancy, nursing, childhood). Conversely, a patient may not be motivated or sufficiently organized to participate actively in behavioral treatment. Explicit patient preference is also important. Some patients prefer the simplicity of taking a daily medication. Others find the act of taking multiple pills an independent source of distress and perceived poor health. Previous responsiveness to medications or behavioral treatment can also be a guide to treatment selection.

As headaches become more frequent and/or disabling, and particularly for chronic daily headache, the practice has been to combine prophylactic medication, a tapering from acute medications (when overuse is suspected), intravenous dihydroergotamine (for status migrainosus), and behavioral and, if indicated, physical modalities into a multidisciplinary program (e.g., Lake, Saper, Madden, & Kreeger, 1993). Significant psychiatric comorbidity may also require a more intensive, combined approach (K. A. Holroyd, Lipchik, & Penzien, 1998). Indeed, for inpatient treatment, depression and functional impairment do not seem to be negative prognostic factors, and older age and medication overuse may even be favorable signs (Saper, Lake, & Kreeger, 1994). Thus, in the little evidence so far available, the same factors that impede single modality treatment may actually facilitate progress in a multimodal program.

Thus, there is some basis for stratifying patients to inpatient or outpatient treatment ("**stratified care**"). Holroyd et al. suggest that to distinguish among outpatient therapies, a stepped care approach may also be useful: Patients with tension-type headache, for example, might simply receive group training in relaxation skills. For those not acquiring the skills, additional training and/or surface EMG biofeedback would be included, followed, if needed, by stress management and/or medication prophylaxis. In this way, more involved, higher cost interventions would accumulate only for those patients shown to require them.

When an empirical basis for treatment matching is unavailable, stepped care provides a rational way of allocating therapies in a cost effective manner. However, stepped care may not be optimal. For patients who do not respond to low intensity therapy, more effective interventions are postponed (Lipton, Stewart, A. M. Stone, Láinez, & J. P. C. Sawyer, 2000). And by engaging treatments serially, we lose the increased effectiveness that may come from combining them (Duckro, W. Richardson, J. E. Marshall, Cassabaum, & G. Marshall, 1999). Thus, research clarifying which patients will benefit from which treatments remains quite important (K. A. Holroyd, Lipchik, & Penzien, 1998).

CHAPTER 17

Long-Term Outcome and Future Directions

Nietzsche was . . . plagued with migraines, as many as 120 attacks per year. . . . He starved himself and led an austere life. Starvation, of course, aggravates headaches, and as time went on, his headaches worsened. By age forty-five years, he was insane, and some historians believe this was caused by his headaches. Others believe that his "insane" behavior caused his headaches. Either way, we know that Nietzsche strongly influenced history, and migraine headaches strongly influenced Nietzsche"

—J. M. Jones (1999, p. 629)

LONG-TERM OUTCOME

We have seen in Chapter 14 that behavioral treatment for migraines and tension-type headaches seems to be well supported empirically. However, in a typical outcome study, the follow-up period ranges from a few weeks to one year post-treatment. As Blanchard, et al. have pointed out, one year is a rather brief interval compared with the natural history of the headaches, which is measured in decades (Blanchard, Appelbaum, Guarnieri, Morrill, & Dentinger, 1987). Thus, we turn in this chapter to those studies in which the investigators recontacted their research participants two, three, and even ten years after the completion of treatment.

Of course in examining these results, there is the question of spontaneous remission (Blanchard, 1987). Perhaps any group of headache patients will be markedly improved after a few years, regardless of treatment. However, Blanchard notes that in the sparse data available there is no suggestion of spontaneous remission in chronic headaches over at least three years.

Program Outcome Surveys

The earliest long-term studies were based on surveys mailed by researchers at the large headache clinics, to people who had been patients there years before. For example, Diamond and coworkers sent questionnaires to 556 former patients of the Diamond Headache Clinic, of whom 407, or 73 percent, responded (Diamond, Medina, Diamond-Falk, & DeVeno, 1979). For all of these patients the treatment had consisted of thermal biofeedback, frontalis EMG biofeedback, autogenics training and progressive muscle relaxation exercises. And the results were encouraging. Of the respondents who had been treated between 3 and 5 years earlier, 63 percent felt that the therapy had had some sort of lasting benefit, and nearly 21 percent felt that it had provided "permanent relief." "Permanent relief" is not operationalized in the article, but it seems to mean "cure." And given that the patients had proved refractory both to care by their regular physicians (or they would not have been referred) and to medication management at the Diamond Clinic, an over 20 percent cure rate is rather impressive. There is a hint, though, in this early study, that the results might not truly be permanent. As shown in Table 17–1, there is a steady decline in the proportion of subjects endorsing "permanent relief," from 38 percent at c. 1 year to 21 percent at 3–5 years. Younger participants and females seemed to have better long-term outcomes.

A second study from the Diamond Clinic, on a new cohort of 693 former biofeedback-relaxation training patients, gave similar results. Of the initial pool of patients, 395 (57 percent) returned a mailed survey, and of the respondents, 65 percent felt they had been able to maintain their gains, and 56 percent reported having decreased or eliminated their headache medications (Diamond & Montrose, 1984). These patients had been treated up to four years earlier. As in the earlier study, younger patients and females seemed to have better long-term results. Patients who were severely depressed, habituated to symptomatic medications, or, in most cases, who were over 50 years of age, were excluded from the study.

Needless to say, the results are impressive. However, the conclusions we can draw are limited by the methodology. The 1979 survey was not anonymous, and presumably some of the patients were still being seen at the clinic for long-term follow-up. In the second, anonymous survey, the results still depended on the patients' ability to recall their pain levels from four or five years prior. Pain recall can be quite unreliable over a period of six months, and we must presume that this problem is only compounded over time. Also, of course, we do not know how the people who did not return their surveys fared. Presumably, treatment successes are more favorably disposed towards the program, and more likely to return the questionnaire.

W. B. Smith circumvented this last problem by using a telephone survey of 318 former biofeedback patients (W. B. Smith, 1987). All patients had received thermal and frontalis EMG biofeedback, and some had received EMG biofeedback at other sites as well. Patients also learned about triggers and were encouraged to decrease their medication use. Some received psychotherapy as an additional treatment. Patients were grouped according to the number of biofeedback sessions they had received, and the length of time that had elapsed since treatment. When the therapy had included at least seven biofeedback sessions, nearly all patients felt they had improved by 75–100 percent, even two or more years post-treatment. There was no indication that the biofeedback lost effectiveness over time (see Table 17–2).

In this study, in which differential subject attrition was prevented, the maintenance of gains over 2 or more years appears excellent, with no effect for the amount of time that had elapsed since training. There seems to be a strong effect for the number of treatment sessions. However, the patients who received no biofeedback sessions in fact had been offered the sessions and refused them. Patients with 6 or fewer sessions in some cases had terminated biofeedback early. Thus, the active treatment effects are confounded with patient expectations and motivation (W. B. Smith, 1987).

TABLE 17–1
Long-Term Outcome: Retrospective Questionnaire Data (Diamond, et al., 1979)

Time Since Training	% Who Felt It Had Lasting Effect	% Reporting Permanent Relief
3–18 months	80.9%	37.5%
19–36 months	79.2%	30.6%
37–62 months	62.6%	20.6%

Note. Adapted from "The Value of Biofeedback in the Treatment of Chronic Headache: A Five-Year Retrospective Study," by S. Diamond, J. Medina, J. Diamond-Falk, and T. De Veno, 1979, *Headache, 19*, p. 94. Copyright 1979 by the American Headache Society. Adapted with permission.

TABLE 17–2
Long-Term Outcome: Retrospective Telephone Survey (W. B. Smith, 1987)

	Number of Months Since Last Contact With Practice		
	3–12	13–24	25+
Number of Biof. Sessions	Percent Who Felt They Were 75–100% Improved		
0	−11% (N = 34)[a]	−7% (N = 36)	31% (N = 32)
1	33% (N = 25)	24% (N = 24)	36% (N = 24)
2–6	72% (N = 23)	68% (N = 24)	70% (N = 23)
7+	91% (N = 25)	89% (N = 25)	86% (N = 23)

Note. From "Biofeedback and Relaxation Training: The Effect on Headache and Associated Symptoms," by W. B. Smith, 1987, *Headache, 27*, p. 512. Copyright 1987 by the American Headache Society. Reprinted with permission.
[a]Negative percentages indicate an increase in headache frequency.

This points to another limitation of the studies we have reviewed so far in this chapter. Unlike the controlled outcome studies emphasized in Chapter 14, there has been no random assignment to treatments. And the study by Smith, like those by Diamond, relies on the subjects' recall of their prior pain levels.

As a final example, we may cite a report by Adler and Adler (1984), who examined migraine frequency a full 10–12 years after therapy had ended. Now, for most of the patients, the authors had conducted psychodynamic therapy, into which biofeedback had been integrated. That is, patients were not merely taught to relax to a high-level criterion (95 °F); they were taught to maintain that degree of relaxation while discussing emotionally difficult topics. And the patients used the machine readings—the signs of increased anxiety—during therapy sessions to gain insight into which material was emotionally relevant. The 53 patients who received this combination therapy reported on average an 84 percent reduction in headache frequency at the ten year follow-up. A matched group of 15 migraineurs who received only relaxation training and thermal biofeedback were also improved, but on average their headache frequency was reduced by only 34 percent. Still, this is indeed a noticeable improvement a decade after treatment had ended.

Adler and Adler's study is generally described as retrospective, although in my own reading of it, it sounds like global reports of headache frequency at follow-up were compared with the original headache frequency. The report is brief, though, and unclear on this point. One limitation that definitely seems present is that all data were collected through a direct interview by the original therapist, and hence patients may have felt motivated to relate positive results.

Prospective Program Outcome Studies

A key advance in rigor is found in Reich's (1989) study of treatment results from a pain management program in Mineola, New York. He specifically used random assignment to treatments and prospective headache monitoring. That is, participants completed a headache diary 6 times a day for 4 weeks, before treatment, after treatment, and at 8, 24, and 36 months post-treatment.

There were four conditions: Group R received relaxation training, hypnosis, or cognitive therapy, singly or in combination. Group B received thermal biofeedback (for migraine) or EMG biofeedback from the frontalis, trapezius, and/or paracervical muscles (for muscle contraction headache). Group E was treated with electrical stimulation and/or a TENS, unit. Group M's treatment was multimodal; that is, it included treatments from two or more of the other groups.

For patients with muscle contraction headache, all treatments brought about a reduction in headache frequency and intensity, and apparently in medication use. Biofeedback, however, was

TABLE 17–3
Long-Term Outcome: Prospective Randomized Trial (Reich, 1989)

Group	N	*Number of Headache Hours per Week*		
		Pre-Treatment	*Post-Treatment*	*36 Months*
Biofeedback	78	31.1	1.3	1.5
Relaxation	78	29.6	10.2	14.7

Note. Data from "Non-Invasive Treatment of Vascular and Muscle Contraction Headache: A Comparative Longitudinal Clinical Study," by B. A. Reich, 1989, *Headache*, 29, p. 37. Copyright 1989 by the American Headache Society. Adapted with permission.

TABLE 17–4
Long-Term Changes in Medication Use (Reich, 1989)

	Pre-Treatment	*Post-Treatment*	*36 Months*
Taking Prescribed Meds	88%	11%	<10%
Taking OTC Meds	100%	10%	<10%

Note. Data from "Non-Invasive Treatment of Vascular and Muscle Contraction Headache: A Comparative Longitudinal Clinical Study," by B. A. Reich, 1989, *Headache*, 29, p. 36. Copyright 1989 by the American Headache Society. Adapted with permission.

the most successful intervention and relaxation training was the least successful. Multimodal therapy and the electrical modalities had success rates intermediate between biofeedback and relaxation. (All results are statistically significant, to which the large sample size of course contributes). Thus, comparing pretreatment with 36-month follow-up, the biofeedback group showed a 95 percent reduction in the number of headache hours per week. The relatively less successful relaxation group showed a 50 percent reduction during this same time period (see Table 17–3). The chronicity of the headaches (whether or not the disorder had been present for at least 2 years) did not affect treatment outcome.

Across both types of headache and all four treatment groups there was a marked decline in the proportion of patients using medications (see Table 17–4). At baseline, all patients had been using over-the-counter preparations, and nearly all had been taking prescribed medications. Fewer than 10 percent of patients were using either type of pharmacotherapy at 36-month follow-up.

In the study, only those patients who participated at all five assessment periods are included. Thus, we do not know the amount of subject attrition in the various treatment categories. Over 36 months, participants can leave a study for many reasons, but presumably patients who found the treatment unsuccessful would be less likely to stay involved. Of course, if this process did occur, the overall effectiveness of treatment would be overestimated. Presumably, statements about trends over time are on somewhat firmer ground.

Clinical Research Groups

University-based research projects have similarly provided long-term outcome data. In particular, we may note a series of long-term follow-ups conducted by Blanchard and associates, as part of their extensive program of studies on the behavioral treatment of headaches.

In one study, patients were followed two years after undergoing brief treatment (3–10 sessions) for either migraine or tension headaches (Blanchard, Appelbaum, Guarnieri, Neff, Andrasik,

Jaccard, & Barron, 1988). Results were derived from prospective headache-diary monitoring, and are shown in Table 17–5. For both types of headache, treatment gains seem to consolidate over the first year after treatment, to an approximately 50 percent reduction in headache index. There is essentially no further change between the one- and two-year follow-ups.

The results for tension-type headache are qualified by a differential tendency of patients who obtained less reduction in headaches with treatment to drop out prior to follow-up. However, data for these subjects were excluded at all time points. Also, Blanchard et al. suggest that it is the maintenance of gains by successful subjects (rather than the "persistence of failure") that is most interesting in long-term follow-up studies. Moreover, Lisspers and Öst note that long-term follow-up of only treatment successes will result in an underestimate of the degree to which change endures (Lisspers & Öst, 1990). The reason is statistical artifact. Because the treatment successes are an extreme group, there will inevitably be some regression to the mean due simply to intrinsic unreliability of measurement. No differential drop-out was seen among migraine patients.

A five-year outcome study was reported by the same group, of patients who had received relaxation training, supplemented as necessary with biofeedback, for migraine, tension, or mixed headaches (Blanchard, Appelbaum, Guarnieri, Morrill, & Dentinger, 1987). The participants had been seen for weekly follow-up sessions for the first six months. Also, they had the option of receiving a booster session at each one-year follow-up. Improvement was measured prospectively by means of a 4-week headache diary at each time point.

The results, especially the absence of an upward trend-line, are quite encouraging, and all the more so when we factor in that the patients generally reported little medication use at the 5-year mark. On average, patients' headache index values at each yearly follow-up were at least 50 percent lower than prior to treatment (see Table 17–6).

The primary limitation of this study is the small sample size, such that replication by other research groups would be valuable. And, as in the earlier study, initial treatment failures tended to refuse long-term follow-up, so that their data was excluded at all time points. In total, there had been 38 treatment successes still available at 1-year follow-up, and of these, 21 were still available and willing to participate at 5 years.

TABLE 17–5
Two-Year Outcome: Prospective Data (Blanchard, et al., 1988)

Time	Headache Intensity X Duration (M±SD)
Tension-Type Headache	
Pre-Treatment	4.64 ± 3.81
Post-Treatment	2.81 ± 3.39
1 Year Follow-up	2.59 ± 3.19
2 Year Follow-up	2.37 ± 2.17
Migraine	
Pre-Treatment	3.60 ± 2.85
Post-Treatment	2.07 ± 2.14
1 Year Follow-up	1.42 ± 1.62
2 Year Follow-up	1.40 ± 1.59

Note. Adapted from "Two Studies of the Long-Term Follow-Up of Minimal Therapist Contact Treatments of Vascular and Tension Headache," by E. B. Blanchard, K. A. Appelbaum, P. Guarnieri, D. F. Neff, F. Andrasik, J. Jaccard, and K. D. Barron, 1988, *Journal of Consulting and Clinical Psychology*, 56, p. 430. Copyright 1988 by the American Psychological Association. Adapted with permission.

TABLE 17–6
Five-Year Outcome: Prospective Data (Blanchard, et al., 1987)

	N	Baseline	Post-Tx	Year 1	Year 2	Year 3	Year 4	Year 5
				Headache Index				
Migraine & Mixed	12	2.89	1.04	1.03	1.30	1.37	1.43	0.60
Tension	9	2.22	0.52	0.38	0.90	1.04	0.60	0.37

Note. Adapted from "Five Year Prospective Follow-Up on the Treatment of Chronic Headache with Biofeedback and/or Relaxation," by E. B. Blanchard, K. A. Appelbaum, P. Guarnieri, B. Morrill, and M. P. Dentinger, 1987, *Headache, 27*, p. 581. Copyright 1987 by the American Headache Society. Adapted with permission.

TABLE 17–7
Five-Year Outcome: Prospective Data (Lisspers and Öst, 1990)

	Pre-Treatment	Post-Treatment	6 Months	4–6 Years
		Time of Measurement		
Total Headache Activity	2.78	1.74	1.38	1.45
% Reduction From Baseline		38%	50%	48%
% of Clinical Successes[a]		36%	53%	60%
Medication Index	0.93	0.41	0.51	0.44

Note. Adapted from "Long-Term Follow-Up of Migraine Treatment: Do the Effects Remain up to Six Years?," 1990, *Behaviour Research and Therapy, 28*, p. 317. Copyright 1990 by Pergamon Press Inc.

[a]Percent of subjects attaining at least a 50% reduction in headache activity from baseline.

Thus, we have preliminary, reassuring results that for patients who are initially successful, the success persists, with no sign of abating after 5 years. Ideally, however, we would be able to get beyond the vexing problem of long-term subject retention.

In two investigations, this problem seems to have been solved. The first, by Lisspers and Öst (1990), was a prospective study of migraineurs who had been treated with thermal biofeedback, blood volume pulse biofeedback, or relaxation training. Of their 63 participants, 50 (79 percent) completed four weeks of follow-up headache diary an average of 5 years and 2 months after treatment. Moreover, the 21 percent who were lost to follow-up did not differ from the remaining 79 percent in headache activity at baseline, at post-treatment, or at 6-month follow-up. Thus, both in severity of their condition and in their treatment response, the subjects available at 5 year follow-up seem representative of the sample as a whole.

Now, in the 5 years following the conclusion of treatment, the subjects had had no booster sessions or other personal contacts at the clinic. How much, then, were they able to maintain their gains? Results are given in Table 17–7, and as can be seen they are quite encouraging.

Participants had recorded their pain four times a day for four weeks pretreatment, and then again at post-treatment and at each of the two follow-up periods. Total Headache Activity refers to the average daily sum of pain ratings over the particular four-week interval. The percent of clinical successes refers to the percentage of subjects who achieved at least a 50 percent reduction in total headache activity. The medication index was computed as the number of over-the-counter analgesic pills consumed, plus twice the number of ergot pills (which were thus regarded as having twice the potency of an aspirin or an acetaminophen).

Now, all of the post-treatment measures shown above were significantly different from baseline, but there were no significant differences among follow-up periods. Indeed, there is no evidence of even a numeric decline in efficacy over the five years. Whether measured by total headache activity (48 percent lower), or by medication use (53 percent lower), or by the proportion of subjects who were clinically improved (60 percent), the results at 5 years are nearly the same as those at 6 months, and better than the results immediately post-treatment.

Similar data are reported by Sorbi and associates, who had taught either relaxation or cognitive stress management skills to 29 people with migraines (Sorbi, Tellegen, & Du Long, 1989). The participants kept 8-week headache diaries on four occasions: baseline, post-treatment, 8-month follow-up, and 3-year follow-up. At 3 years, only 5 (17 percent) of the subjects were lost to follow-up, and their scores did not differ from those of the remaining 24 subjects at any of the prior periods. Their outcomes, where "percent change" is in comparison to pretreatment levels, are shown in Table 17–8.

There is no significant change and, indeed, no numeric change between the 8-month and 3-year follow-up periods. All variables improved by about 30–55 percent. In general, medication use declined commensurately with the headaches. Thus, the results of Sorbi, et al. seem equivalent to those of Lispers and Öst.

We should add that there were few significant changes at any time point for migraine intensity or duration; almost all of the improvement is in terms of migraine frequency. This is part of a mass of data suggesting that a migraine, once triggered, is an all-or-none phenomenon.

LONG-TERM OUTCOME IN CHILDREN

Because chronic headaches often first emerge in childhood, and can remain troublesome for years or decades, it is especially important to know if treatment will be of lasting benefit in children. Bussone and coworkers have addressed this question for episodic tension-type headache, reporting long-term results from a clinical series treated sparingly: 10 sessions of progressive relaxation and frontalis EMG biofeedback over 5 weeks, without home practice. Participants, ages 7–17, completed a 4-week headache diary at baseline, and again at 1, 3, 6, 9, 12, and 36 months, with a very brief refresher course available at each of the first 5 time points.

We saw in Chapter 14 that in the controlled version of this study, the placebo group maintained a 60 percent improvement, while the biofeedback group progressed on to an 86 percent improvement over the year following treatment. In the clinical series, the results are slightly different. Subjects improve with treatment, maintain their improvements over the first year, and then continue to improve over the next 2 years. In all, the number of headache days per month

TABLE 17–8
Long-Term Outcome: Relaxation Training vs. Stress Management (Sorbi, et al., 1989)

	Group	*Post-Treatment*		*8-Month Follow-Up*		*3-Year Follow-Up*	
		N	*Percent Change*	*N*	*Percent Change*	*N*	*Percent Change*
Migraine	Relaxation Training	13	−40%	12	−27%	10	−38%
Frequency	Stress Management	16	−31%	16	−36%	14	−36%
All HA	Relaxation Training	13	−39%	12	−56%	10	−56%
Frequency	Stress Management	16	−38%	16	−47%	14	−45%

Note. HA = Headache. Adapted from "Long-Term Effects of Training in Relaxation and Stress-Coping in Patients with Migraine: A 3-Year Follow-Up," by M. Sorbi, B. Tellegen, and A. Du Long, 1989, *Headache*, 29, p. 114. Copyright 1989 American Headache Society. Adapted with permission.

All values are significantly different from baseline at the .05 level or better, except for relaxation training at 8-month follow-up.

decreases by 60 percent for females and by 85 percent for males over the first year. After 3 years the number of monthly headaches is down by 98 percent for females and 90 percent for males compared with baseline (Grazzi, Andrasik, D'Amico, Leone, Moschiano, & Bussone, 2001).

A limitation in this study is the attrition rate: 6 of 54 subjects did not complete treatment originally, and 10 of the remaining 48 could not be reached at 3 years (30 percent incomplete or lost to follow-up). Baseline data for these subjects were the same as for the subjects who gave follow-up data. Of greater significance, of course, is the lack of a control group, and hence the uncertainty about how much of the long-term improvement might be due to spontaneous remission.

Engel et al. attempted to circumvent this limitation (J. M. Engel, Rapoff, & Pressman, 1992). Originally, they randomized 20 subjects to receive autogenics relaxation, progressive muscle relaxation, the two forms of relaxation together, or no treatment (waiting list control). After the study, none of the control subjects opted for relaxation training, which provided an opportunity to continue looking at study effects long-term. Specifically, subjects were recontacted 51 months, on average, post-treatment, and again completed a 4-week headache diary. In the statistical analysis, the three active treatments outperform the control group on number of headache-free days and peak headache severity (J. M. Engel, Rapoff, & Pressman, 1992). However, the analysis seems to collapse across time, and hence blend long-term follow-up with the results at 1-, 3-, 6-, and 12-months post-treatment. Graphically, there appears to be maintenance or further improvement of treatment gains over the 51 months for patients who received progressive muscle relaxation, with or without autogenics. At 51 months, the patients who received autogenics alone, and the waiting list controls, were little changed from baseline. Thus, although the data analysis does not seem to tease out the effects at 51 months, the spontaneous remission rate in this small study was very low. It may be quite relevant, however, that 3 of the 4 control group patients had either migraines or mixed migraine-tension-type headaches.

PREDICTING LONG-TERM OUTCOME

Needless to say, it is more important to know who will have enduring success from behavioral treatment than to know who will benefit immediately. Two investigators have tried tentatively to answer the prediction question.

In one such effort, Hudzinski and Levenson mailed questionnaires to 114 (adult) patients who had completed relaxation training and frontalis EMG biofeedback approximately 20 months earlier (Hudzinski & Levenson, 1985). All of the patients had been diagnosed with muscle contraction headaches, at least 4 per week for the 4 months preceding treatment. Patients with severe depression, habituation to medications, or physical pathology (other than myofascial pain) were excluded. Now, of the 114 patients, 74 (65 percent) responded, and among them, improvement was strongly related to an internal locus of control in regard to their pain. That is, patients who believed that their pain was under their control were more likely to have long-term treatment gains. The weakness in this study is that locus of control was assessed only at follow-up. As the authors note, one can hypothesize that the treatment gains produced the belief in control, rather than the other way around.

The second effort is also retrospective, although it will be reported here because of its implications for future studies. At the 3-year follow-up in the study by Sorbi et al., participants were interviewed by their former therapists, about their rehearsal, application, and maintenance of the skills learned in treatment. (Presumably this was after the headache diaries had been collected.) From Table 17–8, there was no difference in overall effectiveness between the relaxation training and cognitive stress management groups. However, for relaxation training, maintenance of gains seemed to correlate negatively with the degree of external life stresses encountered since treatment, positively with the effectiveness of relaxation skills in coping with the stresses, and positively with the preservation of relaxation skills. For the stress management group, the degree of post-treatment life stresses did not correlate with outcome. Rather, outcome was correlated positively with degree of skills maintenance, and with self-motivation for skills maintenance (Sorbi, Tellegen, & Du Long, 1989).

A still-unresolved question in the biofeedback literature is the degree to which home practice is needed. Sorbi et al. provide a two-part answer. Very few of their subjects reported that they still rehearsed their skills three years after treatment. However, most of their subjects reported applying their skills at least weekly. Application of skills correlated positively with success at follow-up, as indeed has been noted by others (Lake & Pingel, 1988). However, rehearsal correlated *negatively* with outcome; it seems to have been a fall-back strategy for people whose skills were not working. Sorbi, et al. suggest that it is these two meanings of the word "practice," and their opposing relationships to success, that explains the diverging results elsewhere on whether home practice is useful.

A different answer is given by Blanchard's group, whose subjects reported "only occasional non-systematic use of the techniques they learned five years ago" (Blanchard, Appelbaum, Guarnieri, Morrill, & Dentinger, 1987, p. 582). For these patients, it is suggested, the headache cycle was broken. They no longer needed to practice regularly because they were no longer chronic headache patients.

FUTURE DIRECTIONS

The field, of course, is far from closed. Let us examine briefly the terrain ahead, beginning with those regions closest to clinical application, and continuing on to longer range questions in need of further research.

Efforts to increase access to behavioral treatment will, and of course should, continue. For sophisticated patients, home-based treatment materials should be published and studied as a step towards developing empirically supported self-help guides. Moreover, educating primary care providers will be crucial, both for encouraging appropriate referrals and perhaps for administering brief group interventions in-office (e.g., Andrasik, Grazzi, Usai, D'Amico, Leone, & Bussone, 2003). Logically, primary care office visits can be an opportunity to reinforce healthy pain coping, by supporting continued involvement in meaningful non-pain activities, by encouraging the precise formulation of questions underlying pain related anxiety, and in depressed patients by prompting activity and appropriate exercise. However, this step depends on primary care providers understanding the psychological dimensions of the pain experience.

Greater attention should be paid to disability, emotional reactions to pain, and similar quality-of-life issues, when evaluating the impact of headaches and treatment modalities (Holroyd, 2002).

Approximately 1 in 7 headache clinic patients meets diagnostic criteria for cervicogenic headache, with which both neck tenderness (Sjaastad, Fredriksen, & Pfaffenrath, 1998) and surface EMG elevations in response to stress (Bansevicius & Sjaastad, 1996) have been associated. In one formulation, the pain is instigated by traction on the dura mater of the upper cervical cord by the rectus capitis muscle (Alix & D. Bates, 1999; Hack, 1998). Extending to cervicogenic headache the research program of surface EMG treatment that has been so successful in tension-type headache seems a reasonable step.

The role of psychophysiological variables in headaches needs to be delineated more clearly. For tension-type headache, biofeedback process studies, typically on people with the chronic form of the disorder, have suggested that an increase in self-efficacy, rather than a decrease in muscle tension, is the active ingredient in treatment. On the other hand, ergonomic studies, often relatively early after pain onset, point to subtle muscle tension difficulties, such as prolonged activation of low threshold motor units, in the genesis of musculoskeletal pain. Preliminary work suggests that within-subject variability in the EMG signal may be a moderating variable (Rokicki, Houle, Dhingra, Weinland, Urban, & Bhalla, 2003). Thus, tension-type headache may include people for whom muscle tension is relevant, and others for whom central sensitization is the key underlying variable.

Similarly, we have seen that for migraines, the theory that they are simply a vascular response to stress is no longer tenable. However, for some patients stress-related vasoconstriction may function as a powerful migraine trigger. An altered neural response to stimulation, depletion of brain energy reserves, central pain sensitization, and perhaps altered platelet function, may each be the predominant variable in a different subset of patients. Dividing the current diagnostic categories into etiological subgroups may help shed light on the role of psychophysiology, and permit a more incisive treatment matching.

The theory that tension-type headaches are analogous to phantom limb pain—generated in the cortex due to a mismatch between motor intention and absent or limited visual and somatosensory feedback from muscle contraction, is of theoretical and practical interest (see A. J. Harris, 1999). The adaptation of classical Jacobsonian relaxation as a form of sensory discrimination training, with visual feedback from a mirror to enhance the discrimination learning, could be studied as an addition to current techniques.

Cluster headache deserves more behavioral research because of the marked suffering caused by this disorder. Epidemiological studies should clarify whether the increased risk associated with current smoking is equivalent to the risk of having formerly smoked. Circumstantial evidence that tobacco is playing a causal but reversible role would of course make smoking cessation a part of the treatment package. The role of stress and letdown in triggering attacks, and the potential role of stress management, needs to be better defined. Also, some cluster headache sufferers show side-to-side temperature differences at the forehead, both within and outside of cluster periods, suggesting a permanent, local sympathetic dysfunction which could predispose to further attacks (Drummond, 1990). Cephalic pulse volume biofeedback, which presumably entails a voluntary increase in pericranial sympathetic tone, could be studied as an interictal, preventive strategy. It seems a useful empirical question whether deep, slow breathing to improve gas exchange in the lungs, perhaps combined with heart rate variability biofeedback, will be useful when hypoxia is a trigger.

More generally, cephalic pulse volume biofeedback seems appropriate for further study. For if indeed its underlying mechanism is an increase in sympathetic tone, its place in the control of migraine may be distinct from that of relaxation training and other forms of biofeedback.

We have caught glimpses of the physiological and psychological processes that participate in the transition from acute to chronic pain. However, little is known about how these two types of processes interrelate. Because central sensitization most likely develops over minutes, hours, and days, and because alterations in descending pain modulation are unlikely to be evident for days or weeks, acute laboratory studies of healthy subjects will probably be of limited utility. Rather, we must follow people with different psychological reactions to pain for several months, beginning with their first presentation to a doctor or emergency room after injury.

Several psychophysical measures reflect the degree of central sensitization:

(a)   A decrease in power law exponent for pain ratings as a function of stimulus intensity. The exponent decreases because, with sensitization, pain emerges at lower stimulus intensities, making the stimulus-response curve less positively accelerated.

(b)   Greater temporal summation, i.e., a steeper rise in "second pain" as stimulation is repeated at short intervals, than in control subjects. Recall that following a brief nociceptive stimulus there is a short, pricking pain (first pain), followed by a longer, often aching pain approximately 1 sec later (second pain). People can learn to distinguish these two pains.

(c)   A greater spread of pain, for example from hand to arm to shoulder during the cold pressor test.

(d)   And of course a decrease in pain threshold.

These measures are appropriate intermediate endpoints for studying the impact of psychological variables and psychological treatment on chronic pain (Janke, K. A. Holroyd, & Romanek, 2004). Presumably, interventions with ameliorative or curative promise will cause a decrease in these psychophysical markers far sooner than improvement is perceived in the pain itself. Effective behavioral interventions could then be examined in headache types for which psychological variables have been under-studied, such as cluster headache and posttraumatic headache.

For as we have seen in Chapters 2 and 3, psychological treatments are not just a way of coping with pain, they seem to get at some of the mechanisms of pain itself. The great unfinished project in pain research is to see how far behavioral treatments can take us in eliminating chronic pain. That this goal might be achievable is hinted in Blanchard's explanation for the enduring success of his research participants—the headache cycle was broken. They no longer needed to practice regularly because they were no longer chronic headache patients.

They were no longer chronic headache patients! The possibility of eliminating chronic pain has flitted in and out of this book—in Hölzl's and Fordyce's operant models, in Vlaeyen's exposure therapy, in Pavlov's early counterconditioning, in Paul Martin's desensitization to triggers, in Crawford's and Daly and Wulff's use of hypnosis . . . and landed just beyond the periphery of our vision. Of course our pharmaceutical companies are investing a tremendous effort in the pursuit of this Holy Grail, and so should psychologists. And someday, perhaps, somebody will find this ancient book, and read it not as a manual, or as a progress report, or as a battle plan, but simply as a record of how people once lived.

Glossary

5-Hydroxytryptamine (5-HT).   The chemical name for the neurotransmitter serotonin. Among other effects, serotonin is involved in constriction and dilation of blood vessels, nausea, depression, sleep, excitatory and inhibitory descending control of pain, processing of pain from the head region, and gating of other sensory information.

5-Hydroxytryptophan (5-HTP).   A derivative of the amino acid tryptophan, 5-HTP is a precursor of the neurotransmitter serotonin, and has been studied in migraine prophylaxis.

Aβ Fibers.   Large diameter sensory nerves, covered with a myelin sheath. Aβ fibers usually transmit information on nonpainful levels of pressure.

Aδ Fibers.   Small diameter, myelinated sensory fibers innervating the skin. Aδ fibers primarily convey information about noxious events, such as high levels of pressure, to the central nervous system. Pain mediated by Aδ fibers tends to be a precisely localized, rapid, brief, pricking sensation.

Absorption.   Sustained, effortless, highly focused attention.

ACE Inhibitors.   A class of blood pressure medications that block the enzyme (angiotensin-converting enzyme) that produces angiotensin II.

Acetylcholine.   A neurotransmitter, used in particular by the parasympathetic branch of the autonomic nervous system, and at the neuromuscular junction.

Algometer.   A device for measuring sensitivity to pressure-type pain. Algometers usually consist of a pressure meter attached to a rod that ends in a rubber tip. The rod is pressed into the skin until pain threshold or tolerance is reached, and the corresponding pressure is read off.

Allodynia.   Altered sensation, in which a non-noxious stimulus, such as light pressure or cool water, is experienced as painful. Allodynia is generally more distressing than ordinary pain.

Alpha-2 Adrenoreceptors.   A type of receptor for the neurotransmitter norepinephrine. On blood vessels, α_2 receptors mediate vasoconstriction. In the central nervous system, α_2 receptors tend to be inhibitory, including in pain pathways.

AMPA Receptor.   A type of receptor for the neurotransmitter glutamate. Changes in the strength and number of AMPA-type receptors are thought to be the basis for such processes as learning, memory, and central pain sensitization.

Amphetamines.   Stimulant drugs that block the reuptake of norepinephrine and dopamine, increasing their concentration in the synapse.

Amygdala.   An almond-shaped structure just medial to the forward pole of the temporal lobe. The amygdala is part of the limbic system, and seems to be important in fear, aggression, and learning fear associations (fear conditioning).

Angiotensin II.   A chemical produced in the kidneys, brain, and vasculature. Angiotensin II raises blood pressure by constricting blood vessels, lowering sodium excretion, and by facilitating signals from the sympathetic nervous system. Angiotensin II may play a role in migraines.

Anterior Cingulate Cortex.   The forward part of the cingulate gyrus, an inner lobe of the brain. Portions of anterior cingulate cortex seem to be involved in unpleasant emotional tone, and in prioritizing competing emotional stimuli.

Arginine.   An amino acid, found principally in plant-based foods such as nuts. Arginine is the precursor of nitric oxide, a neurotransmitter and smooth muscle relaxant produced in the body.

Associative Tolerance.   Loss of effectiveness of a drug due to learned physiological responses that counteract the drug. The component of drug tolerance that depends on classical conditioning.

Automatic Thoughts.   Appraisals of situations or oneself that take place in a rapid, overlearned manner, often without conscious awareness. Automatic thoughts are prone to cognitive distortions, and may contribute to depression, anxiety, and maladaptive personality traits.

Autonomic Instability.   Exaggerated responsiveness of the autonomic nervous system.

Autonomic Nervous System (ANS).   The branch of the nervous system that controls the cardiovasculature, viscera, energy storage and release, and other automatic processes. The sympathetic and parasympathetic nervous systems are branches of the ANS.

Autoreceptors.   Receptors for a neurotransmitter, found on the same presynaptic cell that is secreting the neurotransmitter. Autoreceptors allow the presynaptic cell to "read" the amount of neurotransmitter in the synapse and adjust subsequent secretion accordingly.

Autosomal Dominant.   A classic inheritance pattern in which a trait is transmitted by a single, non-sex-linked, dominant gene. If one parent has the trait, each child has a 50 percent chance of inheriting it.

Baroreceptors.   Receptors in the aorta and carotid arteries that are sensitive to blood pressure, conveying the information to the brain.

Basal Ganglia.   Deep brain structures involved in the control of movement. The basal ganglia may also play a role in pain perception.

Beck Depression Inventory.   A reliable and well validated questionnaire that quantifies clinical depression by asking about presence and degree of somatic, mood, and cognitive symptoms.

Beta-Blockers.   Antagonists of β-adrenoreceptors, found in the sympathetic nervous system. Beta-blockers are used to treat hypertension, and also show efficacy in preventing migraines.

Biofeedback.   The therapeutic technique of teaching control over a physiological process by giving accurate, real-time, machine-based feedback about the process. For example, muscle relaxation skills can be acquired by learning to reduce muscle tension displayed on a gauge or computer screen.

Blood-Brain Barrier.   The relative impermeability of capillary walls in most regions of the brain to substances, including many drugs, circulating in the blood. In general, water soluble substances cannot, and fat soluble substances can, pass through the blood-brain barrier.

Body Schema.   The mental representation of one's body.

Bogus Pipeline.   In psychology experiments, an intervention by which subjects are led to believe that false responding can be detected, e.g., through a fake lie detector.

Bradykinin.   A chemical, produced by damaged tissue, which stimulates nearby nociceptors and dilates local blood vessels.

Brain stem.   A region of the brain comprised of the medulla, pons, midbrain, and possibly the hypothalamus and thalamus. The brain stem contains a number of nuclei, or cell groups, involved in pain processing.

Brodmann Areas.   The small divisions of the cortex proposed by Korbinian Brodmann in 1909, based on subtle variations in the way neuronal cell bodies are layered. Not surprisingly, these structurally distinct regions later turned out to have different functions as well (L. W. Swanson, 2003).

Bruxism.   Jaw clenching (by day) or grinding (at night), thought to contribute to myofascial pain in the jaw region. Jaw clenching during the day seems to be a stress-related behavior. The role of stress in nocturnal bruxism is uncertain.

C Fibers.   Small diameter, unmyelinated sensory fibers innervating the skin. C fibers primarily convey information about noxious levels of temperature, pressure, or chemical stimulation to the central nervous system. Pain mediated by C fibers tends to be a sustained, somewhat diffuse burning or aching sensation.

Calcitonin Gene-Related Peptide (CGRP).   A peptide, secreted by the nerve endings of C fibers, that contributes to the neurogenic inflammation of blood vessels in migraine. In part, CGPR works indirectly, by stimulating the release of histamine by mast cells.

Calcium Channel Antagonists (Calcium Channel Blockers).   Drugs that prevent the influx of calcium into cardiac and smooth muscle cells. Calcium channel blockers prevent arterial spasms and seem to affect neurotransmission.

Catastrophization.   A response to stresses characterized by helplessness, rumination, and an exaggerated sense of negative consequences. In chronic pain, catastrophizing seems to be a risk factor for depression, disability, and increased pain.

Caudal.   Towards the "tail." In the central nervous system of humans, this is the direction from prefrontal cortex through the thalamus and hypothalamus, the brain stem, and down the spine.

Central Pain Syndrome.   A state of persistent pain due to damage in the central nervous system, often the thalamus.

Cervicogenic Headache.   A headache in which the pain is referred from, or spreads from, the neck.

Channelopathy.   A disorder due to alterations in the functioning of ion channels. Typically, channelopathies involve changes in the excitability of neurons.

Cholecystokinin.   A peptide neurotransmitter. In the gastrointestinal tract it signals satiety. In the central nervous system it is used in pathways that oppose the effects of endorphins and opiate medications.

Chronic Pain Syndrome.   The combination of chronic pain, distress, and disability. In chronic pain syndrome, deficits in pain coping are thought to contribute to the impact of the pain, and possibly to the pain itself, through behavioral (e.g., activity avoidance) and cognitive- emotional (e.g., catastrophizing, anxious vigilance to pain) mechanisms.

Cognitive Distortions.   Characteristic biases or errors in appraising situations or oneself, that lead to emotional responses rather than effective problem solving. Typical examples include over-simplified, black-and-white thinking, and overgeneralization from a single negative event.

Cognitive Therapy.   A form of psychotherapy in which one reduces distress and increases adaptive functioning by modifying beliefs, appraisals, and problem solving.

Cold Pressor Task.   A procedure in which a subject is asked to immerse their hand or arm in ice water. The cold pressor task is used as an experimental intervention to raise blood pressure, or for producing an ischemic-like pain.

Conditioned Taste Aversion.   Aversion to a food, learned when the food is followed by nausea. Conditioned taste aversion is an unusually rapid form of classical (Pavlovian) conditioning.

Confirmatory Bias.   Selectively perceiving or assigning importance to instances that support one's beliefs.

Construct Validity.   In psychometric theory, the extent to which a scale is measuring the intended property. Evidence for construct validity accrues when the scale correlates with similar constructs, does not correlate with divergent constructs, and relates to independent variables in the way expected of the construct.

Conversion Disorder.   Symptoms or deficits in sensory or voluntary motor function that are thought to be initiated or exacerbated by psychological factors.

Coping.   As per Lazarus and Folkman (1984), the cognitive and behavioral activities by which a person seeks to manage stressful environmental demands and/or the emotions generated by those demands.

Corticotropin-Releasing Factor (CRF; also called Corticotropin-Releasing Hormone).   A polypeptide hormone secreted by the hypothalamus in response to stress. Corticotropin-releasing factor causes the pituitary to produce adrenocorticotropic hormone (ACTH), which in turn stimulates the adrenal cortex to produce cortisol, a key part of the stress response. CRF is also used as a neurotransmitter in the locus coeruleus and the dorsal horn, and may regulate the activity of mast cells.

Cortisol.   A hormone secreted by the adrenal cortex. Stress causes a sharp increase in cortisol release, which raises blood glucose levels, suppresses immune functioning, and activates the sympathetic nervous system, among other effects.

Cross-tolerance.   The tendency for reduced effectiveness of one drug, from repeated administration, to also reduce the effectiveness of another drug.

Cytokines.   Small proteins, secreted mostly by white blood cells, which help coordinate the immune response. Certain cytokines attract, stimulate, induce proliferation of, or otherwise affect other white blood cells, and help to regulate the inflammatory response.

Degranulation.   Large-scale secretion of histamine and other chemicals by mast cells.

Diffuse Noxious Inhibitory Controls (DNIC).   A reflexive decrease in sensitivity, caused by a painful stimulus, for pain elsewhere in the body. DNIC is mediated by endorphinergic pathways. In DNIC, pain of moderate severity is especially attenuated.

Discriminative Stimulus.   In behavior theory, an environment or event that increases the probability of a behavior by signaling that the behavior is likely to be reinforced. The reinforcement may be positive (reward) or negative (escape or avoidance).

Dissociation.   A usually reversible alteration in an aspect of consciousness due to psychological factors. Examples include loss of autobiographical memory (psychogenic amnesia), personal identity (dissociative identity disorder and fugue), or aspects of sensory or motor functioning (conversion).

Diving Reflex.   A set of automatic adjustments made by mammals in response to immersion of the face, or to cooling of the forehead. The diving reflex resembles the relaxation response in some respects (e.g., decreased heart rate) but not others (peripheral vasoconstriction in diving vs. vasodilation during relaxation).

Dorsal Horn.   Part of the grey matter of the spinal cord, the dorsal horn provides early, sophisticated processing of somatosensory information, including nociception. It is the first place where somatosensory nerves connect with the central nervous system. The dorsal horn is highly interconnected with brain stem nuclei, with which it exchanges bi-directional influence.

Dorsal Raphe Nucleus.   A group of serotonin-containing neurons, in the brain stem close to midline, with projections to higher brain centers. The dorsal raphe nucleus seems to be involved in sleep and dreaming, aggression, the control of blood flow to the brain, and the generation of migraine attacks.

Effect Size.   A standardized measure of the impact of an independent variable on a dependent variable. For a 2-group treatment study, effect size is usually calculated as $(M_T - M_C)/S_C$, where M_T is the mean of the treatment group, M_C is the mean of the control group, and S_C is the standard deviation of the control group.

Electromyography (EMG).   Recording the electrical activity of a muscle. In surface EMG, the recording electrodes are placed on the skin, to gauge the force of muscle contraction. In needle EMG, the electrode is inserted into a muscle to obtain diagnostic information from a single motor unit.

Endothelin.   A relatively small molecule (a 21-amino acid polypeptide) produced by the inner lining of blood vessels, causing the vessels to constrict. Endothelin helps limit bleeding after an injury. It also helps regulate cerebral blood flow and may play a role in migraines.

Endorphins.   A group of peptide neurotransmitters used in certain descending pain inhibitory pathways. The endorphins include leu- and met-enkephalin, dynorphin, and beta-endorphin. They are thought to play a role in stress-induced analgesia, diffuse noxious inhibitory controls, and certain forms of placebo pain reduction.

Enkephalins.   A group of peptide neurotransmitters involved in descending pain control. They are functionally related to the endorphins and are often subsumed under them.

Enmeshment.   In family therapy, overidentification among family members, such that individual identities are lost.

Entorhinal Cortex.   A small fold in the inner (medial), basal part of the temporal lobe. Entorhinal cortex is part of the input pathway to an adjacent fold, the hippocampus, important in memory formation.

Enzyme Induction.   The increase in activity of an enzyme when its substrate has been plentiful. Enzyme induction is one potential mechanism underlying drug tolerance. In general, enzymes that are free in the cellular fluid, and not those that are bound to membranes, show induction.

Epinephrine.   Also known as adrenaline. A stress hormone produced by the adrenal medulla. Epinephrine participates in a number of aspects of the fight-or-flight response, including increased heart rate and stroke volume, dilation of arteries in the heart and skeletal muscles, release of glucose from the liver, bronchodilation, and decreased gastric motility.

Event-Related Potential.   Slight but reproducible changes in the EEG signal that follow the presentation of a stimulus. Event-related potentials are divided into components such as N100, a negative shift in voltage occurring roughly 100 msec after the stimulus.

Evoked Potential.   Those event-related potentials thought to be largely determined by the sensory characteristics of the eliciting stimulus. Event-related potentials that depend more on a person's response to the stimulus, or on their cognitive set, would not be considered evoked potentials.

Exteroceptive Suppression Reflex (ESR).   A reflexive decrease in jaw-closing muscle activity in response to a noxious stimulus near the mouth. A nociceptive jaw-opening reflex. The ESR is comprised of early (ES1) and late (ES2) phases.

Extravasation.   Leakage. In migraine, plasma proteins extravasate into the dura mater, causing it to swell and become irritated.

Feverfew.   A bushy, flowering plant, native to Europe, whose leaves have been used as a migraine preventive.

Fibromyalgia.   A syndrome of chronic, widespread soft-tissue pain, with tenderness of at least 11 of 18 characteristic points on the body.

Fourier Analysis.   A mathematical formula for analyzing a complex waveform into its component frequencies.

Gate Control Model.   A model of pain processing in the dorsal horn of the spinal cord, proposed by Ronald Melzack and Patrick Wall. In the theory, large-diameter nerve fibers, which convey information on non-noxious levels of pressure, trigger inhibitory processes that tend to block pain transmission.

Gene Polymorphism.   A variation in the structure of a gene, occurring with some frequency in the population. (Rare variations are usually termed "mutations" instead.) Polymorphisms can involve deletion or insertion of a base pair from the gene's DNA sequence, or the substitution of one base pair by another.

Glutamate.   An excitatory neurotransmitter used throughout the central nervous system, including in pain processing.

Glycine.   An inhibitory neurotransmitter, found particularly in the spinal cord.

Graded Exposure.   A therapeutic technique in which an irrational fear is overcome by purposefully encountering and habituating to progressively more fear-provoking instances.

Hardiness.   A resistance to the effects of stress, derived from a tendency to see the stresses as challenges (vs. threats) and as controllable, and from a commitment to a cause greater than oneself.

Hassles.   Minor daily stresses. Because of their high frequency, hassles are thought to have considerable cumulative impact on stress-related disorders, especially if the hassles interact with areas of personal vulnerability.

Histamine.   An inflammatory chemical, released by mast cells, especially in injured tissue, that causes pain sensitization, vasodilation, and swelling. Histamine also constricts the bronchia, lowers blood pressure, triggers gastric secretion, and functions as a neurotransmitter.

Hydrophilic.   Water soluble.

Hyperalgesia.   Heightened sensitivity to pain. Hyperalgesia may be localized, e.g., to a site of injury, or widespread, e.g., in certain infections and in syndromes such as fibromyalgia.

Hyperpathia.   The abnormal persistence of pain after the inciting stimulus has been withdrawn. Generally also includes hyperalgesia.

Hypnosis.   A condition of deep relaxation, focused attention, suspension of critical judgment, and increased suggestibility. Especially in individuals of high hypnotic susceptibility, hypnotic suggestions of analgesia can produce marked reductions in acute pain. The underlying neurophysiology seems to show considerable individual differences.

Hypoalgesia.   Diminished sensitivity to pain.

Imaginal Desensitization.   A form of graded exposure, in which vivid images of a feared object or situation are paired with deep relaxation.

Infarct.   Tissue death caused by insufficient blood supply.

Insula.   A region of cortex, buried behind the lateral (Sylvian) fissure, medial to the temporal and frontal lobes.

Interictal.   Between attacks; during the interval between migraines.

Internal Consistency.   In classical psychological test theory, the degree to which a scale is reliable, precise, and free of random error.

Item Response Theory.   An approach to psychological test construction in which the probability of endorsing an item is modeled as a function of the underlying trait. For example, on an aptitude test, the probability of passing an easy item would rise sharply at low levels of ability. Knowing this function for each item allows one to fine-tune the discriminative power of the test.

Intrafusal Fibers.   Small skeletal muscle fibers that have, at their center, nerve endings sensing the amount and speed of muscle contraction. Intrafusal fibers are the main constituent of muscle spindles.

Ischemia.   A reduction in local blood flow to a level that impairs tissue viability.

Kinesiophobia.   In chronic pain, a fearful avoidance of movement or activity.

Life Events.   Significant occurrences in a person's life that are, on average, stressful, because they require a large psychosocial readjustment. Examples can be either positively or negatively toned, and include marriage, promotion, divorce, and death of a family member.

Lisinopril.   A blood pressure medication that works by blocking the enzyme that produces angiotensin II (angiotensin-converting enzyme).

Locus Coeruleus.   Literally, the "blue place," from how it appears in dissections (Lance, 1998), the locus coeruleus is a brain stem nucleus that forms part of the sympathetic nervous system. Among other effects, the locus coeruleus raises the level of activation at the cerebral cortex.

Locus of Control.   A generalized belief about the degree to which a desired outcome depends on one's own behavior. People with an internal locus of control believe that their behavior plays a key role. They seem to be more resilient to stress and more problem-focused in their coping than individuals with an external locus of control.

Macrophages.   Large immune system cells that derive from white blood cells, reside in the tissues, and destroy pathogens by engulfing them.

Magnetic Resonance Spectroscopy (MRS).   A noninvasive technique, performed along with magnetic resonance imaging, to shed light on the chemical composition of tissues in the body. In MRS, one studies the absorption and release of radiowave energy by the nuclei of hydrogen atoms. The amount of absorbed energy depends on the number of hydrogen nuclei, and the frequency of absorbed energy depends on which atoms are close to the hydrogen. Thus, different molecules have different spectra or signatures.

Masking.   Blocking of perception of one stimulus by another. By studying the effects of different types of masking stimuli, perception can be divided into non-interacting components or "channels."

Mast Cells.   Cells that resemble white blood cells, but that reside in tissues such as skin and mucous membranes, and around blood vessels. When stimulated, mast cells secrete histamine, serotonin, heparin, and other chemicals, and are involved in inflammation, especially allergic inflammation.

Mechanical Allodynia.   The experience of innocuous levels of pressure as painful.

Mechanoreceptors.   Receptors, particularly in the skin, muscles, and joints, that respond to the level of applied pressure.

Meta-analysis.   Statistically combining the results of separate investigations to determine the presence and magnitude of an effect. Meta-analysis is often used to examine whether or to what extent a particular treatment works.

Migraine.   A disorder characterized by discrete attacks of moderate-to-severe pulsating head pain, nausea, sometimes vomiting, and intolerance of light, sound, odors, and even minor exertion.

Migraine Generator.   A group of brain stem nuclei, including the locus coeruleus, the solitary tract nucleus, and the dorsal raphe nucleus, whose activity is thought to produce migraine episodes. Among migraine treatments, only sleep seems to reduce activity in the migraine generator region.

Miosis.   Constriction of the pupil. When it occurs in only one eye, it raises the possibility of an impairment of the local sympathetic nerves on the affected side.

Mitochondria.   The organelles within cells that utilize glucose to produce high energy phosphate compounds. These compounds are then used by the cell to drive chemical reactions. Mitochondria have their own DNA, and hence are the source of certain genetic diseases.

MMPI.   Minnesota Multiphasic Personality Inventory. A broad-based, well validated psychometric instrument used to predict symptomatology and personality functioning.

Modeling.   Teaching a new skill or competency through demonstration. Learning the mechanics, appropriateness, or value of a skill through observation.

Monoamines.   A chemical formed by removing certain atoms (the carboxyl group) from an amino acid. A number of important neurotransmitters are monoamines, including dopamine, norepinephrine, serotonin, and histamine.

Muscle Spindles.   Sensory receptors within muscles that detect stretch (the amount and velocity of muscle lengthening), contributing to awareness of body position and helping to regulate muscle tone. Possibly, muscle spindles may sometimes generate a pain signal, and may be the anatomical basis for trigger points.

Myocardial Infarction.   Heart attack; the loss of heart muscle due to an interruption in its blood supply.

Myofascial Pain Syndrome.   A syndrome in which pain from a muscle or its surrounding fascia, stiff, painful movement, and trigger point activity are prominent.

N-Acetylaspartate (NAA).   A brain chemical, involved in the production of myelin, synthesis of proteins, and processing of neurotransmitters. Because NAA is present almost exclusively in mature, living neurons, and because it can be detected via magnetic resonance spectroscopy, it provides a noninvasive index of neuronal integrity in a given region.

Neural Networks.   Models of brain functioning in which a mental process is represented as a pattern of activation across nodes, or a change in the strength of inconnections among nodes. Thus, a memory trace might be represented as a pattern of activation, and learning might be modeled as a change in interconnections. Usually, the nodes are meant to be analogous to neurons, the inconnections to synapses, and activation is meant to resemble neural firing rates.

Neuralgia.   Intense, paroxysmal, recurrent pain in the distribution of a nerve. The pain usually has a stabbing, lancinating quality.

Neuromuscular Junction.   The part of the muscle where motor nerves synapse on muscle fibers. When a motor nerve fires, it releases acetylcholine at the neuromuscular junction, initiating muscle contraction.

Neuropathy.   Disease or damage affecting peripheral, cranial, or autonomic nerves.

Neuropeptide.   A molecule, comprised of amino acid units, released by nerve cells when they fire. As neurotransmitters, neuropeptides have long-lasting effects on the post-synaptic cell. Neuropeptides may also stimulate mast cells of the immune system and smooth muscle cells of the blood vessels.

Nitric Oxide.   A small, gaseous molecule. It is produced by nerve cells as a neurotransmitter, including along pain pathways. It is also produced by the inner lining of blood vessels as a vasodilator, and by cells throughout the body as a defense against pathogens, especially viruses.

NMDA Receptor.   A type of receptor for the neurotransmitter glutamate. Stimulation of NMDA- type receptors helps trigger long-term changes in the synapse, thought to underlie such processes as learning, memory, and central pain sensitization.

Nocebo Effect.   The elicitation of pain or other symptoms by an inert treatment, presumably through expectancy or classical conditioning.

Nociceptive.   Pertaining to the transduction and processing of information about noxious stimuli. Nociceptive processes may or may not give rise to the conscious experience of pain, depending on such variables as the state of the organism.

Nociceptive Flexion Reflex.   A reflexive withdrawal, e.g., of a limb, from a noxious stimulus.

Nonsteroidal Anti-inflammatory Drugs (NSAIDs).   A class of medications that block prostaglandin synthesis by inhibiting the cyclooxygenase enzyme. Aspirin was the first NSAID.

Norepinephrine.   A neurotransmitter found in particular in the sympathetic nervous system. Peripheral effects of norepinephrine include facets of the fight-or-flight response: increased heart rate and stroke volume, constriction of arteries and blood vessels in the skin, bronchodilation, and decreased gastric motility. Also known as noradrenaline.

Odds Ratio.   Odds are the probability an event will occur, divided by the probability the event will not occur. Thus, if the probability of contracting a disease is .75, the odds of contracting the disease are .75/.25, or 3 to 1.When a study has two or more conditions, the ratio of the odds in one condition to the odds in another condition tells the comparative risk associated with the two conditions. Odds ratios are often used to describe the degree to which exposure to a trigger or risk factor increases the probability of contracting a disease.

Oligemia.   A modest reduction in blood flow, too small to inhibit the functioning or threaten the viability of the affected tissue. Migrainous aura may be associated with a spreading cortical oligemia thought to reflect a spreading depression of neural activity.

On Cells.   Neurons in the rostroventromedial medulla (RVM) that seem to facilitate nociceptive transmission in the spinal cord.

On-center, Off-surround.   An organization of a neuron's receptive field in which stimulation of the center of the field activates the neuron, while stimulation of the periphery inhibits the neuron.

Oxidative Stress.   In a cell, a condition in which there is increased exposure to highly reactive electron-drawing molecules (free radicals) or impaired defenses against these molecules, leading to cellular damage. Certain transition metals, such as iron, can catalyze this damage.

Pacing.   In pain management, moderating and patterning activity, so that rest breaks are used to prevent flare-ups.

Pain.   As per the International Association for the Study of Pain: "An unpleasant sensory and emotional experience associated with actual or potential tissue damage, or described in terms of such damage" (Merskey & Bogduk, 1994, p. 210). Thus, pain has both sensory and affective qualities. Note, too, that pain is a percept: Tissue damage does not always cause pain, and pain need not arise from tissue damage.

Pain Behaviors.   Actions such as wincing, grimacing, grunting, limping, bracing, and guarding, which communicate pain. In acute conditions, pain behaviors express pain, of course. In some theories, pain behaviors can become functionally autonomous in chronic pain, and independently increase pain or disability.

Paresthesia.   A tingling, pins-and-needles sensation. It may be part of a migraine aura, or caused by nerve damage or medications that affect nerve function, or it may be the temporary result of compression (as when one's foot falls asleep).

Peptide.   A molecule comprised of two or more amino acids strung together. Those peptides used as neurotransmitters generally consist of 5–10 amino acid units.

Periaqueductal Gray.   A region in the midbrain, near the cerebral aqueduct. Neurons in the periaqueductal gray are involved in aggression and in inhibiting pain transmission.

Phantom Limb Pain.   Pain experienced in an extremity that has already been amputated.

Phonophobia.   Painful aversion to sound.

Photophobia.   Painful aversion to light.

Phytoestrogens.   Plant-derived flavonoids that have activity at estrogen receptors. Phytoestrogens also seem to affect androgen metabolism.

Post-Herpetic Neuralgia.   Persistent nerve pain following shingles, a rash caused by the chickenpox virus.

Posttraumatic Stress Disorder (PTSD).   An anxiety disorder produced by exposure to or witnessing of an event that caused or threatened serious physical harm or death. Symptoms of PTSD include persistent reexperiencing of the trauma (e.g., in distressing dreams or intrusive recollections), avoidance of stimuli associated with the trauma, and persistent increased arousal.

Power Function.   A mathematical equation of the form $P = S^X$. In many sensory modalities, the perceived intensity (P) of a stimulus is a power function of the stimulus' physical intensity (S). The exponent, X, is different for different sensory modalities.

Priming.   The increase in a particular response to a stimulus from prior exposure to the same or different stimulus. For example, exposure to pictures depicting physical harm may increase subsequent pain in a laboratory experiment.

Problem Solving Therapy.   A clinical intervention in which one seeks to reduce distress, buffer the negative impact of environmental demands, and maximize functioning by teaching fundamental skills for handling difficult situations, especially social situations.

Prostaglandins.   Locally acting hormones, derived from a fatty acid (arachidonic acid), that sensitize nerve endings, facilitate pain transmission, and contribute to inflammation. They are involved in other processes as well, such as regulation of blood coagulability.

Psychophysics.   The quantitative study of the relationship between the physical characteristics of a stimulus and the resulting sensory or perceptual experience. The equation giving pain intensity as a function of stimulus temperature is an example of a psychophysical result.

Psychophysiology.   The study of the influence of psychological variables, such as thoughts or emotions, on physiological processes. The effects of fear on heart rate or blood vessel diameter, and the effects of depression on immune functioning, are in the domain of psychophysiology.

Ptosis.   A drooping, loss of strength, in the upper eyelid.

R-III Nociceptive Reflex.   A withdrawal reflex triggered by stimulation of small diameter sensory nerves in a muscle. Because RIII is a spinal reflex, its magnitude can provide information on sensitization of very early pain-processing structures, especially in the dorsal horn.

Receptive Field.   The area of the retina, skin, cochlea, or other sensory apparatus, to which a given neuron responds.

Reflex Sympathetic Dystrophy.   A syndrome, typically of a limb, involving intense pain, guarding, changes in skin texture, sensitivity to brushing or stroking, and often swelling, temperature changes, and abnormal sweating. Officially termed Complex Regional Pain Syndrome (CRPS) Type I. When nerve damage can be demonstrated, the condition is termed causalgia, or CRPS II.

Retroperitoneal.   At the back of the abdominal cavity.

Rostral.   Towards the beak. In the human central nervous system, this is the direction from the coccyx (tailbone), up the spine and brain stem, and through the hypothalamus and thalamus to prefrontal cortex.

Schema.   In cognitive psychology, a coherent, organized internal representation of knowledge whose activation underlies expectation, perception, memory, and problem solving.

Self-Efficacy.   The belief that one has the capability in a given area to effect a desired outcome. The belief that problems in an area are surmountable, and that one's efforts will ultimately meet with success. Self-efficacy is thought to lead to positive affect, persistence, and mastery of tasks, and a willingness to take on challenges that lead to growth.

Serotonin.   *See* 5-Hydroxytryptamine.

Skin Conductance Level (SCL).   The degree to which skin, particularly at the palm, allows the passage of a very small electric current. SCL reflects the activity of eccrine sweat glands, which are innervated by the sympathetic nervous system. The psychological correlate of SCL is mental activity, which is raised by such factors as novelty, interest, hypervigilance, and stress.

Skin Conductance Responses.   Small, brief increases in the skin's electrical conductance, often in response to a stimulus. The SCR is a component of orienting and defensive responses.

Solitary Tract Nucleus (STN).   A group of neurons in the medulla involved in processing visceral sensory information and in autonomic responding. Part of the parasympathetic nervous system, the STN seems to be involved in the nausea and vomiting associated with migraine.

Stepped Care.   A strategy in which treatment begins with a low intensity intervention, and escalates until a good response is achieved.

Sternocleidomastoid.   A large muscle, extending diagonally down the side of the neck, used for turning and for bowing the head (cervical rotation and flexion).

Stratified Care.   An intervention strategy in which individuals are allocated to treatments of different intensities based on the severity or intrusiveness of their symptoms.

Stress.   As per Lazarus and Folkman (1984), a transaction or relationship with the environment in which the demands are seen as endangering well being by taxing or exceeding one's coping resources. In this model, stress can be reduced by increasing one's coping resources or by changing one's appraisals, as appropriate.

Stress-Induced Analgesia.   A temporary but sometimes profound reduction in pain sensitivity during and after a severe stressor.

Stress Management.   Techniques that increase coping, typically by changing how stressors are appraised, by increasing one's skills for resolving them, and by managing arousal (e.g., relaxation skills).

Substance P.   A neurotransmitter with long-lasting effects on the receiving (post-synaptic) cell. Substance P is involved in neurotransmission from C fibers into the dorsal horn, and in triggering the neurogenic inflammation of cranial blood vessels in migraine and cluster headache.

Substantia Gelatinosa.   Lamina II (the next-to-outermost layer) of the dorsal horn of the spinal cord. The substantia gelatinosa is dense with interneurons, and is thought to be the site of local pain processing in the spine.

Tender Point.   A small area in soft tissue that is painful to moderate pressure. Certain tender points are felt to be characteristic of fibromyalgia. Unlike trigger points, tender points need not refer pain or cause autonomic symptoms.

TENS (Transcutaneous Electrical Nerve Stimulation).   A method of pain control in which an electrical stimulus is applied to the skin, from a small device worn on the patient's belt. The effects of TENS seem to be mediated in part by endorphinergic pathways. In particular, low frequency TENS shows cross-tolerance with morphine.

Thought Suppression.   Deliberately attempting to exclude a particular thought or experience from consciousness. Sustained thought suppression is very difficult and often produces the opposite effect.

Tinnitus.   An illusory ringing, rushing, or buzzing sound in the ears.

Transcranial Doppler.   The determination of blood flow velocity in a cranial artery from changes in the frequency of ultrasound wave reflected back by the blood. If the amount of blood flow remains constant, velocity can be used to infer blood vessel diameter.

Transcranial Magnetic Stimulation (TMS).   Application of strong magnetic pulses from a coil positioned near the head. The pulses cause nerve cells in the cerebral cortex to fire, which can be detected by the subject as, e.g., flashes of light, or by machine as, e.g., changes in muscle tension. TMS can be used to study cortical excitability, inhibition, and facilitation, and conduction along motor pathways. Experimentally, repetitive pulses of TMS have been proposed as a psychiatric treatment, for altering brain function in specific regions.

Transformed Migraine.   A type of chronic daily headache in which episodic migraine has evolved into frequent tension-type headaches with migrainous flare-ups.

Trigeminal Nucleus Caudalis.   A region in the lower medulla, just above the spine, in which nociceptive information from the head is first processed. The trigeminal nucleus caudalis is analogous to, and an extension of, the dorsal horn of the spine.

Trigger Points.   Small, irritable regions of muscle, located in taut bands, that are highly pain sensitive. When pressed, trigger points refer pain or other symptoms (e.g., numbness, or change in blood flow) in characteristic patterns. Certain trigger points can also cause autonomic symptoms such as dizziness or nausea.

Triptan.   Any of a number of antimigraine drugs that stimulate two types of serotonin receptors: 1B (constricting cranial arteries) and 1D (blocking neurogenic inflammation of the blood vessels and possibly inhibiting pain transmission in the trigeminal nucleus). A selective 5-$HT_{1B/D}$ receptor agonist.

Type A Behavior Pattern.   A generalized approach characterized by intense achievement motivation, competitiveness, time pressure, and proneness to anger.

Tyramine.   A substance found in certain foods, derived from the amino acid tyrosine. In the body, tyramine seems to function as a dopamine and norepinephrine reuptake inhibitor, and probably also as a neurotransmitter.

Vertigo.   The sensation that one's surroundings are spinning, tilting, or otherwise in movement.

Wide Dynamic Range Neurons.   Neurons in the dorsal horn that respond to both noxious levels of pressure and mild, innocuous pressure. Because wide dynamic range neurons receive both types of input, they are thought to be involved in pain sensitization to innocuous pressure.

Zygapophyseal Joints.   The hinges between vertebrae that allow the spine to bend. Also called facet joints.

References

Aaron, L. A., Burke, M. M., & Buchwald, D. (2000). Overlapping conditions among patients with chronic fatigue syndrome, fibromyalgia, and temporomandibular disorder. *Archives of Internal Medicine, 160,* 221–227.

Abdel-Dayem, H. M., Abu-Judeh, H., Kumar, M., Atay, S., Naddaf, S., El-Zeftawy, H., & Luo, J. (1998). SPECT brain perfusion abnormalities in mild or moderate traumatic brain injury. *Clinical Nuclear Medicine, 23,* 309–317.

Abu-Arafeh, I. (2001). Chronic tension-type headache in children and adolescents. *Cephalalgia, 21,* 830–836.

Abu-Arafeh, I., & Callaghan, M. (2004). Short migraine attacks of less than 2 h duration in c children and adolescents. *Cephalalgia, 24,* 333–338.

Abu-Arefeh, I., & Russell, G. (1994). Prevalence of headache and migraine in schoolchildren. *British Journal of Medicine, 309,* 765–769.

Abu-Arafeh, I., & Russell, G. (1995a). Cyclical vomiting syndrome in children: A population-based study. *Journal of Pediatric Gastroenterology and Nutrition, 21,* 454–458.

Abu-Arafeh, I., & Russell, G. (1995b). Paroxysmal vertigo as a migraine equivalent in children: A population-based study. *Cephalalgia, 15,* 22–25.

Achterberg, J. (1984). Imagery and medicine: Psychophysiological speculations. *Journal of Mental Imagery, 8,* 1–14.

Ad Hoc Committee on Classification of headache. (1962). Classification of headache. *Journal of the American Medical Association, 179,* 717–718.

Adams, R. D., Victor, M., & Ropper, A. H. (1997). *Principles of Neurology* (6th ed.). New York: McGraw-Hill.

Adelman, L. C., Adelman, J. U., Von Seggern, R., & Mannix, L. K. (2000). Venlafaxine extended release (XR) for the prophylaxis of migraine and tension-type headache: A retrospective study in a clinical setting. *Headache, 40,* 572–580.

Adelman, J. U., Lipton, R. B., Ferrari, M. D., Diener, H.-C., McCarroll, K. A., Vandormael, K., & Lines, C. R. (2001). Comparison of rizatriptan and other triptans on stringent measures of efficacy. *Neurology, 57,* 1377–1383.

Ader, R. (1997). The role of conditioning in pharmacotherapy. In A. Harrington (Ed.), *The placebo effect: An interdisciplinary exploration* (pp. 138–165). Cambridge, MA: Harvard University Press.

Adler, A. (1931). *What life should mean to you* (A. Porter, Ed.). Boston: Little, Brown & Company.

Adler, C. S., & Adler, S. M. (1976). Biofeedback-psychotherapy for the treatment of headaches: A 5-year follow-up. *Headache, 16,* 189–191.

Adler, C. S., & Adler, S. M. (1984). A 10 year follow-up with control group of psychotherapy and physiological feedback for migraine. *Headache, 24,* 167.

Adler, C. S., & Adler, S. M. (1987). Psychodynamics of migraine: A developmental perspective. In C. S. Adler, S. M. Adler, & R. C. Packard (Eds.), *Psychiatric aspects of headache* (pp. 158–180). Baltimore, MD: Williams and Wilkins.

Adler, C. S., Adler, S. M., & Friedman, A. P. (1987). A historical perspective on psychiatric thinking about headache. In C. S. Adler, S. M. Adler, & R. C. Packard (Eds.), *Psychiatric aspects of headache* (pp. 3–21). Baltimore, MD: Williams and Wilkins.

Adly, C., Straumarus, J., & Chesson, A. (1992). Fluoxetine prophylaxis of migraine. *Headache, 32,* 101–104.

Affleck, G., Tennen, H., Urrows, S., & Higgins, P. (1994). Person and contextual features of daily stress reactivity: Individual differences in relations of undesirable daily events with mood disturbance and chronic pain intensity. *Journal of Personality and Social Psychology, 66*, 329–340.

Afra, J., Mascia, A., Gérard, P., Maertens de Noordhout, A., & Schoenen, J. (1998). Interictal cortical excitability in migraine: A study using transcranial magnetic stimulation of motor and visual cortex. *Annals of Neurology, 44*, 209–215.

Afra, J., Proietti-Cecchini, A., DePasqua, V., Albert, A., & Schoenen, J. (1998). Visual evoked potentials during long periods of pattern-reversal stimulation in migraine. *Brain, 121*, 233–241.

Aghabeigi, B., Feinmann, C., Glover, V., Goodwin, B., Hannah, P., Harris, M., Sandler, M., & Wasil, M. (1993). Tyramine conjugation deficit in patients with chronic idiopathic temporomandibular joint and orofacial pain. *Pain, 54*, 159–163.

Ahles, T. A., King, A., & Martin, J. E. (1984). EMG biofeedback during dynamic movement as a treatment for tension headache. *Headache, 24*, 41–44.

Ahn, A. H., & Basbaum, A. I. (2005). Where do triptans act in the treatment of migraine? *Pain, 115*, 1–4.

Aida, S. (2005). The challenge of preemptive analgesia. *Pain: Clinical Updates, 13*(2), 1–4.

Aitken, P. G., Tombaugh, G. C., Turner, D. A., & Somjen, G. G. (1998). Similar propagation of SD and hypoxic SD-like depolarization in rat hippocampus recorded optically and electrically. *Journal of Neurophysiology, 80*, 1514–1521.

Åkesson, I., Hansson, G.-Å., Balogh, I., Moritz, U., & Skerfving, S. (1997). Quantifying work load in neck, shoulders and wrists in female dentists. *International Archives of Occupational and Environmental Health, 69*, 461–474.

Aktekin, B., Yaltkaya, K., Ozkaynak, S., & Oguz, Y. (2001). Recovery cycle of the blink reflex and exteroceptive suppression of temporalis muscle activity in migraine and tension-type headache. *Headache, 41*, 142–149.

Al'Absi, M., Petersen, K. L., & Wittmers, L. E. (2002). Adrenocortical and hemodynamic predictors of pain perception in men and women. *Pain, 96*, 197–204.

Al-Absi, M., & Rokke, P. D. (1991). Can anxiety help us tolerate pain? *Pain, 46*, 43–51.

Albertyn, J., Barry, R., & Odendaal, C. L. (2004). Cluster headache and the sympathetic nerve. *Headache, 44*, 183–185.

Alden, A. L., Dale, J. A., & DeGood, D. E. (2001). Interactive effects of the affect quality and directional focus of mental imagery on pain analgesia. *Applied Psychophysiology and Biofeedback, 26*, 117–126.

Alfvén, G., de la Torre, B., & Uvnäs-Moberg, K. (1994). Depressed concentrations of oxytocin and cortisol in children with recurrent abdominal pain of non-organic origin. *Acta Paediatrica, 83*, 1076–1080.

Ali, Z., Raja, S. N., Wesselmann, U., Fuchs, P. N., Meyer, R. A., & Campbell, J. N. (2000). Intradermal injection of norepinephrine evokes pain in patients with sympathetically maintained pain. *Pain, 88*, 161–168.

Alix, M. E., & Bates, D. K. (1999). A proposed etiology of cervicogenic headache: The neurophysiologic basis and anatomic relationship between the dura mater and the rectus posterior capitis minor muscle. *Journal of Manipulative and Physiological Therapeutics, 22*, 534–539.

Allen, A. M., Moeller, I., Jenkins, T. A., Zhuo, J., Aldred, G. P., Chai, S. Y., & Mendelsohn, F. A. O. (1998). Angiotensin receptors in the nervous system. *Brain Research Bulletin, 47*, 17–28.

Allen, K. D., & Shriver, M. D. (1997). Enhanced performance feedback to strengthen biofeedback treatment outcome with childhood migraine. *Headache, 37*, 169–173.

Allen, K. D., & Shriver, M. D. (1998). Role of parent-mediated pain behavior management strategies in biofeedback treatment of childhood migraines. *Behavior Therapy, 29*, 477–490.

Allen, M. T., & Crowell, M. D. (1990). The effects of paced respiration on cardiopulmonary responses to laboratory stressors. *Journal of Psychophysiology, 4*, 357–368.

Allen, M. T., Shelley, K. S., & Boquet, A. J., Jr. (1992). A comparison of cardiovascular and autonomic adjustments to three types of cold stimulation tasks. *International Journal of Psychophysiology, 13*, 59–69.

Almeida, A., Cobos, A., Tavares, I., & Lima, D. (2002). Brain afferents to the medullary dorsal reticular nucleus: A retrograde and anterograde tracing study in the rat. *European Journal of Neuroscience, 16*, 81–95.

Altura, B. M., & Altura, B. T. (1978). Magnesium and vascular tone and reactivity. *Blood Vessels, 15*, 5–16.

Amanzio, M., & Benedetti, F. (1999). Neuropharmacological dissection of placebo analgesia: Expectation-activated opioid systems versus conditioning-activated specific subsystems. *Journal of Neuroscience, 19*, 484–494.

Ambrosini, A., de Noordhout, A. M., & Schoenen, J. (2001). Neuromuscular transmission in migraine: A single-fiber EMG study in clinical subgroups. *Neurology, 56*, 1038–1043.

Ambrosini, A., Pierelli, F., & Schoenen, J. (2003). Acetazolamide acts on neuromuscular transmission abnormalities found in some migraineurs. *Cephalalgia, 23*, 75–78.

Ambrosini, A., Vandenheede, M., Rossi, P., Aloj, F., Sauli, E., Pierelli, F., & Schoenen, J. (2005). Suboccipital injection with a mixture of rapid- and long-acting steroids in cluster headache: A double-blind placebo-controlled study. *Pain, 118*, 92–96.

American Council for Headache Education. (1994). *Migraine: The complete guide.* New York: Dell.

American Psychiatric Association. (1994). *Diagnostic and statistical manual of mental disorders* (4th ed.). Washington, DC: Author.

Amit, Z., & Galina, Z. H. (1986). Stress-induced analgesia: Adaptive pain suppression. *Physiological Reviews, 66*, 1091–1120.

Anderson, C. D., & Franks, R. D. (1981). Migraine and tension headache: Is there a physiological difference? *Headache, 21*, 63–71.

Anderson, C. D., Stoyva, J. M., & Vaughn, L. J. (1982). A test of delayed recovery following stressful stimulation in four psychosomatic disorders. *Journal of Psychosomatic Research, 26*, 571–580.

Anderson, J. A. (1995). Mechanisms in adverse reactions to food: The brain *Allergy, 50* (20, suppl.), 78–81.

Anderson, J. A., & Rosenfeld, E. (1998). *Talking nets: An oral history of neural networks.* Cambridge, MA: MIT Press.

Andersson, G., Lundström, P., & Ström, L. (2003). Internet-based treatment of headache: Does telephone contact add anything? *Headache, 43*, 353–361.

Andersson, K. E., & Vinge, E. (1990). Beta-adrenoceptor blockers and calcium antagonists in the prophylaxis and treatment of migraine. *Drugs, 39*, 355–373.

Andersson, P. G. (1973). BC-105 and deseril in migraine prophylaxis: A double-blind study. *Headache, 13*, 68–73.

Andrasik, F., Blanchard, E. B., Arena, J. G., Saunders, N. L., & Barron, K. D. (1982). Psychophysiology of recurrent headache: Methodological issues and new empirical findings. *Behavior Therapy, 13*, 407–429.

Andrasik, F., Grazzi, L., Usai, S., D'Amico, D., Leone, M., & Bussone, G. (2003). Brief neurologist-administered behavioral treatment of pediatric episodic tension-type headache. *Neurology, 60*, 1215–1216.

Andrasik, F., & Holroyd, K. A. (1980). A test of specific and nonspecific effects in the biofeedback treatment of tension headache. *Journal of Consulting and Clinical Psychology, 48*, 575–586.

Andrasik, F., & Holroyd, K. A. (1983). Specific and nonspecific effects in the biofeedback treatment of tension headache: 3-year follow-up. *Journal of Consulting and Clinical Psychology, 51*, 634–636.

Andreassi, J. L. (1995). *Psychophysiology: Human behavior and physiological response* (3rd ed.). Hillsdale, NJ: Lawrence Erlbaum Associates.

Andreychuk, T., & Schriver, C. (1975). Hypnosis and biofeedback in the treatment of migraine headache. *International Journal of Clinical and Experimental Hypnosis, 23*, 172–183.

Angus-Leppan, H., Lambert, G. A., & Michalicek, J. (1997). Convergence of occipital nerve and superior sagittal sinus input in the cervical spinal cord of the cat. *Cephalalgia, 17*, 625–630.

Ansell, E., Fazzone, T., Festenstein, R., Johnson, E. S., Thavapalan, M., Wilkinson, M., & Wozniak, I. (1988). Nimodipine in migraine prophylaxis. *Cephalalgia, 8*, 269–272.

Anthony, M. (1992). Headache and the greater occipital nerve. *Clinical Neurology and Neurosurgery, 94*, 297–301.

Anthony, M. (2000). Cervicogenic headache: Prevalence and response to local steroid therapy. *Clinical and Experimental Rheumatology, 18*(2, Suppl. 19), s59–s64.

Anthony, M., & Lance, J. W. (1969). Monoamine oxidase inhibition in the treatment of migraine. *Archives of Neurology, 21*, 263–268.

Antonaci, F., Sand, T., & Lucas, G. A. (1998). Pressure algometry in healthy subjects: Inter-examiner variability. *Scandinavian Journal of Rehabilitation Medicine, 30*, 3–8.

Antonaci, F., & Sjaastad, O. (1992). Hemicrania continua: A possible symptomatic case, due to mesenchymal tumor. *Functional Neurology, 7*, 471–474.

Antozzi, C., Garavaglia, B., Mora, M., Rimoldi, M., Morandi, L., Ursino, E., et al. (1994). Late-onset riboflavin responsive myopathy with combined multiple acyl coenzyme: A dehydrogenase and respiratory chain deficiency. *Neurology, 44*, 2153–2158.

Anzola, G. P., Magoni, M., Guindani, M., Rozzini, L., & Dalla Volta, G. (1999). Potential source of cerebral embolism in migraine with aura: A transcranial doppler study. *Neurology, 52*, 1622–1625.

Apkarian, A. V., Sosa, Y., Krauss, B. R., Thomas, P. S., Fredrickson, B. E., Levy, R. E., Harden, R. N., & Chialvo, D. R. (2004). Chronic pain patients are impaired on an emotional decision-making task. *Pain, 108*, 129–136.

Apkarian, A. V., Sosa, Y., Sonty, S., Levy, R. M., Harden, R. N., Parrish, T. B., & Gitelman, D. R. (2004). Chronic back pain is associated with decreased prefrontal and thalamic gray matter density. *Journal of Neuroscience, 24*, 10410–10415.

Apkarian, A. V., Stea, R. A., & Bolanowski, S. J. (1994). Heat-induced pain diminishes vibrotactile perception: A touch gate. *Somatosensory and Motor Research, 11*, 259–267.

Arena, J. G., & Blanchard, E. B. (1996). Biofeedback and relaxation therapy for chronic pain disorders. In R. J. Gatchel & D. C. Turk (Eds.), *Psychological approaches to pain management: A practitioner's handbook* (pp. 179–230). New York: Guilford.

Arena, J. G., Blanchard, E. B., Andrasik, F., Appelbaum, K., & Myers, P. E. (1985). Psychophysiological comparisons of three kinds of headache subjects during and between headache states: Analysis of post-stress adaptation periods. *Journal of Psychosomatic Research, 29*, 427–441.

Arena, J. G., Bruno, G. M., Hannah, S. L., & Meador, K. J. (1995). A comparison of frontal electromyographic biofeedback training, trapezius electromyographic biofeedback training, and progressive muscle relaxation therapy in the treatment of tension headache. *Headache, 35*, 411–419.

Arena, J. G., Bruno, G. M., Rozantine, G. S., & Meador, K. J. (1997). A comparison of tension headache sufferers and nonpain controls on the State-Trait Anger Expression Inventory: An exploratory study with implications for applied psychophysiologists. *Applied Psychophysiology and Biofeedback, 22*, 209–214.

Arena, J. G., Hannah, S. L., Bruno, G. M., Smith, J. D., & Meador, K. J. (1991). Effect of movement and position on muscle activity in tension headache sufferers during and between headaches. *Journal of Psychosomatic Research, 35*, 187–195.

Arena, J. G., Sherman, R. A., Bruno, G. M., & Smith, J. D. (1990). The relationship between situational stress and phantom limb pain: Cross-lagged correlational data from six month pain logs. *Journal of Psychosomatic Research, 34*, 71–77.

Arezzo, J. C. (2002). Possible mechanisms for the effects of botulinum toxin on pain. *Clinical Journal of Pain, 18* (6, Supplement), s125–s132.

Arnold, L. M., Lu, Y., Crofford, L. J., Wohlreich, M., Detke, M. J., Iyengar, S., & Goldstein, D. J. (2004). A double-blind, multicenter trial comparing duloxetine with placebo in the treatment of fibromyalgia patients with or without major depressive disorder. *Arthritis and Rheumatism, 50*, 2974–2984.

Arntz, A., & Peters, M. (1995). Chronic low back pain and inaccurate predictions of pain: Is being too tough a risk factor for the development and maintenance of chronic pain? *Behaviour Research and Therapy, 33*, 49–53.

Arntz, A., Rauner, M., & van den Hout, M. (1995). "If I feel anxious, there must be danger": *Ex-consequentia* reasoning in inferring danger in anxiety disorders. *Behaviour Research and Therapy, 33*, 917–927.

Aromaa, M., Rautava, P., Helenius, H., & Sillanpää, M. L. (1998). Factors of early life as predictors of headache in children at school entry. *Headache, 38*, 23–30.

Aromaa, M., Sillanpää, M. L., Rautava, P., & Helenius, H. (1998). Childhood headache at school entry: A controlled clinical study. *Neurology, 50*, 1729–1736.

Aromaa, M., Sillanpää, M., Rautava, P., & Helenius, H. (2000). Pain experience of children with headache and their families: A controlled study. *Pediatrics, 106*, 270–275.

Asghari, M. A., & Nicholas, M. K. (1999). Personality and adjustment to chronic pain. *Pain Reviews, 6*, 85–97.

Ashina, M., Bendtsen, L., Jensen, R., Lassen, L. H., Sakai, F., & Olesen, J. (1999). Possible mechanisms of action of nitric oxide synthase inhibitors in chronic tension-type headache. *Brain, 122*, 1629–1635.

Ashina, M., Bendtsen, L., Jensen, R., Schifter, S., & Olesen, J. (2000). Evidence for increased plasma levels of calcitonin gene-related peptide in migraine outside of attacks. *Pain, 86*, 133–138.

Asmundson, G. J. G., Coons, M. J., Taylor, S., & Katz, J. (2002). PTSD and the experience of pain: Research and clinical implications of shared vulnerability and mutual maintenance models. *Canadian Journal of Psychiatry, 47*, 930–937.

Asmundson, G. J. G., Norton, P. J., & Veloso, F. (1999). Anxiety sensitivity and fear of pain in patients with recurring headaches. *Behaviour Research and Therapy, 37*, 703–713.

Asmundson, G. J. G., Wright, K. D., Norton, P. J., & Veloso, F. (2001). Anxiety sensitivity and other emotionality traits in predicting headache medication use in patients with recurring headaches. Implications for abuse and dependency. *Addictive Behaviors, 26*, 827–840.

Athwal, B. S., & Lennox, G. G. (1996). Acetazolamide responsiveness in familial hemiplegic migraine. *Annals of Neurology, 40*, 820–821.

Aurora, S. K., Ahmad, B. K., Welch, K. M. A., Bdardhwaj, P., & Ramadan, N. M. (1998). Transcranial magnetic stimulation confirms hyperexcitability of occipital cortex in migraine. *Neurology, 50*, 1111–1114.

Avicenna. (1930). Canon of medicine. In: O. C. Gruner, *A treatise on the Canon of medicine of Avicenna, incorporating a translation of the first book*. New York: AMS Press. (Original work published 11th century.)

Bakal, D. A. (1982). *The psychobiology of chronic headache*. New York: Springer Publishing Company.

Bakal, D., Demjen, S., & Duckro, P. N. (1994). Chronic daily headache and the elusive nature of somatic awareness. In R. C. Grzesiak & D. S. Ciccone (Eds.), *Psychological vulnerability to chronic pain*. New York: Springer Publishing Company.

Baldi, J. C., Aoina, J. L., Oxenham, H. C., Bagg, W., & Doughty, R. N. (2003). Reduced exercise arteriovenous O_2 difference in Type 2 diabetes. *Journal of Applied Physiology, 94*, 1033–1038.

Balottin, U., Nicoli, F., Pitillo, G., Ginevra, O. F., Borgatti, R., & Lanzi, G. (2004). Migraine and tension headache in children under 6 years of age. *European Journal of Pain, 8*, 307–314.

Bandell-Hoekstra, I. E., Abu-Saad, H. H., Passchier, J., Frederiks, C. M., Feron, F. J., & Knipschild, P. (2001). Prevalence and characteristics of headache in Dutch schoolchildren. *European Journal of Pain, 5*, 145–153.

Bandler, R., Price, J. L., & Keay, K. A. (2000). Brain mediation of active and passive emotional coping. In E. A. Mayer & C. B. Saper (Eds.), *The biological basis for mind body interactions. Progress in Brain Research, 122*, 333–349.

Bandura, A., O'Leary, A., Taylor, C. B., Gauthier, J., & Gossard, D. (1987). Perceived self-efficacy and pain control: Opioid and nonopioid mechanisms. *Journal of Personality and Social Psychology, 53*, 563–571.

Banks, S. L., Jacobs, D. W., Gevirtz, R., & Hubbard, D. R. (1998). Effects of autogenic relaxation training on electromyographic activity in active myofascial trigger points. *Journal of Musculoskeletal Pain, 6*, 23–32.

Bansevicius, D., & Sjaastad, O. (1996). Cervicogenic headache: The influence of mental load on pain level and EMG of shoulder-neck and facial muscles. *Headache, 36*, 372–378.

Bär, K.-J., Brehm, S., Boettger, M. K., Boettger, S., Wagner, G., & Sauer, H. (2005). Pain perception in major depression depends on pain modality. *Pain, 117*, 97–103.

Barlow, C. F. (1994). Migraine in the infant and toddler. *Journal of Child Neurology, 9*, 92–94.

Barlow, D. H. (1983). Announcement. *Behavior Therapy, 14*, 455–456.

Barnes, V. A., Treiber, F. A., Turner, J. R., Davis, H., & Strong, W. B. (1999). Acute effects of Transcendental Meditation on hemodynamic functioning in middle-aged adults. *Psychosomatic Medicine, 61*, 525–531.

Baron, J. C. (2001). Perfusion thresholds in human cerebral ischemia: Historical perspective and therapeutic implications. *Cerebrovascular Diseases, 11*(Suppl. 1), 2–8.

Barton, K. A., & Blanchard, E. B. (2001). The failure of intensive self-regulatory treatment with chronic daily headache: A prospective study. *Applied Psychophysiology and Biofeedback, 26*, 311–318.

Barton, P. M., & Hayes, K. C. (1996). Neck flexor muscle strength, efficiency, and relaxation times in normal subjects and subjects with unilateral neck pain and headache. *Archives of Physical Medicine and Rehabilitation, 77*, 680–687.

Baskin, S. M. (2001). Comments on Barton and Blanchard. *Applied Psychophysiology and Biofeedback, 26*, 329–330.

Basmajian, J. V., & De Luca, C. J. (1985). *Muscles alive: Their functions revealed by electromyography* (3rd ed.). Baltimore, MD: Williams & Wilkins.

Bathien, N. (1971). Reflexes spinaux chez l'homme et niveaux d'attention. *Electroencephalography and Clinical Neurophysiology, 30*, 32–37.

Bathien, N., & Hugelin, A. (1969). Reflexes monosynaptiques et polysynaptiques de l'homme au cours de l'attention. *Electroencephalography and Clinical Neurophysiology, 26*, 604–612.

Battelli, L., Black, K. R., & Wray, S. H. (2002). Transcranial magnetic stimulation of visual area V5 in migraine. *Neurology, 58*, 1066–1069.

Battistella, P. A., Bordin, A., Cernetti, R., Broetto, S., Corra, S., Piva, E., & Plebani, M. (1996). β-endorphin in plasma and monocytes in juvenile headache. *Headache, 36*, 91–94.

Battistella, P. A., Ruffilli, R., Cernetti, R., Pettenazzo, A., Baldin, L., Bertoli, S., & Zacchello, F. (1993). A placebo-controlled crossover trial using trazodone in pediatric migraine. *Headache, 33*, 36–39.

Bayer, T. L., Baer, P. E., & Early, C. (1991). Situational and psychophysiological factors in psychologically induced pain. *Pain, 44,* 45–50.

Bear, M. F., Connors, B. W., & Paradiso, M. A. (2001). *Neuroscience: Exploring the brain* (2nd ed.). Baltimore, MD: Lippincott Williams & Wilkins.

Beardwood, C. J., Abrahams, A., & Jordi, P. M. (1986). The effect of exposure to positive space charge on aversive responses to noxious stimuli in rats. *Life Sciences, 39,* 2359–2369.

Beck, A. T. (1976). *Cognitive therapy and the emotional disorders.* New York: International Universities Press.

Beck, A. T., Epstein, N., Brown, G., & Steer, R. A. (1988). An inventory for measuring clinical anxiety: Psychometric properties. *Journal of Consulting and Clinical Psychology, 56,* 893–897.

Beck, A. T., Rush, A. J., Shaw, B. F., & Emery, G. (1979). *Cognitive therapy of depression.* New York: Guilford.

Beck, A. T., Ward, C. H., Mendelson, M., Mock, J., & Erlbaugh, J. (1961). An inventory for measuring depression. *Archives of General Psychiatry, 4,* 53–63.

Beck, J. S. (1995). *Cogntive therapy: Basics and beyond.* New York: Guilford.

Beckham, J. C., Crawford, A. L., Feldman, M. E., Kirby, A. C., Hertzberg, M. A., Davidson, J. R. T., & Moore, S. D. (1997). Chronic Posttraumatic Stress Disorder and chronic pain in Vietnam combat veterans. *Journal of Psychosomatic Research, 43,* 379–389.

Beecher, H. K. (1946). Pain in men wounded in battle. *The Bulletin of the U.S. Army Medical Department, 5,* 445–454.

Behan, P. O. (1978). Isometheptene compound in the treatment of vascular headache. *The Practitioner, 221,* 937–939.

Behar, E., Alcaine, O., Zuellig, A. R., & Borkovec, T. D. (2003). Screening for generalized anxiety disorder using the Penn State Worry Questionnaire: A receiver operating characteristic analysis. *Journal of Behavior Therapy and Experimental Psychiatry, 34,* 25–43.

Belforte, J. E., Magariños-Azcone, C., Armando, I., Buño, W., & Pazo, J. H. (2001). Pharmacological involvement of the calcium channel blocker flunarizine in dopamine transmission at the striatum. *Parkinsonism and Related Disorders, 8,* 33–40.

Bellamy, R. (1997). Compensation neurosis. *Clinical Orthopedics and Related Research, 336,* 94–106.

Belton, O., Byrne, D., Kearney, D., Leahy, A., & Fitzgerald, D. J. (2000). Cyclooxygenase-1 and -2-dependent prostacyclin formation in patients with atherosclerosis. *Circulation, 102,* 840–845.

Bendtsen, L. (2003). Amitriptyline in the treatment of primary headaches. *Expert Review of Neurotherapeutics, 3,* 165–173.

Bendtsen, L., & Jensen, R. (2004). Mirtazapine is effective in the prophylactic treatment of chronic tension-type headache. *Neurology, 62,* 1706–1711.

Bendtsen, L., Jensen, R., Brennum, J, Arendt-Nielsen, L., & Olesen, J. (1996). Exteroceptive suppression of temporalis muscle activity is normal in chronic tension-type headache and not related to actual headache state. *Cephalalgia, 16,* 251–256.

Bendtsen, L., Jensen, R., & Olesen, J. (1996a). Amitriptyline, a combined serotonin and noradrenaline reuptake inhibitor, reduces exteroceptive suppression of temporal muscle activity in patients with chronic tension-type headache. *Electroencephalography and Clinical Neurophysiology, 101,* 418–422.

Bendtsen, L., Jensen, R., & Olesen, J. (1996b). Qualitatively altered nociception in chronic myofascial pain. *Pain, 65,* 259–264.

Bendtsen, L., Jensen, R., & Olesen, J. (1996c). A non-selective (amitriptyline), but not a selective (citalopram), serotonin reuptake inhibitor is effective in the prophylactic treatment of chronic tension-type headache. *Journal of Neurology, Neurosurgery, and Psychiatry, 61,* 285–290.

Benedetto, C., Allais, G., Ciochetto, D., & De Lorenzo, C. (1997). Pathophysiological aspects of menstrual migraine. *Cephalalgia, 17*(Suppl. 20), 32–34.

Bengtsson, A., & Bengtsson, M. (1988). Regional sympathetic blockade in primary fibromyalgia. *Pain, 33* (Suppl.), 161–167.

Benson, H. (1984). *Beyond the relaxation response.* New York: Times Books.

Benson, H., Klemchuk, H. P., & Graham, J. R. (1974). The usefulness of the relaxation response in the therapy of headache. *Headache, 14,* 49–52.

Bereiter, D. A., Stanford, L. R., & Barker, D. J. (1980). Hormone-induced enlargement of receptive fields in trigeminal mechanoreceptive neurons. II. Possible mechanisms. *Brain Research, 184,* 411–423.

Berenbaum, H. (1996). Childhood abuse, alexithymia and personality disorder. *Journal of Psychosomatic Research, 41,* 585–595.

Berg-Johnsen, J., Haugstad, T. S., & Langmoen, I. A. (1998). Glutamate in the human brain: Possible roles in synaptic transmission and ischemia. *Progress in Brain Research, 116,* 287–302.

Berkley, K . J., & Holdcroft, A. (1999). Sex and gender differences in pain. In P. D. Wall & R. Melzack (Eds.), *Textbook of pain* (4th ed., pp. 951–965). New York: Churchill-Livingstone.

Berkovic, S. F. (2000). Paroxysmal movement disorders and epilepsy: Links across the channel [Editorial]. *Neurology, 55,* 169–170.

Bernasconi, A., Andermann, F., Bernasconi, N., Reutens, D. C., & Dubeau, F. (2001). Lateralizing value of peri-ictal headache: A study of 100 patients with partial epilepsy. *Neurology, 56,* 130–132.

Bernstein, D. A., Borkovec, T. D., & Hazlett-Stevens, H. (2000). *New directions in progressive relaxation training: A guidebook for helping professionals.* Westport, CT: Praeger.

Bernstein, E., & Putnam, F. (1986). Development, reliability, and validity of a dissociation scale. *Journal of Nervous and Mental Disease, 174,* 727–735.

Berntson, G. G., Bigger, J. T., Jr., Eckberg, D. L., Grossman, P., Kaufmann, P. G., Malik, M., et al. (1997). Heart rate variability: Origins, methods, and interpretive caveats. *Psychophysiology, 34,* 623–648.

Berntson, G. G., & Cacioppo, J. T. (2000). From homeostasis to allodynamic regulation. In J. T. Cacioppo, L. G. Tassinary, & G. G. Berntson (Eds.), *Handbook of psychophysiology* (2nd ed., pp. 459–481). New York: Cambridge University Press.

Berntson, G. G., Cacioppo, J. T., & Quigley, K. S. (1993). Respiratory sinus arrhythmia: Autonomic origins, physiological mechanisms, and psychophysiological implications. *Psychophysiology, 30,* 183–196.

Berntzen, D., & Götestam, K. G. (1987). Effects of on-demand versus fixed interval schedules in the treatment of chronic pain with analgesic compounds. *Journal of Consulting and Clinical Psychology, 55,* 213–217.

Berry, H. (2000). Chronic whiplash syndrome as a functional disorder. *Archives of Neurology, 57,* 592–594.

Berry, H. (2001). In reply. *Archives of Neurology, 58,* 681.

Beutler, L. E., Engle, D., Oro'-Beutler, M. E., Daldrup, R., & Meredith, K. (1986). Inability to express intense affect: A common link between depression and pain? *Journal of Consulting and Clinical Psychology, 54,* 752–759.

Bianchi, A., Pitari, G., Amenta, V., Giuliano, F., Gallina, M., Costa, R., & Ferlito, S. (1996). Endothelial, haemostatic, and haemorheological modifications in migraineurs. *Artery, 22*(2), 93–100.

Bic, Z., Blix, G. G., Hopp, H. P., & Leslie, F. M. (1998). In search of the ideal treatment for migraine headache. *Medical Hypotheses, 50,* 1–7.

Bic, Z., Blix, G. G., Hopp, H. P., Leslie, F. M., & Schell, M. J. (1999). The influence of a low-fat diet on incidence and severity of migraine headaches. *Journal of Women's Health and Gender-Based Medicine, 8,* 623–630.

Bigal, M. E., Sheftell, F. D., Rapoport, A. M., Tepper, S. J., Weeks, R., & Baskin, S. M. (2003). MMPI personality profiles in patients with primary chronic daily headache: A case-control study. *Neurological Sciences, 24,* 103–110.

Bille, B. (1962). Migraine in school children. *Acta Paediatrica Scandinavia, 51* (Suppl. 136), 1–151.

Bille, B. (1997). A 40-year follow-up of school children with migraine. *Cephalalgia, 17,* 488–491.

Binder, L. M., & Rohling, M. L. (1996). Money matters: A meta-analytic review of the effects of financial incentives on recovery after closed head injury. *American Journal of Psychiatry, 153,* 7–10.

Binzer, M., & Kullgren, G. (1998). Motor conversion disorder: A prospective 2- to 5-year follow-up study. *Psychosomatics, 39,* 519–527.

Blanchard, E. B. (1987). Long-term effects of behavioral treatment of chronic headache. *Behavior Therapy, 18,* 375–385.

Blanchard, E. B. (1992). Psychological treatment of benign headache disorders. *Journal of Consulting and Clinical Psychology, 60,* 537–551.

Blanchard, E. B. (1998). Headache. In E. A. Blechman & K. Brownell (Eds.), *Behavioral medicine and women: A comprehensive handbook* (pp. 654–658). New York: Guilford.

Blanchard, E. B., & Andrasik, F. (1982). Psychological assessment and treatment of headache: Recent developments and emerging issues. *Journal of Consulting and Clinical Psychology, 50,* 859–879.

Blanchard, E. B., & Andrasik, F. (1985). *Management of chronic headaches: A psychological approach.* New York: Pergamon Press.

Blanchard, E. B., Andrasik, F., Ahles, T. A., Teders, S. J., & O'Keefe, D. (1980). Migraine and tension headache: A meta-analytic review. *Behavior Therapy, 11,* 613–631.

Blanchard, E. B., Andrasik, F., Arena, J. G., Neff, D. F., Jurish, S. E., Teders, S. J., Barron, K. D., & Rodichok, L. D. (1983). Nonpharmacologic treatment of chronic headache: Prediction of outcome. *Neurology, 33,* 1596–1603.

Blanchard, E. B., Andrasik, F., Arena, J. G., Neff, D. F., Saunders, N. L., Jurish, S. E., Teders, S. J., & Rodichok, L. D. (1983). Psychophysiological responses as predictors of response to behavioral treatment of chronic headache. *Behavior Therapy, 14*, 357–374.

Blanchard, E. B., Andrasik, F., Evans, D. D., Neff, D. F., Appelbaum, K. A., & Rodichok, L. D. (1985). Behavioral treatment of 250 chronic headache patients: A clinical replication series. *Behavior Therapy, 16*, 308–327.

Blanchard, E. B., Andrasik, F., Jurish, S. E., & Teders, S. J. (1982). The treatment of cluster headache with relaxation and thermal biofeedback. *Biofeedback and Self-Regulation, 7*, 185–191.

Blanchard, E. B., Andrasik, F., Neff, D. F., Arena, J. G., Ahles, T. A., Jurish, S. E., Pallmeyer, T. P., Saunders, N. L., & Teders, S. J. (1982). Biofeedback and relaxation training with three kinds of headache: Treatment effects and their prediction. *Journal of Consulting and Clinical Psychology, 50*, 562–575.

Blanchard, E. B., Andrasik, F., Neff, D. F., Teders, S. J., Pallmeyer, T. P., Arena, J. G., Jurish, S. E., Saunders, N. L., Ahles, T. A., & Rodichok, L. D. (1982). Sequential comparisons of relaxation training and biofeedback in the treatment of three kinds of chronic headache or, the machines may be necessary some of the time. *Behaviour Research and Therapy, 20*, 469–481.

Blanchard, E. B., Appelbaum, K. A., Guarnieri, P., Morrill, B., & Dentinger, M. P. (1987). Five year prospective follow-up on the treatment of chronic headache with biofeedback and/or relaxation. *Headache, 27*, 580–583.

Blanchard, E. B., Appelbaum, K. A., Guarnieri, P., Neff, D. F., Andrasik, F., Jaccard, J., & Barron, K. D. (1988). Two studies of the long-term follow-up of minimal therapist contact treatments of vascular and tension headache. *Journal of Consulting and Clinical Psychology, 56*, 427–432.

Blanchard, E. B., Appelbaum, K. A., Radnitz, C. L., Jaccard, J., & Dentinger, M. P. (1989). The refractory headache patient—I. Chronic, daily, high intensity headache. *Behaviour Research and Therapy, 27*, 403–410.

Blanchard, E. B., Appelbaum, K. A., Radnitz, C. L., Michultka, D., Morrill, B., Kirsch, C., Hillhouse, J., Evans, D. D., Guarnieri, P., Attanasio, V., Andrasik, F., Jaccard, J., & Dentinger, M. P. (1990). Placebo-controlled evaluation of abbreviated progressive muscle relaxation and of relaxation combined with cognitive therapy in the treatment of tension headache. *Journal of Consulting and Clinical Psychology, 58*, 210–215.

Blanchard, E. B., Appelbaum, K. A., Radnitz, C. L., Morrill, B., Michultka, D., Kirsch, C., Guarnieri, P., Hillhouse, J., Evans, D. D., Jaccard, J., & Barron, K. D. (1990). A controlled evaluation of thermal biofeedback and thermal biofeedback combined with cognitive therapy in the treatment of vascular headache. *Journal of Consulting and Clinical Psychology, 58*, 216–224.

Blanchard, E. B., Kim, M., Hermann, C., Steffek, B. D., et al. (1994). The role of perception of success in the thermal biofeedback treatment of vascular headache. *Headache Quarterly, 5*, 231–236.

Blanchard, E. B., Morrill, B., Wittrock, D. A., Scharff, L., & Jaccard, J. (1989). Hand temperature norms for headache, hypertension, and irritable bowel syndrome. *Biofeedback and Self-Regulation, 14*, 319–331.

Blanchard, E. B., Nicholson, N. L., Radnitz, C. L., Steffek, B. D., Appelbaum, K. A., & Dentinger, M. P. (1991). The role of home practice in thermal biofeedback. *Journal of Consulting and Clinical Psychology, 59*, 507–512.

Blanchard, E. B., Peters, M. L., Hermann, C., Turner, S. M., Buckley, T. C., Barton, K., & Dentinger, M. P. (1997). Direction of temperature control in the thermal biofeedback treatment of vascular headache. *Applied Psychophysiology and Biofeedback, 22*, 227–245.

Blaszczynski, A. P. (1984). Personality factors in classical migraine and tension headache. *Headache, 24*, 238–244.

Blau, J. N. (1992). Migraine: Theories of pathogenesis. *Lancet, 339*, 1202–1207.

Blau, J. N. (1995). Migraine with aura and migraine without aura are not different entities. *Cephalalgia, 15*, 186–190.

Blau, J. N., & Engel, H. O. (1999). A new cluster headache precipitant: Increased body heat. *Lancet, 354*, 1001–1002.

Blau, J. N., & MacGregor, E. A. (1994). Migraine and the neck. *Headache, 34*, 88–90.

Blau, J. N., & Thavapalan, M. (1988). Preventing migraine: A study of precipitating factors. *Headache, 28*, 481–483.

Blersch, W., Schulte-Mattler, W. J., Przywara, S., May, A., Bigalke, H., & Wohlfarth, K. (2002). Botulinum toxin A and the cutaneous nociception in humans: A prospective, double-blind, placebo-controlled, randomized study. *Journal of the Neurological Sciences, 205*, 59–63.

Block, A., Kremer, E., & Gaylor, M. (1980). Behavioral treatment of chronic pain: The spouse as a discriminative cue for pain behavior. *Pain, 9*, 243–252.

Blockmans, D., Persoons, P., Van Houdenhove, B., Lejeune, M., & Bobbaers, H. (2003). Combination therapy with hydrocortisone and fludrocortisone does not improve symptoms in chronic fatigue syndrome: A randomized, placebo-controlled, double-blind, crossover study. *American Journal of Medicine, 114*, 736–741.

Blumenthal, L. S., & Fuchs, M. (1961). Muscle relaxation in the treatment of headache. *Headache, 1*(2), 8–20.

Bogaards, M. C., & ter Kuile, M. M. (1994). Treatment of recurrent tension headache: A meta-analytic review. *Clinical Journal of Pain, 10*, 174–190.

Bogduk, N. (1997). Headache and the neck. In P. J. Goadsby & S. D. Silberstein (Eds.), *Headache* (pp. 369–381). Newton, MA: Butterworth-Heinemann.

Bogduk, N. (2004). Role of anesthesiologic blockade in headache management. *Current Pain and Headache Reports, 8*, 399–403.

Bogduk, N., & Marsland, A. (1986). On the concept of third occipital headache. *Journal of Neurology, Neurosurgery, and Psychiatry, 49*, 775–780.

Bohotin, V., Fumal, A., Vandenheede, M., Bohotin, C., & Schoenen, J. (2003). Excitability of visual V1-V2 and motor cortices to single transcranial magnetic stimuli in migraine: A reappraisal using a figure-of-eight coil. *Cephalalgia, 23*, 264–270.

Bohotin, V., Fumal, A., Vandenheede, M., Gérard, P., Bohotin, C., Maertens de Noordhout, A., & Schoenen, J. (2002). Effects of repetitive transcranial magnetic stimulation on visual evoked potentials in migraine. *Brain, 125*, 912–922.

Bolanowski, S. J., Maxfield, L. M., Gescheider, G. A., & Apkarian, A. V. (2000). The effects of stimulus location on the gating of touch by heat- and cold-induced pain. *Somatosensory and Motor Research, 17*, 195–204.

Boles, R. G., Chun, N., Senadheera, D., & Wong, L.-J. C. (1997). Cyclic vomiting syndrome and mitochondrial DNA mutations. *Lancet, 350*, 1299–1300.

Boles, R. G., & Williams, J. C. (1999). Mitochondrial disease and cyclic vomiting syndrome. *Digestive Disease and Science, 44*(Suppl.), 103S–107S.

Boline, P. D., Kassak, K., Bronfort, G., Nelson, C., & Anderson, A. V. (1995). Spinal manipulation vs. amitriptyline for the treatment of chronic tension-type headaches: A randomized clinical trial. *Journal of Manipulative and Physiological Therapeutics, 18*, 148–154.

Bonney, I. M., Foran, S. E., Marchand, J. E., Lipkowski, A. W., & Carr, D. B. (2004). Spinal antinociceptive effects of AA501, a novel chimeric peptide with opioid receptor agonist and tachykinin receptor antagonist moieties. *European Journal of Pharmacology, 488*, 91–99.

Bonuccelli, U., Nuti, A., Lucetti, C., Pavese, N., Dell'Agnello, G., & Muratorio, A. (1996). Amitriptyline and dexamethasone combined treatment in drug-induced headache. *Cephalalgia, 16*, 197–200.

Bonuso, S., Di Stasio, E., Marano, E., Covelli, V., Testa, N., Tetto, A., & Buscaino, G. A. (1994). The antimigraine effect of ergotamine: A role for alpha-adrenergic blockade? *Acta Neurologica (Napoli), 16*, 1–10.

Boorstin, D. J. (1983). *The discoverers*. New York: Vintage Books.

Boring, E. G. (1932). Max von Frey: 1852–1932. *American Journal of Psychology, 44*, 584–586.

Boring, E. G. (1942). *Sensation and perception in the history of experimental psychology*. New York: Appleton-Century-Crofts.

Boring, E. G. (1950). *A history of experimental psychology* (2nd ed.). Englewood Cliffs, NJ: Prentice-Hall.

Boring, E. G. (1966). Editor's introduction. In: G. Fechner, *Elements of psychophysics*, vol. 1 (D. H. Howes & E. G. Boring, Eds., H. E. Adler, Trans.). New York: Holt, Rinehart & Winston.

Borowsky, B., Adham, N., Jones, K. A., Raddatz, R., Artymyshyn, R., Ogozalek, K. L., Durkin, M. M., Lakhlani, P. P., Bonini, J. A., Pathirana, S., Boyle, N., Pu, X., Kouranova, E., Lichtblau, H., Ochoa, F. Y., Branchek, T. A., & Gerald, C. (2001). Trace amines: Identification of a family of mammalian G protein-coupled receptors. *Proceedings of the National Academy of Sciences (USA), 98*, 8966–8971.

Borsook, D., Burstein, R., & Becerra, L. (2004). Functional imaging of the human trigeminal system: Opportunities for new insights into pain processing in health and disease. *Journal of Neurobiology, 61*, 107–125.

Boscarino, J. A. (1996). Posttraumatic Stress Disorder, exposure to combat, and lower plasma cortisol among Vietnam veterans: Findings and clinical implications. *Journal of Consulting and Clinical Psychology, 64*, 191–201.

Boscarino, J. A. (2004). Posttraumatic stress disorder and physical illness: Results from clinical and epidemiologic studies. *Annals of the New York Academy of Sciences, 1032*, 141–153.

Boucher, T. J., Okuse, K., Bennett, D. L. H., Munson, J. B., Wood, J. N., & McMahon, S. B. (2000). Potent analgesic effects of GDNF in neuropathic pain states. *Science, 290*, 124–127.

Bouhassira, D., Bing, Z., & Le Bars, D. (1990). Studies of the brain structures involved in diffuse noxious inhibitory controls: The mesencephalon. *Journal of Neurophysiology, 64*, 1712–1723.

Bovim, G., & Sand, T. (1992). Cervicogenic headache, migraine without aura and tension-type headache. Diagnostic blockade of greater occipital and supraorbital nerves. *Pain, 32*, 43–48.

Bower, G. H. (1981). Mood and memory. *American Psychologist, 36*, 129–148.

Bowsher, D. (1997). The effects of pre-emptive treatment of postherpetic neuralgia with amitriptyline: A randomized, double-blind, placebo-controlled trial. *Journal of Pain and Symptom Management, 13*, 327–331.

Boyce, P., Parker, G., Barnett, B., Cooney, M., & Smith, F. (1991). Personality as a vulnerability factor to depression. *British Journal of Psychiatry, 159*, 106–114.

Boylan, L. S., & Sackeim, H. A. (2000). Magnetoelectric brain stimulation in the assessment of brain physiology and pathophysiology. *Clinical Neurophysiology, 111*, 504–512.

Bracha, H. S., Ralston, T. C., Williams, A. E., Yamashita, J. M., & Bracha, A. S. (2005). The clenching-grinding spectrum and fear circuitry disorders: Clinical insights from the neuroscience/paleoanthropology interface. *CNS Spectrums, 10*, 311–318.

Bradley, L. A. (1996). Cognitive-behavioral therapy for chronic pain. In R. J. Gatchel & D. C. Turk (Eds.), *Psychological approaches to pain management: A practitioner's handbook* (pp. 131–147). New York: Guilford Press.

Brandes, J. L., Saper, J. R., Diamond, M., Couch, J. R., Lewis, D. W., Schmitt, J., Neto, W., Schwabe, S., & Jacobs, D. (2004). Topiramate for migraine prevention: A randomized controlled trial. *JAMA, 291*, 965–973.

Brandt, J., Celentano, D., Stewart, W., Linet, M., & Folstein, M. F. (1990). Personality and emotional disorder in a community sample of migraine headache sufferers. *American Journal of Psychiatry, 147*, 303–308.

Bresalier, R. S., Sandler, R. S., Quan, H., Bolognese, J. A., Oxenius, B., Horgan, K., et al. (2005). Cardiovascular events associated with rofecoxib in a colorectal adenoma chemoprevention trial. *New England Journal of Medicine, 352*, 1092–1102.

Breslau, N., & Andreski, P. (1995). Migraine, personality and psychiatric comorbidity. *Headache, 35*, 382–386.

Breslau, N., Chilcoat, H. D., & Andreski, P. (1996). Further evidence on the link between migraine and neuroticism. *Neurology, 47*, 663–667.

Breslau, N., & Davis, G. C. (1993). Migraine, physical health and psychiatric disorder: a prospective epidemiologic study in young adults. *Journal of Psychiatric Research, 27*, 211–221.

Breslau, N., Davis, G. C., Schultz, L. R., & Peterson, E. L. (1994). Migraine and major depression: A longitudinal study. *Headache, 34*, 387–393.

Breslau, N., Lipton, R. B., Stewart, W. F., Schultz, L. R., & Welch, K. M. A. (2003). Comorbidity of migraine and depression: investigating potential etiology and prognosis. *Neurology, 60*, 1308–1312.

Breuer, J., & Freud, S. (1893–1895/1957). *Studies on hysteria* (J. Strachey, Trans.). New York: Basic Books.

Brilla, R., Evers, S., Soros, P., & Husstedt, I. W. (1998). Hemicrania continua in an HIV-infected outpatient. *Cephalalgia, 18*, 287–288.

Brøsen, K. (1998). Differences in interactions of SSRIs. *International Clinical Psychopharmacology, 13*(Suppl. 5), s45–s47.

Brown, G. K. (1990). A causal analysis of chronic pain and depression. *Journal of Abnormal Psychology, 99*, 127–137.

Brown, G. K., & Nicassio, P. M. (1987). Development of a questionnaire for the assessment of active and passive coping strategies in chronic pain patients. *Pain, 31*, 53–64.

Brown, T. A., O'Leary, T. A., & Barlow, D. H. (2001). Generalized anxiety disorder. In D. H. Barlow (Ed.), *Clinical handbook of psychological disorders: A step-by-step treatment manual* (3rd ed., pp. 154–208). New York: Guilford.

Brown, T. H., Ganong, A. H., Kairiss, E. W., Keenan, C. L., & Kelso, S. R. (1989). Long-term potentiation in two synaptic systems of the hippocampal brain slice. In J. H. Byrne & W. O. Berry (Eds.), *Neural models of plasticity: Experimental and theoretical approaches*. San Diego, CA: Academic Press.

Bruehl, S., Burns, J. W., Chung, O. Y., Ward, P., & Johnson, B. (2002). Anger and pain sensitivity in chronic low back pain patients and pain-free controls: The role of endogenous opioids. *Pain, 99*, 223–233.

Bruehl, S., Chung, O. Y., & Burns, J. W. (2003). Differential effects of expressive anger regulation on chronic pain intensity in CRPS and non-CRPS limb pain patients. *Pain, 104*, 647–654.

Brunton, T. L. (1886). *On disorders of digestion: Their consequences and treatment.* London: Macmillan & Co.

Bryson, H. M., & Wilde, M. I. (1996). Amitriptyline: A review of its pharmacological properties and therapeutic use in chronic pain states. *Drugs and Aging, 8*, 459–476.

Buchan, P., Keywood, C., Wade, A., & Ward, C. (2002). Clinical pharmacokinetics of frovatriptan. *Headache, 42* (Suppl. 2), s54–s62.

Buchan, P., Wade, A., Ward, C., Oliver, S. D., Stewart, A. J., & Freestone, S. (2002). Frovatriptan: A review of drug-drug interactions. *Headache, 42* (Suppl. 2), s63–s73.

Buchgreitz, L., Lyngberg, A. C., Bendtsen, L., & Jensen, R. (2006). Frequency of headache is related to sensitization: A population study. *Pain, 123*, 19–27.

Buchner, H., Reinartz, U., Waberski, T. D., Gobbele, R., Noppeney, U., & Scherg, M. (1999). Sustained attention modulates the immediate effect of de-afferentation on the cortical representation of the digits: Source localization of somatosensory evoked potentials in humans. *Neuroscience Letters, 260*, 57–60.

Budd, K. S., & Kedesky, J. H. (1989). Investigation of environmental factors in pediatric headache. *Headache, 29*, 569–573.

Budzinski, J. W., Foster, B. C., Vandenhoek, S., & Arnason, J. T. (2000). An in vitro evaluation of human cytochrome P450 3A4 inhibition by selected commercial herbal extracts and tinctures. *Phytomedicine, 7*, 273–282.

Budzynski, T. H., Stoyva, J. M., & Adler, C. S. (1970). Feedback induced muscle relaxation: Application to tension headache. *Journal of Behavioral Therapy and Experimental Psychiatry, 1*, 205–211.

Budzynski, T. H., Stoyva, J. M., Adler, C. S., & Mulhaney, D. J. (1973). EMG biofeedback and tension headache: A controlled outcome study. *Psychosomatic Medicine, 35*, 484–496.

Bulut, S., Berilgen, M. S., Baran, A., Tekatas, A., Atmaca, M., & Mungen, B. (2004). Venlafaxine versus amitriptyline in the prophylactic treatment of migraine: Randomized, double-blind, crossover study. *Clinical Neurology and Neurosurgery, 107*, 44–48.

Bureš, J., Burešová, O., & Křivánek, J. (1974). *The mechanism and applications of Leão's spreading depression of electroencephalographic activity.* New York: Academic Press.

Burgess, S. E., Gardell, L. R., Ossipov, M. H., Malan, T. P., Jr., Vanderah, T. W., Lai, J., & Porreca, F. (2002). Time-dependent descending facilitation from the rostral ventromedial medulla maintains, but does not initiate, neuropathic pain. *Journal of Neuroscience, 22*, 5129–5136.

Burke, B. E., Olson, R. D., & Cusack, B. J. (2002). Randomized, controlled trial of phytoestrogen in the prophylactic treatment of menstrual migraine. *Biomedicine and Pharmacotherapy, 56*, 283–288.

Burnier, M., & Brunner, H. R. (2000). Angiotensin II receptor antagonists. *Lancet, 355*, 637–645.

Burns, J. W. (1997). Anger management style and hostility: Predicting symptom-specific physiological reactivity among chronic low back pain patients. *Journal of Behavioral Medicine, 20*, 505–522.

Burns, J. W. (2000). Repression predicts outcome following multidisciplinary treatment of chronic pain. *Health Psychology, 19*, 75–84.

Burns, J. W., Johnson, B. J., Mahoney, N., Devine, J., & Pawl, R. (1996). Anger management style, hostility and spouse responses: Gender differences in predictors of adjustment among chronic pain patients. *Pain, 64*, 445–453.

Burns, J., Higdon, L., Mullen, J., Lansky, D., & Mei Wei, J. (1999). Relationships among patient hostility, anger expression, depression, and the working alliance in a work hardening program. *Annals of Behavioral Medicine, 21*, 77–82.

Burns, J. W., Sherman, M. L., Devine, J., Mahoney, N., & Pawl, R. (1995). Association between workers' compensation and outcome following multidisciplinary treatment for chronic pain: Roles of mediators and moderators. *Clinical Journal of Pain, 11*, 94–102.

Burstein, R., Cutrer, M. F., & Yarnitsky, D. (2000). The development of cutaneous allodynia during a migraine attack: Clinical evidence for the sequential recruitment of spinal and supraspinal nociceptive neurons in migraine. *Brain, 123*, 1703–1709.

Burstein, R., Jakubowski, M., & Levy, D. (2005). Anti-migraine action of triptans is preceded by transient aggravation of headache caused by activation of meningeal nociceptors. *Pain, 115*, 21–28.

Burton, A. K., Waddell, G., Tillotson, K. M., & Summerton, N. (1999). Information and advice to patients with back pain can have a positive effect. A randomized controlled trial of a novel educational booklet in primary care. *Spine, 24*, 2484–2491.

Bussone, G., Grazzi, L., D'Amico, D., Leone, M., & Andrasik, F. (1998). Biofeedback-assisted relaxation training for young adolescents with tension-type headache: A controlled study. *Cephalalgia, 18*, 463–467.

Bussone, G., Leone, M., Peccarisi, C., Micieli, G., Granella, F., Magri, M., Manzoni, G. C., & Nappi, G. (1990). Double blind comparison of lithium and verapamil in cluster headache prophylaxis. *Headache, 30*, 411–417.

Butchko, H. H. (1997). Safety of aspartame [letter]. *Lancet, 349*, 1105.

Buzzi, M. G., Dimitriadou, V., Theoharides, T. C., & Moskowitz, M. A. (1992). 5-Hydroxytryptamine receptor agonists for the abortive treatment of vascular headaches block mast cell, endothelial and platelet activation within the rat dura mater after trigeminal stimulation. *Brain Research, 583*, 137–149.

Cacioppo, J. T., Berntson, G. G., Binkley, P. F., Quigley, K. S., Uchino, B. N., & Fieldstone, A. (1994). Autonomic cardiac control. II. Noninvasive indices and basal response as revealed by autonomic blockades. *Psychophysiology, 31*, 586–598.

Cacioppo, J. T., Rourke, P. A., Marshall-Goodell, B. S., Tassinary, L. G., & Baron, R. S. (1990). Rudimentary physiological effects of mere observation. *Psychophysiology, 27*, 177–186.

Cahn, T., & Cram, J. R. (1980). Changing measurement instrument at follow-up: A potential source of error. *Biofeedback and Self-Regulation, 5*, 265–273.

Caldji, C., Tannenbaum, B., Sharma, S., Francis, D., Plotsky, P. M., & Meaney, M. J. (1998). Maternal care during infancy regulates the development of neural systems mediating the expression of fearfulness in the rat. *Proceedings of the National Academy of Sciences (USA), 95*, 5335–5340.

Calejesan, A. A., Kim, S. J., & Zhuo, M. (2000). Descending facilitatory modulation of a behavioral nociceptive response by stimulation in the adult rat anterior cingulate cortex. *European Journal of Pain, 4*, 83–96.

Callaghan, M., & Abu-Arafeh, I. (2001). Chronic posttraumatic headache in children and adolescents. *Developmental Medicine and Child Neurology, 43*, 819–822.

Callahan, C. D. (2000). Stress, coping, and personality hardiness in patients with temporomandibular disorders. *Rehabilitation Psychology, 45*, 38–48.

Callaway, J. E., Arezzo, J. C., & Grethlein, A. J. (2002). Botulinum toxin type B: An overview of its biochemistry and preclinical pharmacology. *Disease-a-Month, 48*, 367–383.

Cameron, O. G., Modell, J. G., & Hariharam, M. (1990). Caffeine and human cerebral blood flow: A positron emission tomography study. *Life Sciences, 47*, 1141–1146.

Campbell, J., Lahuerta, J., & Bowsher, D. (1996). Quantitative assessment of somatosensory function. *British Journal of Therapy and Rehabilitation, 3*, 135–141.

Campbell, J. K., Penzien, D. B., & Wall, E. M. (2000). *Evidence-based guidelines for migraine headache: Behavioral and physical treatments*. Retrieved April 11, 2004, from American Academy of Neurology Web site: http://www.aan.com/professionals/practice/pdfs/gl0089.pdf

Campbell, J. N., & Sciubba, D. M. (2005). Neurosurgical approaches to the treatment of pain. In: M. Pappagallo (Ed.), *The neurological basis of pain* (pp. 631–639). New York: McGraw-Hill.

Canavero, S., & Bonicalzi, V. (2002). Therapeutic extradural cortical stimulation for central and neuropathic pain: A review. *Clinical Journal of Pain, 18*, 48–55.

Cannon, W. B., & Gray, H. (1914). Factors affecting the coagulation time of blood: II. The hastening or retarding of coagulation by adrenalin injections. *American Journal of Physiology, 34*, 232–242.

Cao, M., Zhang, S., Wang, K., Wang, Y., & Wang, W. (2002). Personality traits in migraine and tension-type headaches: A five-factor model study. *Psychopathology, 35*, 254–258.

Caputi, C., & Firetto, V. (1997). Therapeutic blockade of greater occipital and supraorbital nerves in migraine patients. *Headache, 37*, 174–179.

Carbajal, R., Chauvet, X., Couderc, S., & Olivier-Martin, M. (1999). Randomised trial of analgesic effects of sucrose, glucose, and pacifiers in term neonates. *British Medical Journal, 319*, 1393–1397.

Carlson, C. R., Collins, F. L. Jr., Nitz, A. J., Sturgis, E. T., & Rogers, J. L. (1990). Muscle stretching as an alternative relaxation training procedure. *Journal of Behavior Therapy and Experimental Psychiatry, 21*, 29–38.

Carlson, C. R., Okeson, J. P., Falace, D. A., Nitz, A. J., & Anderson, D. (1991). Stretch-based relaxation and the reduction of EMG activity among masticatory muscle pain patients. *Journal of Craniomandibular Disorders, 5*, 205–212.

Carlsson, J., Larsson, B., & Mark, A. (1996). Psychosocial functioning in schoolchildren with recurrent headaches. *Headache, 36*, 77–82.

Carr-Hill, R., Jenkins-Clarke, S., Dixon, P., et al. (1998). Do minutes count? Consultation lengths in general practice. *Journal of Health Service Research and Policy, 3*, 207–213.

Carter, R. L., Feuerstein, M., & Love, J. T. (1986). Repeated measures regression: An application to the analysis of mood and chronic pain. *Computational Statistics and Data Analysis, 4*, 131–140.

Carver, C. S., Scheier, M. F., & Weintraub, J. K. (1989). Assessing coping strategies: A theoretically based approach. *Journal of Personality and Social Psychology, 56*, 267–283.

Cassidy, E. M., Tomkins, E., Dinan, T., Hardiman, O., & O'Keane, V. (2003). Central 5-HT receptor hyper-sensitivity in migraine without aura. *Cephalalgia, 23*, 29–34.

Caterina, M. J., & Julius, D. (2001). The vanilloid receptor: A molecular gateway to the pain pathway. *Annual Review of Neuroscience, 24*, 487–517.

Caterina, M. J., Schumacher, M. A., Tominaga, M., Rosen, T. A., Levine, J. D., & Julius, D. (1997). The capsaicin receptor: A heat-activated ion channel in the pain pathway. *Nature, 389*, 816–824.

Catterall, W. A., & Mackie, K. (2001). Local anesthetics. In J. G. Hardman, L. E. Limbird, P. B. Molinoff, R. W. Ruddon, & A. G. Gilman (Eds.), *Goodman and Gilman's pharmacological basis of therapeutics* (pp. 367–384). New York: Macmillan.

Caudill, M. (1995). *Managing pain before it manages you*. New York: Guilford.

Centers for Disease Control. (1984). Evaluation of consumer complaints related to aspartame use. *MMWR, 33*, 605–607.

Century Dictionary. (1890). New York: The Century Company.

Cesar, J. M., Garćcia-Avello, A., Vecino, A. M., Sastre, J. L., & Alvarez-Cermeño, J. C. (1995). Increased levels of plasma von Willebrand factor in migraine crisis. *Acta Neurologica Scandinavia, 91*, 412–413.

Chance, W. T., Krynock, G. M., & Rosecrans, J. M. (1978). Antinociception following lesion-induced hyper-emotionality and conditioned fear. *Pain, 4*, 243–252.

Chandran, P., & Sluka, K. A. (2003). Development of opioid tolerance with repeated transcutaneous electrical nerve stimulation administration. *Pain, 102*, 195–201.

Chapman, R. C., Nakamura, Y., & Flores, L. Y. (1999). Chronic pain and consciousness: A constructivist perspective. In R. J. Gatchel & D. C. Turk (Eds.), *Psychosocial factors in pain: Critical perspectives* (pp. 35–55). New York: Guilford Press.

Chen, T. C., & Leviton, A. (1990). Asthma and eczema in children born to women with migraine. *Archives of Neurology, 47*, 1227–1230.

Cheng, T. M. W., Cascino, T. L., & Onofrio, B. M. (1993). Comprehensive study of diagnosis and treatment of trigeminal neuralgia secondary to tumors. *Neurology, 43*, 2298–2302.

Chervin, R. D., Zallek, S. N., Lin, X., Hall, J. M., Sharma, N., & Hedger, K. M. (2000). Sleep disordered breathing in patients with cluster headache. *Neurology, 54*, 2302–2306.

Cheshire, W. P., Abashian, S. W., & Mann, J. D. (1994). Botulinum toxin in the treatment of myofascial pain syndrome. *Pain, 59*, 65–69.

Chesterton, L. S., Barlas, P., Foster, N. E., Lundeberg, T., Wright, C. C., & Baxter, G. D. (2002). Sensory stimulation (TENS): Effects of parameter manipulation on mechanical pain thresholds in healthy human subjects. *Pain, 99*, 253–262.

Cheunsuang, O., & Morris, R. (2000). Spinal lamina I neurons that express neurokinin 1 receptors: Morphological analysis. *Neuroscience, 97*, 335–345.

Chibnall, J. T., & Duckro, P. N. (1994). Post-traumatic stress disorder in chronic post-traumatic headache patients. *Headache, 34*, 357–361.

Chikanza, I. C., Petrou, P., Kingsley, G., et al. (1992). Defective hypothalamic pituitary adrenal response to immune and inflammatory stimuli in patients with rheumatoid arthritis. *Arthritis and Rheumatism, 35*, 1281–1288.

Chioza, B., Wilkie, H., Nashef, L., Blower, J., McCormick, D., Sham, P., Asherson, P., & Makoff, A. J. (2001). Association between the α_{1a} calcium channel gene CACNA1A and idiopathic generalized epilepsy. *Neurology, 56*, 1245–1246.

Choi, B., & Rowbotham, M. C. (1997). Effect of adrenergic receptor activation on post-herpetic neuralgia pain and sensory disturbances. *Pain, 69*, 55–63.

Christenfeld, N. (1997). Memory for pain and the delayed effects of distraction. *Health Psychology, 16*, 327–330.

Chronicle, E. P., & Mulleners, W. M. (1994). Might migraine damage the brain? *Cephalalgia, 14*, 415–418.

Chudler, E. H., & Dong, W. K. (1995). The role of the basal ganglia in nociception and pain. *Pain, 60*, 3–38.

Chugani, D. C., Niimura, K., Chaturvedi, S., Muzik, O., Fakhouri, M., Lee, M. L., & Chugani, H. T. (1999). Increased brain serotonin synthesis in migraine. *Neurology, 53*, 1473–1479.

Chutkow, J. G. (1981). The neurophysiologic function of magnesium: An update. *Magnesium Bulletin, 1a*, 11–20.

Ciccone, D. S., Elliott, D. K., Chandler, H. K., Nayak, S., & Raphael, K. G. (2005). Sexual and physical abuse in women with fibromyalgia syndrome: A test of the trauma hypothesis. *Clinical Journal of Pain, 21*, 378–386.

Cioffi, D., & Holloway, J. (1993). Delayed costs of suppressed pain. *Journal of Personality and Social Psychology, 64*, 274–282.

Claghorn, J. L., Mathew, R. J., Largen, J. W., & Meyer, J. S. (1981). Directional effects of skin temperature self-regulation on regional cerebral blood flow in normal subjects and migraine patients. *American Journal of Psychiatry, 138*, 1182–1187.

Clark, S., Tindall, E., & Bennett, R. M. (1985). A double blind crossover trial of prednisone vs. placebo in the treatment of fibrositis. *Journal of Rheumatology, 12*, 980–983.

Cleland, P. G., Barnes, D., Elrington, G. M., Loizou, L. A., & Rawes, G. D. (1997). Studies to assess if pizotifen prophylaxis improves migraine beyond the benefit offered by acute sumatriptan therapy alone. *European Neurology, 38*, 31–38.

Clemente, C. D. (1997). *Anatomy: A regional atlas of the human body* (4th ed.). Baltimore, MD: Williams and Wilkins.

Clemmey, P. A., & Nicassio, P. M. (1997). Illness self-schemas in depressed and nondepressed rheumatoid arthritis patients. *Journal of Behavioral Medicine, 20*, 273–290.

Cliff, N. (1993). What is and isn't measurement. In G. Keren & C. Lewis (Eds.), *A handbook for data analysis in the behavioral sciences: Methodological issues*. Hillsdale, NJ: Lawrence Erlbaum Associates.

Coderre, T. J., Katz, J., Vaccarino, A. L., & Melzack, R. (1993). Contribution of central neuroplasticity to pathological pain: Review of clinical and experimental evidence. *Pain, 52*, 259–285.

Codignola, A., Tarroni, P., Clementi, F., et al. (1993). Calcium channel subtypes controlling serotonin release from human small cell lung carcinoma cell lines. *Journal of Biological Chemistry, 268*, 26240–26247.

Coggeshall, R. E., Lekan, H. A., White, F. A., & Woolf, C. J. (2001). A-fiber sensory input induces neuronal cell death in the dorsal horn of the adult rat spinal cord. *Journal of Comparative Neurology, 435*, 276–282.

Cohen, J. (1960). A coefficient of agreement for nominal scales. *Educational and Psychological Measurement, 20*, 37–46.

Cohen, J. (1988). *Statistical power analysis for the behavioral sciences* (Rev. ed.). Hillsdale, NJ: Erlbaum.

Cohen, M. J., Rickles, W. H., & McArthur, D. L. (1978). Evidence for physiological response stereotypy in migraine headache. *Psychosomatic Medicine, 40*, 344–354.

Cohen, R. A., Williamson, D. A., Monguillot, J. E., Hutchinson, P. C., Gottlieb, J., & Waters, W. F. (1983). Psychophysiological response patterns in vascular and muscle-contraction headaches. *Journal of Behavioral Medicine, 6*, 93–107.

Cohen, S., Doyle, W. J., Skoner, D. P., Fireman, P., Gwaltney, J. M., Jr., & Newsom, J. T. (1995). State and trait negative affect as predictors of objective and subjective symptoms of respiratory viral infections. *Journal of Personality and Social Psychology, 68*, 159–169.

Cohen, S., Hamrick, N., Rodriguez, M. S., Feldman, P. J., Rabin, B. S., & Manuck, S. B. (2000). The stability of and intercorrelations among cardiovascular, immune, endocrine, and psychological reactivity. *Annals of Behavioral Medicine, 22*, 171–179.

Comer, M. B. (2002). Pharmacology of the selective 5-HT$_{1B/1D}$ agonist frovatriptan. *Headache, 42*(Suppl. 2), s47–s53.

Compas, B. E. (1987). Coping with stress during childhood and adolescence. *Psychological Bulletin, 101*, 393–403.

Compas, B. E., Davis, G. E., Forsythe, C. J., & Wagner, B. M. (1987). Assessment of major and daily stressful events during adolescence: The Adolescent Perceived Events Scale. *Journal of Consulting and Clinical Psychology, 55*, 534–541.

Compas, B. E., Haaga, D. A. F., Keefe, F. J., et al. (1998). Sampling of empirically supported psychological treatments from health psychology: Smoking, chronic pain, cancer, and bulimia nervosa. *Journal of Consulting and Clinical Psychology, 66*, 89–112.

Compton, P., Charuvastra, V. C., & Ling, W. (2001). Pain intolerance in opioid-maintained former opiate addicts: Effect of long-acting maintenance agent. *Drug and Alcohol Dependence, 63*, 139–146.

Connally, G. H., & Sanders, S. H. (1991). Predicting low back pain patients' response to lumbar sympathetic nerve blocks and interdisciplinary rehabilitation: The role of pretreatment overt pain behaviour and cognitive coping strategies. *Pain, 44*, 139–146.

Connolly, J. F., Gawel, M., & Clifford, R. F. (1982). Migraine patients exhibit abnormalities in the visual evoked potential. *Journal of Neurology, Neurosurgery, and Psychiatry, 45*, 464–467.

Connors, M. J. (1995). Cluster headache: A review. *Journal of the American Osteopathic Association, 95*, 533–539.

Cooke, L. J., Rose, M. S. & Becker, W. J. (2000). Chinook winds and migraine headache. *Neurology, 54*, 302–307.

Cornwell, N., & Clarke, L. (1991). Dietary modification in patients with migraine and tension-type headache. *Cephalalgia, 11*(Suppl. 11), 142–143.

Cortelli, P., Pierangeli, G., Parchi, P., Contin, M., Baruzzi, A., & Lugaresi, E. (1991). Autonomic nervous system function in migraine without aura. *Headache, 31*, 457–462.

Cortright, D. N., & Szallasi, A. (2004). Biochemical pharmacology of the vanilloid receptor TRPV1. An update. *European Journal of Biochemistry, 271*, 1814–1819.

Costa, P. T., & McCrae, R. R. (1985). Hypochondriasis, neuroticism, and aging: When are somatic complaints unfounded? *American Psychologist, 40*, 19–28.

Costa e Silva, J. A., Alvarez, N., Mazzotti, G., Gattaz, W. F., Ospina, J., Larach, V., et al. (2001). Olanzapine as alternative therapy for patients with haloperidol-induced extrapyramidal symptoms: Results of a multicenter, collaborative trial in Latin America. *Journal of Clinical Psychopharmacology, 21*, 375–381.

Couch, J. R., & Bearss, C. (2001). Chronic daily headache in the posttrauma syndrome: Relation to extent of head injury. *Headache, 41*, 559–564.

Couch, J. R., & Hassanein, R. S. (1979). Amitriptyline in migraine prophylaxis. *Archives of Neurology, 36*, 695–699.

Coughtrie, M. W. H., Jones, A. L., & Roberts, R. C. (1994). Migraine as a chemical-induced syndrome—the influence of sulphation, diet and genetics. In F. C. Rose (Ed.), *New advances in headache research.* (3rd ed., pp. 137–144). London: Smith-Gordon and Company, Ltd.

Couturier, E. G. M., Laman, D. M., van Duijn, M. A. J., & van Duijn, H. (1997). Influence of caffeine and caffeine withdrawal on headache and cerebral blood flow velocities. *Cephalalgia, 17*,188–190.

Cox, B. J., & McWilliams, L. A. (2002). Mood and anxiety disorders in relation to chronic pain: Evidence from the National Comorbidity Study. *Pain Research and Management*, 5(Suppl. A), 11A.

Craig, A. D. (1998). A new version of the thalamic disinhibition hypothesis of central pain. *Pain Forum, 7*, 1–14.

Craig, A. D., & Dostrovsky, J. O. (1999). Medulla to thalamus. In P. D. Wall & R. Melzack (Eds.), *Textbook of pain* (4th ed., pp. 183–214). New York: Churchill Livingstone.

Cram, J. R. (1999). Dynamic surface electromyographic evaluations for cervical flexion studies. *American Journal of Pain Management, 9*, 60–66.

Cram, J. R., & Engstrom, D. (1986). Patterns of neuromuscular activity in pain and non-pain patients. *Clinical Biofeedback and Health: An International Journal. 9*, 106–116.

Cram, J. R., & Garber, A. (1986). The relationship between narrow and wide bandwidth filter settings during an EMG scanning procedure. *Biofeedback and Self-Regulation, 11*, 105–114.

Cram, J. R., Kasman, G. S., & Holtz, J. (1998). *Introduction to surface electromyography*. Gaithersburg, MD: Aspen Publishers.

Cram, J. R., & Rommen, D. (1989). Effects of skin preparation on data collected using an EMG muscle-scanning procedure. *Biofeedback and Self-Regulation, 14*, 75–82.

Crawford, H. J., Knebel, T., Kaplan, L., Vendemia, J. M. C., Xie, M., Jamison, S., & Pribram, K. H. (1998). Hypnotic analgesia: 1. Somatosensory event-related potential changes to noxious stimuli and 2. Transfer learning to reduce chronic low back pain. *International Journal of Clinical and Experimental Hypnosis, 46*, 92–132.

Crawford, H. J., Knebel, T., & Vendemia, J. M. C. (1998). The nature of hypnotic analgesia: Neurophysiological foundation and evidence. *Contemporary Hypnosis, 15*, 22–33.

Crider, A. B., & Glaros, A. G. (1999). A meta-analysis of EMG biofeedback treatment of temporomandibular disorders. *Journal of Orofacial Pain, 13*, 29–37.

Crimlisk, H. L., Bhatia, K., Cope, H., David, A., Marsden, C. D., & Ron, M. A. (1998). Slater revisited: 6 year follow up study of patients with medically unexplained motor symptoms. *British Medical Journal, 316*, 582–586.

Critchley, E. M. R. (1996). Migraine. *Journal of Neurology, Neurosurgery, and Psychiatry, 60*, 338, 448, & 585.

Critchley, H. D., Melmed, R. N., Featherstone, E., Mathias, C. J., & Dolan, R. J. (2001). Brain activity during biofeedback relaxation: A functional neuroimaging investigation. *Brain, 124*, 1003–1012.

Crofford, L. J., Pillemer, S. R., Kalogeras, K. T., Cash, J. M., Michelson, D., Kling, M. A., Sternberg, E. M., Gold, P. W., Chrousos, G. P., & Wilder, R. L. (1994). Hypothalamic- pituitary-adrenal axis perturbations in patients with fibromyalgia. *Arthritis and Rheumatism, 37*, 1583–1592.

Crombez, G., Baeyens, F., & Eelen, P. (1997). Changes in facial EMG activity related to painful heat stimuli on the hand. *Journal of Psychophysiology, 11*, 256–262.

Crombez, G., Eccleston, C., Baeyens, F., & Eelen, P. (1997). Habituation and the interference of pain with task performance. *Pain, 70*, 149–154.

Crombez, G., Eccleston, C., Baeyens, F., & Eelen, P. (1998b). Attentional disruption is enhanced by the threat of pain. *Behaviour Research and Therapy, 36*, 195–204.

Crombez, G., Eccleston, C., Baeyens, F., & Eelen, P. (1998a). When somatic information threatens, pain catastrophizing enhances attentional interference. *Pain, 75*, 187–198.

Crombez, G., Vervaet, L., Baeyens, F., Lysens, R., & Eelen, P. (1996). Do pain expectancies cause pain in chronic low back patients? A clinical investigation. *Behaviour Research and Therapy, 34*, 919–925.

Crookshank, F. G. (1926). *Migraine and other common neuroses: A psychological study*. London: Kegan Paul, Trench, Trubner & Co.

Crotogino, J., Feindel, A., & Wilkinson, F. (2001). Perceived scintillation rate of migraine aura. *Headache, 41*, 40–48.

Csikszentmihalyi, M., & Larson, R. (1987). Validity and reliability of the experience-sampling method. *Journal of Nervous and Mental Disease, 175*, 526–536.

Curatolo, M., Petersen-Felix, S., Arendt-Nielsen, L., Giani, C., Zbinden, A. M., & Radanov, B. P. (2001). Central hypersensitivity in chronic pain after whiplash injury. *Clinical Journal of Pain, 17*, 306–315.

Currà, A., Modugno, N., Inghilleri, M., Manfredi, M., Hallett, M., & Berardelli, A. (2002). Transcranial magnetic stimulation techniques in clinical investigation. *Neurology, 59*, 1851–1859.

Curtis, A. L., Florin-Lechner, S. M., Pavcovich, L. A., & Valentino, R. J. (1997). Activation of the locus coeruleus noradrenergic system by intracoerulear microinfusion of corticotropin-releasing factor: Effects on discharge rate, cortical norepinephrine levels and cortical electroencephalographic activity. *Journal of Pharmacology and Experimental Therapeutics, 281*, 163–172.

Curtis, A. L., Pavcovich, L. A., & Valentino, R. J. (1999). Long-term regulation of locus ceruleus sensitivity to corticotropin-releasing factor by swim stress. *Journal of Pharmacology and Experimental Therapeutics, 289*, 1211–1219.

Curtis, D. R., & Watkins, J. C. (1961). Analogues of glutamic acid and γ-amino-*n*-butyric acids having potent actions on mammalian neurones. *Nature, 191*, 1010–1011.

Cutrer, F. M., Mitsikostas, D. D., Ayata, G., & Sanchez del Rio, M. (1999). Attenuation by butalbital of capsaicin-induced c-fos-like immunoreactivity in trigeminal nucleus caudalis. *Headache, 39*, 697–704.

Cutrer, F. M., O'Donnell, A., & del Rio, M. S. (2000). Functional neuroimaging: Enhanced understanding of migraine pathophysiology. *Neurology, 55*(Suppl. 2), S36–S45.

Cytovitch, I. S., & Folkman, N. F. (1917). Pléthysmographie, comme méthode d'enregistrement des réflexes conditionnels chez l'homme. *Comptes Rendus des Séances de la Société de Biologie et de ses Filiales, 80*, 762–764.

Dahlöf, C. G. H., Dodick, D., Dowson, A. J., & Pascual, J. (2002). How does almotriptan compare with other triptans? A review of data from placebo-controlled clinical trials. *Headache, 42*, 99–113.

Dahlöf, C., & Lines, C. (1999). Rizatriptan: A new 5-HT$_{1B/1D}$ receptor agonist for the treatment of migraine. *Expert Opinion on Investigational Drugs, 8*, 671–685.

Dahlöf, C. G. H., Lipton, R. B., McCarroll, K. A., Kramer, M. S., Lines, C. R., & Ferrari, M. D. (2000). Within-patient consistency of response of rizatriptan for treating migraine. *Neurology, 55*, 1511–1516.

Dalessio, D. J., Kunzel, M., Sternbach, R., & Sovak, M. (1979). Conditioned adaptation-relaxation reflex in migraine therapy. *Journal of the American Medical Association, 242*, 2102–2104.

Dalton, K. (1975). Food intake prior to a migraine attack—Study of 2313 spontaneous attacks. *Headache, 15*, 188–193.

Daly, E., & Wulff, J. (1987). Treatment of a post-traumatic headache. *British Journal of Medical Psychology, 60*, 85–88.

Damen, L., Bruijn, J., Koes, B. W., Berger, M. Y., Passchier, J., & Verhagen, A. P. (2006). Prophylactic treatment of migraine in children. Part 1. A systematic review of non-pharmacological trials. *Cephalalgia, 26*, 373–383.

D'Amico, D., Usai, S., Grazzi, L., Rigamonti, A., Solari, A., Leone, M., & Bussone, G. (2003). Quality of life and disability in primary chronic daily headaches. *Neurological Sciences, 24* (Suppl. 2), s97–s100.

D'Andrea, G., Cananzi, A. R., Perini, F., & Hasselmark, L. (1995). Platelet models and their possible usefulness in the study of migraine pathogenesis. *Cephalalgia, 15*, 265–271.

D'Andrea, G., Terrazzino, S., Fortin, D., Cocco, P., Balbi, T., & Leon, A. (2003). Elusive amines and primary headaches: Historical background and prospectives. *Neurological Sciences, 24*(Suppl. 2), s65–s67.

D'Andrea, G., Terrazzino, S., Leon, A., Fortin, D., Perini, F., Granella, F., & Bussone, G. (2004). Elevated levels of circulating trace amines in primary headaches. *Neurology, 62*, 1701–1705.

Danziger, N., Fournier, E., Bouhassira, D., Michaud, D., De Broucker, T., Santarcangelo, E., Carli, G., Chertock, L., & Willer, J. C. (1998). Different strategies of modulation can be operative during hypnotic analgesia: A neurophysiological study. *Pain, 75*, 85–92.

Dao, T. T. T., Knight, K., & Ton-That, V. (1998). Modulation of myofascial pain by the reproductive hormones: A preliminary report. *Journal of Prosthetic Dentistry, 79*, 663–670.

Dar, R., Ariely, D., & Frenk, H. (1995). The effect of past-injury on pain threshold and tolerance. *Pain, 60*, 189–193.

Dauer, W. T., Burke, R. E., Greene, P., & Fahn, S. (1998). Current concepts on the clinical features, aetiology and management of idiopathic cervical dystonia. *Brain, 121*, 547–560.

Davidoff, R. A. (1998). Trigger points and myofascial pain: Toward understanding how they affect headaches. *Cephalalgia, 18*, 436–448.

Davis, C. M., Brickett, P., Stern, R. M., & Kimball, W. H. (1978). Tension in the two frontales: Electrode placement and artifact in the recording of forehead EMG. *Psychophysiology, 15*, 591–593.

Dawson, M. E., Schell, A. M., & Filion, D. L. (2000). The electrodermal system. In J. T. Cacioppo, L. G. Tassinary, & G. G. Berntson (Eds.), *Handbook of psychophysiology* (2nd ed., pp. 200–223). New York: Cambridge University Press.

Dawson-Basoa, M. E., & Gintzler, A. R. (1996). Estrogen and progesterone activate spinal kappa-opiate receptor analgesic mechanisms. *Pain, 64*, 169–177 and 608–615.

De Almeida, R. M. M., Nikulina, E. M., Faccidomo, S., Fish, E. W., & Miczek, K. A. (2001). Zolmitriptan—a 5-HT$_{1B/D}$ agonist, alcohol, and aggression in mice. *Psychopharmacology, 157*, 131–141.

De Benedittis, G., & Lorenzetti, A. (1992). The role of stressful life events in the persistence of primary headache: Major events vs. daily hassles. *Pain, 51*, 35–42.

De Benedittis, G., Lorenzetti, A., & Pieri, A. (1990). The role of stressful life events in the onset of chronic primary headache. *Pain, 40*, 65–75.

De Boer, T. (1996). The pharmacologic profile of mirtazapine. *Journal of Clinical Psychiatry, 57*(Suppl. 4), 19–25.

de Bruijn-Kofman, A. T., van de Wiel, H., Groenman, N. H., Sorbi, M. J., & Klip, E. (1997). Effects of a mass media behavioral treatment for chronic headache: A pilot study. *Headache, 37*, 415–420.

Deffenbacher, J. L., Dahlen, E. R., Lynch, R. S., Morris, C. D., & Gowensmith, W. N. (2000). An application of Beck's cognitive therapy to general anger reduction. *Cognitive Therapy and Research, 24*, 689–697.

Deffenbacher, J. L., Oetting, E. R., Huff, M. E., Cornell, G. R., & Dallager, C. J. (1996). Evaluation of two cognitive-behavioral approaches to general anger reduction. *Cognitive Therapy and Research, 20*, 551–573.

De Fusco, M., Marconi, R., Silvestri, L., Atorino, L., Rampoldi, L., Morgante, L., et al. (2003). Haploinsufficiency of ATP1A2 encoding the Na$^+$/K$^+$ pump alpha2 subunit associated with familial hemiplegic migraine type 2. *Nature Genetics, 33*, 192–196.

DeGood, D. E., Manning, D. C., & Middaugh, S. J. (1997). *The headache and neck pain workbook: An integrated mind and body program.* Oakland, CA: New Harbinger Publications.

De Laat, A., Svensson, P., & Macaluso, G. M. (1998). Are jaw and facial reflexes modulated during clinical or experimental orofacial pain? *Journal of Orofacial Pain, 12*, 260–271.

De Leeuw, R., Bertoli, E., Schmidt, J. E., & Carlson, C. R. (2005). Prevalence of post-traumatic stress disorder symptoms in orofacial pain patients. *Oral Surgery, Oral Medicine, Oral Pathology, Oral Radiology, and Endodontics, 99*, 558–568.

De Luca, C. J. (1979). Physiology and mathematics of myoelectric signals. *IEEE Transactions on Biomedical Engineering, BME-26*, 313–325.

De Pascalis, V., Magurano, M. R., & Bellusci, A. (1999). Pain perception, somatosensory event-related potentials and skin conductance responses to painful stimuli in high, mid, and low hypnotizable subjects: Effects of differential pain reduction strategies. *Pain, 83*, 499–508.

de Tommaso, M. (2005). Central nervous system excitability in migraine: Who is right? *Pain, 118*, 1–2.

De Weerdt, C. J., Bootsma, H. P. R., & Hendriks, H. (1996). Herbal medicines in migraine prevention: Randomized double-blind placebo-controlled crossover trial of a feverfew preparation. *Phytomedicine, 3*, 225–230.

De Wied, M., & Verbaten, M. N. (2001). Affective pictures processing, attention, and pain tolerance. *Pain, 90*, 163–172.

Del Bone, E., & Poggioni, M. (1987). Typical and atypical cluster headache in childhood [Abstract]. *Cephalalgia, 7*(Suppl. 6), 128–130.

Deleu, D., & Hanssens, Y. (2000). Current and emerging second-generation triptans in acute migraine therapy: A comparative review. *Journal of Clinical Pharmacology, 40*, 687–700.

Del Sette, M., Angeli, S., Leandri, M., Ferriero, G., Bruzzone, G. L., Finocchi, C., & Gandolfo, A. (1998). Migraine with aura and right-to-left shunt on transcranial doppler: A case-control study. *Cerebrovascular Diseases, 8*, 327–330.

Delva, N. J., Horgan, S. A., & Hawken, E. R. (2000). Valproate prophylaxis for migraine induced by selective serotonin reuptake inhibitors. *Headache, 40*, 248–251.

Derby, R. Jr. (1996). Point of view. *Spine, 21*, 1744–1745.

Derbyshire, S. W. G., Jones, A. K. P., Gyulai, F., Clark, S., Townsend, D., & Firestone, L. L. (1997). Pain processing during three levels of noxious stimulation produces differential patterns of central activity. *Pain, 73*, 431–445.

Descartes, R. (1960). *Discourse on method and meditations* (L. J. Lafleur, Trans.). Indianapolis, IN: Bobbs-Merrill Educational Publishing. (Original work published 1637).

DeVane, C. L. (1998). Differential pharmacology of newer antidepressants. *Journal of Clinical Psychiatry, 59* (Suppl. 20), 85–93.

Devor, M. (2001). Obituary: Patrick David Wall, 1925–2001. *Pain, 94*, 125–129.

Di Trapani, G., Mei, D., Marra, C., Mazza, S., & Capuano, A. (2000). Gabapentin in the prophylaxis of migraine: A double-blind randomized placebo-controlled study. *Clinica Terapeutica, 151*, 145–148.

Diamond, S. (1993). Tension-type headaches. In D. J. Dalessio & S. D. Silberstein (Eds.), *Wolff's Headache and Other Head Pain*, 6th ed. New York: Oxford University Press.

Diamond, S. (1999). Migraine headache. In M. L. Diamond & G. D. Solomon (Eds.), *Diamond and Dalessio's The practicing physician's approach to headache* (6th ed., pp. 46–70). Philadelphia: W. B. Saunders.

Diamond, S., & Franklin, M. A. (2001). *Conquering your migraine*. New York: Simon and Schuster.

Diamond, S., & Freitag, F. G. (2001). The use of ibuprofen plus caffeine to treat tension-type headache. *Current Pain and Headache Reports, 5*, 472–478.

Diamond, S., Freitag, F. G., & Nursall, A. (1990). The effects of weather on migraine frequency in Chicago. *Headache Quarterly, 1*(2), 136–145.

Diamond, S., Medina, J., Diamond-Falk, J., & De Veno, T. (1979). The value of biofeedback in the treatment of chronic headache: A five-year retrospective study. *Headache, 19*, 90–96.

Diamond, S., & Montrose, D. (1984). The value of biofeedback in the treatment of chronic headache: A four-year retrospective study. *Headache, 24*, 5–18.

Diaz-Mitoma, F., Vanast, W. J., & Tyrrell, D. L. J. (1987). Increased frequency of Epstein-Barr virus excretion in patients with new daily persistent headaches. *Lancet, 1*, 411–415.

Dib, M., Massiou, H., Weber, M., Henry, P., Garcia-Acosta, S., & Bousser, M. G. (2002). Efficacy of oral ketoprofen in acute migraine. *Neurology, 58*, 1660–1665.

Dickens, C., McGowan, L., & Dale, S. (2003). Impact of depression on experimental pain perception: A systematic review of the literature with meta-analysis. *Psychosomatic Medicine, 65*, 369–375.

Didion, J. (1979). In bed. In: *The white album*. New York: Farrar, Straus, and Giroux.

Diener, H. C. (2000). Flunarizine for migraine prophylaxis. In H. C. Diener (Ed.), *Drug treatment of migraine and other headaches* (pp. 269–278). Basel: Karger.

Diener, H. C., Dichgans, J., Scholz, E., Geiselhart, S., Gerber, W. D., & Bille, A. (1989). Analgesic-induced chronic headache: Long term results of withdrawal therapy. *Journal of Neurology, 236*, 9–14.

Diener, H. C., Haab, J., Peters, C., Ried, S., Dichgans, J., & Pilgrim, A. (1991). Subcutaneous sumatriptan in the treatment of headache during withdrawal from drug-induced headache. *Headache, 31*, 205–209.

Diener, H. C., Kaube, H., & Limmroth, V. (1998). A practical guide to the management and prevention of migraine. *Drugs, 56*, 811–824.

Diener, H. C., & Klein, K. (1996). The first comparison of the efficacy and safety of 311C90 and sumatriptan in the treatment of migraine. *Functional Neurology, 11*, 152.

Diener, H.-C., Tfelt-Hansen, P., Dahlöf, C., Láinez, M. J. A., Sandrini, G., Wang, S.-J., et al. (2004). Topiramate in migraine prophylaxis: Results from a placebo-controlled trial with propranolol as an active control. *Journal of Neurology, 251*, 943–950.

Dieppe, P. A., Ebrahim, S., Martin, R. M., & Jüni, P. (2004). Lessons from the withdrawal of rofecoxib. *British Medical Journal, 329*, 867–868.

Dillmann, J., Miltner, W. H., & Weiss, T. (2000). The influence of semantic priming on event-related potentials to painful laser-heat stimuli in humans. *Neuroscience Letters, 284*, 53–56.

Dimitriadou, V., Buzzi, M. G., Moskowitz, M. A., & Theoharides, T. C. (1991). Trigeminal sensory fiber stimulation induces morphological changes reflecting secretion in rat dura mater cells. *Neuroscience, 44*, 97–112.

Dirnagl, U., Iadecora, C., & Moskowitz, M. A. (1999). Pathobiology of *ischaemic* stroke: An integrated view. *Trends in Neurosciences, 22*(9), 391–397.

Dodick, D. W. (2002a). Is there a preferred triptan? *Headache, 42*, 1–7.

Dodick, D. W. (2002b). Patient perceptions and treatment preferences in migraine management. *CNS Drugs, 16* (Suppl. 1), 19–24.

Dodick, D. W., & Campbell, J. K. (2001). Cluster headache: Diagnosis, management, and treatment. In S. D. Silberstein, R. B. Lipton, & D. J. Dalessio (Eds.), *Wolff's headache and other head pain* (7th ed., pp. 283–309). New York: Oxford University Press.

Dohrenwend, B. P., Raphael, K. G., Marbach, J. J., & Gallagher, R. M. (1999). Why is depression comorbid with chronic myofascial face pain? A family study test of alternative hypotheses. *Pain, 83*, 183–192.

Domino, E. F. (1974). Centrally acting skeletal-muscle relaxants. *Archives of Physical Medicine and Rehabilitation, 55*, 369–373.

Domino, J., & Haber, J. (1987). Prior physical and sexual abuse in women with chronic headache: Clinical correlates. *Headache, 27*, 310–314.

Donaldson, C. C. S., Skubick, D. L., Clasby, R. G., & Cram, J. R. (1994). The evaluation of trigger-point activity using dynamic EMG techniques. *American Journal of Pain Management, 4*(3), 118–122.

Dooley, D. J., Donovan, C. M., Meder, W. P., et al. (2002). Preferential action of gabapentin and pregabalin at P/Q-type voltage-sensitive calcium channels: Inhibition of K^+-evoked [^3H]-norepinephrine release from rat neocortical slices. *Synapse, 45*, 171–190.

Dooley, J., & Bagnell, A. (1995). The prognosis and treatment of headaches in children—A ten year follow-up. *Canadian Journal of Neurological Sciences, 22*, 47–49.

Dora, B., Balkan, S., & Tercan, E. (2003). Normalization of high interictal cerebrovascular reactivity in migraine without aura by treatment with flunarizine. *Headache, 43*, 464–469.

Doubell, T. P., Mannion, R. J., & Woolf, C. J. (1999). The dorsal horn: State-dependent sensory processing, plasticity and the generation of pain. In P. D. Wall & R. Melzack (Eds.), *Textbook of pain* (4th ed., pp. 165–181). New York: Churchill Livingstone.

Dowman, R. (2001). Attentional set effects on spinal and supraspinal responses to pain. *Psychophysiology, 38*, 451–464.

Drangsholt, M., & LeResche, L. (1999). Temporomandibular disorder pain. In I. K. Crombie (Ed.), *Epidemiology of pain* (pp. 203–233). Seattle: IASP Press.

Dreier, J. P., Kleeberg, J., Petzold, G., Priller, J., Windmüller, O., Orzechowski, H.-D., Lindauer, U., Heinemann, U., Einhäupl, K. M., & Dirnagl, U. (2002). Endothelin-1 potently induces Leão's cortical spreading depression *in vivo* in the rat: A model for an endothelial trigger of migrainous aura? *Brain, 125*, 102–112.

Droogleever Fortuyn, H. A., van Broekhoven, F., Span, P. N., Backstrom, T., Zitman, F. G., & Verkes, R. J. (2004). Effects of Ph.D. examination stress on allopregnanolone and cortisol plasma levels and peripheral benzodiazepine receptor density. *Psychoneuroendocrinology, 29*, 1341–1344.

Drossman, D. A. (1994). Physical and sexual abuse and gastrointestinal illness: What is the link? *American Journal of Medicine, 97*, 105–107.

Drottning, M., Staff, P. H., Levin, L., & Malt, U. F. (1995). Acute emotional response to common whiplash predicts subsequent pain complaints. *Nordic Journal of Psychiatry, 49*, 293–299.

Drummond, P. D. (1982). Extracranial and cardiovascular reactivity in migrainous subjects. *Journal of Psychosomatic Research, 26*, 317–331.

Drummond, P. D. (1984). Extracranial vascular changes during headache, exercise and stress. *Journal of Psychosomatic Research, 28*, 133–138.

Drummond, P. D. (1985). Vascular responses in headache-prone subjects during stress. *Biological Psychology, 21*, 11–25.

Drummond, P. D. (1990a). Dissociation between pain and autonomic disturbances in cluster headache. *Headache, 30,* 505–508.

Drummond, P. D. (1990b). Disturbances in ocular sympathetic function and facial blood flow in unilateral migraine headache. *Journal of Neurology, Neurosurgery, and Psychiatry, 53,* 121–125.

Drummond, P. D. (1991). Effects of body heating and mental arithmetic on facial sweating and blood flow in unilateral migraine headache. *Psychophysiology, 28,* 172–176.

Drummond, P. D. (1997). Photophobia and autonomic responses to facial pain in migraine. *Brain, 120,* 1857–1864.

Drummond, P. D., & Anderson, M. (1992). Visual field loss after attacks of migraine with aura. *Cephalalgia, 12,* 349–352.

Drummond, P. D., & Lance, J. W. (1983). Extracranial vascular changes and the source of pain in migraine headache. *Annals of Neurology, 13,* 32–37.

Drummond, P. D., & Quah, S. H. (2001). The effect of expressing anger on cardiovascular reactivity and facial blood flow in Chinese and Caucasians. *Psychophysiology, 38,* 190–196.

Dubey, K., Balani, D. K., & Pillai, K. K. (2003). Potential adverse interaction between aspirin and lisinopril in hypertensive rats. *Human and Experimental Toxicology, 22,* 143–147.

Dubner, R. (1991). Neuronal plasticity and pain following peripheral tissue inflammation or nerve injury. In M. R. Bond, J. E. Charlton & C. J. Woolf (Eds.), *Pain research and clinical management, Vol. 4,* Proceedings of the VIth World Congress on Pain (pp. 263–276). New York: Elsevier.

Dubois, B., Levy, R., Verin, M., Teixeira, C., Agid, Y., & Pillon, B. (1995). Experimental approach to prefrontal functions in humans. In J. Grafman, K. J. Holyoak, & F. Boller (Eds.), *Structure and functions of the human prefrontal cortex* (pp. 41–60). New York: New York Academy of Sciences. [*Annals of the New York Academy of Sciences*, vol. 769.]

Dubuisson, D. (1999). Nerve root disorders and arachnoiditis. In P. D. Wall & R. Melzack (Eds.), *Textbook of pain* (4th ed., pp. 851–878). London: Churchill Livingstone.

Duckro, P. N., & Chibnall, J. T. (1999). Chronic posttraumatic headache. In A. R. Block, E. F. Kremer, & E. Fernandez (Eds.), *Handbook of pain syndromes: Biopsychosocial perspectives* (pp. 303–320). Mahwah, NJ: Lawrence Erlbaum Associates.

Duckro, P. N., Chibnall, J. T., & Greenberg, M. S. (1995). Myofascial involvement in chronic post-traumatic headache. *Headache Quarterly: Current Treatment and Research, 6,* 34–38.

Duckro, P. N., Chibnall, J. T., & Tomazic, T. J. (1995). Anger, depression, and disability: A path analysis of relationships in a sample of chronic posttraumatic headache patients. *Headache, 35,* 7–9.

Duckro, P. N., Richardson, W. D., Marshall, J. E., Cassabaum, S., & Marshall, G. (1999). *Taking control of your headaches.* New York: Guilford.

Duncan, G. H., Bushnell, M C., Bates, R., & Dubner, R. (1987). Task-related responses of monkey medullary dorsal horn neurons. *Journal of Neurophysiology, 57,* 289–310.

Dunn, T. G., Ponsor, S., Weil, N., & Utz, S. W. (1986). The learning process in biofeedback: Is it feedforward or feedback? *Biofeedback and Self-Regulation, 11,* 143–156.

Dunne, E. L., Moss, S. J., & Smart, T. G. (1998). Inhibition of $GABA_A$ receptor function by tyrosine kinase inhibitors and their inactive analogues. *Molecular and Cellular Neurosciences, 12,* 300–310.

Dworkin, R. H., Handlin, D. S., Richlin, D. M., Brand, L., & Vannucci, C. (1985). Unraveling the effects of compensation, litigation, and employment on treatment response in chronic pain. *Pain, 23,* 49–59.

Dworkin, S. F. (1996). Longitudinal course of behavioral and physical findings in temporomandibular disorders. *Journal of Musculoskeletal Pain, 4*(4), 135–144.

Dworkin, S. F. (1999). Temporomandibular disorders: A problem in dental health. In R. J. Gatchel & D. C. Turk (Eds.), *Psychosocial factors in pain: Critical perspectives* (pp. 213–226). New York: Guilford.

Dworkin, S. F., Huggins, K. H., LeResche, L., Von Korff, M., Howard, J., Truelove, E., & Sommers, E. (1990). Epidemiology of signs and symptoms in temporomandibular disorders: Clinical signs in cases and controls. *Journal of the American Dental Association, 120,* 273–281.

Dworkin, S. F., & LeResche, L. (Eds.). (1992). Research diagnostic criteria for temporomandibular disorders: Review, criteria, examinations and specifications, critique. *Journal of Craniomandibular Disorders: Facial and Oral Pain, 6,* 301–355.

Dworkin, S. F., Turner, J. A., Wilson, L., Massoth, D., Whitney, C., Huggins, K. H., Burgess, J., Sommers, E., & Truelove, E. (1994). Brief group cognitive-behavioral intervention for temporomandibular disorders. *Pain, 59,* 175–187.

Dwyer, A., April, C., & Bogduk, N. (1990). Cervical zygapophyseal joint pain patterns I: A study in normal volunteers. *Spine, 15,* 453–457.

Dyb, G., Holmen, T. L., & Zwart, J.-A. (2006). Analgesic overuse among adolescents with headache: The Head-HUNT-Youth Study. *Neurology, 66*, 198–201.

D'Zurilla, T. J., & Nezu, A. M. (1999). *Problem-solving therapy: A social competence approach to clinical intervention* (2nd ed.). New York: Springer.

Eaves, L. J., Eysenck, H. J., & Martin, N. G. (1989). *Genes, culture and personality: An empirical approach.* London: Academic Press.

Ebersberger, A., Schaible, H.-G., Averbeck, B., & Richter, F. (2001). Is there a correlation between spreading depression, neurogenic inflammation, and nociception that might cause migraine headache? *Annals of Neurology, 49*, 7–13.

Eccleston, C. (1994). Chronic pain and attention: A cognitive approach. *British Journal of Clinical Psychology, 33*, 535–547.

Eccleston, C., & Crombez, G. (1999). Pain demands attention: A cognitive-affective model of the interruptive function of pain. *Psychological Bulletin, 125*, 356–366.

Eccleston, C., Crombez, G., Aldrich, S., & Stannard, C. (1997). Attention and somatic awareness in chronic pain. *Pain, 72*, 209–215.

Edes, B., & Dallenbach, K. M. (1936). The adaptation of pain aroused by cold. *American Journal of Psychology, 48*, 307–315.

Edmeads, J. (1988). The cervical spine and headache. *Neurology, 38*, 1874–1878.

Edmeads, J., & Mackell, J. A. (2002). The economic impact of migraine: An analysis of direct and indirect costs. *Headache, 42*, 501–509.

Edvinsson, L. (1982). Sympathetic control of cerebral circulation. *Trends in Neuroscience, 5*, 425–429.

Edvinsson, L. (1991). Innervation and effects of dilatory neuropeptides on cerebral vessels. New aspects. *Blood Vessels, 28*, 35–45.

Edvinsson, L. (2001). Aspects on the pathophysiology of migraine and cluster headache. *Pharmacology and Toxicology, 89*, 65–73.

Edvinsson, L., Olesen, I. J., Kingman, T. A., McCulloch, J., & Uddman, R. (1995). Modification of vasoconstrictor responses in cerebral blood vessels by lesioning of the trigeminal nerve: Possible involvement of CGRP. *Cephalalgia, 15*, 373–383.

Edwards, L. C., & Pearce, S. A. (1994). Word completion in chronic pain: Evidence for schematic representation of pain? *Journal of Abnormal Psychology, 103*, 379–382.

Eekers, P. J. E., & Koehler, P. J. (2001). Naratriptan prophylactic treatment in cluster headache. *Cephalalgia, 21*, 75–76.

Egermark, I., Carlsson, G. E., & Magnusson, T. (2001). A 20-year longitudinal study of subjective symptoms of temporomandibular disorders from childhood to adulthood. *Acta Odontologica Scandinavica, 59*, 40–48.

Ehde, D. M., & Holm, J. E. (1992). Stress and headache: Comparison of migraine, tension, and headache-free subjects. *Headache Quarterly, 3*, 54–60.

Eimer, B. N., & Freeman, A. (1998). *Pain management psychotherapy: A practical guide*. New York: Wiley.

Eisenach, J. C. (2000). Preemptive hyperalgesia, not analgesia? *Anesthesiology, 92*, 308–309.

Eisenberg, E., Chistyakov, A. V., Yudashkin, M., Kaplan, B., Hafner, H., & Feinsod, M. (2005). Evidence for cortical hyperexcitability of the affected limb representation area in CRPS: A psychophysical and transcranial magnetic stimulation study. *Pain, 113*, 99–105.

Eisenberg, R. S. (2005). Learning the value of drugs—Is rofecoxib a regulatory success story? *New England Journal of Medicine, 352*, 1285–1287.

Eisenberger, N. I., & Lieberman, M. D. (2004). Why rejection hurts: A common neural alarm system for physical and social pain. *Trends in Cognitive Sciences, 8*, 294–300.

Eisenberger, N. I., Lieberman, M. D., & Williams, K. D. (2003). Does rejection hurt? An FMRI study of social exclusion. *Science, 302*, 290–292.

Ekbom, K. (1975). Alprenolol for migraine prophylaxis. *Headache, 15*, 129–132.

Ekbom, K., & Hardebo, J. E. (2002). Cluster headache: Aetiology, diagnosis and management. *Drugs, 62*, 61–69.

Ekbom, K., Krabbe, A., Micelli, G., Prusinski, A., Cole, J. A., Pilgrim, A. J., & Noronha, D. (1995). Cluster headache attacks treated for up to three months with subcutaneous sumatriptan (6 mg). *Cephalalgia, 15*, 230–236.

Ekbom, K., Svensson, D. A., Traff, H., & Waldenlind, E. (2002). Age at onset and sex ratio in cluster headache: Observations over three decades. *Cephalalgia, 22*, 94–100.

Ekbom, K., & Zetterman, M. (1977). Oxprenolol in the treatment of migraine. *Acta Neurologica Scandinavica, 56*, 181–184.

Elenbaas, J. K. (1980). Centrally acting oral skeletal muscle relaxants. *American Journal of Hospital Pharmacy, 37*, 1313–1323.

Elkind, M. S., & Elkind, A. H. (1999). Post-traumatic headache. In M. L. Diamond & G. D. Solomon (Eds.), *Diamond and Dalessio's The practicing physician's approach to headache* (6th ed., pp. 137–150). Philadelphia: W. B. Saunders Company.

Ellemberg, D., Hammarrenger, B., Lepore, F., Roy, M.-S., & Guillemot, J.-P. (2001). Contrast dependency of VEPs as a function of spatial frequency: The parvocellular and magnocellular contributions to human VEPs. *Spatial Vision, 15*, 99–111.

Ellertsen, B., & Hammerborg, D. (1982). Psychophysiological response patterns in migraine patients. *Cephalalgia, 2*, 19–24.

Ellertsen, B., Nordby, H., Hammerborg, D., & Thorlacius, S. (1987). Psychophysiologic response patterns in migraine before and after temperature biofeedback. Prediction of treatment outcome. *Cephalalgia, 7*, 109–124.

Elser, J. M., & Woody, R. C. (1990). Migraine headache in the infant and young child. *Headache, 30*, 366–368.

Elwan, O., Abdella, M., El Bayad, A. B., & Hamdy, S. (1991). Hormonal changes in headache patients. *Journal of the Neurological Sciences, 106*, 75–81.

Embretson, S. E., & Reise, S. P. (2000). *Item response theory for psychologists*. Mahwah, NJ: Lawrence Erlbaum Associates.

Engel, G. L. (1977). The need for a new medical model: A challenge for biomedicine. *Science, 196*, 129–136.

Engel, J. M., Rapoff, M. A., & Pressman, A. R. (1992). Long-term follow-up of relaxation training for pediatric headache disorders. *Headache, 32*, 152–156.

Engel, P. A. (2002). New onset migraine associated with use of soy isoflavone supplements. *Neurology, 59*, 1289–1290.

Enoka, R. M., Rankin, L. L., Joyner, M. J., & Stuart, D. G. (1988). Fatigue-related changes in neuromuscular excitability of rat hindlimb muscles. *Muscle and Nerve, 11*, 1123–1132.

Erichsen, J. E. (1866). *On railway and other injuries of the nervous system*. London: Walton and Maberly.

Etminan, M., Levine, M. A. H., Tomlinson, G., & Rochon, P. A. (2002). Efficacy of angiotensin II receptor antagonists in preventing headache: A systematic overview and meta-analysis. *American Journal of Medicine, 112*, 642–646.

Evans, F. J. (1977). The placebo control of pain: A paradigm for investigating nonspecific effects in psychotherapy. In J. P. Brady, J. Mendels, W. R. Reiger, & M. T. Orne (Eds.), *Psychiatry: Areas of promise and advancement* (pp. 249–271). New York: Plenum.

Evans, R. W., & Rozen, T. D. (2001). Etiology and treatment of new daily persistent headache. *Headache, 41*, 830–832.

Evers, S., Bauer, B., Suhr, B., Voss, H., Frese, A., & Husstedt, I.-W. (1999). Cognitive processing is involved in cluster headache but not in chronic paroxysmal hemicrania. *Neurology, 53*, 357–363.

Evers, S., Suhr, B., Bauer, B., Grotemeyer, K.-H., & Husstedt, I.-W. (1999). A retrospective long-term analysis of the epidemiology and features of drug-induced headache. *Journal of Neurology, 246*, 802–809.

Eysenck, H. J. (1967). *The biological basis of personality*. Springfield, IL: C. C. Thomas.

Eysenck, H. J. (1991). *Smoking, personality, and stress: Psychosocial factors in the prevention of cancer and coronary heart disease*. New York: Springer-Verlag.

Fabiani, M., Gratton, G., & Coles, M. G. H. (2000). Event-related brain potentials: Methods, theory, and applications. In J. T. Cacioppo, L. G. Tassinary, & G. G. Berntson (Eds.), *Handbook of psychophysiology* (2nd ed., pp. 53–84). New York: Cambridge University Press.

Fadeyi, M. O., & Adams, Q. M. (2002). Use of botulinum toxin type B for migraine and tension headaches. *American Journal of Health-System Pharmacy, 59*, 1860–1862.

Fairbanks, C. A., Stone, L. S., Kitto, K. F., Nguyen, H. O., Posthumus, I. J., & Wilcox, G. L. (2002). Alpha(2C)-adrenergic receptors mediate spinal analgesia and adrenergic-opioid synergy. *Journal of Pharmacology and Experimental Therapeutics, 300*, 282–290.

Fanciullacci, M. (1979). Iris adrenergic impairment in idiopathic headache. *Headache, 19*, 8–13.

Fanselow, M. S. (1994). Neural organization of the defensive behavior system responsible for fear. *Psychonomic Bulletin Review, 1*, 429–438.

Faraci,, F. M., & Heistad, D. D. (1998). Regulation of the cerebral circulation: Role of endothelium and potassium channels. *Physiological Reviews, 78*, 53–97.

Farago, M., Szabo, C., Dora, E., Horvath, I., & Kovach, A. G. (1991). Contractile endothelium-dependent dilatatory responses of cerebral arteries at various extracellular magnesium concentrations. *Journal of Cerebral Blood Flow and Metabolism, 11*, 161–164.

Farmer, K., Cady, R., Bleiberg, J., Reeves, D., Putnam, G., O'Quinn, S., & Batenhorst, A. (2001). Sumatriptan nasal spray and cognitive function during migraine: Results of an open-label study. *Headache, 41*, 377–384.

Farthing, G. W., Venturino, M., & Brown, S. W. (1984). Suggestion and distraction in the control of pain: Test of two hypotheses. *Journal of Abnormal Psychology, 93*, 266–276.

Farthing, G. W., Venturino, M., Brown, S. W., & Lazar, J. D. (1997). Internal and external distraction in the control of cold-pressor pain as a function of hypnotizability. *International Journal of Clinical and Experimental Hypnosis, 45*, 433–446.

Faymonville, M. E., Laureys, S., Degueldre, C., Del Fiore, G., Luxen, A., Franck, G., Lamy, M., & Maquet, P. (2000). Neural mechanisms of antinociceptive effects of hypnosis. *Anesthesiology, 92*, 1257–1267.

Fearon, P., & Hotopf, M. (2001). Relation between headache in childhood and physical and psychiatric symptoms in adulthood: National birth cohort study. *British Medical Journal, 322*, 1145–1148.

Fechner, G. T. (1966). *Elements of psychophysics* (Trans. by H. E. Adler, D. H. Howes, & E. G. Boring). New York: Holt, Rinehart, and Winston. (Original work published 1860).

Fehrenbacher, J. C., Taylor, C. P., & Vasko, M. R. (2003). Pregabalin and gabapentin reduce release of substance P and CGRP from rat spinal tissues only after inflammation or activation of protein kinase C. *Pain, 105*, 133–141.

Feinstein, A., Ouchterlony, D., Somerville, J., & Jardine, A. (2001). The effects of litigation on symptom expression: A prospective study following mild traumatic brain injury. *Medicine, Science and the Law, 41*, 116–121.

Fenichel, O. (1945). *The psychoanalytic theory of neurosis*. New York: W. W. Norton and Company.

Ferguson, L. R. (2001). Role of plant polyphenols in genomic stability. *Mutation Research, 475*, 89–111.

Ferguson, R. (2000). Using the Beck Anxiety Inventory in primary care. In: M. E. Maruish (Ed.), *Handbook of psychological assessment in primary care settings* (pp. 509–535). Mahwah, NJ: Lawrence Erlbaum Associates.

Fernandez, E., & Turk, D. C. (1989). The utility of cognitive coping strategies for altering pain perception: A meta-analysis. *Pain, 38*, 123–135.

Ferrari, M. D. (1998a). The economic burden of migraine to society. *Pharmacoeconomics, 13*, 667–676.

Ferrari, M. D. (1998b). Migraine. *Lancet, 351*, 1043–1051.

Ferrari, M. D., Goadsby, P. J., Roon, K. I., & Lipton, R. B. (2002). Triptans (serotonin, 5-$HT_{1B/1D}$ agonists) in migraine: Detailed results and methods of a meta-analysis of 53 trials. *Cephalalgia, 22*, 633–658.

Ferrari, M. D., Odink, J., Tapparelli, C., Van Kempen, G. M. J., Pennings, E. J. M., & Bruyn, G. W. (1989). Serotonin metabolism in migraine. *Neurology, 39*, 1239–1242.

Ferrari, M. D., Roon, K. I., Lipton, R. B., & Goadsby, P. J. (2001). Oral triptans (serotonin 5-$HT_{1B/1D}$ agonists) in acute migraine treatment: A meta-analysis of 53 trials. *Lancet, 358*, 1668–1675.

Ferreira, S. H., Lorenzetti, B. B., Bristow, A. F., & Poole, S. (1988). Interleukin-1 beta as a potent hyperalgesic agent antagonized by a tripeptide analogue. *Nature, 334*, 698–700.

Fetrow, C. W., & Avila, J. R. (2001). *Professional's handbook of complementary and alternative medicines* (2nd ed.). Springhouse, PA: Springhouse.

Feuerstein, M., Bortolussi, L., Houle, M., & Labbé, E. (1983). Stress, temporal artery activity, and pain in migraine headache: A prospective analysis. *Headache, 23*, 296–304.

Feuerstein, M., Bush, C., & Corbisiero, R. (1982). Stress and chronic headache: A psychophysiological analysis of mechanisms. *Journal of Psychosomatic Research, 26*, 167–182.

Feuerstein, M., Carter, R. L., & Papciak, A. S. (1987). A prospective analysis of stress and fatigue in recurrent low back pain. *Pain, 31*, 333–344.

Fields, H. L. (1996). Treatment of trigeminal neuralgia. *New England Journal of Medicine, 334*, 1125–1126.

Fields, H. L. (1997). Pain modulation and headache. In P. J. Goadsby & S. D. Silberstein (Eds.), *Headache* (pp. 39–57). Boston: Butterworth-Heinemann.

Fields, H. L. (2000). Pain modulation: Expectation, opioid analgesia and virtual pain. In E. A. Mayer & C. B. Saper (Eds.), *The biological basis for mind body interactions. Progress in Brain Research, 122*, 245–253.

Fields, H. L. (2001, July 1). Pain modulating networks in headache pathogenesis. Invited lecture to the 10th Congress of the International Headache Society (IHC 2001). New York City.

Filippi, G. M., Errico, P., Santarelli, R., Bagolini, B., & Manni, E. (1993). Botulinum A toxin effects on rat jaw muscle spindles. *Acta Otolaryngologica, 113*, 400–404.

Fillingim, R. B., Wilkinson, C. S., & Powell, T. (1999). Self-reported abuse history and pain complaints among young adults. *Clinical Journal of Pain, 15*, 85–91.

Finneson, B. E. (1969). *Diagnosis and management of pain syndromes.* Philadelphia: W. B. Saunders.

Fioroni, L., Martignoni, E., & Facchinetti, F. (1995). Changes of neuroendocrine axes in patients with menstrual migraine. *Cephalalgia, 15*, 297–300.

Fiske, S. T., & Taylor, S. E. (1991). *Social cognition* (2nd ed.). New York: McGraw-Hill.

Flor, H., & Birbaumer, N. (1991). Comprehensive assessment and treatment of chronic back pain patients without physical disabilities. In M. Bond (Ed.), *Proceedings of the VIth World Congress on Pain* (pp. 229–234). Amsterdam: Elsevier.

Flor, H., & Birbaumer, N. (1993). Comparison of the efficacy of electromyographic biofeedback, cognitive-behavioral therapy, and conservative medical interventions in the treatment of chronic musculoskeletal pain. *Journal of Consulting and Clinical Psychology, 61*, 653–658.

Flor, H., Birbaumer, N., Schugens, M. M., & Lutzenberger, W. (1992). Symptom-specific psychophysiological responses in chronic pain patients. *Psychophysiology, 29*, 452–460.

Flor, H., Birbaumer, N., Schulte, W., & Roos, R. (1991). Stress-related electromyographic responses in patients with chronic temporomandibular pain. *Pain, 46*, 145–152.

Flor, H., Braun, C., Elbert, T., & Birbaumer, N. (1997). Extensive reorganization of primary somatosensory cortex in chronic back pain patients. *Neuroscience Letters, 224*, 5–8.

Flor, H., Breitenstein, C., Birbaumer, N., & Fürst, M. (1995). A psychophysiological analysis of spouse solicitousness towards pain behaviors, spouse interaction, and pain perception. *Behavior Therapy, 26*, 255–272.

Flor, H., Denke, C., Schaefer, M., & Grüsser, S. (2001). Effect of sensory discrimination training on cortical reorganisation and phantom limb pain. *Lancet, 357*, 1763–1764.

Flor, H., Elbert, T., Knecht, S., Wienbruch, C., Pantev, C., Birbaumer, N., Larbig, W., & Taub, E. (1995). Phantom-limb pain as a perceptual correlate of cortical reorganization following arm amputation. *Nature, 375*, 482–484.

Flor, H., Fuerst, M., & Birbaumer, N. (1999). Deficient discrimination of EMG levels and overestimation of perceived tension in chronic pain patients. *Applied Psychophysiology and Biofeedback, 24*, 55–66.

Flor, H., Knost, B., & Birbaumer, N. (1997). Processing of pain- and body-related verbal material in chronic pain patients: Central and peripheral correlates. *Pain, 73*, 413–421.

Flor, H., Knost, B., & Birbaumer, N. (2002). The role of operant conditioning in pain: An experimental investigation. *Pain, 95*, 111–118.

Flor, H., Schugens, M. M., & Birbaumer, N. (1992). Discrimination of muscle tension in chronic pain patients and healthy controls. *Biofeedback and Self-Regulation, 17*, 165–177.

Flor, H., & Turk, D. C. (1989). Psychophysiology of chronic pain: Do chronic pain patients exhibit symptom-specific psychophysiological responses? *Psychological Bulletin, 105*, 215–259.

Fogle, L. L., & Glaros, A. G. (1995). Contributions of facial morphology, age, and gender to EMG activity under biting and resting conditions: A canonical correlation analysis. *Journal of Dental Research, 74*, 1496–1500.

Folkers, K., & Simonsen, R. (1995). Two successful double-blind trials with coenzyme Q_{10} (vitamin Q_{10}) on muscular dystrophies and neurogenic atrophies. *Biochimica Biophysica Acta, 1271*, 281–286.

Folstein, M. F., Folstein, S. E., & McHugh, P. R. (1975). "Mini-mental State." A practical method for grading the cognitive state of patients for the clinician. *Journal of Psychiatric Research, 12*, 189–198.

Ford, A. (1964). *John James Audubon.* Norman, OK: University of Oklahoma Press.

Fordyce, W. E. (1976). *Behavioral methods for chronic pain and illness.* St. Louis, MO: Mosby.

Fordyce, W. E. (1979). Environmental factors in the genesis of low back pain. In J. Bonica, J. Liebeskind, & V. Albe-Fessard (Eds.), *Advances in pain research and therapy* (Vol. 3, pp. 659–666). New York: Raven Press.

Fordyce, W. E. (1988). Pain and suffering: A reappraisal. *American Psychologist, 43*, 276–283.

Forman, S. G., (1993). *Coping skills interventions for children and adolescents.* San Francisco: Jossey-Bass.

Foster, B. C., Vandenhoek, S., Hana, J., Krantis, A., Akhtar, M. H., Bryan, M., Budzinski, J. W., Ramputh, A., & Arnason, J. T. (2003). In vitro inhibition of human cytochrome P450-mediated metabolism of marker substrates by natural products. *Phytomedicine, 10*, 334–342.

Foster, P. S. (2004). Use of the Calmset 3 biofeedback/relaxation system in the assessment and treatment of chronic nocturnal bruxism. *Applied Psychophysiology and Biofeedback, 29*, 141–147.

Fothergill, J. (1784). Remarks on that complaint commonly known under the name of the sick- headach [sic] (Read Dec. 14, 1778). *Medical Observations and Inquiries, 6*, 103–137.

Fozard, J. R., & Kalkman, H. O. (1994). 5-Hydroxytriptamine (5-HT) and the initiation of migraine: New perspectives. *Naunyn-Schmiedeberg's Archives of Pharmacology, 350*, 225–229.

Fragoso, Y. D. (1997). Reduction of migraine attacks during the use of warfarin. *Headache, 37*, 667–668.

France, C. R. (1999). Decreased pain perception and risk for hypertension: Considering a common physiological mechanism. *Psychophysiology, 36*, 683–692.

France, C. R., France, J. L., al' Absi, M., Ring, C., & McIntyre, D. (2002). Catastrophizing is related to pain ratings, but not nociceptive flexion reflex threshold. *Pain, 99*, 459–463.

Frankenstein, U. N., Richter, W., McIntyre, M. C., & Remy, F. (2001). Distraction modulates anterior cingulate gyrus activations during the cold pressor test. *Neuroimage, 14*, 827–836.

Fredholm, B. B. (1995). Adenosine, adenosine receptors and the actions of caffeine. *Pharmacology and Toxicology, 76*, 93–101.

Fredriksen, T. A., Fougner, R., Tangerud, A., & Sjaastad, O. (1989). Cervicogenic headache: Radiological investigations concerning head and neck. *Cephalalgia, 9*, 139–146.

Freedman, R. R. (1987). Long-term effectiveness of behavioral treatments for Raynaud's disease. *Behavior Therapy, 18*, 387–399.

Freedman, R. R. (1993). Raynaud's disease and phenomenon. In R. J. Gatchel & E. B. Blanchard (Eds.) *Psychophysiological disorders: Research and clinical applications.* Washington, DC: American Psychological Association.

Freedman, R. R., Sabharwal, S. C., Ianni, P., Desai, N., Wenig, P., & Mayes, M. (1988). Nonneural beta-adrenergic vasodilating mechanism in temperature biofeedback. *Psychosomatic Medicine, 50*, 394–401.

Freeman, M. D. (2001). Are Demolition Derby drivers a valid proxy for the population at risk for whiplash injury? *Archives of Neurology, 58*, 680–681.

Freeman, R., & Rutkove, S. (2000). Syncope. In: O. Appenzeller (Ed.), *Handbook of clinical neurology (vol. 75): the autonomic nervous system. Part II. Dysfunctions* (pp. 203–228). New York: Elsevier.

Freitag, F. G., Collins, S. D., Carlson, H. A., Goldstein, J., Saper, J., Silberstein, S., Mathew, N., Winner, P. K., Deaton, R., & Sommerville, K. (2002). A randomized trial of divalproex sodium extended-release tablets in migraine prophylaxis. *Neurology, 58*, 1652–1659.

French, D. J., Gauthier, J. G., Roberge, C., Bouchard, S., & Nouwen, A. (1997). Self-efficacy in the thermal biofeedback treatment of migraine sufferers. *Behavior Therapy, 28*, 109–125.

French, D. J., Holroyd, K. A., Pinell, C., Malinoski, P. T., O'Donnell, F., & Hill, K. R. (2000). Perceived self-efficacy and headache-related disability. *Headache, 40*, 647–656.

Fresco, D. M., Mennin, D. S., Heimberg, R. G., & Turk, C. L. (2003). Using the Penn State Worry Questionnaire to identify individuals with generalized anxiety disorder: A receiver operating characteristic analysis. *Journal of Behavior Therapy and Experimental Psychiatry, 34*, 283–291.

Freud, S. (1925/1963). *An autobiographical study* (J. Strachey, Trans.). New York: W. W. Norton & Co.

Freund, B. J., & Schwartz, M. (2000). Treatment of chronic cervical-associated headache with botulinum toxin A: A pilot study. *Headache, 40*, 231–236.

Friberg, L. (1996). Migraine pathophysiology and its relation to cerebral hemodynamic changes. In F. C. Rose (Ed.), *Towards migraine 2000* (pp. 101–109). New York: Elsevier.

Friberg, L., Nicolic, I., Olesen, J., Iversen, H., Sperling, B., Lassen, N. A., & Tfelt-Hansen, P. (1991). Interictal SPECT studies of rCBF in migraine patients suggesting abnormal, patchy vascular regulation. *Cephalalgia, 11*(Suppl. 11), S40–S41.

Friberg, L., Olesen, J., Iverson, H. K., & Sperling, B. (1991). Migraine pain associated with middle cerebral artery dilation: Reversal by sumatriptan. *Lancet, 338*, 13–17.

Fridlund, A. J., & Cacioppo, J. T. (1986). Guidelines for human electromyographic research. *Psychophysiology, 23*, 567–589.

Friederich, M., Trippe, R. H., Özcan, M., Weiss, T., Hecht, H., & Miltner, W. H. R. (2001). Laser-evoked potentials to noxious stimulation during hypnotic analgesia and distraction of attention suggest different brain mechanisms of pain control. *Psychophysiology, 38*, 768–776.

Friedman, A. P. (1972). The headache in history, literature, and legend. *Bulletin of the New York Academy of Medicine, 48*, 661–681.

Friedman, A. P., von Storch, T. J. C., & Merritt, H. H. (1954). Migraine and tension headaches: A clinical study of two thousand cases. *Neurology, 4*, 773–788.

Friedman, D. I. (1999). Pseudotumor cerebri. *Neurosurgical Clinics of North America, 10*, 609–621.

Frishberg, B. M., Rosenberg, J. H., Matchar, D. B., McCrory, D. C., Pietrzak, M. P., Rozen, T. D., & Silberstein, S. D. (2000). *Evidence-based guidelines in the primary care setting: Neuroimaging in patients with nonacute headache.* Retrieved April 11, 2004, from American Academy of Neurology web site: *http://www.aan.com/*professionals/practice/pdfs/gl0088.pdf

Fromm-Reichmann, F. (1937). Contribution to the psychogenesis of migraine. *Psychoanalytic Review, 24*, 26–33.

Fruhstorfer, H., Gross, W., & Selbmann, O. (2001). Von Frey hairs: New materials for a new design. *European Journal of Pain, 5*, 341–342.

Fruhstorfer, H., Lindblom, U., & Schmidt, W. G. (1976). Method for quantitative estimation of thermal thresholds in patients. *Journal of Neurology, Neurosurgery, and Psychiatry, 39*, 1071–1075.

Fumal, A., Laureys, S., Di Clemente, L., Boly, M., Bohotin, V., Vandenheede, M., et al. (2006). Orbitofrontal cortex involvement in chronic analgesic-overuse headache evolving from episodic migraine. *Brain, 129*, 543–550.

Furmanski, A. R. (1952). Dynamic concepts of migraine. *Archives of Neurology and Psychiatry, 67*, 23–31.

Furue, H., Katafuchi, T., & Yoshimura, M. (2004). Sensory processing and functional reorganization of sensory transmission under pathological conditions in the spinal dorsal horn. *Neuroscience Research, 48*, 361–368.

Fusco, B. M., Colantoni, O., & Giacovazzo, M. (1997). Alteration of central excitation circuits in chronic headache and analgesic misuse. *Headache, 37*, 486–491.

Fuster, J. M. (1997). *The prefrontal cortex: Anatomy, physiology, and neuropsychology of the frontal lobe* (3rd ed.). Philadelphia: Lippincott-Raven.

Gaab, J., Baumann, S., Budnoik, A., Gmünder, H., Hottinger, N., & Ehlert, U. (2005). Reduced activity and enhanced negative feedback sensitivity of the hypothalamus-pituitary-adrenal axis in chronic whiplash-associated disorder. *Pain, 119*, 219–224.

Gabai, I. J., & Spierings, E. L. (1989). Prophylactic treatment of cluster headache with verapamil. *Headache, 29*, 167–168.

Gabrielli, M., Santarelli, L., Addolorato, G., Foschi, G., Cristiana, D. C., & Gasbarrini, A. (2002). High prevalence of antiendothelial cell antibodies in migraine. *Headache, 42*, 385–386.

Gaist, D., Pedersen, L., Madsen, C., Tsiropoulos, I., Bak, S., Sindrup, S., et al. (2005). Long-term effects of migraine on cognitive function. A population-based study of Danish twins. *Neurology, 64*, 600–607.

Gallagher, R. M., & Myers, P. (1996). Referral delay in back pain patients on worker's compensation: Costs and policy implications. *Psychosomatics, 37*, 270–284.

Gallai, V., Sarchielli, P., Carboni, F., Benedetti, P., Mastropaolo, C., & Puca, F. (1995). Applicability of the 1988 IHS criteria to headache patients under the age of 18 years attending 21 Italian headache clinics. *Headache, 35*, 146–153.

Gallai, V., Sarchielli, P., Firenze, C., Trequattrini, A., Paciaroni, M., Usai, F., & Palumbo, R. (1994). Endothelin 1 in migraine and tension-type headache. *Acta Neurologica Scandinavica, 89*, 47–55.

Galli, S. J., & Lantz, C. S. (1999). Allergy. In W. E. Paul (Ed.), *Fundamental immunology* (4th ed., pp. 1127–1174). Philadelphia, PA: Lippincott-Raven.

Gannon, L. R., Haynes, S. N., Cuevas, J., & Chavez, R. (1987). Psychophysiological correlates of induced headaches. *Journal of Behavioral Medicine, 10*, 411–423.

Gannon, L. R., Haynes, S. N., Safranek, R., & Hamilton, J. (1981). A psychophysiological investigation of muscle-contraction and migraine headache. *Journal of Psychosomatic Research, 25*, 271–280.

Gannon, L., & Sternbach, R. A. (1971). Alpha enhancement as a treatment for pain: A case study. *Journal of Behavior Therapy and Experimental Psychiatry, 2*, 209–213.

Garcia-Monco, J. C., & Mateo, I. (2005). Migraine, epilepsy, and brain neuronal hyperexcitation: A response. *Headache, 45*, 89–90.

Gardea, M. A., Gatchel, R. J., & Mishra, K. D. (2001). Long-term efficacy of biobehavioral treatment of temporomandibular disorders. *Journal of Behavioral Medicine, 24*, 341–359.

Gardell, L. R., Wang, R., Burgess, S. E., Ossipov, M. H., Vanderah, T. W., Malan, T. P. Jr., Lai, J., & Porreca, F. (2002). Sustained morphine exposure induces a spinal dynorphin-dependent enhancement of excitatory transmitter release from primary afferent fibers. *Journal of Neuroscience, 22*, 6747–6755.

Gardner, K., Barmada, M. M., Ptacek, L. J., & Hoffman, E. P. (1997). A new locus for hemiplegic migraine maps to chromosome 1q31. *Neurology, 49*, 1231–1238.

Gatchel, R. J., Garofalo, J. P., Ellis, E., & Holt, C. (1996). Major psychological disorders in acute and chronic TMD: An initial examination. *Journal of the American Dental Association, 127*, 1365–1374.

Gaudet, R. J., & Kessler, I. I. (1987). Transparently blinded trials of methysergide. *New England Journal of Medicine, 316*, 279–280.

Gauthier, J., Côté, G., & French, D. (1994). The role of home practice in the thermal biofeedback treatment of migraine headache. *Journal of Consulting and Clinical Psychology, 62*, 180–184.

Gauthier, J. G., Fournier, A.-L., & Roberge, C. (1991). The differential effects of biofeedback in the treatment of menstrual and nonmenstrual migraine. *Headache, 31*, 82–90.

Gauthier, J. G., Ivers, H., & Carrier, S. (1996). Nonpharmacological approaches in the management of recurrent headache disorders and their comparison and combination with pharmacotherapy. *Clinical Psychology Review, 6*, 543–571.

Gawel, M., Burkitt, M., & Rose, F. C. (1979). The platelet release reaction during migraine attacks. *Headache, 19*, 323–327.

Gawel, M. J., & Ichise, M. (1994). The cavernous sinus in cluster headache. In F. C. Rose (Ed.), *New advances in headache research* (3rd edition, pp. 221–223). London: Smith-Gordon.

Gawel, M. J., Kreeft, J., Nelson, R. F., Simard, D., & Arnott, W. S. (1992). Comparison of the efficacy and safety of flunarizine to propranolol in the prophylaxis of migraine. *Canadian Journal of Neurological Sciences, 19*, 340–345.

Gawel, M. J., & Rothbarth, P. J. (1992). Occipital nerve block in the management of headache and cervical pain. *Cephalalgia, 12*, 9–13.

Gay, M.-C., Philippot, P., & Luminet, O. (2002). Differential effectiveness of psychological interventions for reducing osteoarthritis pain: A comparison of Erickson hypnosis and Jacobson relaxation. *European Journal of Pain, 6*, 1–16.

Geary, G. G., Krause, D. N., & Duckles, S. P. (1998). Estrogen reduces myogenic tone through a nitric oxide-dependent mechanism in rat cerebral arteries. *American Journal of Physiology, 275*(1 Pt 2), H292–H300.

Geddes, L. A. (1998). *Medical device accidents: with illustrative cases*. Boca Raton: CRC Press.

Geenen, R., Jacobs, J. W. G., & Bijlsma, J.W. J. (2002). Evaluation and management of endocrine dysfunction in fibromyalgia. *Rheumatic Diseases Clinics of North America, 28*, 389–404.

Geisser, M. E., Roth, R. S., & Robinson, M. E. (1997). Assessing depression among persons with chronic pain using the Center for Epidemiological Studies Depression Scale and the Beck Depression Inventory: A comparative analysis. *Clinical Journal of Pain, 13*, 163–170.

Gelkopf, M. (1997). Laboratory pain and styles of coping with anger. *Journal of Psychology, 131*, 121–123.

Gelmers, H. J. (1993). Nimodipine, a new calcium antagonist, in the prophylactic treatment of migraine. *Headache, 23*, 106–109.

Gentle, M. J., & Tilston, V. L. (1999). Reduction in peripheral inflammation by changes in attention. *Physiology and Behavior, 66*, 289–292.

Géraud, G., Keywood, C., & Senard, J. M. (2003). Migraine headache recurrence: Relationship to clinical, pharmacological, and pharmacokinetic properties of triptans. *Headache, 43*, 376–388.

Géraud, G., Spierings, E. L. H., & Keywood, C. (2002). Tolerability and safety of frovatriptan with short- and long-term use for treatment of migraine and in comparison with sumatriptan. *Headache, 42*(Suppl. 2), s93–s99.

Gerber, W. D., Miltner, W., & Niederberger, U. (1988). The role of behavioral and social factors in the development of drug-induced headache. In H.-C. Diener & M. Wilkinson (Eds.), *Drug-induced headache* (pp. 65–74). New York: Springer-Verlag.

Gerber, W. D., & Schoenen, J. (1998). Biobehavioral correlates in migraine: The role of hypersensitivity and information-processing dysfunction. *Cephalalgia, 18*(Suppl. 21), 5–11.

Gershon, A. A., Dannon, P. N., & Grunhaus, L. (2003). Transcranial magnetic stimulation in the treatment of depression. *American Journal of Psychiatry, 160*, 835–845.

Gershon, E. S., & Buchsbaum, M. S. (1977). A genetic study of average evoked response augmentation/ reduction in affective disorders. In C. Shagass, S. Gershon, & A. J. Friedhoff (Eds.), *Psychopathology and brain dysfunction*. New York: Raven.

Gervais, R. O., Fitzsimmons, G. W., & Thomas, N. R. (1989). Masseter and temporalis electromyographic activity in asymptomatic, subclinical, and temporomandibular joint dysfunction patients. *Journal of Craniomandibular Practice, 7*, 52–57.

Gescuk, B. D., Lang, S., & Kornetsky, C. (1995). Chronic escapable footshock causes a reduced response to morphine in rats as assessed by local cerebral metabolic rates. *Brain Research, 701*, 279–287.

Gessel, A. H. (1989). Edmund Jacobson, M.D., Ph.D.: The founder of scientific relaxation. *International Journal of Psychosomatics, 36*(1–4), 5–14.

Gevirtz, R. N., Glaros, A. G., Hopper, D., & Schwartz, M. S. (1995). Temporomandibular disorders. In: M. S. Schwartz (Ed.), *Biofeedback: A practitioner's guide* (2nd ed., pp. 411–428). New York: Guilford Press.

Ghione, S. (1996). Hypertension-associated hypalgesia. Evidence in experimental animals and humans, pathophysiological mechanisms, and potential clinical consequences. *Hypertension, 28*, 494–504.

Ghose, K., Coppen, A., & Carrol, D. (1977). Intravenous tyramine response in migraine before and during treatment with indoramin. *British Medical Journal, 1*, 1191–1193.

Ghose, K., & Turner, P. (1977). The menstrual cycle and the tyramine pressor response test. *British Journal of Clinical Pharmacology, 4*, 500–502.

Giardino, N. D., Glenny, R. W., Borson, S., & Chan, L. (2003). Respiratory sinus arrhythmia is associated with efficiency of pulmonary gas exchange in healthy humans. *American Journal of Physiology: Heart and Circulatory Physiology, 284*, H1585–H1591.

Giardino, N. D., & Lehrer, P. M. (2000). Behavioral conditioning and idiopathic environmental intolerance. *Occupational Medicine: State of the Art Reviews, 15*, 519–528.

Giglio, J. A., Bruera, O. C., & Leston, J. A. (1995). Influence of transformation factors on chronic daily headache. *Headache, 35*(Suppl. 14), 165.

Gil, K. M., Carson, J. W., Sedway, J. A., Porter, L. S., Schaeffer, J. J. W., & Orringer, E. (2000). Follow-up of coping skills training in adults with sickle cell disease: Analysis of daily pain and coping practice diaries. *Health Psychology, 19*, 85–90.

Gil, K. M., Keefe, F. J., Crisson, J. E., & Van-Dalfsen, P. J. (1987). Social support and pain behavior. *Pain, 29*, 209–217.

Gilkey, S. J., Ramadan, N. M., Aurora, T. K., & Welch, K. M. (1997). Cerebral blood flow in chronic posttraumatic headache. *Headache, 37*, 583–587.

Gillis, M. M., Haaga, D. A. F., & Ford, G. T. (1995). Normative values for the Beck Anxiety Inventory, Fear Questionnaire, Penn State Worry Questionnaire, and Social Phobia and Anxiety Inventory. *Psychological Assessment, 7*, 450–455.

Gintzler, A. R., & Liu, N. J. (2001). The maternal spinal cord: Biochemical and physiological correlates of steroid-activated antinociceptive processes. *Progress in Brain Research, 133*, 83–97.

Giolas, M. H., & Sanders, B. (1992). Pain and suffering as a function of dissociation level and instructional set. *Dissociation, 5*, 205–209.

Gjerstad, J., Tjølsen, A., & Hole, K. (2001). Induction of long-term potentiation of single wide dynamic range neurones in the dorsal horn is inhibited by descending pathways. *Pain, 91*, 263–268.

Gladstein, J., & Holden, E. W. (1996). Chronic daily headache in children and adolescents: A 2 year prospective study. *Headache, 36*, 349–351.

Gladstein, J., Holden, E. W., Peralta, L., & Raven, M. (1993). Diagnoses and symptom patterns in children presenting to a pediatric headache clinic. *Headache, 33*, 497–500.

Gladstein, J., Holden, E. W., Winner, P., Linder, S., & the Pediatric Committee of the American Association for the Study of Headache. (1997). Chronic daily headache in children and adolescents: Current status and recommendations for the future. *Headache, 37*, 626–629.

Glaros, A. G. (1996). Awareness of physiological responding under stress and nonstress conditions in temporomandibular disorders. *Biofeedback and Self-Regulation, 21*, 261–272.

Glaros, A. G., & Glass, E. G. (1993). Temporomandibular disorders. In R. J. Gatchel & E. B. Blanchard (Eds.), *Psychophysiological disorders: Research and clinical applications* (pp. 299–356). Washington, DC: American Psychological Association.

Glaros, A. G., Tabacchi, K. N., & Glass, E. G. (1998). Effect of parafunctional clenching on TMD pain. *Journal of Orofacial Pain, 12*, 145–152.

Glover, V., Pattichis, K., Jarman, J., Peatfield, R., & Sandler, M. (1994). How does red wine cause migraine? In F. C. Rose (Ed.), *New advances in headache research* (3rd ed., pp. 145–150). London: Smith-Gordon and Company, Ltd.

Goa, K. L., Balfour, J. A., & Zuanetti, G. (1996). Lisinopril. A review of its pharmacology and clinical efficacy in the early management of acute myocardial infarction. *Drugs, 52*, 564–588.

Goadsby, P. J. (1995). Cerebral mechanisms relevant to migraine. In B. Bromm & J. E. Desmedt (Eds.), *Pain and the brain: From nociception to cognition* (*Advances in Pain Research and Therapy*, Vol. 22, pp. 423–437). New York: Raven Press.

Goadsby, P. J. (1997a). Current concepts of the pathophysiology of migraine. *Neurologic Clinics, 15*(1), 27–42.

Goadsby, P. J. (1997b). Is the mechanism of action of dihydroergotamine unique? *Clinical update on dihydroergotamine.* Dumont, NJ: Center for Bio-Medical Communication, Inc.

Goadsby, P. J. (1998). A triptan too far? *Journal of Neurology, Neurosurgery and Psychiatry, 64*, 143–147.

Goadsby, P. J. (1999). Chronic tension-type headache: Where are we? [Editorial]. *Brain, 122*, 1611–1612.

Goadsby, P. J., & Edvinsson, L. (1991). Sumatriptan reverses the changes in calcitonin gene-related peptide seen in the headache phase of migraine. *Cephalalgia, 11*(Suppl. 11), 3–4.

Goadsby, P. J., & Edvinsson, L. (1993). The trigeminovascular system and migraine: Studies characterizing cerebrovascular and neuropeptide changes seen in humans and cats. *Annals of Neurology, 33*, 48–56.

Goadsby, P. J., & Edvinsson, L. (1994). Human in vivo evidence of trigeminovascular activation in cluster headache. Neuropeptide changes and effects of acute attacks therapies. *Brain, 117*, 427–434.

Goadsby, P. J., Edvinsson, L., & Ekman, R. (1990). Vasoactive peptide release in the extracerebral circulation of humans during migraine headache. *Annals of Neurology, 28*, 183–187.

Goadsby, P. J., & Hoskin, K. L. (1996). Inhibition of trigeminal neurons by intravenous administration of the serotonin (5HT)-1-D receptor agonist zolmitriptan (311C90): Are brain stem sites a therapeutic target in migraine? *Pain, 67*, 355–359.

Goadsby, P. J., & Knight, Y. E. (1997a). Direct evidence for central sites of action of zolmitriptan (311C90): An autoradiographic study in cat. *Cephalalgia, 17*, 153–158.

Goadsby, P. J., & Knight, Y. E. (1997b). Naratriptan inhibits trigeminal neurons after intravenous administration through an action at the serotonin ($5HT_{1B/1D}$) receptors. *British Journal of Pharmacology, 122*, 918–922.

Goadsby, P. J., & Lipton, R. B. (1997). A review of paroxysmal hemicranias, SUNCT syndrome and other short-lasting headaches with autonomic feature, including new cases. *Brain, 120*, 193–209.

Göbel, H., Hamouz, V., Hansen, C., et al. (1994). Chronic tension-type headache: Amitriptyline reduces clinical headache duration and experimental pain sensitivity but does not alter pericranial muscle activity readings. *Pain, 59*, 241–249.

Göbel, H., Heinze, A., Heinze-Kuhn, K., & Austermann, K. (2001). Botulinum toxin A in the treatment of headache syndromes and pericranial pain syndromes. *Pain, 91*, 195–199.

Göder, R., Fritzer, G., Kapsokalyvas, A., Kropp, P., Niederberger, U., Strenge, H., Gerber, W. D., & Aldenhoff, J. B. (2001). Polysomnographic findings in nights preceding a migraine attack. *Cephalalgia, 21*, 31–37.

Goldenberg, D. L. (1999). Fibromyalgia syndrome a decade later: What have we learned? *Archives of Internal Medicine, 159*, 777–785.

Goldin, A. L., Barchi, R. L., Caldwell, J. H., Hofmann, F., Howe, J. R., Hunter, J. C., et al. (2000). Nomenclature of voltage-gated sodium channels. *Neuron, 28*, 365–368.

Goldscheider, A. (1889). Untersuchungen über den Muskelsinn. *Archiv für Anatomie und Physiologie (Liepzig), 3*, 369–502.

Goldstein, B. H. (1999). Temporomandibular disorders: A review of current understanding. *Oral Surgery, Oral Medicine, Oral Pathology, Oral Radiology, & Endodontics, 88*, 379–385.

Goldstein, D. J., Lu, Y., Detke, M. J., Wiltse, C., Mallinckrodt, C., & Demitrack, M. A. (2004). Duloxetine in the treatment of depression: A double-blind placebo-controlled comparison with paroxetine. *Journal of Clinical Psychopharmacology, 24*, 389–399.

Goldstein, D. J., Roon, K. I., Offen, W. W., Ramadan, N. M., Phebus, L. A., Johnson, K. W., Schaus, J. M., & Ferrari, M. D. (2001). Selective serotonin 1F ($5-HT_{1F}$) receptor agonist LY334370 for acute migraine: A randomised controlled trial. *Lancet, 358*, 1230–1234.

Gomersall, J. D., & Stuart, A. (1973). Amitriptyline in migraine prophylaxis: Changes in pattern of attacks during a controlled clinical trial. *Journal of Neurology, Neurosurgery, and Psychiatry, 36*, 684–690.

Gonzalez-Heydrich, I., & Peroutka, S. (1990). Serotonin receptor and re-uptake site: Pharmacologic significance. *Journal of Clinical Psychiatry, 51* (April Supplement), 5–12.

Good, P. A., Taylor, R. H., & Mortimer, M. J. (1991). The use of tinted glasses in childhood migraine. *Headache, 31*, 533–536.

Gooden, B. A. (1994). Mechanism of the human diving response. *Integrative Physiological and Behavioral Science, 29*, 6–16.

Gorassini, M. A., Knash, M. E., Harvey, P. J., Bennett, D. J., & Yang, J. F. (2004). Role of motoneurons in the generation of muscle spasms after spinal cord injury. *Brain, 127*, 2247–2258.

Gordon, J. H., & Diamond, B. I. (1981). Antagonism of dopamine supersensitivity by estrogen: Neurochemical studies in an animal model of tardive dyskinesia. *Biological Psychiatry, 16*, 365–371.

Gorecki, J., Hirayama, T., Dostrovsky, J. O., Tasker, R. R., & Lenz, F. A. (1989). Thalamic stimulation and recording in patients with deafferentation and central pain. *Stereotactic and Functional Neurosurgery, 52*, 219–226.

Gotoh, F., Komatsumoto, S., Araki, N., & Gomi, S. (1984). Noradrenergic nervous activity in migraine. *Archives of Neurology, 41*, 951–955.

Goudswaard, P., Passchier, J., & Orlebeke, J. F. (1988). EMG in common migraine: Changes in absolute and proportional EMG levels during real-life stress. *Cephalalgia, 8*, 163–174.

Govind, J., King, W., Bailey, B., & Bogduk, N. (2003). Radiofrequency neurotomy for the treatment of third occipital headache. *Journal of Neurology, Neurosurgery and Psychiatry, 74*, 88–93.

Gracely, R. H. (1995). Hypnosis and hierarchical pain control systems. *Pain, 60,* 1–2.

Gracely, R. H. (1999). Studies of pain in human subjects. In P. D. Wall & R. Melzack (Eds.) *Textbook of pain* (4th ed., pp. 385–407). New York: Churchill Livingstone.

Gracely, R. H., Geisser, M. E., Giesecke, T., Grant, M. A. B., Petzke, F., Williams, D. A., & Clauw, D. J. (2004). Pain catastrophizing and neural responses to pain among persons with fibromyalgia. *Brain, 127,* 835–843.

Grachev, I. D., Fredrickson, B. E., & Apkarian, A. V. (2000). Abnormal brain chemistry in chronic back pain: An in vivo proton magnetic resonance spectroscopy study. *Pain, 89,* 7–18.

Graff-Radford, S. B., Jaeger, B., & Reeves, J. L. (1986). Myofascial pain may present clinically as occipital neuralgia. *Neurosurgery, 19,* 610–613.

Graham, J. R., & Wolff, H. G. (1938). Mechanism of migraine headache and action of ergotamine tartrate. *Archives of Neurology and Psychiatry, 39,* 737–763.

Gramling, S. E., Grayson, R. L., Sullivan, T. N., & Schwartz, S. (1997). Schedule-induced masseter EMG in facial pain subjects vs. no-pain controls. *Physiology and Behavior, 61,* 301–309.

Gramling, S. E., Neblett, J., Grayson, R., & Townsend, D. (1996). Temporomandibular disorder: Efficacy of an oral habit reversal treatment program. *Journal of Behaviour Therapy and Experimental Psychiatry, 27,* 245–255.

Granados-Soto, V., Teran-Rosales, F., Rocha-Gonzalez, H. I., Reyes-Garcia, G., Medina-Santillan, R., Rodriguez-Silverio, J., & Flores-Murrieta, F. J. (2004). Riboflavin reduces hyperalgesia and inflammation but not tactile allodynia in the rat. *European Journal of Pharmacology, 492,* 35–40.

Granfors, M. T., Backman, J. T., Neuvonen, M., Ahonen, J., & Neuvonen, P. J. (2004). Fluvoxamine drastically increases concentrations and effects of tizanidine: A potentially hazardous interaction. *Clinical and Pharmacological Therapeutics, 75,* 331–341.

Grant, E. N., Wagner, R., & Weiss, K. B. (1999). Observations on emerging patterns of asthma in our society. *Journal of Allergy and Clinical Immunology, 104,* S1–S9.

Gray, J. A. (1982). *The neuropsychology of anxiety: An enquiry into the functions of the septo-hippocampal system.* New York: Oxford University Press.

Gray, J. A., & McNaughton, N. (2000). *The neuropsychology of anxiety.* New York: Oxford University Press.

Grazzi, L., Andrasik, F., D'Amico, D., Leone, M., Moschiano, F., & Bussone, G. (2001). Electromyographic biofeedback-assisted relaxation training in juvenile episodic tension-type headache: Clinical outcome at three-year follow-up. *Cephalalgia, 21,* 798–803.

Grazzi, L., Andrasik, F., D'Amico, D., Leone, M., Usai, S., Kass, S. J., & Bussone, G. (2002). Behavioral and pharmacologic treatment of transformed migraine with analgesic overuse: Outcome at 3 years. *Headache, 32,* 483–490.

Greenough, C. G., & Fraser, R. D. (1989). The effects of compensation on recovery from low-back injury. *Spine, 14,* 947–955.

Greenwood, K. A., Thurston, R., Rumble, M., Waters, S. J., & Keefe, F. J. (2003). Anger and persistent pain: Current status and future directions. *Pain, 103,* 1–5.

Gregg, T. R., & Siegel, A. (2001). Brain structures and neurotransmitters regulating aggression in cats: Implications for human aggression. *Progress in Neuropsychopharmacology and Biological Psychiatry, 25,* 91–140.

Grisart, J. M., & Van der Linden, M. (2001). Conscious and automatic uses of memory in chronic pain patients. *Pain, 94,* 305–313.

Grisel, J. E., Wiertelak, E. P., Watkins, L. R., & Maier, S. F. (1994). Route of morphine administration modulates conditioned analgesic tolerance and hyperalgesia. *Pharmacology, Biochemistry and Behavior, 49,* 1029–1035.

Groth-Marnat, G., & Fletcher, A. (2000). Influence of neuroticism, catastrophizing, pain duration, and receipt of compensation on short-term response to nerve block treatment for chronic back pain. *Journal of Behavioral Medicine, 23,* 339–350.

Grubb, B. P. (2005). Neurocardiogenic syncope. *New England Journal of Medicine, 352,* 1004–1010.

Grunau, R. V. E., Whitfield, M. F., & Petrie, J. H. (1994). Pain sensitivity and temperament in extremely low-birth-weight premature toddlers and preterm and full-term controls. *Pain, 58,* 341–346.

Grunau, R. V. E., Whitfield, M. F., Petrie, J. H., & Fryer, E. L. (1994). Early pain experience, child and family factors, as precursors of somatization: A prospective study of extremely premature and fullterm children. *Pain, 56,* 353–359.

Grusser, S. M., Winter, C., Muhlnickel, W., Denke, C., Karl, A., Villringer, K., & Flor, H. (2001). The relationship of perceptual phenomena and cortical reorganization in upper extremity amputees. *Neuroscience, 102,* 263–272.

Grzesiak, R. C., Ury, G. M., & Dworkin, R. H. (1996). Psychodynamic psychotherapy with chronic pain patients. In R. J. Gatchel & D. C. Turk (Eds.), *Psychological approaches to pain management: A practitioner's handbook* (pp. 148–178). New York: Guilford Press.

Guarnieri, P., Radnitz, C. L., & Blanchard, E. B. (1990). Assessment of dietary risk factors in chronic headache. *Biofeedback and Self-Regulation, 15*, 15–25.

Guest, G. H., & Drummond, P. D. (1992). Effect of compensation on emotional state and disability in chronic back pain. *Pain, 48*, 125–130.

Guglielmi, R. S., & Roberts, A. H. (1994). Volitional vasomotor lability and vasomotor control. *Biological Psychology, 39*, 29–44.

Guidetti, V., Bruni, O., Cerutti, R., et al. (1991). How and why childhood headache and migraine differ from that of adults. In V. Gallai & V. Guidetti (Eds.), *Juvenile headache*. Excerpta Medica, International Congress Series 969 (pp. 27–32). Amsterdam: Elsevier.

Guidetti, V., Galli, F., Fabrizi, P., Giannantoni, A. S., Napoli, L., Bruni, O., & Trillo, S. (1998). Headache and psychiatric comorbidity: Clinical aspects and outcome in an 8-year follow-up study. *Cephalalgia, 18*, 455–462.

Guidetti, V., Ottaviano, S., & Pagliarini, M. (1984). Childhood headache risk: Warning signs and symptoms present during the first six months of life. *Cephalalgia, 4*, 237–242.

Guignard, B., Bossard, A. E., Coste, C., Sessler, D. I., Lebrault, C., Alfonsi, P., Fletcher, D., & Chauvin, M. (2000). Acute opioid tolerance: Intraoperative remifentanil increases postoperative pain and morphine requirement. *Anesthesiology, 93*, 409–417.

Guiloff, R. J., & Fruns, M. (1988). Limb pain in migraine and cluster headache. *Journal of Neurology, Neurosurgery, and Psychiatry, 51*, 1022–1031.

Guyton, A. C., & Hall, J. E. (2000). *Textbook of medical physiology* (10th ed.). Philadelphia: W. B. Saunders Co.

Guyuron, B., Tucker, T., & Davis, J. (2002). Surgical treatment of migraine headaches. *Plastic and Reconstructive Surgery, 109*, 2183–2189.

Haan, J., Terwindt, G. M., & Ferrari, M. D. (1997). Genetics of migraine. *Neurologic Clinics, 15*(1), 43–60.

Haas, D. C. (1997). Posttraumatic headache [letter]. *Neurology, 48*, 1735.

Haase, C. G., & Diener, H.-C. (1998). Transcranial Doppler ultrasonographic features during drug withdrawal from drug-induced headache. A transcranial Doppler follow-up study. *Headache, 38*, 679–683.

Hack, G. (1998). Cervicogenic headache: New anatomical discovery provides the missing link. *Chiropractic Reports, 12*(3), 1–3.

Haddock, C. K., Rowan, A. B., Andrasik, F., Wilson, P. G., Talcott, G. W., & Stein, R. J. (1997). Home-based behavioral treatments for chronic benign headache: A meta-analysis of controlled trials. *Cephalalgia, 17*, 113–118.

Hadjistavropoulos, H. D., Hadjistavropoulos, T., & Quine, A. (2000). Health anxiety moderates the effects of distraction versus attention to pain. *Behaviour Research and Therapy, 38*, 425–438.

Hadjistavropoulos, T. (1999). Chronic pain on trial: The influence of litigation and compensation on chronic pain syndromes. In A. R. Block, E. F. Kremer, & E. Fernandez (Eds.), *Handbook of pain syndromes: Biopsychosocial perspectives* (pp. 59–76). Mahwah, NJ: Lawrence Erlbaum Associates.

Hagen, K., Vatten, L., Stovner, L. J., Zwart, J. A., Krokstad, S., & Bovim, G. (2002). Low socio-economic status is associated with increased risk of frequent headache: a prospective study of 22,718 adults in Norway. *Cephalalgia, 22*, 672–679.

Haggerty, J. J. Jr. (1983). The psychosomatic family: An overview. *Psychosomatics, 24*, 615–623.

Hahn, R. A. (1997). The nocebo phenomenon: Scope and Foundations. In A. Harrington (Ed.), *The placebo effect: An interdisciplinary exploration* (pp. 56–76). Cambridge, MA: Harvard University Press.

Haimart, M., Pradalier, A., Launay, J. M., Dreux, C., & Dry, J. (1987). Whole blood and plasma histamine in common migraine. *Cephalalgia, 7*, 39–42.

Haldeman, S., & Dagenais, S. (2001). Cervicogenic headaches: A critical review. *Spine Journal, 1*, 31–46.

Hall, G. S. (1912). *Founders of modern psychology*. New York: D. Appleton and Company.

Hämäläinen, M. L., Hoppu, K., & Santavuori, P. (1997). Sumatriptan for migraine attacks in children: A randomized placebo-controlled study. Do children with migraine attacks respond to oral sumatriptan differently from adults? *Neurology, 48*, 1100–1103.

Hamel, E., & Saxena, P. R. (2000). 5-Hydroxytryptamine involvement in migraine. In J. Olesen, P. Tfelt-Hansen & K. M. A. Welch (Eds.), *The headaches* (2nd ed., pp. 319–324). Philadelphia: Lippincott Williams & Wilkins.

Hammill, J. M., Cook, T. M., & Rosecrance, J. C. (1996). Effectiveness of a physical therapy regimen in the treatment of tension-type headache. *Headache, 36*, 149–153.

Hanington, E. (1967). Preliminary report on tyramine headache. *British Medical Journal, 1*, 550–551.

Hanington, E. (1983). Migraine. In M. H. Lessof (Ed.), *Clinical reactions to food* (pp. 155–180). New York: John Wiley and Sons.

Hanington, E., & Harper, A. M. (1968). The role of tyramine in the aetiology of migraine and related studies on the cerebral and extracerebral circulations. *Headache, 8*, 84–97.

Hanington, E., Jones, R. J., Amess, J. A. L., & Wachowicz, B. (1981). Migraine: A platelet disorder. *Lancet, ii*, 720–723.

Hannerz, J., & Jogestrand, T. (1998). Is chronic tension-type headache a vascular headache? The relation between chronic tension-type headache and cranial hemodynamics. *Headache, 38*, 668–675.

Hans, M., Luvisetto, S., Williams, M. E., Spagnolo, M., Urrutia, A., Tottene, A., Brust, P. F., Johnson, E. C., Harpold, M. M., Stauderman, K. A., & Pietrobon, D. (1999). Functional consequences of mutations in the human α_{1A} calcium channel subunit linked to familial hemiplegic migraine. *Journal of Neuroscience, 19*, 1610–1619.

Hansson, P., & Lundeberg, T. (1999). Transcutaneous electrical nerve stimulation, vibration and acupuncture as pain-relieving measures. In P. D. Wall & R. Melzack (Eds.), *Textbook of pain* (4th edition, pp. 1341–1351). New York: Churchill Livingstone.

Hardebo, J. E. (1991). Activation of pain fibers to the internal carotid artery intracranially may cause the pain and local signs of reduced sympathetic and enhanced parasympathetic activity in cluster headache. *Headache, 31*, 314–320.

Hardebo, J. E. (1994). Sumatriptan constricts the intracranial internal carotid artery: Probable curative action in attacks of cluster headache. In F. C. Rose (Ed.), *New advances in headache research* (3rd ed., pp. 245–252). London: Smith-Gordon.

Hardebo, J. E., Messeter, K., & Ryding, E. (1989). Observations on mechanisms behind the beneficial effect of oxygen in cluster headache. In F. C. Rose (Ed.), *New advances in headache research* (pp. 221–228). London: Smith-Gordon.

Harer, C., & von Kummer, R. (1991). Cerebrovascular CO_2 reactivity in migraine: Assessment by transcranial Doppler ultrasound. *Journal of Neurology, 238*, 23–26.

Hargreaves, R. J., & Shepheard, S. L. (1999). Pathophysiology of migraine—new insights. *Canadian Journal of Neurological Science, 26*(Suppl. 3), S12–S19.

Harkins, S. W., Price, D. D., & Braith, J. (1989). Effects of extraversion and neuroticism on experimental pain, clinical pain, and illness behavior. *Pain, 36*, 209–218.

Harris, A. J. (1999). Cortical origin of pathological pain. *Lancet, 354*, 1464–1466.

Harris, J. A., Westbrook, R. F., Duffield, T. Q., & Bentivoglio, M. (1995). Fos expression in the spinal cord is suppressed in rats displaying conditioned hypoalgesia. *Behavioral Neuroscience, 109*, 320–328.

Harrison, R. (1975). Psychological testing in headache: A review. *Headache, 15*, 177–185.

Hart, J. D., & Cichanski, K. A. (1981). A comparison of frontal EMG biofeedback and neck EMG biofeedback in the treatment of muscle-contraction headache. *Biofeedback and Self-Regulation, 6*, 63–74.

Harter, S. L., & Vanecek, R. J. (2000). Cognitive assumptions and long-term distress in survivors of childhood abuse, parental alcoholism, and dysfunctional family environments. *Cognitive Therapy and Research, 24*, 445–472.

Harvey, A. G., & Bryant, R. A. (1998). The role of valence in attempted thought suppression. *Behaviour Research and Therapy, 36*, 757–763.

Harvey, A. G., & McGuire, B. E. (2000). Suppressing and attending to pain-related thoughts in chronic pain patients. *Behaviour Research and Therapy, 38*, 1117–1124.

Harvey, J. R. (1998). *Total relaxation: Healing practices for body, mind and spirit.* New York: Kodansha International.

Hassinger, H. J., Semenchuk, E. M., & O'Brien, W. H. (1999). Cardiovascular responses to pain and stress in migraine. *Headache, 39*, 605–615.

Havanka-Kanniainen, H., Hokkanen, E., & Myllylä, V. V. (1985). Efficacy of nimodipine in the prophylaxis of migraine. *Cephalalgia, 5*, 39–43.

Hawranko, A. A., & Smith, D. J. (1999). Stress reduces morphine's antinociceptive potency: Dependence upon spinal cholecystokinin processes. *Brain Research, 824*, 251–257.

Hay, K. M., Mortimer, M. J., Barker, D. C., Debney, C. M., & Good, P. A. (1994). 1044 women with migraine: The effect of environmental stimuli. *Headache, 34*, 166–168.

Haynes, S. N., Gannon, L. R., Bank, J., Shelton, D., & Goodwin, J. (1990). Cephalic blood flow correlates of induced headaches. *Journal of Behavioral Medicine, 13*, 467–480.

Head, H., & Holmes, G. (1911). Sensory disturbances from cerebral lesions. *Brain, 34*, 102–154.

Headache Classification Committee of the International Headache Society. (1988). Classification and diagnostic criteria for headache disorders, cranial neuralgias and facial pain. *Cephalalgia, 7*(Suppl. 8), 1–96.

Headache Classification Subcommittee of the International Headache Society. (2004). International classification of headache disorders (2nd ed.). *Cephalalgia, 24*(Suppl. 1).

Heath, M. E., & Downey, J. A. (1990). The cold face test (diving reflex) in clinical autonomic assessment: Methodological considerations and repeatability of responses. *Clinical Science, 78*, 139–147.

Hegerl, U., & Juckel, G. (1993). Intensity dependence of auditory evoked potentials as an indicator of central serotoninergic neurotransmission: A new hypothesis. *Biological Psychiatry, 33*, 173–187.

Heim, C., Ehlert, U., & Hellhammer, D. H. (2000). The potential role of hypocortisolism in the pathophysiology of stress-related bodily disorders. *Psychoneuroendocrinology, 25*, 1–35.

Heim, C., Ehlert, U., Hanker, J. P., & Hellhammer, D. H. (1998). Abuse-related posttraumatic stress disorder and alterations of the hypothalamic-pituitary-adrenal axis in women with chronic pelvic pain. *Psychosomatic Medicine, 60*, 309–318.

Heinrich, T. W. (2004). Medically unexplained symptoms and the concept of somatization. *Wisconsin Medical Journal, 103*, 83–87.

Helson, H. (1964). *Adaptation-level theory: An experimental and systematic approach to behavior.* New York: Harper and Row.

Helm-Hylkema, H. v. d., Orlebeke, J. F., Enting, L. A., Thijssen, J. H. H., & van Ree, J. (1990). Effects of behaviour therapy on migraine and plasma β-endorphin in young migraine patients. *Psychoneuroendocrinology, 15*, 39–45.

Hemingway, M. A., Biedermann, H.-J., & Inglis, J. (1995). Electromyographic recordings of paraspinal muscles: Variations related to subcutaneous tissue thickness. *Biofeedback and Self-Regulation, 20*, 39–49.

Henderson, A. (1911). *George Bernard Shaw: His life and works.* Cincinnati: Stewart & Kidd Company.

Henderson, W. R., & Raskin, N. H. (1972). "Hot-dog" headache: Individual susceptibility to nitrite. *Lancet, 2*, 1162–1163.

Hendler, N. H., & Kozikowski, J. G. (1993). Overlooked physical diagnoses in chronic pain patients involved in litigation. *Psychosomatics, 34*, 494–501.

Henry, P., Daubech, J. F., Lucas, J., & Gagnon, M. (1988). Dependence on analgesic medication in chronic headache sufferers: Psychological analysis. In H.-C. Diener & M. Wilkinson (Eds.), *Drug-induced headache* (pp. 75–79). New York: Springer-Verlag.

Hering, R., Couturier, E. G. M., & Steiner, T. J. (1992). Weekend migraine in men [letter]. *Lancet, 339*, 67.

Hering, R., & Steiner, T. J. (1991). Abrupt outpatient withdrawal of medication in analgesic-abusing migraineurs. *Lancet, 337*, 1442–1443.

Hering-Hanit, R. (2000). Alteration in nature of cluster headache during subcutaneous administration of sumatriptan. *Headache, 40*, 41–44.

Hering-Hanit, R., & Gadoth, N. (2003). Caffeine-induced headache in children and adolescents. *Cephalalgia, 23*, 332–335.

Hermann, C., Blanchard, E. B., & Flor, H. (1997). Biofeedback treatment for pediatric migraine: Prediction of treatment outcome. *Journal of Consulting and Clinical Psychology, 65*, 611–616.

Hermann, C., Kim, M., & Blanchard, E. B. (1995). Behavioral and prophylactic pharmacological intervention studies of pediatric migraine: An exploratory meta-analysis. *Pain, 60*, 239–256.

Hershey, A. D., Tang, Y., Powers, S. W., Kabbouche, M. A., Gilbert, D. L., Glauser, T. A., & Sharp, F. R. (2004). Genomic abnormalities in patients with migraine and chronic migraine: Preliminary blood gene expression suggests platelet abnormalities. *Headache, 44*, 994–1004.

Herwig, U., Padberg, F., Unger, J., Spitzer, M., Schönfeldt-Lecouna, C. (2001). Transcranial magnetic stimulation in therapy studies: Examination of the reliability of "standard" coil positioning by neuronavigation. *Biological Psychiatry, 50*, 58–61.

Heyneman, N. E., Fremouw, W. J., Gano, D., Kirkland, F., & Heiden, L. (1990). Individual differences and the effectiveness of different coping strategies for pain. *Cognitive Therapy and Research, 14*, 63–77.

Hickling, E. J., & Blanchard, E. B. (1992). Post-traumatic stress disorder and motor vehicle accidents. *Journal of Anxiety Disorders, 6*, 285–291.

Hickling, E. J., Blanchard, E. B., Schwarz, S. P., & Silverman, D. J. (1992). Headaches and motor vehicle accidents: Results of the psychological treatment of post-traumatic headache. *Headache Quarterly, 3*(3), 285–289.

Hickling, E. J., Blanchard, E. B., Silverman, D. J., & Schwarz, S. P. (1992). Motor vehicle accidents, headaches and post-traumatic stress disorder: Assessment findings in a consecutive series. *Headache, 32*, 147–151.

Hicks, R. A., & Conti, P. A. (1991). Nocturnal bruxism and self reports of stress-related symptoms. *Perceptual and Motor Skills, 72,* 1182.

Hilgard, E. R. (1986). *Divided consciousness: Multiple controls in human thought and action* (expanded ed.). New York: Wiley.

Hilgard, E. R., & Hilgard, J. R. (1983). *Hypnosis in the relief of pain* (rev. ed.). Los Altos, CA: William Kaufman.

Hines, E. A. Jr., & Brown, G. E. (1932). Standard stimulus for measuring vasomotor reactions. Its application in the study of hypertension. *Proceedings of the Staff Meeting of the Mayo Clinic, 7,* 332–335.

Hines, E. A. Jr., & Brown, G. E. (1933). Standard test for measuring variability of blood pressure: Its significance as index of prehypertensive state. *Annals of Internal Medicine, 7,* 209–217.

Hines, M. E. (1999). Posttraumatic headaches. In N. R. Varney & R. J. Roberts (Eds.), *The evaluation and treatment of mild traumatic brain injury* (pp. 375–410). Mahwah, NJ: Lawrence Erlbaum Associates.

Hirota, K., Smart, D., & Lambert, D. G. (2003). The effects of local and intravenous anesthetics on recombinant rat VR1 vanilloid receptors. *Anesthesia and Analgesia, 96,* 1656–1660.

Hirsch, M. S., & Liebert, R. M. (1998). The physical and psychological experience of pain: The effects of labeling and cold pressor temperature on three pain measures in college women. *Pain, 77,* 41–48.

Hodzic, A., Veit, R., Karim, A. A., Erb, M., & Godde, B. (2004). Improvement and decline in tactile discrimination behavior after cortical plasticity induced by passive tactile coactivation. *Journal of Neuroscience, 24,* 442–446.

Hoelscher, T. J., & Lichstein, K. L. (1983). Blood volume pulse biofeedback treatment of chronic cluster headache. *Biofeedback and Self-Regulation, 8,* 533–541.

Hoffman, R. E., & Cavus, I. (2002). Slow transcranial magnetic stimulation, long-term depotentiation, and brain hyperexcitability disorders. *American Journal of Psychiatry, 159,* 1093–1102.

Holden, E. W., Gladstein, J., Trulsen, M., & Wall, B. (1994). Chronic daily headache in children and adolescents. *Headache, 34,* 508–514.

Holder-Perkins, V., & Wise, T. N. (2001). Somatization disorder. In K. A. Phillips (Ed.), *Somatoform and factitious disorders* (pp. 1–26). Washington, DC: American Psychiatric Publishing.

Hollins, M., Sigurdsson, A., Fillingim, L., & Goble, A. K. (1996). Vibrotactile threshold is elevated in temporomandibular disorders. *Pain, 67,* 89–96.

Holm, J. E., Holroyd, K. A., Hursey, K. G., & Penzien, D. B. (1986). The role of stress in recurrent tension headache. *Headache, 26,* 160–167.

Holm, J. E., Lamberty, K., McSherry, W. C. II, & Davis, P. A. (1997). The stress response in headache sufferers: Physiological and psychological reactivity. *Headache, 37,* 221–227.

Holmes, B., Brogden, R. N., Heel, R. C., Speight, T. M., & Avery, G. S. (1984). Flunarizine: A review of its pharmacodynamic and pharmacokinetic properties and therapeutic use. *Drugs, 27,* 6–44.

Holmes, T. H., & Rahe, R. H. (1967). The Social Readjustment Rating Scale. *Journal of Psychosomatic Research, 11,* 213–218.

Holroyd, J. (1996). Hypnosis treatment of clinical pain: Understanding why hypnosis is useful. *International Journal of Clinical and Experimental Hypnosis, 44,* 33–51.

Holroyd, K. A. (2001). Learning from our treatment failures. *Applied Psychophysiology and Biofeedback, 26,* 319–323.

Holroyd, K. A. (2002). Assessment and psychological management of recurrent headache disorders. *Journal of Consulting and Clinical Psychology, 70,* 656–677.

Holroyd, K. A., & Andrasik, F. (1978). Coping and the self-control of chronic tension headache. *Journal of Consulting and Clinical Psychology, 48,* 1036–1045.

Holroyd, K. A., France, J. L., Cordingley, G. E., Rokicki, L. A., Kvaal, S. A., Lipchik, G. L., & McCool, H. R. (1995). Enhancing the effectiveness of relaxation-thermal biofeedback training with propranolol hydrochloride. *Journal of Consulting and Clinical Psychology, 63,* 327–330.

Holroyd, K. A., Lipchik, G. L., & Penzien, D. B. (1998). Psychological management of recurrent headache disorders: Empirical basis for clinical practice. In K. S. Dobson & K. D. Craig (Eds.), *Best practice: Developing and promoting empirically supported interventions* (pp. 187–236). Newbury Park, CA: Sage Publications.

Holroyd, K. A., Malinoski, P., Davis, M. K., & Lipchik, G. L. (1999). The three dimensions of headache impact: Pain, disability and affective distress. *Pain, 83,* 571–578.

Holroyd, K. A., O'Donnell, F. J., Stensland, M., Lipchik, G. L., Cordingley, G. E., & Carlson, B. W. (2001). Management of chronic tension-type headache with tricyclic antidepressant medication, stress management therapy, and their combination: A randomized controlled trial. *JAMA: Journal of the American Medical Association, 285,* 2208–2215.

Holroyd, K. A., & Penzien, D. B. (1990). Pharmacological versus non-pharmacological prophylaxis of recurrent migraine headache: A meta-analytic review of clinical trials. *Pain, 42,* 1–13.

Holroyd, K. A., Penzien, D. B., & Cordingley, G. E. (1991). Propranolol in the management of recurrent migraine: A meta-analytic review. *Headache, 31,* 333–340.

Holroyd, K. A., Penzien, D. B., Hursey, K. G., Tobin, D. L., Rogers, L., Holm, J.E., & Marcille, P. J. (1984). Change mechanisms in EMG biofeedback training: Cognitive changes underlying improvements in tension headache. *Journal of Consulting and Clinical Psychology, 52,* 1039–1053.

Holroyd, K. A., Penzien, D. B., Rokicki, L. A., & Cordingley, G. E. (1992). Flunarizine vs. propranolol. A meta-analysis of clinical trials. *Headache, 32,* 256.

Holroyd, K. A., Stensland, M., Lipchik, G. L., Hill, K. R., O'Donnell, F. S., & Cordingley, G. (2000). Psychosocial correlates and impact of chronic tension-type headaches. *Headache, 40,* 3–16.

Holzberg, A. D., Robinson, M. E., Geisser, M. E., & Gremillion, H. A. (1996). The effects of depression and chronic pain on psychosocial and physical functioning. *Clinical Journal of Pain, 12,* 118–125.

Hölzl, R., Kleinböhl, D., & Huse, E. (2005). Implicit operant learning of pain sensitization. *Pain, 115,* 12–20.

Honkoop, P. C., Sorbi, M. J., Godaert, G. L., & Spierings, E. L. (1999). High-density assessment of the IHS classification criteria for migraine without aura: A prospective study. *Cephalalgia, 19,* 201–206.

Hooper, L., Brown, T. J., Elliott, R. A., Payne, K., Roberts, C., & Symmons, D. (2004). The effectiveness of five strategies for the prevention of gastrointestinal toxicity induced by non-steroidal anti-inflammatory drugs: Systematic review. *British Medical Journal, 329,* 948–952.

Hori, T., Oka, T., Hosoi, M., Abe, M., & Oka, K. (2000). Hypothalamic mechanisms of pain modulatory actions of cytokines and prostaglandin E2. *Annals of the New York Academy of Sciences, 917,* 106–120.

Horiguchi, T., Snipes, J. A., Kis, B., Shimizu, K., & Busija, D. W. (2005). The role of nitric oxide in the development of cortical spreading depression-induced tolerance to transient focal cerebral ischemia in rats. *Brain Research, 1039,* 84–89.

Horrocks, T. A. (1999). Mease, James. In J. A. Garraty & M. C. Carnes (Eds.), *American national biography* (Vol. 15, pp. 231–232). New York: Oxford University Press.

Hotopf, M., Mayou, R., Wadsworth, M., & Wessely, S. (1999). Childhood risk factors for adults with medically unexplained symptoms: Results from a national birth cohort study. *American Journal of Psychiatry, 156,* 1796–1800.

Hu, J., Milenkovic, N., & Lewin, G. R. (2006). The high threshold mechanotransducer: A status report. *Pain, 120,* 3–7.

Hu, J. W., Sessle, B. J., Raboisson, P., Dallel, R., & Woda, A. (1992). Stimulation of craniofacial muscle afferents induces prolonged facilatory effects in trigeminal nociceptive brain-stem neurones. *Pain, 48,* 53–60.

Hu, X. H., Markson, L. E., Lipton, R. B., Stewart, W. F., & Berger, M. L. (1999). Burden of migraine in the United States: Disability and economic costs. *Archives of Internal Medicine, 159,* 813–818.

Huang, R. Q., Fang, M. J., & Dillon, G. H. (1999). The tyrosine kinase inhibitor genistein directly inhibits $GABA_A$ receptors. *Brain Research. Molecular Brain Research, 67,* 177–183.

Hubbard, D. R. (1996). Chronic and recurrent muscle pain: Pathophysiology and treatment, and review of pharmacologic studies. *Journal of Musculoskeletal Pain, 4,* 123–144.

Hubbard, D. R., & Berkoff, G. (1993). Myofascial trigger points show spontaneous needle EMG activity. *Spine, 18,* 1803–1807.

Hudzinski, L. G., & Lawrence, G. S. (1988). Significance of EMG surface electrode placement models and headache findings. *Headache, 28,* 30–35.

Hudzinski, L. G., & Lawrence, G. S. (1990). EMG surface electrode normative data for muscle contraction headache and biofeedback therapy. *Headache Quarterly, 1,* 224–229.

Hudzinski, L. G., & Lawrence, G. (1992). Normal EMG surface electrode levels for treating myofacial contraction and related headache. *Headache Quarterly, 3,* 415–420.

Hudzinski, L. G., & Levenson, H. (1985). Biofeedback behavioral treatment of headache with locus of control pain analysis: A 20-month retrospective study. *Headache, 25,* 380–386.

Hull, J. G., Van Treuren, R. R., & Virnelli, S. (1987). Hardiness and health: A critique and alternative approach. *Journal of Personality and Social Psychology, 53,* 518–530.

Hunter, J. P., Katz, J., & Davis, K. D. (2003). The effect of tactile and visual sensory inputs on phantom limb awareness. *Brain, 126,* 579–589.

Huntley, G. W., Benson, D. L., & Colman, D. R. (2002). Structural remodeling of the synapse in response to physiological activity. *Cell, 108,* 1–4.

Hurlburt, R. T. (1997). Randomly sampling thinking in the natural environment. *Journal of Consulting and Clinical Psychology, 65*, 941–949.

Hursey, K. G., & Jacks, S. D. (1992). Fear of pain in recurrent headache sufferers. *Headache, 32*, 283–286.

Hurtig, I. M., Raak, R. I., Kendall, S. A., Gerdle, B., & Wahren, L. K. (2001). Quantitative sensory testing in fibromyalgia patients and in healthy subjects: Identification of subgroups. *Clinical Journal of Pain, 17*, 316–322.

Hurwitz, E. L., Aker, P. D., Adams, A. H., Meeker, W. C., & Shekelle, P. G. (1996). Manipulation and mobilization of the cervical spine: A systematic review of the literature. *Spine, 21*, 1746–1760.

Hutcheon, B., & Yarom, Y. (2000). Resonance, oscillation and the intrinsic frequency preferences of neurons. *Trends in Neurosciences, 23*, 216–222.

Iadarola, M. J., Berman, K. F., Zeffiro, T. A., Byas-Smith, M. G., Gracely, R. H., Max, M. B., et al. (1998). Neural activation during acute capsaicin-evoked pain and allodynia assessed with PET. *Brain, 121*, 931–947.

Iezzi, T., Archibald,Y., Barnett, P., Klinck, A., & Duckworth, M. (1999). Neurocognitive performance and emotional status in chronic pain patients. *Journal of Behavioral Medicine, 22*, 205–216.

Ikeda, H., Heinke, B., Ruscheweyh, R., & Sandkühler, J. (2003). Synaptic plasticity in spinal lamina I projection neurons that mediate hyperalgesia. *Science, 299*, 1237–1240.

Ingram, S. L. (2000).Cellular and molecular mechanisms of opioid action. In J. Sandkühler, B. Bromm, & G. F. Gebhart (Eds.), *Nervous system plasticity and chronic pain (Progress in Brain Research, 129*, pp. 483–492). New York: Elsevier.

Isler, H. (1982). Migraine treatment as a cause of chronic migraine. In F. C. Rose (Ed.), *Advances in migraine research and therapy*. New York: Raven Press.

Isler, H. (1992). The Galenic tradition and migraine. *Journal of the History of the Neurosciences, 1*, 227–233.

Isler, H. (1993). Headache classification prior to the Ad Hoc criteria. *Cephalalgia, 13*(Suppl. 12), 9–10.

Isler, H., Agarwalla, P., Würth, G., & Agosti, R. (2005). Migraine in Diderot's *Encyclopedia*: An historical mainstream text. *Cephalalgia, 25*, 1173–1178.

Isojärvi, J. I. T., Laatikainen, T. J., Pakarinen, A. J., Juntunen, K. T. S., Myllylä, V. V. (1993). Polycystic ovaries and hyperandrogenism in women taking valproate for epilepsy. *New England Journal of Medicine, 329*, 1383–1388.

Jackson, E. K. (2001). Renin and angiotensin. In J. G. Hardman, L. E. Limbird, & A. G. Gilman (Eds.), *Goodman and Gilman's the pharmacological basis of therapeutics* (10th ed., pp. 809–841). New York: McGraw-Hill.

Jacobs, B. L., & Azmitia, E. C. (1992). Structure and function of the brain serotonin system. *Physiological Reviews, 72*, 165–229.

Jacobson, E. (1924). The technic of progressive relaxation. *Journal of Nervous and Mental Disease, 60*, 568–578.

Jacobson, E. (1929). *Progressive relaxation*. Chicago: University of Chicago Press.

Jacobson, G. P., Ramadan, N. M., Aggarwal, S. K., & Newman, C. W. (1994). The Henry Ford Hospital Headache Disability Inventory (HDI). *Neurology, 44*, 837–842.

Jacobson, G. P., Ramadan, N. M., Norris, L., & Newman, C. W. (1995). Headache Disability Inventory (HDI): short-term test-retest reliability and spouse perceptions. *Headache, 35*, 534–539.

Jaeger, B. (1994). Differential diagnosis and management of craniofacial pain. In J. I. Ingle & L. K. Bakland (Eds.), *Endodontics* (4th ed., pp. 550–607). Baltimore, MD: Williams and Wilkins.

James, L. D., Thorn, B. E., & Williams, D. A. (1993). Goal specification in cognitive-behavioral therapy for chronic headache pain. *Behavior Therapy, 24*, 305–320.

James, W. (1884). What is an emotion? *Mind, 9*, 188–205.

James, W. (1901). *The principles of psychology*, vol. 1. London: Macmillan and Company.

Jamner, L. D., & Tursky, B. (1987). Syndrome-specific descriptor profiling: A psychophysiological and psychophysical approach. *Health Psychology, 6*, 417–430.

Jamison, R. N., Anderson, K. O., & Slater, M. A. (1995). Weather changes and pain: Perceived influence of local climate on pain complaint in chronic pain patients. *Pain, 61*, 309–315.

Janke, E. A., Holroyd, K. A., & Romanek, K. (2004). Depression increases onset of tension-type headache following laboratory stress. *Pain, 111*, 230–238.

Jankovic, J., Vuong, K. D., & Ahsan, J. (2003). Comparison of efficacy and immunogenicity of original versus current botulinum toxin in cervical dystonia. *Neurology, 60*, 1186–1188.

Janssen, K., & Neutgens, J. (1986). Autogenic training and progressive relaxation in the treatment of three kinds of headache. *Behaviour Research and Therapy, 24*, 199–208.

Janssen, P. A. J., Leysen, J. E., Megens, A. A. H. P., & Awouters, F. H. L. (1999). Does phenylethylamine act as an endogenous amphetamine in some patients? *International Journal of Neuropsychopharmacology, 2,* 229–240.

Janssen, S. A., & Arntz, A. (1996). Anxiety and pain: Attentional and endorphinergic influences. *Pain, 66,* 145–150.

Janssen, S. A., & Arntz, A. (1999). No interactive effects of naltrexone and benzodiazepines on pain during phobic fear. *Behaviour Research and Therapy, 37,* 77–86.

Janssen, S. A., Spinhoven, P., & Brosschot, J. F. (2001). Experimentally induced anger, cardiovascular reactivity, and pain sensitivity. *Journal of Psychosomatic Research, 51,* 479–485.

Jelicic, M., van Boxtel, M. P. J., Houx, P. J., & Jolles, J. (2000). Does migraine headache affect cognitive function in the elderly? Report from the Maastricht Aging Study (MAAS). *Headache, 40,* 715–719.

Jensen, C., Vasseljen, O., & Westgaard, R. H. (1993). The influence of electrode position on bipolar surface electromyogram recordings of the upper trapezius muscle. *European Journal of Applied Physiology and Occupational Physiology, 67,* 266–273.

Jensen, M. P., Turner, J. A., Romano, J. M., & Lawler, B. K. (1994). Relationship of pain-specific beliefs to chronic pain adjustment. *Pain, 57,* 301–309.

Jensen, O. K., Nielsen, F. F., & Vosmar, L. (1990). An open study comparing manual therapy with the use of cold packs in the treatment of post-traumatic headache. *Cephalalgia, 10,* 241–250.

Jensen, R. (1995). Mechanisms of spontaneous tension-type headaches: An analysis of tenderness, pain thresholds and EMG. *Pain, 64,* 251–256.

Jensen, R. (1999a). Pathophysiological mechanisms of tension-type headache: A review of epidemiological and experimental studies. *Cephalalgia, 19,* 602–621.

Jensen, R. (1999b). The tension-type headache alternative. Peripheral pathophysiological mechanisms. *Cephalalgia, 19*(Suppl. 25), 9–10.

Jensen, R., Fuglsang-Frederiksen, A., & Olesen, J. (1994). Quantitative surface EMG of pericranial muscles in headache. A population study. *Electroencephalography and Clinical Neurophysiology, 93,* 335–344.

Jensen, R., & Olesen, J. (1996). Initiating mechanisms of experimentally-induced tension-type headache. *Cephalalgia, 16,* 175–182.

Jensen, R., Rasmussen, B. K., Pedersen, B., Lous, I., & Olesen, J. (1992). Cephalic muscle tenderness and pressure pain threshold in a general population. *Pain, 48,* 197–203.

Jensen, R., Rasmussen, B. K., Pedersen, B., & Olesen, J. (1993). Pericranial tenderness and pressure pain threshold in headache. A population study. *Pain, 52,* 193–199.

Jensen, R., Tuxen, C., & Olesen, J. (1988). Pericranial muscle tenderness and pressure-pain threshold in the temporal region during common migraine. *Pain, 35,* 65–70.

Jeremy, J. Y., Thompson, C. S., Mikhailidis, D. P., & Dandona, P. (1990). Effects of the anti-inflammatory prodrug, nabumetone and its principal active metabolite on rat gastric mucosal, aortic and platelet eicosanoid synthesis, in vitro and ex vivo. *Prostaglandins, Leukotrienes, and Essential Fatty Acids, 41,* 195–199.

Jessell, T. M., & Kelly, D. D. (1991). Pain and analgesia. In E. R. Kandel, J. H. Schwartz, & T. M. Jessell (Eds.), *Principles of neural science* (3rd ed., pp. 385–399). Norwalk, CT: Appleton & Lange.

Jessen, F., Block, W., Träber, F., Keller, E., Flacke, S., Lamerichs, R., Schild, H. H., & Heun, R. (2001). Decrease of *N*-acetylaspartate in the MTL correlates with cognitive decline of AD patients. *Neurology, 57,* 930–932.

Jessup, B. (1978). The role of diet in migraine: Conditioned taste aversion. *Headache, 18,* 229.

Johannes, C. B., Linet, M. S., Stewart, W. F., Celentano, D. D., Lipton, R. B., & Szklo, M. (1995). Relationship of headache to phase of the menstrual cycle among young women: A daily diary study. *Neurology, 45,* 1076–1082.

Johnson, E. S., Kadam, N. P., Hylands, D. M., & Hylands, P. J. (1985). Efficacy of feverfew as prophylactic treatment of migraine. *British Medical Journal, 291,* 569–573.

Johnson, M. H., Breakwell, G., Douglas, W., & Humphries, S. (1998). The effects of imagery and sensory detection distractors on different measures of pain: How does distraction work? *British Journal of Clinical Psychology, 37,* 141–154.

Johnson, M. H., & Petrie, S. M. (1997). The effects of distraction on exercise and cold pressor tolerance for chronic low back pain sufferers. *Pain, 69,* 43–48.

Johnson, P. R., & Thorn, B. E. (1989). Cognitive behavioral treatment of chronic headache: Group versus individual treatment format. *Headache, 29,* 358–365.

Jones, D. A., Rollman, G. B., & Brooke, R. I. (1997). The cortisol response to psychological stress in temporomandibular dysfunction. *Pain, 72,* 171–182.

Jones, A. K. P., Kulkarni, B., & Derbyshire, S. W. G. (2003). Pain mechanisms and their disorders. *British Medical Bulletin, 65,* 83–93.

Jones, J. M. (1999). Great pains: Famous people with headaches. *Cephalalgia, 19,* 627–630.

Josephson, B. R., Singer, J. A., & Salovey, P. (1996). Mood regulation and memory: Repairing sad moods with happy memories. *Cognition and Emotion, 10,* 437–440.

Julius, D., & Basbaum, A. I. (2001). Molecular mechanisms of nociception. *Nature, 413,* 203–210.

Jull, G., Bogduk, N., & Marsland, A. (1988). The accuracy of manual diagnosis for cervical zygapophysial joint pain syndromes. *Medical Journal of Australia, 148,* 233–236.

Junge, A., Dvorak, J., Chomiak, J., Peterson, L., & Graf-Baumann, T. (2000). Medical history and physical findings in football players of different ages and skill levels. *American Journal of Sports Medicine, 28*(5), S16–S21.

Kaas, J. H., Nelson, R. J., Sur, M., Lin, C.-S., & Merzenich, M. M. (1979). Multiple representations of the body within the primary somatosensory cortex of primates. *Science, 204,* 521–523.

Kabat-Zinn, J., Lipworth, L., & Burney, R. (1985). The clinical use of mindfulness meditation for the self-regulation of chronic pain. *Journal of Behavioral Medicine, 8,* 163–190.

Kalkman, H. O. (1994). Is migraine prophylactic activity caused by 5-HT$_{2B}$ or 5-HT$_{2C}$ receptor blockade? *Life Sciences, 54,* 641–644.

Kalmar, J. M., & Cafarelli, E. (1999). Effects of caffeine on neuromuscular function. *Journal of Applied Physiology, 87,* 801–808.

Kane, K., & Taub, A. (1975). A history of local electrical analgesia. *Pain, 1,* 125–138.

Kaniecki, R. G. (1997). A comparison of divalproex with propranolol and placebo for the prophylaxis of migraine without aura. *Archives of Neurology, 54,* 1141–1145.

Kanner, A., Coyne, J. C., Schaefer, C., & Lazarus, R. S. (1981). Comparison of two modes of stress measurement: Daily hassles and uplifts versus major life events. *Journal of Behavioral Medicine, 4,* 1–39.

Kanny, G., Bauza, T., Fremont., S., Guillemin, F., Blaise, A., Daumas, F., Cabanis, J. C., Nicolas, J. P., & Moneret-Vautrin, D. A. (1999). Histamine content does not influence the tolerance of wine in normal subjects. *Allergie et Immunologie (Paris), 31*(2), 45–48.

Kanny, G., Gerbaux, V., Olszewski, A., Frémont, S., Empereur, F., Nabet, F., Cabanis, J. C., & Moneret-Vautrin, D. A. (2001). No correlation between wine intolerance and histamine content of wine. *Journal of Allergy and Clinical Immunology, 107,* 375–378.

Kaplan, P. W. (2004). Reproductive health effects and teratogenicity of antiepileptic drugs. *Neurology, 63*(Suppl. 4), s13–s23.

Karoum, F., Nasrallah H., & Potkin, S. (1979). Mass fragmentography of phenethylamine, *m-* and *p-* tyramine and related amines in plasma, cerebrospinal fluid, urine, and brain. *Journal of Neurochemistry, 33,* 201–212.

Kasper, S. (1996). Treatment options in severe depression. Journal of Clinical Psychiatry, 57, 554–561.

Katsarava, Z., Fritsche, G., Muessig, M., Diener, H.-C., & Limmroth, V. (2001). Clinical features of withdrawal headache following overuse of triptans and other headache drugs. *Neurology, 57,* 1694–1698.

Katsarava, Z., Limmroth, V., Finke, M., Diener, H.-C., & Fritsche, G. (2003). Rates and predictors for relapse in medication overuse headache: A 1-year prospective study. *Neurology, 60,* 1682–1683.

Kaube, H., Hoskin, K. L., & Goadsby, P. J. (1993). Intravenous acetylsalicylic acid inhibits central trigeminal neurons in the dorsal horn of the upper cervical spinal cord in the cat. *Headache, 33,* 541–544.

Kaube, H., May, A., Pfaffenrath, V., & Diener, H.-C. (1994). Sumatriptan misuse in daily chronic headache. *British Medical Journal, 308,* 1573.

Kauhanen, J., Kaplan, G. A., Cohen, R. D., Julkunen, J., & Salonen, J. T. (1996). Alexithymia and risk of death in middle-aged men. *Journal of Psychosomatic Research, 41,* 541–549.

Kawamoto, K., & Matsuda, H. (2004). Nerve growth factor and wound healing. In L. Aloe & L. Calzà (Eds.), *NGF and related molecules in health and disease* (pp. 369–384). New York: Elsevier.

Keefe, F. J., Brown, G. K., Wallston, K. A., & Caldwell, D. S. (1989). Coping with rheumatoid arthritis pain: Catastrophizing as a maladaptive strategy. *Pain, 37,* 51–56.

Keefe, F. J., Caldwell, D. S., Baucom, D., Salley, A., Robinson, E., Timmons, K., Beaupre, P., Weisberg, J., & Helms, M. (1996). Spouse-assisted coping skills training in the management of osteoarthritic knee pain. *Arthritis Care and Research, 9,* 279–291.

Keefe, F. J., Gil, K. M., & Rose, S. C. (1986). Behavioral approaches in the multidisciplinary management of chronic pain: Programs and issues. *Clinical Psychology Review, 6,* 87–113.

Keefe, F. J., Kashikar-Zuck, S., Robinson, E., Salley, A., Beaupre, P., Caldwell, D., Baucom, D., & Haythornthwaite, J. (1997). Pain coping strategies that predict patients' and spouses' ratings of patients' self-efficacy. *Pain, 73,* 191–199.

Keefe, F. J., & Lefebvre, J. C. (1999). Behavioural therapy. In P. D. Wall & R. Melzack (Eds.), *Textbook of pain* (4th ed., pp. 1445–1461). New York: Churchill Livingstone.

Kelly, R., & Smith, B. N. (1981). Posttraumatic syndrome: Another myth discredited. *Journal of the Royal Society of Medicine, 74*, 275–277.

Kemper, R. H. A., Spoelstra, M. B., Meijler, W. J., & Ter Horst, G. J. (1998). Lipopolysaccharide-induced hyperalgesia of intracranial capsaicin sensitive afferents in conscious rats. *Pain, 78*, 181–190.

Kendall, F. P., McCreary, E. K., & Provance, P. G. (1993). *Muscles testing and function: With posture and pain* (4th ed.). Baltimore: Williams & Wilkins.

Kendler, K. S., Neale, M. C., Kessler, R. C., Heath, A. C., & Eaves, L. J. (1993). A longitudinal twin study of personality and major depression in women. *Archives of General Psychiatry, 50*, 853–862.

Kennedy, W. P. (1961). The nocebo reaction. *Medical World, 91*, 203–205.

Kennett, G. A., Lightowler, S., De Biasi, V., Stevens, N. C., Wood, M. D., Tulloch, I. F., & Blackburn, T. P. (1994). Effect of chronic administration of selective 5-hydroxytryptamine and noradrenaline uptake inhibitors on a putative index of 5-$HT_{2C/2B}$ receptor function. *Neuropharmacology, 33*, 1581–1588.

Keogh, E., Hatton, K., & Ellery, D. (2000). Avoidance versus focused attention and the perception of pain: Differential effects for men and women. *Pain, 85*, 225–230.

Kerns, R. D., Turk, D. C., & Rudy, T. E. (1985). The West Haven-Yale Multidimensional Pain Inventory (WHYMPI). *Pain, 23*, 345–356.

Kewman, D., & Roberts, A. H. (1980). Skin temperature biofeedback and migraine headaches: A double-blind study. *Biofeedback and Self-Regulation, 5*, 327–345.

Kewman, D. G., Vaishampayan, N., Zald, D., & Han, B. (1991). Cognitive impairment in musculoskeletal pain patients. *International Journal of Psychiatry in Medicine, 21*, 253–262.

Kharkevich, D. A., & Churukanov, V. V. (1999). Pharmacological regulation of descending cortical control of the nociceptive processing. *European Journal of Pharmacology, 375*, 121–131.

Kiecolt-Glaser, J. K., Marucha, P. T., Atkinson, C., & Glaser, R. (2001). Hypnosis as a modulator of cellular immune dysregulation during acute stress. *Journal of Consulting and Clinical Psychology, 69*, 674–682.

Kiernan, B. D., Dane, J. R., Phillips, L. H., & Price, D. D. (1995). Hypnotic analgesia reduces R-III nociceptive reflex: Further evidence concerning the multifactorial nature of hypnotic analgesia. *Pain, 60*, 39–47.

Kight, M., Gatchel, R. J., & Wesley, L. (1999). Temporomandibular disorders: Evidence for significant overlap with psychopathology. *Health Psychology, 18*, 177–182.

Kihlstrom, J. F. (1998). Dissociations and dissociation theory in hypnosis: Comment on Kirsch and Lynn (1998). *Psychological Bulletin, 123*, 186–191.

Kim, M., & Blanchard, E. B. (1992). Two studies of the non-pharmacological treatment of menstrually-related migraine headaches. *Headache, 32*, 197–202.

King, A. C., & Arena, J. G. (1984). Behavioral treatment of chronic cluster headache in a geriatric patient. *Biofeedback and Self-Regulation, 9*, 201–208.

Kirsch, I., & Lynn, S. J. (1995). The altered state of hypnosis: Changes in the theoretical landscape. *American Psychologist, 50*, 846–858.

Kirsch, I., & Lynn, S. J. (1998). Dissociation theories of hypnosis. *Psychological Bulletin, 123*, 100–115.

Kissel, P., & Barrucand, D. (1974). *Placébos et effet—placébo en médecine*. Paris: Masson.

Kitazono, T., Ibayashi, S., Nagao, T., Kagiyama, T., Kitayama, J., & Fujishima, M. (1998). Role of tyrosine kinase in serotonin-induced constriction of the basilar artery in vivo. *Stroke, 29*, 494–498.

Kitt, C. A., Gruber, K., Davis, M., Woolf, C. J., & Levine, J. D. (2000). Trigeminal neuralgia: Opportunities for research and treatment. *Pain, 85*, 3–7.

Kittrelle, J. P., Grouse, D. S., & Seybold, M. E. (1985). Cluster headache: Local anesthetic abortive agents. *Archives of Neurology, 42*, 496–498.

Kjeldsen, S. E., Weder, A. B., Egan, B., Neubig, R., Zweifler, A. J., & Julius, S. (1995). Effect of circulating epinephrine on platelet function and hematocrit. *Hypertension, 25*, 1096–1105.

Klapper, J. (1997). Divalproex sodium in migraine prophylaxis: A dose-controlled study. *Cephalalgia, 17*, 103–108.

Klopstock, T., May, A., Seibel, P., Papagiannuli, E., Diener, H. C., & Reichmann, H. (1996). Mitochondrial DNA in migraine with aura. *Neurology, 46*, 1735–1738.

Kluger, M. A., Jamner, L. D., & Tursky, B. (1985). Comparison of the effectiveness of biofeedback and relaxation training on hand warming. *Psychophysiology, 22*, 162–166.

Knishkowy, B., Palti, H., Tima, C., Adler, B., & Gofin, R. (1995). Symptom clusters among young adolescents. *Adolescence, 30*, 351–362.

Knost, B., Flor, H., Birbaumer, N., & Schugens, M. M. (1999). Learned maintenance of pain: Muscle tension reduces central nervous system processing of painful stimulation in chronic and subchronic pain patients. *Psychophysiology, 36*, 755–764.

Koban, M., Leis, S., Schultze-Mosgau, S., & Birklein, F. (2003). Tissue hypoxia in complex regional pain syndrome. *Pain, 104*, 149–157.

Kobasa, S. C., Maddi, S. R., & Kahn, S. (1982). Hardiness and health: A prospective study. *Journal of Personality and Social Psychology, 42*, 68–77.

Koehler, P. J., & Isler, H. (2002). The early use of ergotamine in migraine. Edward Woakes' report of 1868, its theoretical and practical background and its international reception. *Cephalalgia, 22*, 686–691.

Koehler, S. M., & Glaros, A. (1988). The effect of aspartame on migraine headache. *Headache, 28*, 10–13.

Koenig, M., Kraus, M., Theek, C., Klotz, E., Gehlen, W., & Heuser, L. (2001). Quantitative assessment of the ischemic brain by means of perfusion-related parameters derived from perfusion CT. *Stroke, 32*, 431–437.

Koeppen, A. S. (1974). Relaxation training for children. *Elementary School Guidance and Counseling, 9*, 14–21.

Kohlenberg, R. J. (1982). Tyramine sensitivity in dietary migraine: A critical review. *Headache, 22*, 30–34.

Kohler, T., & Haimerl, C. (1990). Daily stress as a trigger of migraine attacks: Results of 13 single-subject studies. *Journal of Consulting and Clinical Psychology, 58*, 870–872.

Kolbinson, D. A., Epstein, J. B., & Burgess, J. A. (1996). Temporomandibular disorders, headaches, and neck pain following motor vehicle accidents and the effect of litigation: Review of the literature. *Journal of Orofacial Pain, 10*, 101–125.

Kole-Snijders, A. M. J., Vlaeyen, J. W. S., Goossens, M. E. J. B., Rutten-van Mölken, M. P. M. H., Heuts, P. H. T. G., van Breukelen, G., & van Eek, H. (1999). Chronic low-back pain: What does cognitive coping skills training add to operant behavioral treatment? Results of a randomized clinical trial. *Journal of Consulting and Clinical Psychology, 67*, 931–944.

Kollmitzer, J., Ebenbichler, G. R., & Kopf, A. (1999). Reliability of surface electromyographic measurements. *Clinical Neurophysiology, 110*, 725–734.

Kondo, C. Y., & Canter, A. (1977). True and false electromyographic feedback: Effect on tension headache. *Journal of Abnormal Psychology, 86*, 93–95.

Koopmans, G. T., & Lamers, L. M. (2000). Chronic conditions, psychological distress and the use of psychoactive medications. *Journal of Psychosomatic Research, 48*, 115–123.

Kopp, M., Richter, R., Rainer, J., Kopp-Wilfling, P., Rumpold, G., & Walter, M. H. (1995). Differences in family functioning between patients with chronic headache and patients with chronic low back pain. *Pain, 63*, 219–224.

Koprowska, M., & Romaniuk, A. (1997). Behavioral and biochemical alterations in median and dorsal raphe nuclei lesioned cats. *Pharmacology, Biochemistry and Behavior, 56*, 529–540.

Korn, R. R. (1949). Vasomotor conditioning and the vascular headache: Toward a therapeutic synthesis. *Persona: The Intercollegiate Journal of Psychology, 1*, 51–67.

Korsgaard, A. G. (1995). The tolerability, safety and efficacy of oral sumatriptan 50 mg and 100 mg for the acute treatment of migraine in adolescents. *Cephalalgia, 16*, 98.

Korzan, W. J., Summers, T. R., Ronan, P. J., Renner, K. J., & Summers, C. H. (2001). The role of monoaminergic nuclei during aggression and sympathetic social signaling. *Brain, Behavior, and Evolution, 57*, 317–327.

Kosek, E., Ekholm, J., & Hansson, P. (1996). Modulation of pain thresholds during and following isometric contraction in patients with fibromyalgia and in healthy controls. *Pain, 64*, 415–423.

Kovacs, K., Herman, F., Filep, J., Jelencsik, I., Magyar, K., & Csanda, E. (1990). Platelet aggregation of migraineurs during and between attacks. *Cephalalgia, 10*, 161–165.

Kowacs, P. A., Piovesan, E. J., Werneck, L. C., Fameli, H., & Pereira da Silva, H. (2004). Headache related to a specific screen flickering frequency band. *Cephalalgia, 24*, 408–410.

Kraft, G. H., Johnson, E. W., LaBan, M. M. (1968). The fibrositis syndrome. *Archives of Physical Medicine and Rehabilitation, 49*, 155–168.

Krasuski, J., Horwitz, B., & Rumsey, J. M. (1996). A survey of functional and anatomical neuroimaging techniques. In G. R. Lyon & J. M. Rumsey (Eds.), *Neuroimaging: A window to the neurological foundations of learning and behavior in children* (pp. 25–52). Baltimore, MD: Paul H. Brookes Publishing Company.

Kraus, J. F., McArthur, D. L., & Silberman, T. A. (1994). Epidemiology of mild brain injury. *Seminars in Neurology, 14*, 1–7.

Kröner-Herwig, B., Diergarten, D., Diergarten, D., & Seeger-Siewert, R. (1988). Psychophysiological reactivity of migraine sufferers in conditions of stress and relaxation. *Journal of Psychosomatic Research, 32*, 483–492.

Kröner-Herwig, B., Fritsche, G., & Brauer, H. (1993). The physiological stress response and the role of cognitive coping in migraine patients and non-headache controls. *Journal of Psychosomatic Research, 37*, 467–480.

Kröner-Herwig, B., Mohn, U., & Pothmann, R. (1998). Comparison of biofeedback and relaxation in the treatment of pediatric headache and the influence of parent involvement on outcome. *Applied Psychophysiology and Biofeedback, 23*, 143–157.

Kropp, P., & Gerber, W. D. (1995). Contingent negative variation during migraine attack and interval: Evidence for normalization of slow cortical potentials during the attack. *Cephalalgia, 15*, 123–128.

Kropp, P., & Gerber, W. D. (1998). Prediction of migraine attacks using a slow cortical potential, the contingent negative variation. *Neuroscience Letters, 257*, 73–76.

Kropp, P., Gerber, W. D., Keinath-Specht, A., Kopal, T., & Niederberger, U. (1997). Behavioral treatment in migraine: Cognitive-behavioral therapy and blood-volume-pulse biofeedback: A cross-over study with a two-year followup. *Functional Neurology, 12*, 17–24.

Krueger, A. P., & Reed, E. J. (1976). Biological impact of small air ions. *Science, 193*, 1209–1213.

Kruit, M. C., van Buchem, M. A., Hofman, P. A. M., Bakkers, J. T. N., Terwindt, G. M., Ferrari, M. D., & Launer, L. J. (2004). Migraine as a risk factor for subclinical brain lesions. *JAMA, 291*, 427–434.

Krymchantowski, A. V., & Barbosa, J. S. (2000). Prednisone as initial treatment of analgesic-induced daily headache. *Cephalalgia, 20*, 107–113.

Kudrow, L. (1980). *Cluster headache: Mechanisms and management.* New York: Oxford University Press.

Kudrow, L. (1982). Paradoxical effects of frequent analgesic use. In M. Critchley, A. Friedman, S. Gorini, et al. (Eds.), *Advances in Neurology, 33*, 335–341. New York: Raven Press.

Kudrow, L. (1993). Cluster headache: Diagnosis, management, and treatment. In D. J. Dalessio & S. D. Silberstein (Eds.) *Wolff's Headache and Other Head Pain* (6th ed.). New York: Oxford University Press.

Kudrow, L. (1994). Recent advances in cluster headache research. In F. C. Rose (Ed.), *New advances in headache research* (3rd ed., pp. 193–202). London: Smith-Gordon.

Kudrow, L., & Kudrow, D. B. (1990). Association of sustained oxyhemoglobin desaturation and onset of cluster headache attacks. *Headache, 30*, 474–480.

Kugelmann, R. (2001). Introspective psychology, pure and applied: Henry Rutgers Marshall on pain and pleasure. *History of Psychology, 4*, 34–58.

Kurihara, Y., Kurihara, H., Morita, H., Cao, W. H., Ling, G. Y., Kumada, M., Kimura, S., Nagai, R., Yazaki, Y., & Kuwaki, T. (2000). Role of endothelin-1 in stress response in the central nervous system. *American Journal of Physiology—Regulatory Integrative and Comparative Physiology, 279*, R515–R521.

Kuritzky, A. (1997). Power spectrum analysis on heart rate and diastolic blood pressure variability [editorial commentary]. *Cephalalgia, 17*, 720–721.

Labbe, E. E. (1995). Treatment of childhood migraine with autogenic training and skin temperature biofeedback: A component analysis. *Headache, 35*, 10–13.

LaCroix, J. M., & Gowen, A. H. (1981). The acquisition of autonomic control through biofeedback: Some tests of discrimination theory. *Psychophysiology, 18*, 559–572.

Lai, C., Dean, P., Ziegler, D. K., & Hassanein, R. S. (1989). Clinical and electrophysiological responses to dietary challenge in migraineurs. *Headache, 29*, 180–186.

Lake, A. E. III. (2001). Behavioral and nonpharmacologic treatments of headache. *Medical Clinics of North America, 85*, 1055–1075.

Lake, A. E. III, & Pingel, J. D. (1988). Brief versus extended relaxation: Relationship to improvement at follow-up in mixed headache patients. *Medical Psychotherapy: An International Journal, 1*, 119–129.

Lake, A. E. III, & Saper, J. R. (1988). Prospective outcome evaluation of an accredited inpatient headache program. *Headache, 28*, 315–316.

Lake, A. E. III, Saper, J. R., Hamel, R. L., & Kreeger, C. (1995). Proposal for a multiaxial diagnostic system for headache. *Headache, 35*, 285–286.

Lake, A. E. III, Saper, J. R., Madden, S. F., & Kreeger, C. (1993). Comprehensive inpatient treatment for intractable migraine: A prospective long-term outcome study. *Headache, 33*, 55–62.

Lance, F., Parkes, C., & Wilkinson, M. (1988). Does analgesic abuse cause headaches de novo? *Headache, 28*, 61–62.

Lance, J. W. (1998). *Migraine and other headaches.* East Roseville, Australia: Simon and Schuster (Australia).

Lance, J. W., Anthony, M., & Somerville, B. (1970). Comparative trial of serotonin antagonists in the management of migraine. *British Medical Journal, 2*, 327–330.

Lance, J. W., Lambert, G. A., Goadsby, P. J., & Duckworth, J. W. (1983). Brainstem influences on the cerebral circulation: Experimental data from cat and monkey of relevance to the mechanism of migraine. *Headache, 23*, 258–265.

Lane, J. D. (1994). Neuroendocrine responses to caffeine in the work environment. *Psychosomatic Medicine, 56*, 267–270.

Lane, N. (2005). *Power, sex, suicide: Mitochondria and the meaning of life.* New York: Oxford University Press.

Lang, P. J., Bradley, M. M., & Cuthbert, B. N. (1997). Motivated attention: Affect, activation, and action. In P. J. Lang, R. F. Simons, & M. T. Balaban (Eds.), *Attention and orienting: Sensory and motivational processes* (pp. 97–135). Mahwah, NJ: Lawrence Erlbaum Associates.

Lange, C. G. (1922). The emotions: A psychophysiological study (I. A. Haupt, Trans.). In: K. Dunlap (Ed.), *The emotions* (pp. 33–90). Baltimore: Williams and Wilkins. (Orginal work published 1885)

Langemark, M., Bach, F. W., Ekman, R., & Olesen, J. (1995). Increased cerebrospinal fluid Met-enkephalin immunoreactivity in patients with chronic tension-type headache. *Pain, 63*, 103–107.

Lanzetta, J. T., Cartwright-Smith, J., & Kleck, R. E. (1976). Effects of nonverbal dissimulation on emotional experience and autonomic arousal. *Journal of Personality and Social Psychology, 33*, 354–370.

Lanzi, G., Zambrino, C. A., Balottin, U., Tagliasacchi, M., Vercelli, P., & Termine, C. (1997). Periodic syndrome and migraine in children and adolescents. *Italian Journal of Neurological Sciences, 18*, 283–288.

LaPlanche, J., & Pontalis, J.-B. (1973). *The language of psycho-analysis.* (D. Nicholson-Smith, Trans.) New York: W. W. Norton and Company. (Original work published 1967)

Lapo, I. B., Konarzewski, M., & Sadowski, B. (2003). Effect of cold acclimation and repeated swimming on opioid and nonopioid swim stress-induced analgesia in selectively bred mice. *Physiology and Behavior, 78*, 345–350.

Largen, J. W., Mathew, R. J., Dobbins, K., & Claghorn, J. L. (1981). Specific and non-specific effects of skin temperature control in migraine management. *Headache, 21*, 36–44.

Larson, E. W. (1993). Migraine with typical aura associated with fluoxetine therapy: Case report. *Journal of Clinical Psychiatry, 54*, 235–236.

Larsson, B., & Melin, L. (1988). The psychological treatment of recurrent headache in adolescents—Short-term outcome and its prediction. *Headache, 28*, 187–195.

Larsson, R., Öberg, P. Å., & Larsson, S.-E. (1999). Changes of trapezius muscle blood flow and electromyography in chronic neck pain due to trapezius myalgia. *Pain, 79*, 45–50.

Larsson, R., Zhang, Q., Cai, H., Öberg, P. Å., & Larsson, S.-E. (1998). Psychosocial problems and chronic neck pain: Microcirculation and electromyography of the trapezius muscles at static loads. *Journal of Musculoskeletal Pain, 6*(2), 65–76.

Lashley, K. (1941). Patterns of cerebral integration indicated by the scotomas of migraine. *Archives of Neurology and Psychiatry, 46*, 333–339.

Latham, P. W. (1872). Clinical lectures on nervous or sick headaches. *British Medical Journal*, pp. 305–306 & 336–337.

Laurell, K., Larsson, B., & Eeg-Olofsson, O. (2004). Prevalence of headache in Swedish schoolchildren, with a focus on tension-type headache. *Cephalalgia, 24*, 380–388.

Lauritzen, M. (1994). Pathophysiology of the migraine aura: The spreading depression theory. *Brain, 117*, 199–210.

Lavigne, G. J., Lobbezoo, F., Rompre, P. H., Nielsen, T. A., & Montplaisir, J. (1997). Cigarette smoking as a risk factor or an exacerbating factor for restless legs syndrome and sleep bruxism. *Sleep, 20*, 290–293.

Lea, R. A., Dohy, A., Jordan, K., Quinlan, S., Brimage, P. J., & Griffiths, L. R. (2000). Evidence for allelic association of the dopamine beta-hydroxylase gene (DβH) with susceptibility to typical migraine. *Neurogenetics, 3*, 35–40.

Leão, A. A. P. (1944). Spreading depression of activity in cerebral cortex. *Journal of Neurophysiology, 7*, 379–390.

Leavitt, F. (1990). The role of psychological disturbance in extending disability time among compensable back injured industrial workers. *Journal of Psychosomatic Research, 34*, 447–453.

Lee, H. K., Barbarosie, M., Kameyama, K., Bear, M. F., & Huganir, R. L. (2000). Regulation of distinct AMPA receptor phosphorylation sites during bidirectional synaptic plasticity. *Nature, 405*, 955–959.

Lehnert, H., Schulz, C., & Dieterich, K. (1998). Physiological and neurochemical aspects of corticotropin-releasing factor actions in the brain: The role of the locus coeruleus. *Neurochemical Research, 23*, 1039–1052.

Lehrer, P. M. (1982). How to relax and how not to relax: A re-evaluation of the work of Edmund Jacobson—I. *Behaviour Research and Therapy, 20*, 417–428.

Lehrer, P. M. (1996). Varieties of relaxation methods and their unique effects. *International Journal of Stress Management, 3*, 1–15.

Lehrer, P. M., Batey, D. M., Woolfolk, R. L., Remde, A., & Garlick, T. (1988). The effect of repeated tense-release sequences on EMG and self-report of muscle tension: An evaluation of Jacobsonian and post-Jacobsonian assumptions about progressive relaxation. *Psychophysiology, 25*, 562–569.

Lehrer, P., Sasaki, Y., & Saito, Y. (1999). Zazen and cardiac variability. *Psychosomatic Medicine, 61*, 812–821.

Lehrer, P. M., & Woolfolk, R. L. (1993). Specific effects of stress management techniques. In P. M. Lehrer & R. L. Woolfolk (Eds.), *Principles and practice of stress management* (2nd edition, pp. 481–520). New York: Guilford Press.

Leijdekkers, M. L. A., & Passchier, J. (1990). Prediction of migraine using psychophysiological and personality measures. *Headache, 30*, 445–453.

Lenssinck, M.-L. B., Damen, L., Verhagen, A. P., Berger, M. Y., Passchier, J., & Koes, B. W. (2004). The effectiveness of physiotherapy and manipulation in patients with tension-type headache: A systematic review. *Pain, 112*, 381–388.

Leone, M., Attanasio, A., Croci, D., Ferraris, A., D'Amico, D., Grazzi, L., Nespolo, A., & Bussone, G. (1998). 5-HT$_{1A}$ receptor hypersensitivity in migraine is suggested by the m-chlorophenylpiperazine test. *NeuroReport, 9*, 2605–2608.

Leone, M., Attanasio, A., Croci, D., Filippini, G., D'Amico, D., Grazzi, L., Nespolo, A., & Bussone, G. (2000). The serotonergic agent *m*-chlorophenylpiperazine induces migraine attacks: A controlled study. *Neurology, 55*, 136–139.

Leone, M., & Bussone, G. (1993). A review of hormonal findings in cluster headache: Evidence for hypothalamic involvement. *Cephalalgia, 13*, 309–317.

Leone, M., D'Amico, D., Frediani, F., Moschiano, F., Grazzi, L., Attanasio, A., & Bussone, G. (2000). Verapamil in the prophylaxis of episodic cluster headache: A double-blind study versus placebo. *Neurology, 54*, 1382–1385.

Leone, M., D'Amico, D., Grazzi, L., Attanasio, A., & Bussone, G. (1998). Cervicogenic headache: A critical review of the current diagnostic criteria. *Pain, 78*, 1–5.

Leone, M., D'Amico, D., Moschiano, F., Fraschini, F., & Bussone, G. (1996). Melatonin versus placebo in the prophylaxis of cluster headache: A double-blind pilot study with parallel groups. *Cephalalgia, 16*, 494–496.

Leone, M., Lucini, V., D'Amico, D., Grazzi, L., Moschiano, F., Fraschini, F., & Bussone, G. (1998). Abnormal 24-hour urinary excretory pattern of 6-sulphatoxymelatonin in both phases of cluster headache. *Cephalalgia, 18*, 664–667.

Leone, M., Maltempo, C., Parati, E. A., & Bussone, G. (1994). A unifying concept of neuroendocrine dysfunction in cluster headache. In F. C. Rose (Ed.), *New advances in headache research* (3rd ed., pp. 207–211). London: Smith-Gordon.

Leone, M., Russell, M. B., Rigamonti, A., Attanasio, A., Grazzi, L., D'Amico, D., Usai, S., & Bussone, G. (2001). Increased familial risk of cluster headache. *Neurology, 56*, 1233–1236.

LeResche, L., Saunders, K., Von Korff, M. R., Barlow, W., & Dworkin, S. F. (1997). Use of exogenous hormones and risk of temporomandibular disorder pain. *Pain, 69*, 153–160.

Lerner, M. (1994). *Choices in healing*. Cambridge, Massachusetts: MIT Press.

Lesser, I. M. (1985). Current concepts in psychiatry: Alexithymia. *New England Journal of Medicine, 312*, 690–692.

Levin, M. (2004). Chronic daily headache and the revised International Headache Society classification. *Current Pain and Headache Reports, 8*, 59–65.

Levine, F. M., Krass, S. M., & Padawer, W. J. (1993). Failure hurts: The effects of stress due to difficult tasks and failure feedback on pain report. *Pain, 54*, 335–340.

Levor, R. M., Cohen, M. J., Naliboff, B. D., McArthur, D., & Heuser, G. (1986). Psychosocial precursors and correlates of migraine headache. *Journal of Consulting and Clinical Psychology, 54*, 347–353.

Lewis, T. (1935). Experiments relating to cutaneous hyperalgesia and its spread through somatic fibres. *Clinical Science, 2*, 373–423.

Lewkowski, M. D., Ditto, B., Roussos, M., & Young, S. N. (2003). Sweet taste and blood pressure-related analgesia. *Pain, 106*, 181–186.

Li, A. K., Koroly, M. J., Schattenkerk, M. E., Malt, R. A., & Young, M. (1980). Nerve growth factor: Acceleration of the rate of wound healing in mice. *Proceedings of the National Academy of Sciences (USA), 77*, 4379–4381.

Li, B. U. K. (2001). Cyclic vomiting syndrome: Age-old syndrome and new insights. *Seminars in Pediatric Neurology, 8,* 13–21.

Li, D., & Rozen, T. D. (2002). The clinical characteristics of new daily persistent headache. *Cephalalgia, 22,* 66–69.

Li, J., Simone, D., & Larsson, A. (1999). Wind-up leads to characteristics of central sensitization. *Pain, 79,* 75–82.

Li, P., & Zhuo, M. (1998). Silent glutamatergic synapses and nociception in mammalian spinal cord. *Nature, 393,* 695–698.

Li, Y. Q., Li, H., Kaneko, T., & Mizuno, N. (1999). Substantia gelatinosa neurons in the medullary dorsal horn: An intracellular labeling study in the rat. *Journal of Comparative Neurology, 411,* 399–412.

Li, Y. Q., Takada, M., Matsuzaki, S., Shinonaga, Y., & Mizuno, N. (1993). Identification of periaqueductal gray and dorsal raphe nucleus neurons projecting to both the trigeminal sensory complex and forebrain structures: A flourescent retrograde double-labeling study in the rat. *Brain Research, 623,* 267–277.

Libo, L. N., & Arnold, G. E. (1983). Does training to criterion influence improvement? A follow-up study of EMG and thermal biofeedback. *Journal of Behavioral Medicine, 6,* 397–404.

Licinio, J., & Wong, M.-L. (1997). Pathways and mechanisms for cytokine signaling of the central nervous system. *Journal of Clinical Investigation, 100,* 2941–2947.

Limmroth, V., Kazarawa, Z., Fritsche, G., & Diener, H.-C. (1999). Headache after frequent use of serotonin agonists zolmitriptan and naratriptan. *Lancet, 353,* 378.

Limmroth, V., & Michel, M. C. (2001). The prevention of migraine: A critical review with special emphasis on β-adrenoceptor blockers. *British Journal of Clinical Pharmacology, 52,* 237–243.

Linden, D. J. (1999). The return of the spike: Postsynaptic action potentials and the induction of LTP and LTD. *Neuron, 22,* 661–666.

Linden, W. (1993). The autogenic training method of J. H. Schultz. In P. M. Lehrer and R. L. Woolfolk (Eds.), *Principles and practice of stress management* (2nd ed., pp. 205–229). New York: Guilford Press.

Linden, W., Lenz, J. W., & Stossel, C. (1996). Alexithymia, defensiveness and cardiovascular reactivity to stress. *Journal of Psychosomatic Research, 41,* 575–583.

Linet, M. S., Stewart, W. F., Celentano, D. D., Ziegler, D., & Sprecher, M. (1989). An epidemiologic study of headache among adolescents and young adults. *JAMA, 261,* 2211–2216.

Linton, S. J. (1997). A population-based study of the relationship between sexual abuse and back pain: Establishing a link. *Pain, 73,* 47–53.

Linton, S. J., & Andersson, T. (2000). Can chronic disability be prevented? A randomized trial of a cognitive-behavior intervention for patients with spinal pain. *Spine, 25,* 2825–2831.

Linton, S. J., Lardén, M., & Gillow, Å. M. (1996). Sexual abuse and chronic musculoskeletal pain: Prevalence and psychological factors. *Clinical Journal of Pain, 12,* 215–221.

Lipchik, G. L., Holroyd, K. A., & Nash, J. M. (2002). Cognitive-behavioral management of recurrent headache disorders: A minimal-therapist-contact approach. In D. C. Turk & R. J. Gatchel (Eds.), *Psychological approaches to pain management: A practitioner's handbook* (2nd ed., pp. 365–389). New York: Guilford Press.

Lipp, O. V., Siddle, D. A. T., & Vaitl, D. (1992). Latent inhibition in humans: Single-cue conditioning revisited. *Journal of Experimental Psychology: Animal Behavior Processes, 18,* 115–125.

Lippold, O. C. J. (1967). Electromyography. In P. H. Venables & I. Martin (Eds.) *A manual of psychophysiological methods* (pp. 245–297). Amsterdam: North-Holland.

Lipscombe, S. L., & Prior, T. (2002). Is there any relationship between handedness and unilateral headache in migraine? *Cephalalgia, 22,* 146–148.

Lipsey, M. W., & Wilson, D. B. (2001). *Practical meta-analysis.* Thousand Oaks, CA: Sage Publications.

Lipton, R. B. (2000). Fair winds and foul headaches: Risk factors and triggers of migraine. *Neurology, 54,* 280–281.

Lipton, R. B., Diamond, S., Reed, M., Diamond, M. L., & Stewart, W. F. (2001). Migraine diagnosis and treatment: Results from the American Migraine Study II. *Headache, 41,* 638–645.

Lipton, R. B., Newman, L. C., & Solomon, S. (1988). Aspartame and headache [letter]. *New England Journal of Medicine, 318,* 1200–1201.

Lipton, R. B., Silberstein, S. D., & Stewart, W. F. (1994). An update on the epidemiology of migraine. *Headache, 34,* 319–328.

Lipton, R. B., & Stewart, W. F. (1997). Prevalence and impact of migraine. *Neurologic Clinics, 15*(1), 1–13.

Lipton, R. B., & Stewart, W. F. (1999). Acute migraine therapy: Do doctors understand what patients with migraine want from therapy? *Headache, 39*(Suppl. 2), S20–S26.

Lipton, R. B., Stewart, W. F., Cady, R., Hall, C., O'Quinn, S., Kuhn, T., & Gutterman, D. (2000). Sumatriptan for the range of headaches in migraine sufferers: Results of the Spectrum Study. *Headache, 40*, 783–791.

Lipton, R. B., Stewart, W. F., Diamond, S., Diamond, M. L., & Reed, M. (2001). Prevalence and burden of migraine in the United States: Data from the American Migraine Study II. *Headache, 41*, 646–657.

Lipton, R. B., Stewart, W. F., Ryan, R. E. Jr., Saper, J., Silberstein, S. D., & Sheftell, F. (1998). Efficacy and safety of acetaminophen, aspirin, and caffeine in alleviating migraine headache pain: Three double-blind, randomized, placebo-controlled trials. *Archives of Neurology, 55*, 210–217.

Lipton, R. B., Stewart, W. F., Stone, A. M., Láinez, M. J. A., & Sawyer, J. P. C. (2000). Stratified care vs. step care strategies for migraine: The Disability in Strategies of Care (DISC) Study: A randomized trial. *JAMA, 284*, 2599–2605.

Lishman, W. A. (1988). Physiogenesis and psychogenesis in the 'Postconcussional Syndrome.' *British Journal of Psychiatry, 153*, 160–169.

Lisotto, C., Maggioni, F., Mainardi, F., & Zanchin, G. (2003). Rofecoxib for the treatment of chronic paroxysmal hemicrania. *Cephalalgia, 23*, 318–320.

Lisspers, J., & Öst, L.-G. (1990). Long-term follow-up of migraine treatment: Do the effects remain up to six years? *Behaviour Research and Therapy, 28*, 313–322.

Lisspers, J., Öst, L.-G., & Skagerberg, B. (1992). Clinical effects of biofeedback treatment in migraine: The relation to achieved self-control and pretreatment predictors. *Scandinavian Journal of Behaviour Therapy, 21*, 171–190.

Littlewood, J. T., Gibb, C., Glover, V., Sandler, M., Davies, P. T. G., & Rose, F. C. (1988). Red wine as a cause of migraine. *Lancet, I*, 558–559.

Littlewood, J. T., Glover, V., & Sandler, M. (1985). Red wine contains a potent inhibitor of phenolsulphotransferase. *British Journal of Clinical Pharmacology, 19*, 275–278.

Littlewood, J., Glover, V., Sandler, M., Petty, R., Peatfield, R., & Rose, F. C. (1982). Platelet phenolsulphotransferase deficiency in dietary migraine. *Lancet, I*, 983–986.

Liveing, E. (1872, April 6). Observations on megrim or sick-headache. *British Medical Journal*, pp. 364–366.

Liveing, E. (1873). *On megrim, sick-headache, and some allied disorders: A contribution to the pathology of nerve-storms*. London: J. and A. Churchill.

Llinás, R. R. (2001). *I of the vortex: From neurons to self*. Cambridge, MA: MIT Press.

Loder, E. (2002a). Naratriptan in the prophylaxis of cluster headache. *Headache, 42*, 56–57.

Loder, E. (2002b). What is the evolutionary advantage of migraine? *Cephalalgia, 22*, 624–632.

Loder, E., & Biondi, D. (2003). Disease modification in migraine: A concept that has come of age? *Headache, 43*, 135–143.

Lodi, R., Kemp, G. J., Montagna, P., Pierangeli, G., Cortelli, P., Iotti, S., Radda, G. K., & Barbiroli, B. (1997). Quantitative analysis of skeletal muscle bioenergetics and proton efflux in migraine and cluster headache. *Journal of the Neurological Sciences, 146*, 73–80.

Loeser, J. D. (1982). Concepts of pain. In M. Stanton-Hicks & R. Boas (Eds.), *Chronic low back pain* (pp. 145–148). New York: Raven Press.

Longe, S. E., Wise, R., Bantick, S., Lloyd, D., Johansen-Berg, H., McGlone, F., & Tracey, I. (2001). Counter-stimulatory effects on pain perception and processing are significantly altered by attention: An fMRI study. *NeuroReport, 12*, 2021–2025.

Lord, F. M. (1953). On the statistical treatment of football numbers. *American Psychologist, 8*, 750–751.

Lord, S., Barnsley, L., Wallis, B. J., & Bogduk, N. (1994). Third occipital headache: A prevalence study. *Journal of Neurology, Neurosurgery and Psychiatry, 57*, 1187–1190.

Lord, S. M., Barnsley, L., Wallis, B. J., & Bogduk, N. (1996). Chronic cervical zygapophysial joint pain after whiplash. A placebo-controlled prevalence study. *Spine, 21*, 1737–1744.

Lorenz, J., Kunze, K., & Bromm, B. (1998). Differentiation of conversive sensory loss and malingering by P300 in a modified oddball task. *Neuroreport, 9*, 187–191.

Lorenz, J., Minoshima, S., & Casey, K. L. (2003). Keeping pain out of mind: The role of the dorsolateral prefrontal cortex in pain modulation. *Brain, 126*, 1079–1091.

Löscher, W. (1999). Valproate: A reappraisal of its pharmacodynamic properties and mechanisms of action. *Progress in Neurobiology, 58*, 31–59.

Lous, I., & Olesen, J. (1982). Evaluation of pericranial tenderness and oral function in patients with common migraine, muscle contraction headache and 'combination headache.' *Pain, 12*, 385–393.

Lousberg, R., Schmidt, A. J., & Groenman, N. H. (1992). The relationship between spouse solicitousness and pain behavior: Searching for more experimental evidence. *Pain, 51,* 75–79.

Lousberg, R., Vuurman, E., Lamers, T., Van Breukelen, G., Jongen, E., Rignen, H., et al. (2005). Pain report and pain-related evoked potentials operantly conditioned. *Clinical Journal of Pain, 21,* 262–271.

Love, A. (1987). Depression in chronic low back pain patients: Diagnostic efficiency of three self-report questionnaires. *Journal of Clinical Psychology, 43,* 84–89.

Lowrie, W. (1946). *Religion of a scientist: Selections from Gustav Th. Fechner.* New York: Pantheon Books.

Lu, S. R., Fuh, J. L., Chen, W. T., Juang, K. D., & Wang, S. J. (2001). Chronic daily headache in Taipei, Taiwan: Prevalence, follow-up and outcome predictors. *Cephalalgia, 21,* 980–986.

Lücking, C. H., Oestreich, W., Schmidt, R., & Soyka, D. (1988). Flunarizine vs. propranolol in the prophylaxis of migraine: Two double-blind comparative studies in more than 400 patients. *Cephalalgia, 8,* 21–26.

Ludin, H.-P. (1989). Flunarizine and propranolol in the treatment of migraine. *Headache, 29,* 218–223.

Lumb, B. M. (2002). Inescapable and escapable pain is represented in distinct hypothalamic-midbrain circuits: Specific roles for Adelta- and C-nociceptors. *Experimental Physiology, 87,* 281–286.

Lumley, M. A., Stettner, L., & Wehmer, F. (1996). How are alexithymia and physical illness linked? A review and critique of pathways. *Journal of Psychosomatic Research, 41,* 505–518.

Lundberg, U., Kadefors, R., Melin, B., Palmerud, G., Hassmén, P., Engström, M., & Elfsberg Dohns, I. (1994). Psychophysiological stress and EMG activity of the trapezius muscle. *International Journal of Behavioral Medicine, 1,* 354–370.

Lutzenberger, W., Flor, H., & Birbaumer, N. (1997). Enhanced dimensional complexity of the EEG during memory for personal pain in chronic pain patients. *Neuroscience Letters, 266,* 167–170.

Lutzenberger, W., Preißl, H., & Pulvermüller, F. (1995). Fractal dimension of EEG time series and underlying brain processes. *Biological Cybernetics, 73,* 477–482.

Lynch, M. E. (2001). Antidepressants as analgesics: A review of randomized controlled trials. *Journal of Psychiatry and Neuroscience, 26,* 30–36.

MacGregor, A. J., Griffiths, G. O., Baker, J., & Spector, T. D. (1997). Determinants of pressure pain threshold in adult twins: Evidence that shared environmental influences predominate. *Pain, 73,* 253–257.

MacGregor, E. A. (1997). Menstruation, sex hormones, and migraine. *Neurologic Clinics, 15,* 125–141.

MacQueen, G., Marshall, J., Perdue, M., Siegel, S., & Bienenstock, J. (1989). Pavlovian conditioning of rat mucosal mast cells to secrete rat mast cell protease II. *Science, 243,* 83–85.

Maertens de Noordhout, A., Pepin, J. L., Schoenen, J., & Delwaide, P. J. (1992). Percutaneous magnetic stimulation of the motor cortex in migraine. *Electroencephalography and Clinical Neurophysiology, 85,* 110–115.

Maertens de Noordhout, A., Timsit-Berthier, M., Timsit, M., & Schoenen, J. (1986). Contingent negative variation in headache. *Annals of Neurology, 19,* 78–80.

Magee, J. C., & Johnston, D. (1997). A synaptically controlled, associative signal for Hebbian plasticity in hippocampal neurons. *Science, 275,* 209–213.

Magnusson, J. E., & Becker, W. J. (2003). Migraine frequency and intensity: relationship with disability and psychological factors. *Headache, 43,* 1049–1059.

Magnusson, T., Egermark, I., & Carlsson, G. E. (2000). A longitudinal epidemiologic study of signs and symptoms of temporomandibular disorders from 15 to 35 years of age. *Journal of Orofacial Pain, 14,* 310–319.

Mai, F. (2004). Somatization disorder: A practical review. *Canadian Journal of Psychiatry, 49,* 652–662.

Mailis-Gagnon, A., Giannoylis, I., Downar, J., Kwan, C. L., Mikulis, D. J., Crawley, A. P., Nicholson, K., & Davis, K. D. (2003). Altered cental somatosensory processing in chronic pain patients with "hysterical" anesthesia. *Neurology, 60,* .

Main, A., Dowson, A., & Gross, M. (1997). Photophobia and phonophobia in migraineurs between attacks. *Headache, 37,* 492–495.

Main, A., Vlachonikolis, I., & Dowson, A. (2000). The wavelength of light causing photophobia in migraine and tension-type headache between attacks. *Headache, 40,* 194–199.

Maixner, W., Fillingim, R., Booker, D., & Sigurdsson, A. (1995). Sensitivity of patients with painful temporomandibular disorders to experimentally evoked pain. *Pain, 63,* 341–351.

Maixner, W., Fillingim, R., Sigurdsson, A., Kincaid, S., & Silva, S. (1998). Sensitivity of patients with painful temporomandibular disorders to experimentally evoked pain: Evidence for altered temporal summation of pain. *Pain, 76,* 71–81.

Maizels, M., Scott, B., Cohen, W., & Chen, W. (1996). Intranasal lidocaine for treatment of migraine: A randomized, double-blind, controlled trial. *JAMA, 276,* 319–321.

Malenka, R. C., & Nicoll, R. A. (1999). Long-term potentiation—A decade of progress? *Science, 285,* 1870–1874.

Malmgren, R., & Hasselmark, L. (1988). The platelet and the neuron: Two cells in focus in migraine. *Cephalalgia, 8,* 7–24.

Manfredi, P. L., Shenoy, S., & Payne, R. (2000). Sumatriptan for headache caused by head and neck cancer. *Headache, 40,* 758–760.

Manzoni, G. C. (1997). Male preponderance of cluster headache is progressively decreasing over the years. *Headache, 37,* 587–588.

Manzoni, G. C. (1998). Gender ratio of cluster headache over the years: A possible role of changes in lifestyle. *Cephalalgia, 18,* 138–142.

Manzoni, G. C. (1999). Cluster headache and lifestyle: Remarks on a population of 374 male patients. *Cephalalgia, 19,* 88–94.

Mao, J. (2002). Opioid-induced abnormal pain sensitivity: Implications in clinical opioid therapy. *Pain, 100,* 213–217.

Mao, J., Sung, B., Ji, R. R., & Lim, G. (2002). Neuronal apoptosis associated with morphine tolerance: Evidence for an opioid-induced neurotoxic mechanism. *Journal of Neuroscience, 22,* 7650–7661.

Marchand, S., & Arsenault, P. (2002). Odors modulate pain perception: A gender-specific effect. *Physiology and Behavior, 76,* 251–256.

Marcus, D. A. (1995). Interrelationships of neurochemicals, estrogen, and recurring headache. *Pain, 62,* 129–139.

Marcus, D. A., Nash, J. M., & Turk, D. C. (1994). Diagnosing recurring headaches: IHS criteria and beyond. *Headache, 34,* 329–336.

Marcus, D. A., Scharff, L., Mercer, S., & Turk, D. C. (1998). Nonpharmacological treatment for migraine: Incremental utility of physical therapy with relaxation and thermal biofeedback. *Cephalalgia, 18,* 266–272.

Marcus, D. A., Scharff, L., Mercer, S., & Turk, D. C. (1999). Musculoskeletal abnormalities in chronic headache: A controlled comparison of headache diagnostic groups. *Headache, 39,* 21–27.

Marcus, D. A., Scharff, L., & Turk, D. C. (1995). Nonpharmacological management of headaches during pregnancy. *Psychosomatic Medicine, 57,* 527–535.

Marcus, D. A., Scharff, L., Turk, D., & Gourley, L. M. (1997). A double-blind provocative study of chocolate as a trigger of headache. *Cephalalgia, 17,* 855–862.

Marcus, D. A., & Soso, M. J. (1989). Migraine and stripe-induced visual discomfort. *Archives of Neurology, 46,* 1129–1132.

Marinari, K. T., Leshner, A. I., & Doyle, M. P. (1976). Menstrual cycle status and adrenocortical reactivity to psychological stress. *Psychoneuroendocrinology, 1,* 213–218.

Marinesco, G., & Kreindler, A. (1934). Des réflexes conditionnels. III. Application des reflexes conditionnels à certains problèmes cliniques. *Journal de Psychologie Normale et Pathologique, 31,* 722–791.

Markley, H. G. (1994). Chronic headache: Appropriate use of opiate analgesics. *Neurology, 44*(Suppl. 3), S18–S24.

Markley, H. G., Cheronis, J. C., & Piepho, R. W. (1984). Verapamil in prophylactic therapy of migraine. *Neurology, 34,* 973–976.

Markowitz, J. S., & Patrick, K. S. (1998). Venlafaxine-tramadol similarities. *Medical Hypotheses, 5,* 167–168.

Marlowe, N. (1998). Self-efficacy moderates the impact of stressful events on headache. *Headache, 38,* 662–667.

Marras, W. S., & Davis, K. G. (2001). A non-MVC EMG normalization technique for the trunk musculature: Part 1. Method development. *Journal of Electromyography and Kinesiology, 11,* 1–9.

Marshall, M. E. (1969). Gustav Fechner, Dr. Mises, and the comparative anatomy of angels. *Journal of the History of the Behavioral Sciences, 5,* 39–58.

Marshall, M. E. (1982). Physics, metaphysics, and Fechner's psychophysics. In W. R. Woodward & M. G. Ash (Eds.), *The problematic science: Psychology in nineteenth-century thought.* New York: Praeger Publishers.

Martelletti, P. (2002). Inflammatory mechanisms in cervicogenic headache: An integrative view. *Current Pain and Headache Reports, 6,* 315–319.

Martelletti, P., Lulli, P., Morellini, M., Mariani, B., Pennesi, G., Cappellacci, S., Brioli, G., Giacovazzo, M., & Trabace, S. (1999). Chromosome 6p-encoded HLA-DR2 determinant discriminates migraine without aura from migraine with aura. *Human Immunology, 60,* 69–74.

Martelletti, P., Stirparo, G., & Giacovazzo, M. (1999). Proinflammatory cytokines in cervicogenic headache. *Functional Neurology, 14,* 159–162.

Martelletti, P., & van Suijlekom, H. (2004). Cervicogenic headache: Practical approaches to therapy. *CNS Drugs, 18*, 793–805.

Martelli, M. F., Grayson, R. L., & Zasler, N. D. (1999). Posttraumatic headache: Neuropsychological and psychological effects and treatment implications. *Journal of Head Trauma Rehabilitation, 14*, 49–69.

Martin, B. C., Pathak, D. S., Sharfman, M. I., Adelman, J. U., Taylor, F., Kwong, J., & Jhingran, P. (2000). Validity and reliability of the Migraine-Specific Quality of Life Questionnaire (MSQ Version 2.1). *Headache, 40*, 204–215.

Martin, G. R. (1997). Serotonin receptor involvement in the pathogenesis and treatment of migraine. In P. J. Goadsby & S. D. Silberstein (Eds.) *Headache* (pp. 25–38). Boston: Butterworth-Heinemann.

Martin, J. H. (1991). The collective electrical behavior of cortical neurons: The electroencephalogram and the mechanisms of epilepsy. In E. R. Kandel, J. H. Schwartz, & T. M. Jessell (Eds.), *Principles of neural science* (3rd ed., pp. 777–791). Norwalk, CT: Appleton & Lange.

Martin, N. J., Holroyd, K. A., & Penzien, D. B. (1990). The Headache-Specific Locus of Control Scale: Adaptation to recurrent headaches. *Headache, 30*, 729–734.

Martin, P. R. (1993). *Psychological management of chronic headaches.* New York: Guilford Press.

Martin, P. R. (2000). Headache triggers: To avoid or not to avoid, that is the question. *Psychology and Health, 15*, 801–809.

Martin, P. R. (2001). How do trigger factors acquire the capacity to precipitate headaches? *Behaviour Research and Therapy, 39*, 545–554.

Martin, P. R., Marie, G. V., & Nathan, P. R. (1992). Psychophysiological mechanisms of chronic headaches: Investigation using pain induction and pain reduction procedures. *Journal of Psychosomatic Research, 36*, 137–148.

Martin, P. R., Milech, D., & Nathan, P. R. (1993). Towards a functional model of chronic headaches: Investigation of antecedents and consequences. *Headache, 33*, 461–470.

Martin, P. R., Nathan, P. R., & Milech, D. (1987). The Type A behaviour pattern and chronic headaches. *Behaviour Change, 4*(2), 33–39.

Martin, P. R., & Seneviratne, H. M. (1997). Effects of food deprivation and a stressor on head pain. *Health Psychology, 16*, 310–318.

Martin, P. R., & Teoh, H.-J. (1999). Effects of visual stimuli and a stressor on head pain. *Headache, 39*, 705–715.

Martin, P. R., Todd, J., & Reece, J. (2005). Effects of noise and a stressor on head pain. *Headache, 45*, 1353–1364.

Martín, R., Ribera, C., Moltó, J. M., Ruiz, C., Galiano, L., & Matías-Guiu, J. (1992). Cardiovascular reflexes in patients with vascular headache. *Cephalalgia, 12*, 360–364.

Martínez, F., Castillo, J., Pardo, J., Lema, M., & Noya, M. (1993). Catecholamine levels in plasma and CSF in migraine. *Journal of Neurology, Neurosurgery, and Psychiatry, 56*, 1119–1121.

Marucha, P. T., Kiecolt-Glaser, J. K., & Favagehi, M. (1998). Mucosal wound healing is impaired by examination stress. *Psychosomatic Medicine, 60*, 362–365.

Massiou, H., Tzourio, C., el Amrani, M., & Bousser, M. G. (1997). Verbal scales in the acute treatment of migraine: Semantic categories and clinical relevance. *Cephalalgia, 17*, 37–39.

Matchar, D. B., Young, W. B., Rosenberg, J. H., Pietrzak, M. P., Silberstein, S. D., Lipton, R. B., & Ramadan, N. M. (n.d.). *Evidence-based guidelines for migraine headache in the primary care setting: Pharmacological management of acute attacks.* http://www.aan.com. (Accessed July 3, 2003).

Materazzo, F., Cathcart, S., & Pritchard, D. (2000). Anger, depression, and coping interactions in headache activity and adjustment: A controlled study. *Journal of Psychosomatic Research, 49*, 69–75.

Matharu, M. S., & Goadsby, P. J. (2001). Post-traumatic chronic paroxysmal hemicrania (CPH) with aura. *Neurology, 56*, 273–275.

Matheson, D. W., Toben, T. P., & de la Cruz, D. E. (1988). EMG scanning: Normative data. *Journal of Psychopathology and Behavioral Assessment, 10*, 9–20.

Mathew, N. T. (1981). Prophylaxis of migraine and mixed headache. A randomized controlled study. *Headache, 21*, 105–109.

Mathew, N. T. (1987). Amelioration of ergotamine withdrawal with naproxen. *Headache, 27*, 130–133.

Mathew, N. T. (1993). Chronic refractory headache. *Neurology, 43*(Suppl. 3), S26–S33.

Mathew, N. T. (1997a). Transformed migraine, analgesic rebound, and other chronic daily headaches. *Neurologic Clinics, 15*(1), 167–186.

Mathew, N. T. (1997b). Cluster headache. *Seminars in Neurology, 17*, 313–323.

Mathew, N. T. (1999). Naratriptan: A review. *Expert Opinion on Investigational Drugs, 8*, 687–695.

Mathew, N. T. (2001). Antiepileptic drugs in migraine prevention. *Headache, 41*(Suppl. 1), S18–S24.

Mathew, N. T., Kailasam, J., Gentry, P., & Chernyshev, O. (2000). Treatment of nonresponders to oral suma-triptan with zolmitriptan and rizatriptan: A comparative open trial. *Headache, 40,* 464–465.

Mathew, N. T., Kurman, R., & Perez, F. (1990). Drug induced refractory headache—Clinical features and management. *Headache, 30,* 634–638.

Mathew, N. T., Ravishankar, K., & Sanin, L. C. (1996). Coexistence of migraine and idiopathic intracranial hypertension without papilledema. *Neurology, 46,* 1226–1230.

Mathew, N. T., Saper, J. R., Silberstein, S. D., Rankin, L., Markley, H. G., Solomon, S., Rapoport, A. M., Silber, C. J., & Deaton, R. L. (1995). Migraine prophylaxis with divalproex. *Archives of Neurology, 52,* 281–286.

Mathew, N. T., Stubits, E., & Nigam, M. P. (1982). Transformation of episodic migraine into daily headache: Analysis of factors. *Headache, 22,* 66–68.

Mathew, R. J., Barr, D. L., & Weinman, M. L. (1983). Caffeine and cerebral blood flow. *British Journal of Psychiatry, 143,* 604–608.

Mathew, R. J., & Wilson, W. H. (1985). Caffeine induced changes in cerebral circulation. *Stroke, 16,* 814–817.

Mathew, R. J., Wilson, W. H., Humphreys, D., Lowe, J. V., & Wiethe, K. E. (1997). Cerebral vasodilation and vasoconstriction associated with acute anxiety. *Biological Psychiatry, 41,* 782–795.

Mathiassen, S. E., Winkel, J., & Hägg, G. M. (1995). Normalization of surface EMG amplitude from the upper trapezius muscle in ergonomic studies—A review. *Journal of Electromyography and Kinesiology, 5,* 197–226.

Matser, J. T., Kessels, A. G. H., Jordan, B. D., Lezak, M. D., & Troost, J. (1998). Chronic traumatic brain injury in professional soccer players. *Neurology, 51,* 791–796.

Matser, E. J. T., Kessels, A. G., Lezak, M. D., Jordan, B. D., & Troost, J. (1999). Neuropsychological impairment in amateur soccer players. *Journal of the American Medical Association (JAMA), 282,* 971–973

Mattei, B., Schmied, A., Mazzocchio, R., Decchi, B., Rossi, A., & Vedel, J. P. (2003). Pharmacologically induced enhancement of recurrent inhibition in humans: Effects on motoneurone discharge patterns. *Journal of Physiology, 548,* 615–629.

Mattimoe, D., & Newton, W. (1998). High-dose riboflavin for migraine prophylaxis. *Journal of Family Practice, 47,* 11.

Mauskop, A., & Altura, B. M. (1998). Role of magnesium in the pathogenesis and treatment of migraines. *Clinical Neuroscience, 5,* 24–27.

Mauskop, A., Altura, B. T., Cracco, R. Q., & Altura, B. M. (1995a). Intravenous magnesium sulfate relieves migraine attacks in patients with low serum ionized magnesium levels: A pilot study. *Clinical Science, 89,* 633–636.

Mauskop, A., Altura, B. T., Cracco, R. Q., & Altura, B. M. (1995b). Intravenous magnesium sulfate relieves cluster headaches in patients with low serum ionized magnesium levels. *Headache, 35,* 597–600.

Mauskop, A., & Fox, B. (2001). *What your doctor may not tell you about migraines.* New York: Warner Books.

May, A., Bahra, A., Büchel, C., Frackowiak, R. S. J., & Goadsby, P. J. (1998). Hypothalamic activation in cluster headache attacks. *Lancet, 352,* 275–278.

May, A., Gijsman, H. J., Wallnöfer, A., Jones, R., Diener, H. C., & Ferrari, M. D. (1996). Endothelin antagonist bosentan blocks neurogenic inflammation, but is not effective in aborting migraine attacks. *Pain, 67,* 375–378.

Maytal, J., Young, M., Shechter, A., & Lipton, R. B. (1997). Pediatric migraine and the International Headache Society (IHS) criteria. *Neurology, 48,* 602–607.

Mazur, W. (1998). Phytoestrogen content in foods. *Bailliere's Clinical Endocrinology and Metabolism, 12,* 729–742.

Mazzotta, G., Sarchielli, P., Alberti, A., & Gallai, V. (1999). Intracellular Mg^{++} concentration and electromyographical ischemic test in juvenile headache. *Cephalalgia, 19,* 802–809.

Mazzotta, G., Sarchielli, P., Gaggioli, A., & Gallai, V. (1997). Study of pressure pain and cellular concentration of neurotransmitters related to nociception in episodic tension-type headache patients. *Headache, 37,* 565–571.

McAdam, B. F., Catella-Lawson, F., Mardini, I. A., Kapoor, S., Lawson, J. A., & FitzGerald, G. A. (1999). Systemic biosynthesis of prostacyclin by cyclooxygenase (COX)-2: The human pharmacology of a selective inhibitor of COX-2. *Proceedings of the National Academy of Sciences U.S.A., 96,* 272–277.

McCabe, C. S., Haigh, R. C., Halligan, P. W., & Blake, D. R., (2003). Generating sensory disturbance in healthy controls. *Rheumatology, 42,* 63. (a)

McCabe, C. S., Haigh, R. C., Halligan, P. W., & Blake, D. R. (2003). Distorting proprioception in chronic pain patients exacerbates sensory disturbances—implications for pathology. *Rheumatology, 42*, 145. (b)

McCabe, C. S., Haigh, R. C., Ring, E. F., Halligan, P. W., Wall, P. D., & Blake, D. R. (2003). A controlled pilot study of the utility of mirror visual feedback in the treatment of complex regional pain syndrome (type 1). *Rheumatology, 42*, 97–101.

McCabe, C. S., Haigh, R. C., Shenker, N. G., Lewis, J., & Blake, D. R. (2004). Phantoms in rheumatology. *Novartis Foundation Symposium, 260*, 154–174.

McCaffrey, R. J., Goetsch, V. L., Robinson, J., & Isaac, W. (1986). Differential responsivity of the vaso-motor response system to a "novel" stressor. *Headache, 26*, 240–242.

McCaul, K. D., Monson, N., & Maki, R. H. (1992). Does distraction reduce pain-produced distress among college students? *Health Psychology, 11*, 210–217.

McCaul, K. D., Solomon, S., & Holmes, D. S. (1979). Effects of paced respiration and expectations on physiological and psychological responses to threat. *Journal of Personality and Social Psychology, 37*, 564–571.

McColl, S. L., & Wilkinson, F. (2000). Visual contrast gain control in migraine: Measures of visual corti-cal excitability and inhibition. *Cephalalgia, 20*, 74–84.

McCracken, L. M., & Eccleston, C. (2003). Coping or acceptance: What to do about chronic pain? *Pain, 105*, 197–204.

McCracken, L. M., Gross, R. T., Sorg, P. J., & Edmands, T. A. (1993). Prediction of pain in patients with chronic low back pain: Effects of inaccurate prediction and pain-related anxiety. *Behaviour Research and Therapy, 31*, 647–652.

McCrory, D. C., Matchar, D. B., Gray, R. N., Rosenberg, J. H., & Silberstein, S. D. (n.d.). *Evidence-based guidelines for migraine headache: Overview of program description and methodology.* http://www.aan .com. (Accessed July 3, 2003).

McCrory, D. C., Penzien, D. B., Hasselblad, V., & Gray, R. N. (2001). *Behavioral and physical treatments for tension-type and cervicogenic headache.* Duke University Evidence-Based Practice Center report. Des Moines, IA: Foundation for Chiropractic Education and Research.

McCrory, D. C., Penzien, D. B., Rains, J. C., & Hasselblad, V. (1996). Efficacy of behavioral treatments for migraine and tension-type headache: Meta-analysis of controlled trials. *Headache, 36*, 272.

McCulloch, J., Uddman, R., Kingman, T., & Edvinsson, L. (1986). Calcitonin gene-related peptide: Func-tional role in cerebrovascular regulation. *Proceedings of the National Academy of Sciences (USA), 83*, 5741–5745.

McDermid, A. J., Rollman, G. B., & McCain, G. A. (1996). Generalized hypervigilance in fibromyalgia: Evidence of perceptual amplification. *Pain, 66*, 133–144.

McFarlane, A. C., Atchison, M., Rafalowicz, E., & Papay, P. (1987). Physical symptoms in post-traumatic stress disorder. *Journal of Psychosomatic Research, 38*, 715–726.

McGeer, P. L., Eccles, J. C., & McGeer, E. G. (1978). *Molecular neurobiology of the mammalian brain.* New York: Plenum Press.

McGrady, A., Nadsady, P. A., & Schumann-Brzezinski, C. (1991). Sustained effects of biofeedback-assisted relaxation therapy in essential hypertension. *Biofeedback and Self-Regulation, 16*, 399–411.

McGrady, A., Wauquier, A., McNeil, A., & Gerard, G. (1994). Effect of biofeedback-assisted relaxation on migraine headache and changes in cerebral blood flow velocity in the middle cerebral artery. *Headache, 34*, 424–428.

McGrath, P. A., & Hillier, L. M. (2001). Recurrent headache: Triggers, causes, and contributing factors. In P. A. McGrath & L. M. Hillier (Eds.), *The child with headache: Diagnosis and treatment (Progress in Pain Research and Management, 19*, pp. 77–107). Seattle: IASP Press.

McGrath, P. A., Stewart, D., & Koster, A. L. (2001). Nondrug therapies for childhood headache. In P. A. McGrath & L. M. Hillier (Eds.), *The child with headache: Diagnosis and treatment (Progress in Pain Research and Management, 19*, pp. 129–158). Seattle: IASP Press.

McGrath, P. J. (1999). Clinical psychology issues in migraine headaches. *Canadian Journal of Neurologi-cal Sciences, 26*(Suppl. 3), S33–S36.

McHenry, I. C. (1969). *Garrison's history of neurology.* Springfield, IL: Charles C. Thomas.

McKenzie, R., O'Fallon, A., Dale, J., Demitrack, M., Sharma, G., Deloria, M., et al. (1998). Low-dose hydrocortisone for treatment of chronic fatigue syndrome: A randomized controlled trial. *JAMA, 280*, 1061–1066.

McLachlan, R. S., & Girvin, J. P. (1994). Spreading depression of Leão in rodent and human cortex. *Brain Research, 666*, 133–136.

McNeil, D. W., & Rainwater, A. J. 3rd. (1998). Development of the Fear of Pain Questionnaire—III. *Journal of Behavioral Medicine, 21*, 389–410.

McNulty, W. H., Gevirtz, R. N., Hubbard, D. R., & Berkoff, G. M. (1994). Needle electromyographic evaluation of trigger point response to a psychological stressor. *Psychophysiology, 31*, 313–316.

Meador, K. J., Ray, P. G., Echauz, J. R., Loring, D. W., & Vachtsevanos, G. J. (2002). Gamma coherence and conscious perception. *Neurology, 59*, 847–854.

Mease, J. (1970). *The picture of Philadelphia.* Port Washington, New York: Arno Press. (Original work published 1811)

Mease, J. (1819). *A treatise on the causes, means of prevention, and cure of the sick-headache.* Philadelphia: M. Carey and Son.

Medina, J. (1992). Efficacy of an individualized outpatient program in the treatment of chronic post-traumatic headache. *Headache, 32*, 180–183.

Mei, D., Capuano, A., Vollono, C., Evangelista, M., Ferraro, D., Tonali, P., et al. (2004). Topiramate in migraine prophylaxis: A randomised double-blind versus placebo study. *Neurological Sciences, 25*, 245–250.

Meichenbaum, D. (1977). *Cognitive behavior modification: An integrative approach.* New York: Plenum.

Meier, B., & Lock, J. E. (2003). Contemporary management of patent foramen ovale. *Circulation, 107*, 5–9.

Meier, W., Klucken, M., Soyka, D., & Bromm, B. (1993). Hypnotic hypo- and hyperalgesia: Divergent effects on pain ratings and pain-related cerebral potentials. *Pain, 53*, 175–181.

Meloche, J. P., Bergeron, Y., Bellavance, A., Morand, M., Huot, J., & Belzile, G. (1993). Painful intervertebral dysfunction: Robert Maigne's original contribution to headache of cervical origin. *Headache, 33*, 328–334.

Melzack, R. (1975). The McGill Pain Questionnaire: Major properties and scoring methods. *Pain, 1*, 277–299.

Melzack, R. (1990). Phantom limbs and the concept of a neuromatrix. *Trends in Neuroscience, 13*, 88–92.

Melzack, R., & Casey, K. L. (1968). Sensory, motivational, and central control determinants of pain. A new conceptual model. In D. R. Kenshalo (Ed.), *The skin senses* (pp. 423–443). Springfield, IL: Charles C. Thomas.

Melzack, R., & Wall, P. D. (1965). Pain mechanisms: A new theory. *Science, 150*, 971–979.

Melzack, R., & Wall, P. D. (1996). *The challenge of pain* (Updated 2nd ed.). New York: Penguin Books.

Mendelson, G. (1992). Compensation and chronic pain. *Pain, 48*, 121–123.

Mendizabal, J. E. (1999). Cluster headache. *Archives of Neurology, 56*, 1413–1416.

Mense, S. (1993). Nociception from skeletal muscle in relation to clinical muscle pain. *Pain, 54*, 241–289.

Menzies, R. (1937). Conditioned vasomotor responses in human subjects. *Journal of Psychology, 4*, 75–120.

Mercado, A. C., Carroll, L. J., Cassidy, J. D., & Côté, P. (2005). Passive coping is a risk factor for disabling neck or low back pain. *Pain, 117*, 51–57.

Merikangas, K. R., & Angst, J. (1996). Post-traumatic headache in the Swiss male cohort study. *Schweizer Archiv für Neurologie und Psychiatrie, 147*, 105–108.

Merikangas, K. R., Stevens, D. E., & Angst, J. (1994). Psychopathology and headache syndromes in the community. *Headache, 34*, s17–s22.

Merikangas, K. R., Stevens, D. E., Merikangas, J. R., Katz, C. B. S., Glover, V., Cooper, T., & Sandler, M. (1995). Tyramine conjugation deficit in migraine, tension-type headache, and depression. *Biological Psychiatry, 38*, 730–736.

Merskey, H., & Bogduk, N. (1994). *Classification of chronic pain* (2nd ed.). Seattle: IASP Press.

Merskey, H. & Spear, F. G. (1967). The concept of pain. *Journal of Psychosomatic Research, 11*, 59–67.

Messinger, H. B., Messinger, M. I., Kudrow, L., & Kudrow, L. V. (1994). Handedness and headache. *Cephalalgia, 14*, 64–67.

Metsähonkala, L., Sillanpää, M., & Tuominen, J. (1998). Social environment and headache in 8- to 9-year-old children: A follow-up study. *Headache, 38*, 222–228.

Meyer, J. S., Thornby, J., Crawford, K., & Rauch, G. M. (2000). Reversible cognitive decline accompanies migraine and cluster headaches. *Headache, 40*, 638–646.

Meyer, T. J., Miller, M. L., Metzger, R. L., & Borkovec, T. D. (1990). Development and validation of the Penn State Worry Questionnaire. *Behaviour Research and Therapy, 28*, 487–495.

Meyler, W. J. (1996). Side effects of ergotamine. *Cephalalgia, 16*, 5–10.

Mezei, Z., Kis, B., Gecse, A., Tajti, J., Boda, B., Telegdy, G., & Vecsei, L. (2000). Platelet arachidonate cascade of migraineurs in the interictal phase. *Platelets, 11*, 222–225.

Michultka, D. M., Blanchard, E. B., Appelbaum, K. A., Jaccard, J., & Dentinger, M. P. (1989). The refractory headache patient—II. High medication consumption (analgesic rebound) headache. *Behaviour Research and Therapy, 27*, 411–420.

Micieli, G., Cavallini, A., Bosone, D., Viotti, E., Barzizza, F., Richichi, I., & Nappi, G. (1994). Unbalanced heart rate regulation in cluster headache: A 24 h study. In F. C. Rose (Ed.), *New advances in headache research* (3rd ed., pp. 213–220). London: Smith-Gordon.

Micieli, G., Tassorelli, C., Bosone, D., Cavallini, A., Bellantonio, P., Rossi, F., & Nappi, G. (1995). Increased cerebral blood flow velocity induced by cold pressor test in migraine: A possible basis for pathogenesis? *Cephalalgia, 15*, 494–498.

Micieli, G., Tassorelli, C., Magri, M., Sandrini, G., Cavallini, A., & Nappi, G. (1989). Vegetative imbalance in migraine. A dynamic TV pupillometric evaluation. *Functional Neurology, 4*, 105–111.

Middaugh, S. J., Haythornthwaite, J. A., Thompson, B., Hill, R., Brown, K. M., Freedman, R. R., Attanasio, V., Jacob, R. G., Scheier, M., & Smith, E. A. (2001). The Raynaud's Treatment Study: Biofeedback protocols and acquisition of temperature biofeedback skills. *Applied Psychophysiology and Biofeedback, 26*, 251–278.

Middaugh, S., & Kee, W. G. (1987). Advances in electromyographic monitoring and biofeedback in treatment of chronic cervical and low back pain. In M. G. Eisenberg & R. C. Grzesiak (Eds.), *Advances in clinical rehabilitation* (Vol. 1). New York: Springer.

Middaugh, S. J., Kee, W. G., & Nicholson, J. A. (1994). Muscle overuse and posture as factors in the development and maintenance of chronic musculoskeletal pain. In R. C. Grzesiak & D. S. Ciccone (Eds.), *Psychological vulnerability to chronic pain* (pp. 55–89). New York: Springer.

Middleton, E. Jr., Kandaswami, C., & Theoharides, T. C. (2000). The effects of plant flavonoids on mammalian cells: Implications for inflammation, heart disease, and cancer. *Pharmacological Reviews, 52*, 673–751.

Migliardi, J. R., Armellino, J. J., Friedman, M., Gillings, D. B., & Beaver, W. T. (1994). Caffeine as an analgesic adjuvant in tension headache. *Clinical Pharmacology and Therapeutics, 56*, 576–586.

Migraine-Nimodipine European Study Group (MINES). (1989a). European multicenter trial of nimodipine in the prophylaxis of common migraine (migraine without aura). *Headache, 29*, 633–638.

Migraine-Nimodipine European Study Group (MINES). (1989b). European multicenter trial of nimodipine in the prophylaxis of classic migraine (migraine with aura). *Headache, 29*, 639–642.

Mikamo, K., Takeshima, T., & Takahashi, K. (1989). Cardiovascular sympathetic hypofunction in muscle contraction headache and migraine. *Headache, 29*, 86–89.

Mikuls, T. R., & Moreland, L. W. (2003). Benefit-risk assessment of infliximab in the treatment of rheumatoid arthritis. *Drug Safety, 26*, 23–32.

Millan, M. J. (2002). Descending control of pain. *Progress in Neurobiology, 66*, 355–474.

Miller, J., & Fishman, A. (1961). A serotonin antagonist in the treatment of allergic and allied disorders. *Annals of Allergy, 19*, 164–171.

Miller, W. S. (1925). James Mease. *Annals of Medical History, 7*, 6–30.

Milling, L. S., Kirsch, I., Meunier, S. A., & Levine, M. R. (2002). Hypnotic analgesia and stress inoculation training: Individual and combined effects in analog treatment of experimental pain. *Cognitive Therapy and Research, 26*, 355–371.

Mills, A., Rhodes, P., & Martin, G. R. (1995). [^{3}H]311C90 binding sites in cat brain stem: Implications for migraine treatment. *Cephalalgia, 15*(Suppl. 14), 116.

Mills, P. J., Berry, C. C., Dimsdale, J. E., Nelesen, R. A., & Ziegler, M. G. (1993). Temporal stability of task-induced cardiovascular, adrenergic, and psychological responses: The effects of race and hypertension. *Psychophysiology, 30*, 197–204.

Milner, P. M. (1958). Note on a possible correspondence between scotomas of migraine and spreading depression of Leão. *Electroencephalography and Clinical Neurophysiology, 10*, 705.

Minuchin, S., Rosman, B. L., & Baker, L. (1978). *Psychosomatic families: Anorexia nervosa in context.* Cambridge, MA: Harvard University Press.

Mirza, M., Tutus, A., Erdogan, F., Kula, M., Tomar, A., Silov, G., & Koseoglu, E. (1998). Interictal SPECT with Tc-99m HMPAO studies in migraine patients. *Acta Neurologica Belgica, 98*, 190–194.

Mishra, K. D., Gatchel, R. J., & Gardea, M. A. (2000). The relative efficacy of three cognitive-behavioral treatment approaches to temporomandibular disorders. *Journal of Behavioral Medicine, 23*, 293–309.

Mitchell, C. S., Osborn, R. E., & Grosskreutz, S. R. (1993). Computed tomography in the headache patient: Is routine evaluation really necessary? *Headache, 33*, 82–86.

Mitchell, J. M., Basbaum, A. I., & Fields, H. L. (2000). A locus and mechanism of action for associative morphine tolerance. *Nature Neuroscience, 3*, 47–53.

Mongini, F., Ciccone, G., Deregibus, A., Ferrero, L., & Mongini, T. (2004). Muscle tenderness in different headache types and its relation to anxiety and depression. *Pain, 112*, 59–64.

Mongini, F., Keller, R., Deregibus, A., Raviola, F., Mongini, T., & Sancarlo, M. (2003). Personality traits, depression and migraine in women: A longitudinal study. *Cephalalgia, 23*, 186–192.

Montagna, P., Cortelli, P., Monari, L., Pierangeli, G., Parchi, P., Lodi, R., Iotti, S., Frassineti, C., Zaniol, P., Lugaresi, E., & Barbiroli, B. (1994). ^{31}P-magnetic resonance spectroscopy in migraine without aura. *Neurology, 44*, 666–669.

Montagna, P., Cortelli, P., Pierangeli, G., Monari, L., Mochi, M., Sangiorgi, S., et al. (1994). Abnormal oxidative metabolism in migraine. In F. C. Rose (Ed.), *New advances in headache research* (3rd ed., pp. 151–155). London: Smith-Gordon and Company.

Montgomery, G. H., DuHamel, K. N., & Redd, W. H. (2000). A meta-analysis of hypnotically induced analgesia: How effective is hypnosis? *International Journal of Clinical and Experimental Hypnosis, 48*, 138–153.

Montgomery, G. T. (1994). Slowed respiration training. *Biofeedback and Self-Regulation, 19*, 211–225.

Morandi, E., Anzola, G. P., Angeli, S., Melzi, G., & Onorato, E. (2003). Transcatheter closure of patent foramen ovale: A new migraine treatment? *Journal of Interventional Cardiology, 16*, 39–42.

Morley, S. (1985). An experimental investigation of some assumptions underpinning psychological treatments of migraine. *Behaviour Research and Therapy, 23*, 65–74.

Morley, S., Eccleston, C., & Williams, A. (1999). Systematic review and meta-analysis of randomized controlled trials of cognitive behaviour therapy and behaviour therapy for chronic pain in adults, excluding headache. *Pain, 80*, 1–13.

Morrill, B., & Blanchard, E. B. (1989). Two studies of the potential mechanisms of action in the thermal biofeedback treatment of vascular headache. *Headache, 29*, 169–176.

Morrison, J. (1989). Childhood sexual histories of women with somatization disorder. *American Journal of Psychiatry, 146*, 239–241.

Mortimer, M. J., Kay, J., Gawkrodger, D. J., Jaron, A., & Barker, D. C. (1993). The prevalence of headache and migraine in atopic children: An epidemiological study in general practice. *Headache, 33*, 427–431.

Mortimer, M. J., Kay, J., & Jaron, A. (1992). Epidemiology of headache and childhood migraine in an urban general practice using ad hoc, Vahlquist, and IHS criteria. *Developmental Medicine and Child Neurology, 34*, 1095–1101.

Moseley, G. L. (2004). Graded motor imagery is effective for long-standing complex regional pain syndrome: A randomised controlled trial. *Pain, 108*, 192–198.

Moskowitz, M. A. (1984). The neurobiology of vascular head pain. *Annals of Neurology, 16*, 157–168.

Moskowitz, M. A. (1988). Cluster headache: Evidence for a pathophysiologic focus in the superior pericarotid cavernous sinus plexus. *Headache, 28*, 584–586.

Moskowitz, M. A. (1991). The visceral organ brain: Implications for the pathophysiology of vascular head pain. *Neurology, 41*, 182–186.

Moskowitz, M. A., & Cutrer, F. M. (1997). Attacking migraine headache from beginning to end [Editorial]. *Neurology, 49*, 1193–1195.

Moskowitz, M. A., & Macfarlane, R. (1993). Neurovascular and molecular mechanisms in migraine headaches. *Cerebrovascular and Brain Metabolism Review, 5*, 159–177.

Mosley, T. H., Penzien, D. B., Johnson, C. A., Brantley, P. J., Wittrock, D. A., Andrew, M. E., & Payne, T. J. (1991). Time series analysis of stress and headache. *Cephalalgia, 11*, 306–307.

Moss, R. A. (1987). Oral behavioral patterns in common migraine. *Cranio, 5*, 196–202.

Moss, R. A., Ruff, M. H., & Sturgis, E. T. (1984). Oral behavioral patterns in facial pain, headache and non-headache populations. *Behaviour Research and Therapy, 22*, 683–687.

Moussaoul, S., Duval, P., Lenoir, V., Garret, C., & Kerdelhue, B. (1996). CGRP in the trigeminal nucleus, spinal cord and hypothalamus: Effect of gonadal steroids. *Neuropeptides, 30*, 546–550.

Mulleners, W. M., Chronicle, E. P., Vredeveld, J. W., & Koehler, P. J. (2002). Visual cortex excitability in migraine before and after valproate prophylaxis: A pilot study using TMS. *European Journal of Neurology, 9*, 35–40.

Müller, M., & Somjen, G. G. (2000). Na^{+} and K^{+} concentrations, extra- and intracellular voltages, and the effect of TTX in hypoxic rat hippocampal slices. *Journal of Neurophysiology, 83*, 735–745.

Münchau, A., & Bhatia, K. P. (2000). Uses of botulinum toxin injection in medicine today. *British Medical Journal, 320*, 161–165.

Murphy, D. L., Andrews, A. M., Wichems, C. H., Li, Q., Tohda, M., & Greenberg, B. (1998). Brain serotonin neurotransmission: An overview and update with an emphasis on serotonin subsystem heterogeneity, multiple receptors, interactions with other neurotransmitter systems, and consequent implications for understanding the actions of serotonergic drugs. *Journal of Clinical Psychiatry, 59*(Suppl. 15), 4–12.

Murphy, J. J., Heptinstall, S., & Mitchell, J. R. A. (1988). Randomized double-blind placebo-controlled trial of Feverfew in migraine prevention. *Lancet, 2*(8604), 189–192.

Myers, D. E., Shaikh, Z., & Zullo, T. G. (1997). Hypoalgesic effect of caffeine in experimental ischemic muscle contraction pain. *Headache, 37*, 654–658.

Mylecharane, E. J., & Tfelt-Hansen, P. (2000). Nonsteroidal antiinflammatory and miscellaneous drugs in migraine prophylaxis. In J. Olesen, P. Tfelt-Hansen, & K. M. A. Welch (Eds.), *The headaches* (2nd ed., pp. 489–498). Philadelphia: Lippincott Williams & Wilkins.

Näätänen, R., & Winkler, I. (1999). The concept of auditory stimulus representation in cognitive neuroscience. *Psychological Bulletin, 125*, 826–859.

Nakata, M., Hagner, I.-M., & Jonsson, B. (1993). Trapezius muscle pressure pain threshold and strain in the neck and shoulder regions during repetitive light work. *Scandinavian Journal of Rehabilitation Medicine, 25*, 131–137.

Naliboff, B. D., McCreary, C. P., McArthur, D. L., Cohen, M. J., & Gottlieb, H. J. (1988). MMPI changes following behavioral treatment of chronic low back pain. *Pain, 35*, 271–277.

Nanda, R. N., Johnson, R. H., Gray, J., Keogh, H. J., Melville, I. D. (1978).A double blind trial of acebutolol for migraine prophylaxis. *Headache, 18*, 20–22.

Napier, D. A., Miller, C. M., & Andrasik, F. (1997). Group treatment for recurrent headache. *Advances in Medical Psychotherapy, 9*, 21–31.

Nathan, P. W. (1985). Pain and nociception in the clinical context. *Philosophical Transactions of the Royal Society of London, 308*, 219–226.

Nemiah, J. C. (1996). Alexithymia: Present, past—and future? *Psychosomatic Medicine, 58*, 217–218.

Nestler, E. J., Hyman, S. E., & Malenka, R. C. (2001). *Molecular neuropharmacology: A foundation for clinical neuroscience.* New York: McGraw-Hill.

Neufeld, J. D., Holroyd, K. A., & Lipchik, G. L. (2000). Dynamic assessment of abnormalities in central pain transmission and modulation in tension-type headache sufferers. *Headache, 40*, 142–151.

Newton-John, T. R. O. (2002). Solicitousness and chronic pain: A critical review. *Pain Reviews, 9*, 7–27.

Newman, L. C., & Goadsby, P. J. (2001). Unusual primary headache disorders. In S. D. Silberstein, R. B. Lipton, & D. J. Dalessio (Eds.), *Wolff's headache and other head pain* (7th ed., pp. 310–321). New York: Oxford University Press.

Newman, L., Mannix, L. K., Landy, S., Silberstein, S., Lipton, R. B., Pait Putnam, D. G., Watson, C., Jöbsis, M., Batenhorst, A., & O'Quinn, S. (2001). Naratriptan as short-term prophylaxis of menstrually associated migraine: A randomized, double-blind, placebo-controlled study. *Headache, 41*, 248–256.

Nezu, A. M. (1986). Efficacy of a social problem-solving therapy approach for unipolar depression. *Journal of Consulting and Clinical Psychology, 54*, 196–202.

Ng, J. K., Parnianpour, M., Richardson, C. A., & Kippers, V. (2003). Effect of fatigue on torque output and electromyographic measures of trunk muscles during isometric axial rotation. *Archives of Physical Medicine and Rehabilitation, 84*, 374–381.

Nicholson, R. A., Gramling, S. E., Ong, J. C., & Buenaver, L. (2003). Differences in anger expression between individuals with and without headache after controlling for depression and anxiety. *Headache, 43*, 651–663.

Nicolodi, M., Del Bianco, P. L., & Sicuteri, F. (1997). The way to serotonergic use and abuse in migraine. *International Journal of Clinicial Pharmacology Research, 17*(2/3), 79–84.

Nicolodi, M., Del Bianco, P. L., & Sicuteri, F. (1998). Histamine therapy of chronic daily headache having the features of transformed migraine [abstract]. *Cephalalgia, 18*, 410.

Nicolodi, M., & Sicuteri, F. (1999). Wine and migraine: Compatibility or incompatibility? *Drugs in Experimental and Clinical Research, 25*(2/3), 147–153.

Nilsson, N. (1995). The prevalence of cervicogenic headache in a random population sample of 20–59 year olds. *Spine, 20*, 1884–1888.

Ninan, T. K., & Russell, G. (1992). Respiratory symptoms and atopy in Aberdeen schoolchildren: Evidence from two surveys 25 years apart. *British Medical Journal, 304*, 873–875.

Nisbett, R. E., & Schachter, S. (1966). Cognitive manipulation of pain. *Journal of Experimental Social Psychology, 2*, 227–236.

Nishikawa, T., & Scatton, B. (1985). Inhibitory influence of GABA on central serotonergic transmission: Raphe nuclei as the neuroanatomical site of the GABAergic inhibition of cerebral serotonergic neurons. *Brain Research, 331*, 91–103.

Noll, G., Wenzel, R. R., Schneider, M., Oesch, V., Binggeli, C., Shaw, S., Weidmann, P., & Lüscher, T. F. (1996). Increased activation of sympathetic nervous system and endothelin by mental stress in normotensive offspring of hypertensive parents. *Circulation, 93*, 866–869.

Nussmeier, N. A., Whelton, A. A., Brown, M. T., Langford, R. M., Hoeft, A., Parlow, J. L., et al. (2005). Complications of the COX-2 inhibitors parecoxib and valdecoxib after cardiac surgery. *New England Journal of Medicine, 352*, 1081–1091.

Nuti, A., Lucetti, C., Pavese, N., Dell'Agnello, G., Rossi, G., & Bonuccelli, U. (1996). Long-term follow-up after flunarizine or nimodipine discontinuation in migraine patients. *Cephalalgia, 16*, 337–340.

Nutrition Reviews. (1988). Caffeine can increase brain serotonin levels. *Nutrition Reviews, 46*, 366–367.

Nyklíček, I., & Vingerhoets, A. J. J. M. (2000). Alexithymia is associated with low tolerance to experimental painful stimulation. *Pain, 85*, 471–475.

Obelieniene, D., Schrader, H., Bovim, G., Miseviciene, I., & Sand, T. (1999). Pain after whiplash: A prospective controlled inception cohort study. *Journal of Neurology, Neurosurgery and Psychiatry, 66*, 390–392.

Ochsner, K. N., Ludlow, D. H., Knierim, K., Hanelin, J., Ramachandran, T., Glover, G. C., et al. (2006). Neural correlates of individual differences in pain-related fear and anxiety. *Pain, 120*, 69–77.

Ogden, H., & Schockett, L. (1960). Controlled studies of chlorzoxazone and chlorzoxazone plus acetaminophen in the treatment of myalgia associated with headache. *Southern Medical Journal, 53*, 1415–1418.

Ohayon, M. M., Li, K. K., & Guilleminault, C. (2001). Risk factors for sleep bruxism in the general population. *Chest, 119*, 53–61.

Okazawa, H., Yamauchi, H., Sugimoto, K., Toyoda, H., Kishibe, Y., & Takahashi, M. (2001). Effects of acetazolamide on cerebral blood flow, blood volume, and oxygen metabolism: A positron emission tomography study with healthy volunteers. *Journal of Cerebral Blood Flow and Metabolism, 21*, 1472–1479.

Okifuji, A., Turk, D. C., & Curran, S. L. (1999). Anger in chronic pain: Investigations of anger targets and intensity. *Journal of Psychosomatic Research, 47*, 1–12.

Okifuji, A., Turk, D. C., & Marcus, D. A. (1999). Comparison of generalized and localized hyperalgesia in patients with recurrent headache and fibromyalgia. *Psychosomatic Medicine, 61*, 771–780.

Oldman, A. D., Smith, L. A., McQuay, H. J., & Moore, R. A. (2002). Pharmacological treatments for acute migraine: Quantitative systematic review. *Pain, 97*, 247–257.

Olesen, J. (1990). The classification and diagnosis of headache disorders. *Neurologic Clinics, 8*, 793–799.

Olesen, J. (1991). Clinical and pathophysiological observations in migraine and tension-type headache explained by integration of vascular, supraspinal and myofascial inputs. *Pain, 46*, 125–132.

Oliverio, A., & Castellano, C. (1982). Classical conditioning of stress-induced analgesia. *Physiology and Behavior, 29*, 171–172.

Olness, K., Hall, H., Rozniecki, J. J., Schmidt, W., & Theoharides, T. C. (1999). Mast cell activation in children with migraine before and after training in self-regulation. *Headache, 39*, 101–107.

Olsen, G., Vaughn, T. R., & Ledoux, R. A. (1989). Food induced migraine: Search for immunologic mechanisms. *Journal of Allergy and Clinical Immunology, 83*, 238.

Onghena, P., & Van Houdenhove, B. (1992). Antidepressant-induced analgesia in chronic non-malignant pain: A meta-analysis of 39 placebo-controlled studies. *Pain, 49*, 205–219.

Onishi, N., Sakai, K., & Kogi, K. (1982). Arm and shoulder muscle load in various keyboard operating jobs of women. *Journal of Human Ergology, 11*, 89–97.

Ophoff, R. A., Terwindt, G. M., Vergouwe, M. N., Frants, R. R., & Ferrari, M. D. (1997). Involvement of a Ca^{2+} channel gene in familial hemiplegic migraine and migraine with and without aura. *Headache, 37*, 479–485.

Ophoff, R. A., Terwindt, G. M., Vergouwe, M. N., van Eijk, R., Oefner, P. J., Hoffman, S. M., et al. (1996). Familial hemiplegic migraine and episodic ataxia type-2 are caused by mutations in the Ca2+ channel gene CACNL1A4. *Cell, 87*, 543–552.

Orholm, M., Honore, P. F., & Zeeberg, I. (1986). A randomized general practice group-comparative study of femoxetine and placebo in the prophylaxis of migraine. *Acta Neurologica Scandinavica, 74*, 235–239.

Osman, A., Breitenstein, J. L., Barrios, F. X., Gutierrez, P. M., & Kopper, B. A. (2002). The Fear of Pain Questionnaire—III: Further reliability and validity with nonclinical samples. *Journal of Behavioral Medicine, 25*, 155–173.

Osman, A., Kopper, B. A., Barrios, F. X., Osman, J. R., & Wade, T. (1997). The Beck Anxiety Inventory: Reexamination of factor structure and psychometric properties. *Journal of Clinical Psychology, 53*, 7–14.

Østergaard, S., Russell, M. B., Bendtsen, L., & Olesen, J. (1997). Comparison of first degree relatives and spouses of people with chronic tension headache. *British Medical Journal, 314*, 1092–1093.

Osterhaus, S. O. L., & Passchier, J. (1992). Perception of triggers in young, nonclinical school students with migrainous headaches and tension headaches. *Perceptual and Motor Skills, 75*, 284–286.

Ottosson, A., & Edvinsson, L. (1997). Release of histamine from dural mast cells by substance P and calcitonin gene-related peptide. *Cephalalgia, 17*, 166–174.

Özcan, A., Tulum, Z., Pinar, L., & Başkurt, F. (2004). Comparison of pressure pain threshold, grip strength, dexterity and touch pressure of dominant and non-dominant hands within and between right- and left-handed subjects. *Journal of Korean Medical Sciences, 19*, 874–878.

Packard, R. C. (1979). What does the headache patient want? *Headache, 19*, 370–374.

Packard, R. C., & Ham, L. P. (1997a). Pathogenesis of posttraumatic headache and migraine: A common headache pathway? *Headache, 37*, 142–152.

Packard, R. C., & Ham, L. P. (1997b). EEG biofeedback for post-traumatic headache and cognitive dysfunction: A pilot study. *Headache Quarterly, 8*, 348–352.

Palevitch, D., Earon, G., & Carasso, R. (1997). Feverfew (Tanacetum parthenium) as a prophylactic treatment for migraine: A double-blind placebo-controlled study. *Phytotherapy Research, 11*, 508–511.

Palmer, J. E., & Chronicle, E. P. (1998). Cognitive processing in migraine: A failure to find facilitation in patients with aura. *Cephalalgia, 18*, 125–132.

Panjwani, U., Selvamurthy, W., Singh, S. H., Gupta, H. L., Mukhopadhyay, S., & Thakur, L. (2000). Effect of Sahaja Yoga meditation on auditory evoked potentials (AEP) and visual contrast sensitivity (VCS) in epileptics. *Applied Psychophysiology and Biofeedback, 25*, 1–12.

Pareja, J. A., Caminero, A. B., Franco, E., Casado, J. L., Pascual, J., & Sánchez del Río, M. (2001). Dose, efficacy and tolerability of long-term indomethacin treatment of chronic paroxysmal hemicrania and hemicrania continua. *Cephalalgia, 21*, 906–910.

Parker, G. B., Pryor, D. S., & Tupling, H. (1980). Why does migraine improve during a clinical trial? Further results from a trial of cervical manipulation for migraine. *Australian and New Zealand Journal of Medicine, 10*, 192–198.

Parker, G. B., Tupling, H., & Pryor, D. S. (1978). A controlled trial of cervical manipulation of migraine. *Australian and New Zealand Journal of Medicine, 8*, 589–593.

Parrott, W. G., & Spackman, M. P. (2000). Emotion and memory. In M. Lewis & J. M. Haviland-Jones (Eds.), *Handbook of emotion* (2nd ed., pp. 476–490). New York: Guilford.

Parsons, A. A. (1998). Recent advances in mechanisms of spreading depression. *Current Opinion in Neurology, 11*, 227–231.

Pascual, J. (2001). Almotriptan: Pharmacological differences and clinical results. *Current Medical Research and Opinion, 17*(Suppl. 1), s63–s67.

Pascual, J., Colás, R., & Castillo, J. (2001). Epidemiology of chronic daily headache. *Current Pain and Headache Reports, 5*(6), 529–536.

Passchier, J., Goudswaard, P., & Orlebeke, J. F. (1993). Abnormal extracranial vasomotor response in migraine sufferers to real-life stress. *Journal of Psychosomatic Research, 37*, 405–414.

Passchier, J., Goudswaard, P., Orlebeke, J. F., & Verhage, F. (1988). Migraine and defense mechanisms: Psychophysiological relationships in young females. *Social Science and Medicine, 26*, 343–350.

Passchier, J., van der Helm-Hylkema, H., & Orlebeke, J. F. (1984). Psychophysiological characteristics of migraine and tension headache patients. Differential effects of sex and pain state. *Headache, 24*, 131–139.

Passchier, J., van der Helm-Hylkema, H., & Orlebeke, J. F. (1985). Lack of concordance between changes in headache activity and in psychophysiological and personality variables following treatment. *Headache, 25*, 310–316.

Paterna, S., Di Pasquale, P., D'Angelo, A., Seidita, G., Tuttolomondo, A., Cardinale, A., Maniscalchi, T., Follone, G., Giubilato, A., Tarantello, M., & Licata, G. (2000). Angiotensin-converting enzyme gene deletion polymorphism determines an increase in frequency of migraine attacks in patients suffering from migraine without aura. *European Neurology, 43*, 133–136.

Pattrick, M., Heptinstall, S., & Doherty, M. (1989). Feverfew in rheumatoid arthritis: A double blind, placebo controlled study. *Annals of the Rheumatic Diseases, 48*, 547–549.

Pauli, P., Wiedemann, G., & Nickola, M. (1999). Pain sensitivity, cerebral laterality, and negative affect. *Pain, 80*, 359–364.

Pauls, C. A., & Stemmler, G. (2003). Repressive and defensive coping during fear and anger. *Emotion, 3*, 284–302.

Pavese, N., Giannaccini, G., Betti, L., Ferrari, S., Bonanni, E., Bonuccelli, U., Murri, L., & Lucacchini, A. (2000). Peripheral-type benzodiazepine receptors in human blood cells of patients affected by migraine without aura. *Neurochemistry International, 37*, 363–368.

Pavlov, I. P. (1927/1960). *Conditioned reflexes: An investigation of the physiological activity of the cerebral cortex* (G. V. Anrep, Trans. & Ed.). New York: Dover Publications.

Pearce, J. M. (1995). Cervicogenic headache: A personal view. *Cephalalgia, 15*, 463–469.

Peatfield, R., Littlewood, J. T., Glover, V., Sandler, M., & Rose, F. C. (1983). Pressor sensitivity to tyramine in patients with headache: Relationship to platelet monoamine oxidase and to dietary provocation. *Journal of Neurology, Neurosurgery, and Psychiatry, 46*, 827–831.

Pedersen, T. F., Paulson, O. B., Nielsen, A. H., & Strandgaard, S. (2003). Effect of nephrectomy and captopril on autoregulation of cerebral blood flow in rats. *American Journal of Physiology: Heart and Circulatory Physiology*.

Peikert, A., Wilimzig, C., & Köhne-Volland, R. (1996). Prophylaxis of migraine with oral magnesium: Results from a prospective, multi-center, placebo-controlled and double-blind randomized study. *Cephalalgia, 16*, 257–263.

Penn, A. M. W., Lee, J. W. K., Thuillier, P., et al. (1992). MELAS syndrome with mitochondrial tRNALeu(UUR) mutation: Correlation of clinical state, nerve conduction, and muscle 31P magnetic resonance spectroscopy during treatment with nicotinamide and riboflavin. *Neurology, 42*, 2147–2152.

Pennebaker, J. W. (1982). *The psychology of physical symptoms*. New York: Springer-Verlag.

Pennington, J. A. T. (1998). *Bowes & Church's food values of portions commonly used* (17th ed.). Philadelphia: Lippincott.

Peres, M. F. P., Seabra, M. L. V., Zukerman, E., & Tufik, S. (2000). Cluster headache and melatonin [letter]. *Lancet, 355*, 147.

Peres, M. F. P., & Silberstein, S. D. (2002). Hemicrania continua responds to cyclooxygenase-2 inhibitors. *Headache, 42*, 530–531.

Peres, M. F. P., Silberstein, S. D., Nahmias, S., Shechter, A. L., Youssef, I., Rozen, T. D., & Young, W. B. (2001). Hemicrania continua is not that rare. *Neurology, 57*, 948–951.

Peres, M. P., Stiles, M. A., Oshinsky, M., & Rozen, T. D. (2001). Remitting form of hemicrania continua with seasonal pattern. *Headache, 41*, 592–594.

Peres, M. F. P., Stiles, M. A., Siow, H. C., Rozen, T. D., Young, W. B., & Silberstein, S. D. (2002). Greater occipital nerve blockade for cluster headache. *Cephalalgia, 22*, 520–522.

Peres, M. F. P., Young, W. B., Kaup, A. O., Zukerman, E., & Silberstein, S. D. (2001). Fibromyalgia is common in patients with transformed migraine. *Neurology, 57*, 1326–1328.

Peres, M. F. P., Zukerman, E., Senne Soares, C. A., Alonso, E. O., Santos, B. F. C., & Faulhaber, M. H. W. (2004). Cerebrospinal fluid glutamate levels in chronic migraine. *Cephalalgia, 24*, 735–739.

Perkin, G. D. (1995). Migraine [Neurology in literature]. *Journal of Neurology, Neurosurgery, and Psychiatry, 59*, 486.

Perkin, J. E., & Hartje, J. (1983). Diet and migraine: A review of the literature. *Journal of the American Dietetic Association, 83*, 459–463.

Peroutka, S. J. (2001). Analysis of Internet sites for headache. *Cephalalgia, 21*, 20–24.

Peroutka, S. J. (2002). Sympathetic look at genetic basis of migraine. *Headache, 42*, 378–381.

Persson, A. L., Hansson, G.-Å., Kalliomäki, J., Moritz, U., & Sjölund, B. H. (2000). Pressure pain thresholds and electromyographically defined muscular fatigue induced by a muscular endurance test in normal women. *Clinical Journal of Pain, 16*, 155–163.

Pertovaara, A. (2000). Plasticity in descending pain modulatory systems. In J. Sandkühler, B. Bromm, & G. F. Gebhart (Eds.), *Nervous system plasticity and chronic pain* (*Progress in Brain Research, 129*, pp. 231–242). New York: Elsevier.

Pertovaara, A., & Hämäläinen, H. (1982). Vibrotactile threshold elevation produced by high-frequency transcutaneous electrical nerve stimulation. *Archives of Physical Medicine and Rehabilitation, 63*, 597–600.

Petrovic, P., & Ingvar, M. (2002). Imaging cognitive modulation of pain processing. *Pain, 95*, 1–5.

Petrovic, P., Kalso, E., Petersson, K. M., & Ingvar, M. (2001). Shared processing in the rostral ACC during opioid and placebo treatment [Abstract]. *Neuroscience, 120*, 10.

Petrovic, P., Petersson, K. M., Ghatan, P. H., Stone-Elander, S., & Ingvar, M. (2000). Pain-related cerebral activation is altered by a distracting cognitive task. *Pain, 85*, 19–30.

Pfaffenrath, V., Diener, H.-C., Isler, H., Meyer, C., Scholz, E., Taneri, Z., Wessely, P., Zaiser-Kaschel, H., Haase, W., & Fischer, W. (1994). Efficacy and tolerability of amitriptylinoxide in the treatment of chronic tension-type headache: A multi-centre controlled study. *Cephalalgia, 14*, 149–155.

Pfaffenrath, V., & Kaube, H. (1990). Diagnostics of cervicogenic headache. *Functional Neuology, 5*, 159–164.

Pfaffenrath, V., Wessely, P., Meyer, C., Isler, H. R., Evers, S., Grotemeyer, K. H., Tancri, Z., Soyka, D., Göbel, H., & Fischer, M. (1996). Magnesium in the prophylaxis of migraine—a double-blind, placebo-controlled study. *Cephalalgia, 16*, 436–440.

Pfau, B. T., Li, B. U. K., Murray, R. D., Heitlinger, L. A., McClung, H. J., & Hayes, J. R. (1996). Differentiating cyclic from chronic vomiting patterns in children: Quantitative criteria and diagnostic implications. *Pediatrics, 97*, 364–368.

Philippot, P., Chapelle, G., & Blairy, S. (2002). Respiratory feedback in the generation of emotion. *Cognition and Emotion, 16*, 605–627.

Philips, C. (1977). A psychological analysis of tension headache. In S. Rachman (Ed.), *Contributions to medical psychology* (Vol. 1). Oxford: Pergamon Press.

Philips, H. C. (1987). Avoidance behaviour and its role in sustaining chronic pain. *Behaviour Research and Therapy, 25*, 273–279.

Philips, H. C., & Hunter, M. S. (1982). A psychophysiological investigation of tension headache. *Headache, 22*, 173–179.

Philips, H. C., & Jahanshahi, M. (1985). Chronic pain: An experimental analysis of the effects of exposure. *Behaviour Research and Therapy, 23*, 281–290.

Philips, H. C., & Rachman, S. (1996). *The psychological management of chronic pain: A treatment manual* (2nd ed.). New York: Springer.

Phivthong-ngam, L., Bode-Boger, S. M., Boger, R. H., Bohme, M., Brandes, R. P., Mugge, A., & Frolich, J. C. (1998). Dietary L-arginine normalizes endothelin-induced vascualar contractions in cholesterol-fed rabbits. *Journal of Cardiovascular Pharmacology, 32*, 300–307.

Physicians' Desk Reference. (2004). Montvale, NJ: Thomson PDR.

Picavet, H. S. J., Vlaeyen, J. W. S., & Schouten, J. S. A. G. (2002). Pain catastrophizing and kinesiophobia: Predictors of chronic low back pain. *American Journal of Epidemiology, 156*, 1028–1034.

Pielsticker, A., Haag, G., Zaudig, M., & Lautenbacher, S. (2005). Impairment of pain inhibition in chronic tension-type headache. *Pain, 118*, 215–223.

Pierangeli, G., Parchi, P., Barletta, G., Chiogna, M., Lugaresi, E., & Cortelli, P. (1997). Power spectral analysis of heart rate and diastolic blood pressure variability in migraine with and without aura. *Cephalalgia, 17*, 756–760.

Pillsbury, W. B. (1901). Does the sensation of movement originate in the joint? *American Journal of Psychology, 12*, 346–353.

Pilowsky, I. (1978). Psychodynamic aspects of the pain experience. In R. A. Sternbach (Ed.), *The psychology of pain* (pp. 203–217). New York: Raven Press.

Pincus, T., & Morley, S. (2001). Cognitive-processing bias in chronic pain: A review and integration. *Psychological Bulletin, 127*, 599–617.

Piorecky, J., Becker, W. J., & Rose, M. S. (1997). Effect of chinook winds on the probability of migraine headache occurrence. *Headache, 37*, 153–157.

Pitman, R. K., van der Kolk, B. A., Orr, S. P., & Greenberg, M. S. (1990). Naloxone-reversible analgesic response to combat-related stimuli in posttraumatic stress disorder. *Archives of General Psychiatry, 47*, 541–544.

Pittler, M. H., Vogler, B. K., & Ernst, E. (2003). Feverfew for preventing migraine (Cochrane Review). In: *The Cochrane Library*, Issue 3. Oxford: Update Software.

Plaghki, L., Delisle, D., & Godfraind, J. M. (1994). Heterotopic nociceptive conditioning stimuli and mental task modulate differently the perception and physiological correlates of short CO_2 laser stimuli. *Pain, 57*, 181–192.

Pleger, B., Dinse, H. R., Ragert, P., Schwenkreis, P., Malin, J. P., & Tegenthoff, M. (2001). Shifts in cortical representations predict human discrimination improvement. *Proceedings of the National Academy of Sciences, 98*, 12255–12260.

Pleger, B., Janssen, F., Schwenkreis, P., Völker, B., Maier, C., & Tegenthoff, M. (2004). Repetitive transcranial magnetic stimulation of the motor cortex attenuates pain perception in complex regional pain syndrome type I. *Neuroscience Letters, 356*, 87–90.

Ploghaus, A., Tracey, I., Gati, J. S., Clare, S., Menon, R. S., Matthews, P. M., & Rawlins, J. N. P. (1999). Dissociating pain from its anticipation in the human brain. *Science, 284*, 1979–1981.

Ploghaus, A., Narain, C., Beckmann, C. F., Clare, S., Bantick, S., Wise, R., Matthews, P. M., Rawlins, J. N. P., & Tracey, I. (2001). Exacerbation of pain by anxiety is associated with activity in a hippocampal network. *Journal of Neuroscience, 21*, 9896–9903.

Pogacnik, T., Sega, S., Pecnik, B., & Kiauta, T. (1993). Autonomic function testing in patients with migraine. *Headache, 33*, 545–550.

Polgár, E., Hughes, D. I., Riddell, J. S., Maxwell, D. J., Puskár, Z., & Todd, A. J. (2003). Selective loss of spinal GABAergic or glycinergic neurons is not necessary for development of thermal hyperalgesia in the chronic constriction injury model of neuropathic pain. *Pain, 104*, 229–239.

Pollo, A., Amanzio, M., Arslanian, A., Casadio, C., Maggi, G., & Benedetti, F. (2001). Response expectancies in placebo analgesia and their clinical relevance. *Pain, 93*, 77–84.

Pomeranz, B. (2001). Acupuncture analgesia—basic research. In G. Stux & R. Hammerschlag (Eds.), *Clinical acupuncture: Scientific basis* (pp. 1–28). New York: Springer.

Porreca, F., Burgess, S. E., Gardell, L. R., Vanderah, T. W., Malan, T. P. Jr., Ossipov, M. H., Lappi, D. A., & Lai, J. (2001). Inhibition of neuropathic pain by selective ablation of brainstem medullary cells expressing the mu-opioid receptor. *Journal of Neuroscience, 21*, 5281–5288.

Porreca, F., Ossipov, M. H., & Gebhart, G. F. (2002). Chronic pain and medullary descending facilitation. *Trends in Neurosciences, 25*, 319–325.

Porro, C. A., Baraldi, P., Pagnoni, G., Serafini, M., Facchin, P., maieron, M., & Nichelli, P. (2002). Does anticipation of pain affect cortical nociceptive systems? *Journal of Neuroscience, 22*, 3206–3214.

Porter, J., & Jick, H. (1980). Addiction rare in patients treated with narcotics. *New England Journal of Medicine, 302*, 123.

Potter, P. T., Zautra, A. J., & Reich, J. W. (2000). Stressful events and information processing dispositions moderate the relationship between positive and negative affect: Implications for pain patients. *Annals of Behavioral Medicine, 22*, 191–198.

Powers, S. W., Mitchell, M. J., Byars, K. C., Bentti, A.-L., LeCates, S. L., & Hershey, A. D. (2001). A pilot study of one-session biofeedback training in pediatric headache. *Neurology, 56*, 133.

Pradalier, A., Bakouche, P., Baudesson, G., Delage, A., Cornaille-Lafage, G., Launay, J. M., & Biason, P. (2001). Failure of omega-3 polyunsaturated fatty acids in prevention of migraine: A double-blind study versus placebo. *Cephalalgia, 21*, 818–822.

Premont, R. T., Gainetdinov, R. R., & Caron, M. G. (2001). Following the trace of elusive amines. *Proceedings of the National Academy of Sciences (USA), 98*, 9474–9475.

Price, D. D. (1999). *Psychological mechanisms of pain and analgesia.* Seattle: IASP Press.

Price, D. D. (2000). Psychological and neural mechanisms of the affective dimension of pain. *Science, 288*, 1769–1772.

Price, D. D., & Barrell, J. J. (2000). Mechanisms of analgesia produced by hypnosis and placebo suggestions. *Progress in Brain Research, 122*, 255–271.

Price, D. D., & Fields, H. L. (1997). The contribution of desire and expectation to placebo analgesia: Implications for new research strategies. In A. Harrington (Ed.), *The placebo effect: An interdisciplinary exploration* (pp. 117–137). Cambridge, MA: Harvard University Press.

Price, D. D., Harkins, S. W., & Baker, C. (1987). Sensory-affective relationships among different types of clinical and experimental pain. *Pain, 28*, 297–307.

Price, K. P., & Clarke, L. K. (1979). Classical conditioning of digital pulse volume in migraineurs and normal controls. *Headache, 19*, 328–332.

Pritchard, D. (1995). EMG levels in children who suffer from severe headache. *Headache, 35*, 554–556.

Pryse-Phillips, W. (2002). Evaulating migraine disability: The Headache Impact Test instrument in context. *Canadian Journal of Neurological Sciences, 29*(Suppl. 2), s11–s15.

Puca, F., Genco, S., Prudenzano, M. P., Savarese, M., Bussone, G., D'Amico, D., et al. (1999). Psychiatric comorbidity and psychosocial stress in patients with tension-type headache from headache centers in Italy. The Italian Collaborative Group for the Study of Psychopathological Factors in Primary Headaches. *Cephalalgia, 19*, 159–164.

Quattrone, A., Bono, F., Oliveri, R. L., Gambardella, A., Pirritano, D. Labate, A., et al. (2001). Cerebral venous thrombosis and isolated intracranial hypertension without papilledema in CDH. *Neurology, 57*, 31–36.

Quimby, L. G., Block, S. R., & Gratwick, G. M. (1988). Fibromyalgia: Generalized pain intolerance and manifold symptom reporting. *Journal of Rheumatology, 15*, 1264–1270.

Quintero, L., Moreno, M., Avila, C., Arcaya, J., Maixner, W., & Suarez-Roca, H. (2000). Long-lasting delayed hyperalgesia after subchronic swim stress. *Pharmacology, Biochemistry and Behavior, 67*, 449–458.

Rabasseda, X. (2004). Duloxetine: A new serotonin/noradrenaline reuptake inhibitor for the treatment of depression. *Drugs of Today, 40*, 773–790.

Rachman, S., & Eyrl, K. (1989). Predicting and remembering recurrent pain. *Behaviour Research and Therapy, 27,* 621–635.

Rachman, S., & Lopatka, C. (1988). Accurate and inaccurate predictions of pain. *Behaviour Research and Therapy, 26,* 291–296.

Radanov, B. P., Begré, S., Sturzenegger, M., & Augustiny, K. F. (1996). Course of psychological variables in whiplash injury—a 2-year follow-up with age, gender and education pair-matched patients. *Pain, 64,* 429–434.

Radanov, B. P., Sturzenegger, M., & Di Stefano, G. (1995). Long-term outcome after whiplash injury. A 2-year follow-up considering features of injury mechanism and somatic, radiologic, and psychosocial findings. *Medicine, 74*(5), 281–297.

Radhakrishnan, R., King, E. W., Dickman, J. K., Herold, C. A., Johnston, N. F., Spurgin, M. L., & Sluka, K. A. (2003). Spinal 5-HT$_2$ and 5-HT$_3$ receptors mediate low, but not high, frequency TENS-induced antihyperalgesia in rats. *Pain, 105,* 205–213.

Radloff, L. S. (1977). The CES-D Scale: A self-report depression scale for research in the general population. *Applied Psychological Measurement, 1,* 385–401.

Radnitz, C. L., Blanchard, E. B., & Bylina, J. (1990). A preliminary report of dietary therapy as a treatment for refractory migraine headache. *Headache Quarterly, 1,* 239–243.

Radojevic, V., Nicassio, P. M., & Weisman, M. H. (1992). Behavioral intervention with and without family support for rheumatoid arthritis. *Behavior Therapy, 23,* 13–30.

Radwan, I. A. M., Saito, S., & Goto, F. (2001). High-concentration tetracaine for the management of trigeminal neuralgia: Quantitative assessment of sensory function after peripheral nerve block. *Clinical Journal of Pain, 17,* 323–326.

Rainero, I., Amanzio, M., Vighetti, S., Bergamasco, B., Pinessi, L., & Benedetti, F. (2001). Quantitative EEG responses to ischaemic arm stress in migraine. *Cephalalgia, 21,* 224–229.

Rainero, I., Gallone, S., Valfrè, W., Ferrero, M., Angilella, G., Rivoiro, C., Rubino, E., De Martino, P., Savi, L., Ferrone, M., & Pinessi, L. (2004). A polymorphism of the *hypocretin receptor 2* gene is associated with cluster headache. *Neurology, 63,* 1286–1288.

Rainero, I., Pinessi, L., Salani, G., Valfrè, W., Rivoiro, C., Savi, L., Gentile, S., Giudice, R. L., & Grimaldi, L. M. E. (2002). A polymorphism in the interleukin-1α gene influences the clinical features of migraine. *Headache, 42,* 337–340.

Rains, J. C., & Penzien, D. B. (1996). Precipitants of episodic migraine: Behavioral, environmental, hormonal, and dietary factors. *Headache, 36,* 274–275.

Rains, J. C., Penzien, D. B., & Holroyd, K. A. (1993). Meta-analysis of alternative behavioral treatments for recurrent headache. *Headache, 33,* 271–272.

Rainville, P., Bao, Q. V. H., & Chrétien, P. (2005). Pain-related emotions modulate experimental pain perception and autonomic responses. *Pain, 118,* 306–318.

Rainville, P., Duncan, G. H., Price, D. D., Carrier, B., & Bushnell, M. C. (1997). Pain affect encoded in human anterior cingulate but not somatosensory cortex. *Science, 277,* 968–971.

Raja, M., Altavista, M. C., Azzoni, A., & Albanese, A. (1996). Severe barbiturate withdrawal syndrome in migrainous patients. *Headache, 36,* 119–121.

Raja, S. N., Mayer, R. A., Ringkamp, M., & Campbell, J. N. (1999). Peripheral neural mechanisms of nociception. In P. D. Wall & R. Melzack (Eds.), *Textbook of pain* (4th ed., pp. 11–57). New York: Churchill Livingstone.

Raja, S. N., Abatzis, V., & Frank, S. M. (1998). Role of α–adrenoceptors in neuroma pain in amputees. *Anesthesiology, 89,* A1083.

Ramachandran, V. S., & Rogers-Ramachandran, D. (1996). Synaesthesia in phantom limbs induced with mirrors. *Proceedings of the Royal Society of London, Series B, 263,* 377–386.

Ramadan, N. M. (2001). Comments on 'The failure of intensive self-regulatory treatment with chronic daily headache.' *Applied Psychophysiology and Biofeedback, 26,* 325–327.

Ramadan, N. M., & Keidel, M. (2000). Chronic posttraumatic headache. In: J. Olesen, P. Tfelt-Hansen, & K. M. A. Welch (Eds.), *The headaches* (2nd ed., pp. 771–780). Philadelphia: Lippincott, Williams & Wilkins.

Ramsay, D. S., & Woods, S. C. (1997). Biological consequences of drug administration: Implications for acute and chronic tolerance. *Psychological Review, 104,* 170–193.

Rao, B. S., Das, D. G., Taraknath, V. R., & Sarma, Y. (2000). A double blind controlled study of propranolol and cyproheptadine in migraine prophylaxis. *Neurology India, 48,* 223–226.

Raphael, K. G., Widom, C. S., & Lange, G. (2001). Childhood victimization and pain in adulthood: A prospective investigation. *Pain, 92,* 283–293.

Rapoport, A., & Edmeads, J. (2000). Migraine: The evolution of our knowledge. *Archives of Neurology, 57*, 1221–1223.

Rapoport, A. M., & Silberstein, S. D. (1992). Emergency treatment of headache. *Neurology, 42*(Suppl. 2),43–44.

Rapoport, A. M., & Tepper, S. J. (2001). Triptans are all different. *Archives of Neurology, 58*, 1479–1480.

Rapoport, A. M., Weeks, R. E., Sheftell, F. D., et al. (1985). Analgesic rebound headache: Theoretical and practical implications. *Cephalalgia, 5*(Suppl. 3), 448–449.

Rappaport, N. B., McAnulty, D. P., & Brantley, P. J. (1988). Exploration of the Type A Behavior Pattern in chronic headache sufferers. *Journal of Consulting and Clinical Psychology, 56*, 621–623.

Raskin, N. H. (1982). Psychosomatic illness review: Migraine. *Psychosomatics, 23*, 897–907.

Raskin, N. H. (1986). Repetitive intravenous dihydroergotamine as therapy for intractable migraine. *Neurology, 36*, 995–997.

Raskin, N. H., Hosobuchi, Y., & Lamb, S. (1987). Headache may arise from perturbation of brain. *Headache, 27*, 416–420.

Rasmussen, B. K. (1995a). Epidemiology of headache. *Cephalalgia, 15*, 45–68.

Rasmussen, B. K. (1995b). Migraine with aura and migraine without aura are two different entities. *Cephalalgia, 15*, 183–186.

Rasmussen, B. K. (2001). Epidemiology of headache. *Cephalalgia, 21*, 774–777.

Rasmussen, B. K., Jensen, R., Schroll, M., & Olesen, J. (1991). Epidemiology of headache in a general population—A prevalence study. *Journal of Clinical Epidemiology, 44*, 1147–1157.

Rasmussen, B. K., Jensen, R., Schroll, M., & Olesen, J. (1992). Interrelations between migraine and tension-type headache in the general population. *Archives of Neurology, 49*, 914–918.

Rasmussen, B. K., & Olesen, J. (1992). Migraine with aura and migraine without aura: An epidemiological study. *Cephalalgia, 12*, 221–228.

Rasmussen, P. (1991). Facial pain. IV. A prospective study of 1052 patients with a view of: Precipitating factors, associated symptoms, objective psychiatric and neurological symptoms. *Acta Neurochirurgica (Wien), 108*, 100–109.

Rau, H., Pauli, P., Brody, S., Elbert, T., & Birbaumer, N. (1993). Baroreceptor stimulation alters cortical activity. *Psychophysiology, 30*, 322–325.

Redillas, C., & Solomon, S. (2000). Prophylactic pharmacological treatment of chronic daily headache. *Headache, 40*, 83–102.

Reich, B. A. (1989). Non-invasive treatment of vascular and muscle contraction headache: A comparative longitudinal clinical study. *Headache, 29*, 34–41.

Reiman, E. M., Lane, R. D., Van Petten, C., & Bandettini, P. A. (2000). Positron emission tomography and functional magnetic resonance imaging. In J. T. Cacioppo, L. G. Tassinary, & G. G. Berntson (Eds.) *Handbook of psychophysiology* (2nd ed., pp. 85–118). New York: Cambridge University Press.

Ren, K., & Dubner, R. (2002). Descending modulation in persistent pain: An update. *Pain, 100*, 1–6.

Reynaert, C., Janne, P., Delire, V., Pirard, M., Randour, P., Collard, E., Installe, E., Coche, E., & Cassiers, L. (1995). To control or be controlled? From health locus of control to morphine control during patient-controlled analgesia. *Psychotherapy and Psychosomatics, 64*, 74–81.

Reyners, A. K., Tio, R. A., Vlutters, F. G., van der Woude, G. F., Reitsma, W. D., & Smit, A. J. (2000). Re-evaluation of the cold face test in humans. *European Journal of Applied Physiology, 82*, 487–492.

Reynolds, D. J., & Hovanitz, C. A. (2000). Life event stress and headache frequency revisited. *Headache, 40*, 111–118.

Rhee, H. (2000). Prevalence and predictors of headaches in U.S. adolescents. *Headache, 40*, 528–538.

Rhudy, J. L., & Meagher, M. W. (2000). Fear and anxiety: divergent effects on human pain thresholds. *Pain, 84*, 65–75.

Ribeiro, C. A. F. (2000). L-5-Hydroxytryptophan in the prophylaxis of chronic tension-type headache: A double-blind, randomized, placebo-controlled study. *Headache, 40*, 451–456.

Riley, H. A. (1932). Migraine. *Bulletin of the Neurological Institute of New York, 2*, 429–544.

Ring, C., Harrison, L. K., Winzer, A., Carroll, D., Drayson, M., & Kendall, M. (2000). Secretory immunoglobulin A and cardiovascular reactions to mental arithmetic, cold pressor, and exercise: Effects of alpha-adrenergic blockade. *Psychophysiology, 37*, 634–643.

Rivner, M. H. (2001). The neurophysiology of myofascial pain syndrome. *Current Pain and Headache Reports, 5*, 432–440.

Roatta, S., Windhorst, U., Ljubisavljevic, M., Johansson, H., & Passatore, M. (2002). Sympathetic modulation of muscle spindle afferent sensitivity to stretch in rabbit jaw closing muscles. *Journal of Physiology, 540*, 237–248.

Robbins, L. (1994). Precipitating factors in migraine: A retrospective review of 494 patients. *Headache, 34*, 214–216.

Robbins, L. (1995). Intranasal lidocaine for cluster headache. *Headache, 35*, 83–84.

Robbins, L. (1997). Daily opioids (methadone) for refractory chronic daily headache: Quality of life assessment [abstract]. *Headache, 37*, 328.

Roberts, A. H., Kewman, D. G., & MacDonald, H. (1973). Voluntary control of skin temperature: Unilateral changes using hypnosis and feedback. *Journal of Abnormal Psychology, 82*, 163–168.

Roberts, A. H., Schuler, J., Bacon, J., Zimmerman, R., & Patterson, R. (1975). Individual differences and autonomic control: Absorption, hypnotic susceptibility, and the unilateral control of skin temperature. *Journal of Abnormal Psychology, 84*, 272–279.

Roby-Brami, A., Bussel, B., Willer, J. C., & Le Bars, D. (1987). An electrophysiological investigation into the pain-relieving effects of heterotopic nociceptive stimuli. *Brain, 110*, 1497–1508.

Rocca, M. A., Colombo, B., Inglese, M., Codella, M., Comi, G., & Filippi, M. (2003). A diffusion tensor magnetic resonance imaging study of brain tissue from patients with migraine. *Journal of Neurology, Neurosurgery, and Psychiatry, 74*, 501–503.

Rocca, M. A., Colombo, B., Pratesi, A., Comi, G., & Filippi, M. (2000). A magnetization transfer imaging study of the brain in patients with migraine. *Neurology, 54*, 507–509.

Rocha-González, H. I., Meneses, A., Carlton, S. M., & Granados-Soto, V. (2005). Pronociceptive role of peripheral and spinal 5-HT7 receptors in the formalin test. *Pain, 117*, 182–192.

Rock, I., & Victor, J. (1964). Vision and touch: An experimentally created conflict between the two senses. *Science, 143*, 594–596.

Roerig, S. C., O'Brien, S. M., Fujimoto, J. M., & Wilcox, G. L. (1984). Tolerance to morphine analgesia: Decreased multiplicative interaction between spinal and supraspinal sites. *Brain Research, 308*, 360–363.

Rohling, M. L., Binder, L. M., & Langhinrichsen-Rohling, J. (1995). Money matters: A meta-analytic review of the association between financial compensation and the experience and treatment of chronic pain. *Health Psychology, 14*, 537–547.

Rojahn, J., & Gerhards, F. (1986). Subjective stress sensitivity and physiological responses to an aversive auditory stimulus in migraine and control subjects. *Journal of Behavioral Medicine, 9*, 203–212.

Rokicki, L. A., Holroyd, K. A., France, C. R., Lipchik, G. L., France, J. L., & Kvaal, S. A. (1997). Change mechanisms associated with combined relaxation/EMG biofeedback training for chronic tension headache. *Applied Psychophysiology and Biofeedback, 22*, 21–41.

Rokicki, L. A., Houle, T. T., Dhingra, L. K., Weinland, S. R., Urban, A. M., & Bhalla, R. K. (2003). A preliminary analysis of EMG variance as an index of change in EMG biofeedback treatment of tension-type headache. *Applied Psychophysiology and Biofeedback, 28*, 205–215.

Rolan, P. E., & Martin, G. R. (1998). Zolmitriptan: A new acute treatment for migraine. *Expert Opinion on Investigational Drugs, 7*, 633–652.

Rolke, T., Campbell, K. A., Magerl, W., & Treede, R. D. (2005). Deep pain thresholds in the distal limbs of healthy human subjects. *European Journal of Pain, 9*, 39–48.

Rollnik, J. D., Tanneberger, O., Schubert, M., Schneider, U., & Dengler, R. (2000). Treatment of tension-type headache with botulinum toxin A: A double-blind, placebo-controlled study. *Headache, 40*, 300–305.

Romano, J. M., & Turner, J. A. (1985). Chronic pain and depression: Does the evidence support a relationship? *Psychological Bulletin, 97*, 18–34.

Romano, J. M., Turner, J. A., Friedman, L. S., Bulchroft, R. A., Jensen, M. P., Hops, H., & Wright, S. F. (1992). Sequential analysis of chronic pain behaviors and spouse responses. *Journal of Consulting and Clinical Psychology, 60*, 777–782.

Ron, M. (2001). Explaining the unexplained: Understanding hysteria. *Brain, 124*, 1065–1066.

Rosch, E., & Mervis, C. B. (1975). Family resemblances: Studies in the internal structure of categories. *Cognitive Psychology, 7*, 573–605.

Rosenstiel, A. K., & Keefe, F. J. (1983). The use of coping strategies in chronic low back pain patients: Relationship to patient characteristics and current adjustment. *Pain, 17*, 33–40.

Rossi, L. N., Cortinovis, I., Menegazzo, L., Brunelli, G., Bossi, A., & Macchi, M. (2001). Classification criteria and distinction between migraine and tension-type headache in children. *Developmental Medicine and Child Neurology, 43*, 45–51.

Rosso, T., Aglioti, S. M., Zanette, G., Ischia, S., Finco, G., Farina, S., Fiaschi, A., & Tinazzi, M. (2003). Functional plasticity in the human primary somatosensory cortex following acute lesion of the anterior lateral spinal cord: Neurophysiological evidence of short-term cross-modal plasticity. *Pain, 101*, 117–127.

Rothman, R. B., & Baumann, M. H. (2002). Serotonin releasing agents: Neurochemical, therapeutic and adverse effects. *Pharmacology, Biochemistry and Behavior, 71*, 825–836.

Rothner, A. D. (1978). Headaches in children: A review. *Headache, 18*, 169–175.

Rothner, A., Edwards, K., Kerr, L., et al. (1997). Efficacy and safety of naratriptan tablets in adolescent migraine. *Journal of Neurological Science, 150*, S106.

Rowan, A. B., & Andrasik, F. (1996). Efficacy and cost-effectiveness of minimal therapist contact treatments of chronic headaches: A review. *Behavior Therapy, 27*, 207–234.

Roy, R. (1989). Couple therapy and chronic headache: A preliminary outcome study. *Headache, 29*, 455–457.

Rozanski, A., Blumenthal, J. A., & Kaplan, J. (1999). Impact of psychological factors on the pathogenesis of cardiovascular disease and implications for therapy. *Circulation, 99*, 2192–2217.

Rozen, T. D. (2001). Olanzapine as an abortive agent for cluster headache. *Headache, 41*, 813–816.

Rozen, T. D. (2003). Melatonin as treatment for idiopathic stabbing headache. *Neurology, 61*, 865–866.

Rozen, T. D., Capobianco, D. J., & Dalessio, D. J. (2001). Cranial neuralgias and atypical facial pain. In: S. D. Silberstein, R. B. Lipton, & D. J. Dalessio (Eds.), *Wolff's headache and other head pain* (7th ed., pp. 509–524). New York: Oxford University Press.

Rozen, T. D., Oshinsky, M. L., Gebeline, C. A., Bradley, K. C., Young, W. B., Shechter, A. L., & Silberstein, S. D. (2002). Open label trial of coenzyme Q10 as a migraine preventive. *Cephalalgia, 22*, 137–141.

Rozen, T. D., Swanson, J. W., Stang, P. E., McDonnell, S. K., & Rocca, W. A. (1999). Increasing incidence of medically recognized migraine headache in a United States population. *Neurology, 53*, 1468–1473.

Rozniecki, J. J., Dimitriadou, V., Lambracht-Hall, M., Pang, X., & Theoharides, T. C. (1999). Morphological and functional demonstration of rat dura mater mast cell-neuron interactions in vitro and in vivo. *Brain Research, 849*, 1–15.

Rudiak, D., & Marg, E. (1994). Finding the depth of magnetic brain stimulation: A re-evaluation. *Electroencephalography and Clinical Neurophysiology, 93*, 358–371.

Russell, M. B., Hilden, J., Sørensen, S. A., & Olesen, J. (1993). Familial occurrence of migraine without aura and migraine with aura. *Neurology, 43*, 1369–1373.

Russell, M. B., Iversen, H. K., & Olesen, J. (1994). Improved description of the migraine aura by a diagnostic aura diary. *Cephalalgia, 14*, 107–117.

Russell, M. B., & Olesen, J. (1995). Increased family risk and evidence of genetic factors in migraine. *British Medical Journal, 311*, 541–544.

Sacks, O. (1992). *Migraine* (revised & expanded ed.). New York: Vintage Books.

Salinsky, M. C., Storzbach, D., Spencer, D. C., Oken, B. S., Landry, T., & Dodrill, C. B. (2005). Effects of topiramate and gabapentin on cognitive abilities in healthy volunteers. *Neurology, 64*, 792–798.

Salkovskis, P. M., & Warwick, H. M. (1986). Morbid preoccupations, health anxiety and reassurance: A cognitive-behavioural approach to hypochondriasis. *Behaviour Research and Therapy, 24*, 597–602.

Sallis, R. E., & Jones, K. (2000). Prevalence of headaches in football players. *Medicine and Science in Sports and Exercise, 32*, 1820–1824.

Salonen, R. (1999). Naratriptan. *International Journal of Clinical Practice, 53*, 552–556.

Sanders, S. H. (1996). Operant conditioning with chronic pain: Back to basics. In R. J. Gatchel & D. C. Turk (Eds.), *Psychological approaches to pain management: A practitioner's handbook* (pp. 112–130). New York: Guilford Press.

Sandkühler, J. (2000). Learning and memory in pain pathways. *Pain, 88*, 113–118.

Sandler, M., Li, N.-Y., Jarrett, N., & Glover, V. (1995). Dietary migraine: Recent progress in the red (and white) wine story. *Cephalalgia, 15*, 101–103.

Sandler, M., Youdim, M. H., & Hanington, E. (1974). A phenylethylamine oxidizing defect in migraine. *Nature, 250*, 335–337.

Sándor, P. S., Áfra, J., Ambrosini, A., & Schoenen, J. (2000). Prophylactic treatment of migraine with β-blockers and riboflavin: Differential effects on the intensity dependence of auditory evoked cortical potentials. *Headache, 40*, 30–35.

Sándor, P. S., Di Clemente, L., Coppola, G., Saenger, U., Fumal, A., Magis, D., et al. (2005). Efficacy of coenzyme Q10 in migraine prophylaxis: A randomized controlled trial. *Neurology, 64*, 713–715.

Sandrini, G., Antonaci, F., Pucci, E., Bono, G., & Nappi, G. (1994). Comparative study with EMG, pressure algometry and manual palpation in tension-type headache and migraine. *Cephalalgia, 14*, 451–457.

Sandrini, G., Manzoni, G. C., Zanferrari, C., & Nappi, G. (1993). An epidemiological approach to the nosography of chronic daily headache. *Cephalalgia, 13*(Suppl 12), 72–77.

Sandrini, G., Milanov, I., Malaguti, S., Nigrelli, M. P., Moglia, A., & Nappi, G. (2000). Effects of hypnosis on diffuse noxious inhibitory controls. *Physiology and Behavior, 69*, 295–300.

Sangiorgi, S., Mochi, M., Riva, R., Cortelli, P., Monari, L., Pierangeli, G., & Montagna, P. (1994). Abnormal platelet mitochondrial function in patients affected by migraine with and without aura. *Cephalalgia, 14*, 21–23.

Saper, J. R. (2001). What matters is not the differences between triptans, but the differences between patients. *Archives of Neurology, 58*, 1481–1482.

Saper, J. R., Lake, A. E. III, Cantrell, D., Winner, P. K., White, J., & Cross, V. (2002). Chronic daily headache prophylaxis with tizanidine: A double-blind, placebo-controlled, multicenter outcome study. *Headache, 42*, 470–482.

Saper, J. R., Lake, A. E. III, Hamel, R. L., Lutz, T. E., Branca, B., Sims, D. B., & Kroll, M. M. (2004). Daily scheduled opioids for intractable head pain: Long-term observations of a treatment program. *Neurology, 62*, 1687–1694.

Saper, J. R., Lake, A. E. III, & Kreeger, C. (1994). Comprehensive inpatient treatment for intractable head pain: Patient factors associated with outcome. *Headache, 34*, 314.

Saper, J. R., Lake, A. E. III, & Tepper, S. J. (2001). Nefazodone for chronic daily headache prophylaxis: An open-label study. *Headache, 41*, 465–474.

Saper, J. R., Silberstein, S. D., Lake, A. E. III, & Winters, M. E. (1994). Double blind trial of fluoxetine: Chronic daily headache and migraine. *Headache, 34*, 497–502.

Sarafino, E. P., & Goehring, P. (2000). Age comparisons in acquiring biofeedback control and success in reducing headache pain. *Annals of Behavioral Medicine, 22*, 10–16.

Sarchielli, P., Alberti, A., Floridi, A. L., Mazzotta, G., & Floridi, A. R. (2004). Increased cerebrospinal fluid levels of nerve growth factor and brain-derived neurotrophic factor are not specific for chronic migraine. *Cephalalgia, 24*, 777.

Sarchielli, P., Tognoloni, M., Russo, S., Vulcano, M. R., Feleppa, M., Mala, M., Sartori, M., & Gallai, V. (1996). Variations in the platelet arginine/nitric oxide pathway during the ovarian cycle in females affected by menstrual migraine. *Cephalalgia, 16*, 468–475.

Sargent, J., Solbach, P., Coyne, L., Spohn, H., & Sergerson, J. (1986). Results of a controlled, experimental, outcome study of nondrug treatments for the control of migraine headaches. *Journal of Behavioral Medicine, 9*, 291–323.

Sargent, J., Solbach, P., Damasio, H., Baumel, B., Corbett, J., Eisner, L., et al. (1985). A comparison of naproxen sodium to propranolol hydrochloride and a placebo control for the prophylaxis of migraine headache. *Headache, 25*, 320–324.

Sargent, J., Walters, D., & Green, E. (1973). Psychosomatic self-regulation of migraine headaches. *Seminars in Psychiatry, 5*, 415–428.

Sarlani, E., Farooq, N., & Greenspan, J. D. (2003). Gender and laterality differences in thermosensation throughout the perceptible range. *Pain, 106*, 9–18.

Sartory, G., Müller, B., Metsch, J., & Pothmann, R. (1998). A comparison of psychological and pharmacological treatment of pediatric migraine. *Behaviour Research and Therapy, 36*, 1155–1170.

Sawamoto, N., Honda, M., Okada, T., Hanakawa, T., Kanda, M., Fukuyama, H., et al. (2000). Expectation of pain enhances responses to nonpainful somatosensory stimulation in the anterior cingulate cortex and parietal operculum/posterior insula: An event-related functional magnetic resonance imaging study. *Journal of Neuroscience, 20*, 7438–7445.

Sawynok, J. (1995). Pharmacological rationale for the clinical use of caffeine. *Drugs, 49*, 37–50.

Sawynok, J. (1998). Adenosine receptor activation and nociception. *European Journal of Pharmacology, 347*, 1–11.

Scharff, L., & Marcus, D. A. (1994). Interdisciplinary outpatient group treatment of intractable headache. *Headache, 34*, 73–78.

Scharff, L., & Marcus, D. A. (1999). The association between chocolate and migraine: A review. *Headache Quarterly, 10*, 199–205.

Scharff, L., Marcus, D. A., & Masek, B. J. (2002). A controlled study of minimal-contact thermal biofeedback treatment in children with migraine. *Journal of Pediatric Psychology, 27*, 109–119.

Scharff, L., Turk, D. C., & Marcus, D. A. (1995). Triggers of headache episodes and coping responses of headache diagnostic groups. *Headache, 35*, 397–403.

Schechter, N. L., Bernstein, B. A., Beck, A., Hart, L., & Scherzer, L. (1991). Individual differences in children's response to pain: Role of temperament and parental characteristics. *Pediatrics, 87*, 171–177.

Schepelmann, K., Dannhausen, M., Kötter, I., Schabet, M., & Dichgans, J. (1998). Exteroceptive suppression of temporalis muscle activity in patients with fibromyalgia, tension-type headache, and normal controls. *Electroencephalography and Clinical Neurophysiology, 107*, 196–199.

Scher, A. I., Lipton, R. B., & Stewart, W. (2002). Risk factors for chronic daily headache. *Current Pain and Headache Reports, 6,* 486–491.

Scher, A. I., Stewart, W. F., & Lipton, R. B. (1999). Migraine and headache: A meta-analytic approach. In I. K. Crombie, P. R. Croft, S. J. Linton, L. LeResche, & M. Von Korff (Eds.), *Epidemiology of pain* (pp 159–170). Seattle: IASP Press.

Scher, A. I., Stewart, W. F., & Lipton, R. B. (2002). Snoring and chronic daily headache: Results from the Frequent Headache Epidemiology Study. *Neurology, 58*(Suppl. 3), A332.

Scher, A. I., Stewart, W. F., & Lipton, R. B. (2004). Caffeine as a risk factor for chronic daily headache: A population-based study. *Neurology, 63,* 2022–2027.

Scher, A. I., Stewart, W. F., Ricci, J. A., & Lipton, R. B. (2003). Factors associated with the onset and remission of chronic daily headache in a population-based study. *Pain, 106,* 81–89.

Scher, W., & Scher, B. M. (1992). A possible role for nitric oxide in glutamate (MSG)-induced Chinese Restaurant Syndrome. *Medical Hypotheses, 38,* 185–188.

Schiffman, S. S., Buckley, C. E. III, Sampson. H. A., Massey, E. W., Baraniuk, J. N., Follett, J. V., & Warwick, Z. S. (1987). Aspartame and susceptibility to headache. *New England Journal of Medicine, 317,* 1181–1185.

Schiller, F. (1975). The migraine tradition. *Bulletin of the History of Medicine, 49,* 1–19.

Schmidt, N. B., & Cook, J. H. (1999). Effects of anxiety sensitivity on anxiety and pain during a cold pressor challenge in patients with panic disorder. *Behaviour Research and Therapy, 37,* 313–323.

Schmidt-Wilcke, T., Leinisch, E., Straube, A., Kämpfe, N., Draganski, B., Diener, H. C., et al. (2005). Gray matter decrease in patients with chronic tension type headache. *Neurology, 65,* 1483–1486.

Schmitt, W. J., Slowey, E., Fravi, N., Weber, S., & Burgunder, J. M. (2001). Effect of botulinum toxin A injections in the treatment of chronic tension-type headache: A double-blind, placebo-controlled trial. *Headache, 41,* 658–664.

Schmuck, K., Ullmer, C., Kalkman, H. O., Probst, A., & Lubbert, H. (1996). Activation of meningeal 5-HT$_{2B}$ receptors: An early step in the generation of migraine headache? *European Journal of Neuroscience, 8,* 959–967.

Schoenen, J. (1982). The dendritic organization of the human spinal cord: The dorsal horn. *Neuroscience, 7,* 2057–2087.

Schoenen, J. (1991). EMG activity in pericranial muscles during postural variation and mental activity in healthy volunteers and patients with chronic tension type headache. *Headache, 31,* 321–324.

Schoenen, J. (1993). Exteroceptive suppression of temporalis muscle activity in patients with chronic headache and normal volunteers: Methodology, clinical and pathophysiological relevance. *Headache, 33,* 3–17.

Schoenen, J. (1996a). Deficient habituation of evoked cortical potentials in migraine: A link between brain biology, behavior and trigeminovascular activation? *Biomedicine and Pharmacotherapy, 50,* 71–78.

Schoenen, J. (1996b). Abnormal cortical information processing between migraine attacks. In M. Sandler, M. Ferrari, & S. Harnett (Eds.), *Migraine: Pharmacology and genetics* (pp. 233–253). London: Altman.

Schoenen, J. (1997). Clinical neurophysiology of headache. *Neurologic Clinics, 15*(1), 85–105.

Schoenen, J. (2000). Tension-type headache. In H.-C. Diener (Ed.), *Drug treatment of migraine and other headaches* (pp. 314–321). Basel: Karger.

Schoenen, J., Jacquy, J., & Lenaerts, M. (1998). Effectiveness of high-dose riboflavin in migraine prophylaxis: A randomized controlled trial. *Neurology, 50,* 466–470.

Schoenen, J., Jamart, B., Gerard, P., Lenarduzzi, P., & Delwaide, P. J. (1987). Exteroceptive suppression of temporalis muscle activity in chronic headache. *Neurology, 37,* 1834–1836.

Schoenen, J., Lenarduzzi, P., & Sianard-Gainko, J. (1989). Chronic headaches associated with analgesics and/or ergotamine abuse: A clinical survey of 434 consecutive out patients. In F. C. Rose (Ed.), *New advances in headache research* (pp. 255–259). London: Smith Gordon.

Schoenen, J., Maertens de Noordhout, A., Timsit-Berthier, M., & Timsit, M. (1986). Contingent negative variation and efficacy of beta-blocking agents in migraine. *Cephalalgia, 6,* 229–233.

Schon, F., & Blau, J. N. (1987). Post-epileptic headache and migraine. *Journal of Neurology, Neurosurgery and Psychiatry, 50,* 1148–1152.

Schott, G. D. (2001). Delayed onset and resolution of pain. Some observations and implications. *Brain, 124,* 1067–1076.

Schrader, H., Obelieniene, D., Bovim, G., Surkiene, D., Mickeviciene, D., Miseviciene, I., & Sand, T. (1996). Natural evolution of late whiplash syndrome outside the medicolegal context. *Lancet, 347,* 1207–1211.

Schrader, H., Stovner, L. J., Helde, G., Sand, T., & Bovim, G. (2001). Prophylactic treatment of migraine with angiotensin converting enzyme inhibitor (lisinopril): Randomised, placebo controlled, crossover study. *British Medical Journal, 322,* 1–5.

Schröder, H., & Schröder, C. (1993). Gustav Theodor Fechner during his life-crisis. In H. Schröder, K. Reschke, M. Johnston, & S. Maes (Eds.), *Health psychology: Potential in diversity*. Regensburg: S. Roderer Verlag.

Schulman, J., Leviton, A., Slack, W., Porter, D., & Graham, J. R. (1980). The relationship of headache occurrence to barometric pressure. *International Journal of Biometeorology, 24*(3), 263–269.

Schulte-Mattler, W. J., Krack, P., & BoNTTH Study Group. (2004). Treatment of chronic tension-type headache with botulinum toxin A: A randomized, double-blind, placebo-controlled multicenter study. *Pain, 109,* 110–114.

Schultz, J. H., & Luthe, W. (1959). *Autogenic training: A psychophysiologic approach to psychotherapy.* New York: Grune and Stratton.

Schwartz, B. S., Stewart, W. F., & Lipton, R. B. (1997). Lost workdays and decreased work effectiveness associated with headache in the workplace. *Journal of Occupational and Environmental Medicine, 39,* 320–327.

Schwartz, B. S., Stewart, W. F., Simon, D., & Lipton, R. B. (1998). Epidemiology of tension-type headache. *Journal of the American Medical Association, 279,* 381–383.

Schwartz, L., Slater, M. A., & Birchler, G. R. (1996). The role of pain behaviors in the modulation of marital conflict in chronic pain couples. *Pain, 65,* 227–233.

Schweiger, A., & Parducci, A. (1981). Nocebo: The psychological induction of pain. *Pavlovian Journal of Biological Science, 16,* 140–143.

Scopp, A. L. (1992). Headache triggers: Theory, research, and clinical application—Part I. *Headache Quarterly, 3,* 32–38.

Scott, A. J., & Cadden, S. W. (1996). Suppression of an inhibitory jaw reflex by the anticipation of pain in man. *Pain, 66,* 125–131.

Scott, J., & Huskisson, E. C. (1976). Graphic representation of pain. *Pain, 2,* 175–184.

Scrivani, S. J., Keith, D. A., Mathews, E. S., & Kaban, L. B. (1999). Percutaneous stereotactic differential radiofrequency thermal rhizotomy for the treatment of trigeminal neuralgia. *Journal of Oral and Maxillofacial Surgery, 57,* 104–111.

Sears, R. R. (1932). Experimental study of hypnotic anesthesia. *Journal of Experimental Psychology, 15,* 1–22.

Selby, G., & Lance, J. W. (1960). Observations on 500 cases of migraine and allied vascular headache. *Journal of Neurology, Neurosurgery, and Psychiatry, 23,* 23–32.

Seminowicz, D. A., & Davis, K. D. (2006). Cortical responses to pain in healthy individuals depends on pain catastrophizing. *Pain, 120,* 297–306.

Setchell, K. D. R. (1998). Phytoestrogens: The biochemistry, physiology, and implications for human health of soy isoflavones. *American Journal of Clinical Nutrition, 68*(Suppl.), 1333S–1346S.

Shah, A. K., Guyot, A. M., Ham, S. D., et al. (1991). CT or not to CT: ER evaluation of head trauma. *Neurology, 41*(Suppl. 1), 308.

Shaheen, S. O., Sterne, J. A. C., Songhurst, C. E., & Burney, P. G. J. (2000). Frequent paracetamol use and asthma in adults. *Thorax, 55,* 266–270.

Sharav, Y. (1999). Orofacial pain. In P. D. Wall & R. Melzack (Eds.), *Textbook of pain* (4th ed., pp. 711–737). New York: Churchill Livingstone.

Shechter, A., Stewart, W. F., Silberstein, S. D., & Lipton, R. B. (2002). Migraine and autonomic nervous system function: A population-based, case-control study. *Neurology, 58,* 422–427.

Sheftell, F. D., Rapoport, A. M., & Coddon, D. R. (1999). Naratriptan in the prophylaxis of transformed migraine. *Headache, 39,* 506–510.

Shepherd, A. J. (2001). Increased visual after-effects following pattern adaptation in migraine: A lack of intracortical excitation? *Brain, 124,* 2310–2318.

Sherman, J. J., & Turk, D. C. (2001). Nonpharmacologic approaches to the management of myofascial temporomandibular disorders. *Current Pain and Headache Reports, 5,* 421–431.

Shevel, E., & Spierings, E. H. (2004). Role of the extracranial arteries in migraine headache: A review. *Journal of Craniomandibular Practice, 22,* 132–136.

Shimizu, T., Koja, T., Fujisaki, T., & Fukuda, T. (1981). Effects of methysergide and naloxone on analgesia induced by the peripheral electric stimulation in mice. *Brain Research, 208,* 463–467.

Shmavonian, B. M. (1959). Methodological study of vasomotor conditioning in human subjects. *Journal of Comparative and Physiological Psychology, 52,* 315–321.

Sholz, E., Diener, H. C., & Geiselhart, S. (1988). Does a critical dosage exist in drug-induced headache? In H. C. Diener & M. Wilkinson (Eds.), *Drug-induced headache* (pp. 29–43). New York: Springer-Verlag.

Shutty, M. S. Jr., Cundiff, G., & DeGood, D. E. (1992). Pain complaint and the weather: Weather sensitivity and symptom complaints in chronic pain patients. *Pain, 49*, 199–204.

Siegel, S., Baptista, M. A. S., Kim, J. A., McDonald, R. V., & Weise-Kelly, L. A. (2000). Pavlovian psychopharmacology: the associative basis of tolerance. *Experimental and Clinical Psychopharmacology, 8*, 276–293.

Sifneos, P. E. (1973). The prevalence of "alexithymic" characteristics in psychosomatic patients. *Psychotherapy and Psychosomatics, 22*, 255–262.

Signoretti, S., Marmarou, A., Tavazzi, B., Lazzarino, G., Beaumont, A., & Vagnozzi, R. (2001). N-Acetylaspartate reduction as a measure of injury severity and mitochondrial dysfunction following diffuse traumatic brain injury. *Journal of Neurotrauma, 18*, 977–991.

Silberstein, S. D. (1997). Pharmacology of dihydroergotamine. *Clinical update on dihydroergotamine.* Dumont, NJ: Center for Bio-Medical Communication, Inc.

Silberstein, S. D. (1998). Methysergide. *Cephalalgia, 18*, 421–435.

Silberstein, S. D. (2000). Practice parameter: Evidence-based guidelines for migraine headache (an evidence-based review). *Neurology, 55*, 754–763.

Silberstein, S. D., & Freitag, F. G. (2003). Preventive treatment of migraine. *Neurology, 60*(Suppl. 2), S38–S44.

Silberstein, S. D., & Liption, R. B. (2001). Chronic daily headache, including transformed migraine, chronic tension-type headache, and medication overuse. In S. D. Silberstein, R. B. Lipton, & D. J. Dalessio (Eds.), *Wolff's headache and other head pain* (7th ed., pp. 247–282). New York: Oxford University Press.

Silberstein, S. D., Lipton, R. B., & Goadsby, P. J. (1998). *Headache in clinical practice.* Oxford, UK: Isis Medical Media Ltd.

Silberstein, S. D., Lipton, R. B., Goadsby, P. J., & Smith, R. T. (1999). *Headache in primary care.* Oxford, UK: Isis Medical Media Ltd.

Silberstein, S. D., Lipton, R. B., & Sliwinski, M. (1996). Classification of daily and near-daily headaches: Field trial of revised IHS criteria. *Neurology, 47*, 871–875.

Silberstein, S., Lipton, R. B., Solomon, S., & Mathew, N. (1994). Classification of daily and near-daily headaches: Proposed revisions to the IHS criteria. *Headache, 34*, 1–7.

Silberstein, S., Mathew, N., Saper, J., & Jenkins, S. (2000). Botulinum toxin type A as a migraine preventive treatment. *Headache, 40*, 445–450.

Silberstein, S. D., & McCrory, D. C. (2001). Butalbital in the treatment of headache: History, pharmacology, and efficacy. *Headache, 41*, 953–967.

Silberstein, S. D., & McCrory, D. C. (2003). Ergotamine and dihydroergotamine: History, pharmacology, and efficacy. *Headache, 43*, 144–166.

Silberstein, S. D., & Merriam, G. R. (2000). Physiology of the menstrual cycle. *Cephalalgia, 20*, 148–154.

Silberstein, S. D., Neto, W., Schmitt, J., & Jacobs, D. (2004). Topiramate in migraine prevention: Results of a large controlled trial. *Archives of Neurology, 61*, 490–495.

Silberstein, S. D., Niknam, R., Rozen, T. D., & Young, W. B. (2000). Cluster headache with aura. *Neurology, 54*, 219–221.

Silberstein, S. D., Olesen, J., Bousser, M.-G., Diener, H.-C., Dodick, D., First, M., et al. (2005). The International Classification of Headache Disorders, 2nd Edition (ICHD–II)—revision of criteria for 8.2 *Medication-overuse headache. Cephalalgia, 25*, 460–465.

Silberstein, S. D., Peres, M. F. P., Hopkins, M. M., Shechter, A. L., Young, W. B., & Rozen, T. D. (2002). Olanzapine in the treatment of refractory migraine and chronic daily headache. *Headache, 42*, 515–518.

Silberstein, S. D., & Saper, J. R. (1993). Migraine: Diagnosis and treatment. In D. J. Dalessio and S. D. Silberstein (Eds.), *Wolff's headache and other head pain.* (6th ed.) New York: Oxford University Press.

Silberstein, S. D., Saper, J. R., & Freitag, F. G. (2001). Migraine: Diagnosis and treatment. In S. D. Silberstein, R. B. Lipton, & D. J. Dalessio (Eds.), *Wolff's headache and other head pain* (7th ed., pp. 121–237). New York: Oxford University Press.

Silberstein, S. D., Schulman, E. A., & Hopkins, M. M. (1990). Repetitive intravenous DHE in the treatment of refractory headache. *Headache, 30*, 334–339.

Sillanpää, M., & Anttila, P. (1996). Increasing prevalence of headache in 7-year-old school children. *Headache, 36*, 466–470.

Silverman, K., Evans, S. M., Strain, E. C., & Griffiths, R. R. (1992). Withdrawal syndrome after the double-blind cessation of caffeine consumption. *New England Journal of Medicine, 327*, 1109–1114.

Simons, D. G. (1996). Clinical and etiological update of myofascial pain from trigger points. *Journal of Musculoskeletal Pain, 4*, 93–121.

Simons, D. G., & Mense, S. (1998). Understanding and measurement of muscle tone as related to clinical muscle pain. *Pain, 75*, 1–17.

Singh, G., & Triadafilopoulos, G. (1999). Epidemiology of NSAID induced gastrointestinal complications. *Journal of Rheumatology, 26*(Suppl.), 18–24.

Siniatchkin, M., Averkina, N., & Gerber, W. D. (2006). Relationship between precipitating agents and neurophysiological abnormalities in migraine. *Cephalalgia, 26*, 457–465.

Siniatchkin, M., Gerber, W.-D., Kropp, P., & Vein, A. (1999). How the brain anticipates an attack: A study of neurophysiological periodicity in migraine. *Functional Neurology, 14*, 69–77.

Siniatchkin, M., Hierundar, A., Kropp, P., Kuhnert, R., Gerber, W.-D., & Stephani, U. (2000). Self-regulation of slow cortical potentials in children with migraine: An exploratory study. *Applied Psychophysiology and Biofeedback, 25*, 13–32.

Siniatchkin, M., Kropp, P., Neumann, M., Gerber, W.-D., & Stephani, U. (2000). Intensity dependence of auditory evoked cortical potentials in migraine families. *Pain, 85*, 247–254.

Sjaastad, O., Fredriksen, T. A., & Pfaffenrath, V. (1998). Cervicogenic headache: Diagnostic criteria. *Headache, 38*, 442–445.

Sjaastad, O., & Spierings, E. L. (1984). Hemicrania continua: Another headache absolutely responsive to indomethacin. *Cephalalgia, 4*, 65–70.

Skyba, D. A., Radhakrishnan, R., Rohlwing, J. J., Wright, A., & Sluka, K. A. (2003). Joint manipulation reduces hyperalgesia by activation of monoamine receptors but not opioid or GABA receptors in the spinal cord. *Pain, 106*, 159–168.

Skyhoj, O. T., Friberg, L., & Lassen, N. A. (1987). Ischemia may be the primary cause of the neurological deficits in classic migraine. *Archives of Neurology, 44*, 156–161.

Sliwka, U., Harscher, S., Diehl, R. R., van Schayck, R., Niesen, W. D., & Weiller, C. (2001). Spontaneous oscillations in cerebral blood flow velocity give evidence of different autonomic dysfunctions in various types of headache. *Headache, 41*, 157–163.

Smeets, G., de Jong, P. J., & Mayer, B. (2000). If you suffer from a headache, then you have a brain tumour: Domain-specific reasoning 'bias' and hypochondriasis. *Behaviour Research and Therapy, 38*, 763–776.

Smith, M., Cros, D., & Sheen, V. (2002). Hyperperfusion with vasogenic leakage by fMRI in migraine with prolonged aura. *Neurology, 58*, 1308–1310.

Smith, M. J., Adams, L. F., Schmidt, P. J., Rubinow, D. R., & Wassermann, E. M. (2002). Effects of ovarian hormones on human cortical excitability. *Annals of Neurology, 51*, 599–603.

Smith, M. J., & Jensen, N. M. (1988). The severity model of chronic headache. *Journal of General Internal Medicine, 3*, 396–409.

Smith, W. B. (1987). Biofeedback and relaxation training: The effect on headache and associated symptoms. *Headache, 27*, 511–514.

Smith, W. B., Gracely, R. H., & Safer, M. A. (1998). The meaning of pain: Cancer patients' rating and recall of pain intensity and affect. *Pain, 78*, 123–129.

Smyth, A. E., Hughes, A. E., Bruce, I. N., & Bell, A. L. (1999). A case-control study of candidate vasoactive mediator genes in primary Raynaud's phenomenon. *Rheumatology* (Oxford), *38*, 1094–1098.

Snow, V., Weiss, K., Wall, E. M., & Mottur-Pilson, C. (2002). Pharmacologic management of acute attacks of migraine and prevention of migraine headache. *Annals of Internal Medicine, 137*, 840–849.

Solomon, G. D. (1995). The pharmacology of medications used in treating headache. *Seminars in Pediatric Neurology, 2*, 165–177.

Solomon, G. D. (1999). Classification and mechanism of headache. In M. L. Diamond & G. D. Solomon (Eds.), *Diamond and Dalessio's The practicing physician's approach to headache* (6th ed., pp. 8–15). Philadelphia: W. B. Saunders Company.

Solomon, G. D., Steel, J. G., & Spaccavento, L. J. (1983). Verapamil prophylaxis of migraine: A double-blind, placebo-controlled study. *JAMA, 250*, 2500–2502.

Solomon, S. (1997). Diagnosis of primary headache disorders. *Neurologic Clinics, 15*, 15–26.

Solomon, S., & Färkkilä, M. (2000). The complex chronic patient: Mixed headache and drug overuse. In: J. Olesen, P. Tfelt-Hansen, & K. M. A. Welch (Eds.), *The headaches* (2nd ed., pp. 987–992). Philadelphia: Lippincott, Williams & Wilkins.

Solomon, S. D., McMurray, J. J. V., Pfeffer, M. A., Wittes, J., Fowler, R., Finn, P., et al. (2005). Cardiovascular risk associated with celecoxib in a clinical trial for colorectal adenoma prevention. *New England Journal of Medicine, 352*, 1071–1080.

Somerville, B. W. (1972). The role of estradiol withdrawal in the etiology of menstrual migraine. *Neurology, 22*, 355–365.

Somerville, B. W. (1975). Estrogen-withdrawal migraine. I. Duration of exposure required and attempted prophylaxis by premenstrual estrogen administration. *Neurology, 25*, 239–244.

Somjen, G. G. (2001). Mechanisms of spreading depression and hypoxic spreading depression-like depolarization. *Physiological Reviews, 81*, 1065–1096.

Son, B. C., Kim, M. C., Moon, D. E., & Kang, J. K. (2003). Motor cortex stimulation in a patient with intractable complex regional pain syndrome Type II with hemibody involvement. *Journal of Neurosurgery, 98*, 175–179.

Sorbi, M. J., Maassen, G. H., & Spierings, E. L. H. (1996). A time series analysis of daily hassles and mood changes in the 3 days before the migraine attack. *Behavioral Medicine, 22*, 103–113.

Sorbi, M., Tellegen, B., & Du Long, A. (1989). Long-term effects of training in relaxation and stress-coping in patients with migraine: A 3-year follow-up. *Headache, 29*, 111–121.

Sørensen, L. V. (1992). Preoperative psychological testing with the MMPI at first operation for prolapsed lumbar disc: Five-year follow up. *Danish Medical Bulletin, 39*, 186–190.

Sørensen, L. V., Mors, O., & Skovlund, O. (1987). A prospective study of the importance of psychological and social factors for the outcome after surgery in patients with slipped lumbar disk operated upon for the first time. *Acta Neurochirurgica, 88*, 119–125.

Sosin, D. M., Sniezek, J. E., & Thurman, D. J. (1996). Incidence of mild and moderate brain injury in the United States, 1991. *Brain Injury, 10*, 47–54.

Spalding, A., Vaitkevicius, H., Dill, S., MacKenzie, S., Schmaier, A., & Lockette, W. (1998). Mechanism of epinephrine-induced platelet aggregation. *Hypertension, 31*, 603–607.

Spanos, N. P. (1991). A sociocognitive approach to hypnosis. In S. J. Lynn & J. W. Rhue (Eds.), *Theories of hypnosis: Current models and perspectives* (pp. 324–361). New York: Guilford Press.

Spanos, N. P., Gwynn, M., & Stam, H. J. (1983). Instructional demands and ratings of overt and hidden pain during hypnotic analgesia. *Journal of Abnormal Psychology, 92*, 479–488.

Sparaco, M., Feleppa, M., Lipton, R. B., Rapoport, A. M., & Bigal, M. E. (2006). Mitochondrial dysfunction and migraine: Evidence and hypotheses. *Cephalalgia, 26*, 361–372.

Speckenbach, U., & Gerber, W. D. (1999). Reliability of infrared plethysmography in BVP biofeedback therapy and the relevance for clinical application. *Applied Psychophysiology and Biofeedback, 24*, 261–265

Spiegel, D., Bierre, P., & Rootenberg, J. (1989). Hypnotic alteration of somatosensory perception. *American Journal of Psychiatry, 146*, 749–754.

Spitzer, R. L., Williams, J. B. W., Kroenke, K., Linzer, M., deGruy, F. V. III, Hahn, S. R., et al. (1994). Utility of a new procedure for diagnosing mental disorders in primary care: The PRIME-MD 1000 Study. *JAMA, 272*, 1749–1756.

Srikiatkhachorn, A., Maneesri, S., Govitrapong, P., & Kasantikul, V. (1998). Derangement of serotonin system in migrainous patients with analgesic abuse headache: Clues from platelets. *Headache, 38*, 43–49.

Srikiatkhachorn, A., Suwattanasophon, C., Ruangpattanatawee, U., & Phansuwan-Pujito, P. (2002). 5-HT$_{2A}$ receptor activation and nitric oxide synthesis: A possible mechanism determining migraine attacks. *Headache, 42*, 566–574.

Stacy, M. (2000). Idiopathic cervical dystonia: An overview. *Neurology, 55*(Suppl. 5), S2–S8.

Stang, P., Sternfeld, B., & Sidney, S. (1996). Migraine headache in a prepaid health plan: Ascertainment, demographics, physiological, and behavioral factors. *Headache, 36*, 69–76.

Stang, P., Von Korff, M., & Galer, B. S. (1998). Reduced labor force participation among primary care patients with headache. *Journal of General Internal Medicine, 13*, 296–302.

Staud, R., Vierck, C. J., Cannon, R. L., Mauderli, A. P., & Price, D. D. (2001). Abnormal sensitization and temporal summation of second pain (wind-up) in patients with fibromyalgia syndrome. *Pain, 91*, 165–175.

Steardo, L., Marano, E., Barone, P., Denman, D. W., Monteleone, P., & Cardone, G. (1986). Prophylaxis of migraine attacks with a calcium-channel blocker: Flunarizine versus methysergide. *Journal of Clinical Pharmacology, 26*, 524–528.

Steed, P. A., & Wexler, G. B. (2001). Temporomandibular disorders—traumatic etiology vs. nontraumatic etiology: A clinical and methodological inquiry into symptomatology and treatment outcomes. *Journal of Craniomandibular Practice, 19*, 188–194.

Steiner, T. J., Scher, A. I., Stewart, W. F., Kolodner, K., Liberman, J., & Lipton, R. B. (2003). The prevalence and disability burden of adult migraine in England and their relationships to age, gender and ethnicity. *Cephalalgia, 23*, 519–527.

Steiner, T. J., & Tfelt-Hansen, P. (2000). Antiepileptic drugs in migraine prophylaxis. In J. Olesen, P. Tfelt-Hansen, & K. M. A. Welch (Eds.), *The headaches* (2nd ed., pp. 483–487). Philadelphia: Lippincott Williams & Wilkins.

Stemmler, G., Heldmann, M., Pauls, C. A., & Scherer, T. (2001). Constraints for emotion specificity in fear and anger: The context counts. *Psychophysiology, 38*, 275–291.

Sterling, M., Jull, G., & Wright, A. (2001). Cervical mobilisation: Concurrent effects on pain, sympathetic nervous system activity and motor activity. *Manual Therapy, 6*(2), 72–81.

Stern, R. M., Ray, W. J., & Quigley, K. S. (2001). *Psychophysiological recording* (2nd ed.). New York: Oxford University Press.

Sternberg, E. M. (1997). Neural-immune interactions in health and disease. *Journal of Clinical Investigation, 100*, 2641–2647.

Sternberg, P. E. (1997). Posttraumatic headache [letter]. *Neurology, 48*, 1735.

Sternberg, R. J. (1998). *In search of the human mind* (2nd ed.). Fort Worth, TX: Harcourt Brace College Publishers.

Stewart, W. F., Lipton, R. B., Celentano, D. D., & Reed, M. L. (1992). Prevalence of migraine headache in the United States. Relation to age, income, race, and other sociodemographic factors. *Journal of the American Medical Association, 267*, 64–69.

Stewart, W. F., Lipton, R. B., Dowson, A. J., & Sawyer, J. (2001). Development and testing of the Migraine Disability Assessment (MIDAS) Questionnaire to assess headache-related disability. *Neurology, 56*(Suppl. 1), s20–s28.

Stewart, W. F., Lipton, R. B., Kolodner, K. B., Sawyer, J., Lee, C., & Liberman, J. N. (2000). Validity of the Migraine Disability Assessment (MIDAS) score in comparison to a diary-based measure in a population sample of migraine sufferers. *Pain, 88*, 41–52.

Stewart, W. F., Lipton, R. B., & Liberman, J. (1996). Variation in migraine prevalence by race. *Neurology, 47*, 52–59.

Stewart, W. F., Lipton, R. B., & Simon, D. (1996). Work-related disability: Results from the American Migraine Study. *Cephalalgia, 16*, 231–238.

Stewart, W. F., Lipton, R. B., Simon, D., Liberman, J., & Von Korff, M. (1999). Validity of an illness severity measure for headache in a population sample of migraine sufferers. *Pain, 79*, 291–301.

Stewart, W. F., Lipton, R. B., Whyte, J., Dowson, A., Kolodner, K., Liberman, J. N., & Sawyer, J. (1999). An international study to assess reliability of the Migraine Disability Assessment (MIDAS) score. *Neurology, 53*, 988–994.

Stewart, W. F., Scher, A. I., & Lipton, R. B. (2001). The Frequent Headache Epidemiology Study (FrHE): Stressful life events and risk of chronic daily headache. *Neurology, 56*, A138–A139.

Stock, H. S., Caldarone, B., Abrahamsen, G., Mongeluzi, D., Wilson, M. A., & Rosellini, R. A. (2001). Sex differences in relation to conditioned fear-induced enhancement of morphine analgesia. *Physiology and Behavior, 72*, 439–447.

Storer, R. J., & Goadsby, P. J. (1999). Trigeminovascular nociceptive transmission involves N-methyl-D-aspartate and non-N-methyl-D-aspartate glutamate receptors. *Neuroscience, 90*, 1371–1376.

Storey, J. R., Calder, C. S., Hart, D. E., & Potter, D. L. (2001). Topiramate in migraine prevention: A double-blind, placebo-controlled study. *Headache, 41*, 968–975.

Ström, L., Pettersson, R., & Andersson, G. (2000). A controlled trial of self-help treatment of recurrent headache conducted via the Internet. *Journal of Consulting and Clinical Psychology, 68*, 722–727.

Stronks, D. L., Tulen, J. H. M., Verheij, R., Boomsma, F., Fekkes, D., Pepplinkhuizen, L., Mantel, G. W. H., & Passchier, J. (1998). Serotonergic, catecholaminergic, and cardiovascular reactions to mental stress in female migraine patients. A controlled study. *Headache, 38*, 270–280.

Sturzenegger, M., Radanov, B. P., & Di Stefano, G. (1995). The effect of accident mechanisms and initial findings on the long-term course of whiplash injury. *Journal of Neurology, 242*, 443–449.

Sudoh, Y., Cahoon, E. E., Gerner, P., & Wang, G. K. (2003). Tricyclic antidepressants as long-acting local anesthetics. *Pain, 103*, 49–55.

Suh, J. H., Moreau, R., Heath, S.-H. D., & Hagen, T. M. (2005). Dietary supplementation with (R)-α-lipoic acid reverses the age-related accumulation of iron and depletion of antioxidants in the rat cerebral cortex. *Redox Report, 10*, 52–60.

Sullivan, M. J. L., Bishop, S. R., & Pivik, J. (1995). The Pain Catastrophizing Scale: Development and validation. *Psychological Assessment, 7*, 524–532.

Sullivan, M. J. L., Rouse, D., Bishop, S., & Johnston, S. (1997). Thought suppression, catastrophizing, and pain. *Cognitive Therapy and Research, 21*, 555–568.

Suzuki, R., Morcuende, S., Webber, M., Hunt, S. P., & Dickenson, A. H. (2002). Superficial NK1-expressing neurons control spinal excitability through activation of descending pathways. *Nature Neuroscience, 5*, 1319–1326.

Svensson, P., List, T., & Hector, G. (2001). Analysis of stimulus-evoked pain in patients with myofascial temporomandibular pain disorders. *Pain, 92*, 399–409.

Swanson, L. W. (2003). *Brain architecture: Understanding the basic plan.* New York: Oxford.

Syme, C. A., Gerlach, A. C., Singh, A. K., & Devor, D. C. (2000). Pharmacological activation of cloned intermediate- and small-conductance Ca^{2+}-activated K^+ channels. *American Journal of Physiology. Cell Physiology, 278*, C570–C581.

Symon, D. N. K., & Russell, G. (1986). Abdominal migraine: A childhood syndrome defined. *Cephalalgia, 6*, 223–228.

Szabo, C. P. (1995). Fluoxetine and sumatriptan: Possibly a counterproductive combination. *Journal of Clinical Psychiatry, 56*, 37–38.

Szallasi, A., & Appendino, G. (2004). Vanilloid receptor TRPV1 antagonists as the next generation of painkillers. Are we putting the cart before the horse? *Journal of Medicinal Chemistry, 47*, 2717–2723.

Sztajzel, R., Genoud, D., Roth, S., Mermillod, B., & Le Floch-Rohr, J. (2002). Patent foramen ovale, a possible cause of symptomatic migraine: A study of 74 patients with acute ischemic stroke. *Cerebrovascular Diseases, 13*, 102–106.

Taffi, R., Vignini, A., Lanciotti, C., Luconi, R., Nanetti, L., Mazzanti, L., et al. (2005). Platelet membrane fluidity and peroxynitrite levels in migraine patients during headache-free periods. *Cephalalgia, 25*, 353–358.

Takase, Y., Nakano, M., Tatsumi, C., & Matsuyama, T. (2004). Clinical features, effectiveness of drug-based treatment, and prognosis of new daily persistent headache (NDPH): 30 cases in Japan. *Cephalalgia, 24*, 955–959.

Takeshima, T., & Takahashi, K. (1988). The relationship between muscle contraction headache and migraine: A multivariate analysis study. *Headache, 28*, 272–277.

Tambeli, C. H., Parada, C. A., Levine, J. D., & Gear, R. W. (2002). Inhibition of tonic spinal glutamatergic activity induces antinociception in the rat. *European Journal of Neuroscience, 16*, 1547–1553.

Tataroglu, C., Kanik, A., Sahin, G., Özge, A., Yalçinkaya, D., & Idiman, F. (2002). Exteroceptive suppression patterns of masseter and temporalis muscles in central and peripheral headache disorders. *Cephalalgia, 22*, 444–452.

Taub, E., & Emurian, C. S. (1976). Feedback aided self-regulation of skin temperature with a single feedback locus: I. Acquisition and reversal training. *Biofeedback and Self-Regulation, 1*, 147–167.

Taub, E., & School, P. J. (1978). Some methodological considerations in thermal biofeedback training. *Behavior Research Methods and Instrumentation, 10*, 617–622.

Tayefeh, F., Kurz, A., Sessler, D. I., Lawson, C. A., Ikeda, T., & Marder, D. (1997). Thermoregulatory vasodilation increases the venous partial pressure of oxygen. *Anesthesia and Analgesia, 85*, 657–662.

Taylor, C. P., Gee, N. S., Su, T., et al. (1998). A summary of mechanistic hypotheses of gabapentin pharmacology. *Epilepsy Research, 29*, 233–249.

Taylor, G. J., Bagby, R. M., & Parker, J. D. A. (1991). The alexithymia construct: A potential paradigm for psychosomatic medicine. *Psychosomatics, 32*, 153–164.

Taylor, M. L., Trotter, D. R., & Csuka, M. E. (1995). The prevalence of sexual abuse in women with fibromyalgia. *Arthritis and Rheumatism, 38*, 229–234.

Taylor, S. E. (1981). The interface of cognitive and social psychology. In J. Harvey (Ed.), *Cognition, social behavior, and the environment* (pp. 189–211). Hillsdale, NJ: Lawrence Erlbaum Associates.

Teasell, R. W. (2001). Compensation and chronic pain. *Clinical Journal of Pain, 17* (4, Supplement), S46–S51.

Tellegen, A., & Atkinson, G. (1974). Openness to absorbing and self-altering experiences ("absorption"), a trait related to hypnotic susceptibility. *Journal of Abnormal Psychology, 83*, 268–277.

Tepper, S., Allen, C., Sanders, D., Greene, A., & Boccuzzi, S. (2003). Coprescription of triptans with potentially interacting medications: A cohort study involving 240268 patients. *Headache, 43*, 44–48.

Tepper, S. J., Rapoport, A. M., & Sheftell, F. D. (2002). Mechanisms of action of the $5\text{-HT}_{1B/1D}$ receptor agonists. *Archives of Neurology, 59*, 1084–1088.

ter Kuile, M. M., Spinhoven, P., Linssen, A. C. G., & van Houwelingen, H. C. (1995a). Cognitive coping and appraisal processes in the treatment of chronic headaches. *Pain, 64*, 257–264.

ter Kuile, M. M., Spinhoven, P., & Linssen, A. C. G. (1995b). Responders and nonresponders to autogenic training and cognitive self-hypnosis: Prediction of short- and long-term success in tension-type headache patients. *Headache, 35*, 630–636.

Terrón, J. A. (2002). Is the 5-HT$_7$ receptor involved in the pathogenesis and prophylactic treatment of migraine? *European Journal of Pharmacology, 439*, 1–11.

Tfelt-Hansen, P., Block, G., Dahlof, C., Diener, H. C., Ferrari, M. D., Goadsby, P. J., et al. (2000). Guidelines for controlled trials of drugs in migraine (2nd ed.). *Cephalalgia, 20*, 765–786.

Tfelt-Hansen, P., Lous, I., & Olesen, J. (1981). Prevalence and significance of muscle tenderness during common migraine attacks. *Headache, 21*, 49–54.

Tfelt-Hansen, P., & Saxena, P. R. (2000). 5-HT receptor antagonists in migraine prophylaxis. In H.-C. Diener (Ed.), *Drug treatment of migraine and other headaches* (pp. 279–287). Basel: Karger.

Tfelt-Hansen, P., Saxena, P. R., Dahlöf, C., Pascual, J., Láinez, M., Henry, P., et al. (2000). Ergotamine in the acute treatment of migraine: A review and European consensus. *Brain, 123*, 9–18.

Theoharides, T. C., Spanos, C., Pang, X., Alferes, L., Ligris, K., Letourneau, R., et al. (1995). Stress-induced intracranial mast cell degranulation: A corticotropin-releasing hormone-mediated effect. *Endocrinology, 136*, 5745–5750.

Thie, A., Carvajal-Lizano, M., Schlichting, U., Spitzer, K., & Kunze, K. (1992). Multimodal tests of cerebrovascular reactivity in migraine: A transcranial Doppler study. *Journal of Neurology, 239*, 338–342.

Thie, A., Fuhlendorf, A., Spitzer, K., & Kunze, K. (1990). Transcranial Doppler evaluation of common and classic migraine. Part 1. Ultrasonic features during the headache-free period. *Headache, 30*, 201–208.

Thomaides, T., Karagounakis, D., Spantideas, A., & Katelanis, S. (2003). Transcranial Doppler in migraine attacks before and after treatment with oral zolmitriptan or sumatriptan. *Headache, 43*, 54–58.

Thompson, C. M., Wojno, H., Greiner, E., May, E. L., Rice, K. C., & Selley, D. E. (2004). Activation of G-proteins by morphine and codeine congeners: Insights into the relevance of O- and N-demethylated metabolites at ???- and ???-opioid receptors. *Journal of Pharmacology and Experimental Therapeutics, 308*, 547–554.

Thompson, J. K., & Adams, H. E. (1984). Psychophysiological characteristics of headache patients. *Pain, 18*, 41–52.

Thomsen, L. L., Iversen, H. K., & Olesen, J. (1995). Cerebral blood flow velocities are reduced during attacks of unilateral migraine without aura. *Cephalalgia, 15*, 109–116.

Thomsen, L. L., & Olesen, J. (1998). Nitric oxide theory of migraine. *Clinical Neuroscience, 5*, 28–33.

Thonnard-Neumann, E. (1973). Heparin in migraine headache. *Headache, 13*, 49–64.

Thurman, D. J., Alverson, C., Dunn, K. A., Guerrero, J., & Sniezek, J. E. (1999). Traumatic brain injury in the United States: A public health perspective. *Journal of Head Trauma Rehabilitation, 14*, 602–615.

Tibbetts, V., Charbonneau, J., & Peper, E. (1987). Adjunctive strategies to enhance peripheral warming: Clinical techniques. *Biofeedback and Self-Regulation, 12*, 313–321.

Tietjen, G. E., Al-Qasmi, M. M., Athanas, K., Dafer, R. M., & Khuder, S. A. (2001). Increased von Willebrand factor in migraine. *Neurology, 57*, 334–336.

To, J., Issenman, R., & Kamath, M. V. (1999). Evaluation of neurocardiac signals in pediatrics patients with cyclic vomiting syndrome through power spectral analysis of heart rate variability. *Journal of Pediatrics, 135*, 363–366.

Tobin, D. L., Holroyd, K. A., Baker, A., Reynolds, R. V. C., & Holm, J. E. (1988). Development and clinical trial of a minimal contact, cognitive-behavioral treatment for tension headache. *Cognitive Therapy and Research, 12*, 325–339.

Tocco, G., Maren, S., Shors, T. J., Baudry, M., & Thompson, R. F. (1992). Long-term potentiation is associated with increased [^{3}H]AMPA binding in rat hippocampus. *Brain Research, 573*, 228–234.

Toda, N., & Tfelt-Hansen, P. (2000). Calcium antagonists in migraine prophylaxis. In J. Olesen, P. Tfelt-Hansen, & K. M. A. Welch (Eds.), *The headaches* (2nd ed., pp. 477–482). Philadelphia: Lippincott Williams & Wilkins.

Tomkins, G. E., Jackson, J. L., O'Malley, P. G., Balden, E., & Santoro, J. E. (2001). Treatment of chronic headache with antidepressants: A meta-analysis. *American Journal of Medicine, 111*, 54–63.

Tommerdahl, M., Delemos, K. A., Favorov, O. V., Metz, C. B., Vierck, C. J. Jr., & Whitsel, B. L. (1998). Response of anterior parietal cortex to different modes of same-site skin stimulation. *Journal of Neurophysiology, 80*, 3272–3283.

Torebjork, E. (1985). Nociceptor activation and pain. *Philosophical Transactions of the Royal Society of London. Series B. Biological Sciences, 308*, 227–234.

Torebjörk, H. E., Lundberg, L. E., & LaMotte, R. H. (1992). Central changes in processing of mechanoreceptive input in capsaicin-induced secondary hyperalgesia in humans. *Journal of Physiology, 448*, 765–780.

Torelli, P., Cologno, D., & Manzoni, G. C. (1999). Weekend headache: A retrospective study in migraine without aura and episodic tension-type headache. *Headache, 39*, 11–20.

Trabace, S., Brioli, G., Lulli P., Morellini, M., Giacovazzo, M., Cicciarelli, G., & Martelletti, P. (2002). Tumor necrosis factor gene polymorphism in migraine. *Headache, 42*, 341–345.

Travell, J. G., & Simons, D. G. (1983). *Myofascial pain and dysfunction: The trigger point manual* (Vol. 1., *The upper extremities*). Baltimore: Williams and Wilkins.

Treede, R.-D., Handwerker, H. O., Baumgärtner, U., Meyer, R. A., & Magerl, W. (2004). Hyperalgesia and allodynia: Taxonomy, assessment, and mechanisms. In K. Brune & H. O. Handwerker (Eds.), *Hyperalgesia: Molecular mechanisms and clinical implications*. Seattle: IASP Press.

Treede, R.-D., Kenshalo, D. R., Gracely, R. H., & Jones, A. K. P. (1999). The cortical representation of pain. *Pain, 79*, 105–111.

Treede, R.-D., Rolke, R., Andrews, K., & Magerl, W. (2002). Pain elicited by blunt pressure: Neurobiological basis and clinical relevance. *Pain, 98*, 235–240.

Treiber, F. A., Jackson, R. W., Davis, H., Pollock, J. S., Kapuku, G., Mensah, G. A., & Pollock, D. M. (2000). Racial differences in endothelin-1 at rest and in response to acute stress in adolescent males. *Hypertension, 35*, 722–725.

Treleaven, J., Jull, G., & Atkinson, L. (1994). Cervical musculoskeletal dysfunction in post-concussional headache. *Cephalalgia, 14*, 273–279.

Tricarico, D., Barbieri, M., & Camerino, D. C. (2000). Acetazolamide opens the muscular KCa2+ channel: A novel mechanism of action that may explain the therapeutic effect of the drug in hypokalemic periodic paralysis. *Annals of Neurology, 48*, 304–312.

Triplett, G., Hill, C., Freeman, L., Rajan, U., & Templer, D. I. (1996). Incidence of head injury: Lasting effects among college students and working adults in the general population. *Perceptual and Motor Skills, 83*, 1344–1346.

Tronvik, E., Stovner, L. J., Helde, G., Sand, T., & Bovim, G. (2003). Prophylactic treatment of migraine with an angiotensin II receptor blocker: A randomized controlled trial. *JAMA, 289*, 65–69.

Tsai, G., & Coyle, J. T. (1995). *N*-Acetylaspartate in neuropsychiatric disorders. *Progress in Neurobiology, 46*, 531–540.

Tschannen, T. A., Duckro, P. N., Margolis, R. B., & Tomazic, T. J. (1992). The relationship of anger, depression, and perceived disability among headache patients. *Headache, 32*, 501–503.

Tunis, M. M., & Wolff, H. G. (1953). Studies on headache: Long-term observations of the reactivity of the cranial arteries in subjects with vascular headache of the migraine type. *AMA Archives of Neurology and Psychiatry, 70*, 551–557.

Tunks, E., Crook, J., Norman, G., & Kalaher, S. (1988). Tender points in fibromyalgia. *Pain, 34*, 11–19.

Turk, D. C., & Okifuji, A. (1994). Detecting depression in chronic pain patients: Adequacy of self-reports. *Behaviour Research and Therapy, 32*, 9–16.

Turk, D. C., & Okifuji, A. (2004). Psychological aspects of pain. In C. A. Warfield & Z. H. Bajwa (Eds.), *Principles and practice of pain medicine* (2nd ed., pp. 139–147). New York: McGraw-Hill.

Turk, D. C., & Rudy, T. E. (1987). Towards a comprehensive assessment of chronic pain patients. *Behaviour Research and Therapy, 25*, 237–249.

Turk, D. C., Rudy, T. E., Kubinski, J. A., Zaki, H. S., & Greco, C. M. (1996). Dysfunctional patients with temporomandibular disorders: Evaluating the efficacy of a tailored treatment protocol. *Journal of Consulting and Clinical Psychology, 64*, 139–146.

Turk, D. C., Zaki, H. S., & Rudy, T. E. (1993). Effects of intraoral appliance and biofeedback/stress management alone and in combination in treating pain and depression in patients with temporomandibular disorders. *Journal of Prosthetic Dentistry, 70*, 158–164.

Turner, J. A., & Romano, J. M. (1984). Self-report screening measures for depression in chronic pain patients. *Journal of Clinical Psychology, 40*, 909–913.

Turner, J. A., Whitney, C., Dworkin, S. F., Massoth, D., & Wilson, L. (1995). Do changes in patient beliefs and coping strategies predict temporomandibular disorder treatment outcomes? *Clinical Journal of Pain, 11*, 177–188.

Twenge, J. M. (2000). The age of anxiety? Birth cohort change in anxiety and neuroticism. *Journal of Personality and Social Psychology, 79*, 1007–1021.

Tzourio, C., El Amrani, M., Poirier, O., Nicaud, V., Bousser, M.-G., & Alpérovitch, A. (2001). Association between migraine and endothelin type A receptor (ETA -231 A/G) gene polymorphism. *Neurology, 56*, 1273–1277.

Ulrich, V., Gervil, M., & Olesen, J. (2004). The relative influence of environment and genes in episodic tension-type heache. *Neurology, 62*, 2065–2069.

Ulrich, V., Russell, M. B., Jensen, R., & Olesen, J. (1996). A comparison of tension-type headache in migraineurs and in non-migraineurs: A population-based study. *Pain, 67*, 501–506.

Ulrich-Lai, Y. M., Flores, C. M., Harding-Rose, C. A., Goodis, H. E., & Hargreaves, K. M. (2001). Capsaicin-evoked release of immunoreactive calcitonin gene-related peptide from rat trigeminal ganglion: Evidence for intraganglionic neurotransmission. *Pain, 91*, 219–226.

Uomoto, J. M., Turner, J. A., & Herron, L. D. (1988). Use of the MMPI and MCMI in predicting outcome of lumbar laminectomy. *Journal of Clinical Psychology, 44*, 191–197.

U. S. Congress. (1946). Senate, Committee on Foreign Relations, Subcommittee on S.1875, 79th Congress, 2nd Session, Cancer Research, hearings, July 1–3, 1946. Washington, DC: U. S. Government Printing Office.

Utz, S. W. (1994). The effect of instructions on cognitive strategies and performance in biofeedback. *Journal of Behavioral Medicine, 17*, 291–308.

Vahedi, K., Taupin, P., Djomby, R., El-Amrani, M., Lutz, G., Filipetti, V., Landais, P., Massiou, H., & Bousser, M. G. (2002). Efficacy and tolerability of acetazolamide in migraine prophylaxis: A randomised placebo-controlled trial. *Journal of Neurology, 249*, 206–211.

Vahlquist, B. (1955). Migraine in children. *International Archives of Allergy, 7*, 348–355.

Vahtera, J., Kivimaki, M., Koskenvuo, M., & Pentti, J. (1997). Hostility and registered sickness absences: A prospective study of municipal employees. *Psychological Medicine, 27*, 693–701.

Valeriani, M., Rinalduzzi, S., & Vigevano, F. (2005). Multilevel somatosensory system disinhibition in children with migraine. *Pain, 118*, 137–144.

Valikovics, A., Oláh, L., Fülesdi, B., Káposzta, Z., Ficzere, A., Bereczki, D., & Csiba, L. (1996). Cerebrovascular reactivity measured by transcranial Doppler in migraine. *Headache, 36*, 323–328.

Van Bockstaele, E. J., Bajic, D., Proudfit, H., & Valentino, R. J. (2001). Topographic architecture of stress-related pathways targeting the noradrenergic locus coeruleus. *Physiology and Behavior, 73*, 273–283.

Van Boxtel, A. (2001). Optimal signal bandwidth for the recording of surface EMG activity of facial, jaw, oral, and neck muscles. *Psychophysiology, 38*, 22–34.

Van Boxtel, A., Goudswaard, P., & Schomaker, L. R. B. (1984). Amplitude and bandwidth of the frontalis surface EMG: Effects of electrode parameters. *Psychophysiology, 21*, 699–707.

Van Boxtel, A., & Jessurun, M. (1993). Amplitude and bilateral coherency of facial and jaw-elevator EMG activity as an index of effort during a two-choice serial reaction task. *Psychophysiology, 30*, 589–604.

Van Boxtel, A., & van der Ven, J. R. (1978). Differential EMG activity in subjects with muscle contraction headaches related to mental effort. *Headache, 17*, 233–237.

Van Den Eeden, S. K., Koepsell, T. D., Longstreth, W. T. Jr., van Belle, G., Daling, J. R., & McKnight, B. (1994). Aspartame ingestion and headaches: A randomized crossover trial. *Neurology, 44*, 1787–1793.

van der Naalt, J., van Zomeren, A. H., Sluiter, W. J., & Minderhoud, J. M. (1999). One year outcome in mild to moderate head injury: The predictive value of acute injury characteristics related to complaints and return to work. *Journal of Neurology, Neurosurgery, and Psychiatry, 66*, 207–213.

van Vliet, J. A., Vein, A. A., Le Cessie, S., Ferrari, M. D., & van Dijk, J. G. (2003). Impairment of trigeminal sensory pathways in cluster headache. *Cephalalgia, 23*, 414–419.

Vanast, W. J. (1986). New daily persistent headaches. Definition of a benign syndrome. *Headache, 26*, 318.

VandeCreek, L., & O'Donnell, F. (1992). Psychometric characteristics of the Headache-Specific Locus of Control Scale. *Headache, 32*, 239–241.

Vanderah, T. W., Ossipov, M. H., Lai, J., Malan, T. P. Jr., & Porreca, F. (2001). Mechanisms of opioid induced pain and antinociceptive tolerance: Descending facilitation and spinal dynorphin. *Pain, 92*, 5–9.

Vanderah, T. W., Suenaga, N. M. H., Ossipov, M. H., Malan, T. P. Jr., Lai, J., & Porreca, F. (2001). Tonic descending facilitation from the rostral ventromedial medulla mediates opioid-induced abnormal pain and antinociceptive tolerance. *Journal of Neuroscience, 21*, 279–286.

Vanegas, H., & Schaible, H.-G. (2001). Prostaglandins and cycloxygenases in the spinal cord. *Progress in Neurobiology, 64*, 327–363.

Vanmolkot, K. R., Kors, E. E., Hottenga, J. J., Terwindt, G. M., Haan, J., Hoefnagels, W. A., et al. (2003). Novel mutations in the Na+, K+-ATPase pump gene ATP1A2 associated with familial hemiplegic migraine and benign familial infantile convulsions. *Annals of Neurology, 54*, 360–366.

Vasconcellos, E., Pina-Garza, J. E., Millan, E. J., & Warner, J. S. (1998). Analgesic rebound headache in children and adolescents. *Journal of Child Neurology, 13*, 443–447.

Vasudeva, S., Claggett, A. L., Tietjen, G. E., & McGrady, A. V. (2003). Biofeedback-assisted relaxation in migraine headache: Relationship to cerebral blood flow velocity in the middle cerebral artery. *Headache, 43*, 245–250.

Vaughan, T. R. (1994). The role of food in the pathogenesis of migraine headache. *Clinical Reviews in Allergy, 12*, 167–180.

Vaughan, W. T. (1927). Allergic migraine. *JAMA: Journal of the American Medical Association, 88*, 1383–1386.

Veiersted, K. B., Westgaard, R. H., & Andersen, P. (1993). Electromyographic evaluation of muscular work pattern as a predictor of trapezius myalgia. *Scandinavian Journal of Work, Environment, and Health, 19*, 284–290.

Velly, A. M., Gornitsky, M., & Philippe, P. (2003). Contributing factors to chronic myofascial pain: A case-control study. *Pain, 104*, 491–499.

Vernon, H. (1995). The effectiveness of chiropractic manipulation in the treatment of headache: An exploration in the literature. *Journal of Manipulative and Physiological Therapeutics, 18*, 611–617.

Veves, A., & Sarnow, M. R. (1995). Diagnosis, classification, and treatment of diabetic peripheral neuropathy. *Clinics in Podiatric Medicine and Surgery, 12*, 19–30.

Viane, I., Crombez, G., Eccleston, C., Poppe, C., Devulder, J., Van Houdenhove, B., & De Corte, W. (2003). Acceptance of pain is an independent predictor of mental well-being in patients with chronic pain: Empirical evidence and reappraisal. *Pain, 106*, 65–72.

Viken, R. J., Rose, R. J., Kaprio, J., & Koskenvuo, M. (1994). A developmental genetic analysis of adult personality: Extraversion and neuroticism from 18 to 59 years of age. *Journal of Personality and Social Psychology, 66*, 722–730.

Villemure, C., & Bushnell, M. C. (2002). Cognitive modulation of pain: How do attention and emotion influence pain processing? *Pain, 95*, 195–199.

Villemure, C., Slotnick, B. M., & Bushnell, M. C. (2003). Effects of odors on pain perception: Deciphering the roles of emotion and attention. *Pain, 106*, 101–108.

Visser, W. H., Burggraaf, J., Muller, L. M., Schoemaker, R. C., Fowler, P. A., Cohen, A. F., & Ferrari, M. D. (1996). Pharmacokinetic and pharmacodynamic profiles of sumatriptan in migraine patients with headache recurrence or no response. *Clinical Pharmacology and Therapeutics, 60*, 452–460.

Visser, W. H., Jaspers, N. M. W. H., de Vriend, R. H. M., & Ferrari, M. D. (1996). Risk factors for headache recurrence after sumatriptan: A study in 366 migraine patients. *Cephalalgia, 16*, 264–269.

Vitton, O., Gendreau, M., Gendreau, J., Kranzler, J., & Rao, S. G. (2004). A double-blind placebo-controlled trial of milnacipran in the treatment of fibromyalgia. *Human Psychopharmacology, 19*(Suppl. 1), s27–s35.

Vlaeyen, J. W. S., de Jong, J., Geilen, M., Heuts, P. H. T. G., & van Breukelen, G. (2001). Graded exposure in vivo in the treatment of pain-related fear: A replicated single-case experimental design in four patients with chronic low back pain. *Behaviour Research and Therapy, 39*, 151–166.

Vlaeyen, J. W. S., Kole-Snijders, A. M. J., Boeren, R. G. B., & van Eek, H. (1995). Fear of movement/(re)injury in chronic low back pain and its relation to behavioral performance. *Pain, 62*, 363–372.

Vlaeyen, J. W. S., Seelen, H. A. M., Peters, M., De Jong, P., Aretz, E., Beisiegel, E., & Weber, W. E. J. (1999). Fear of movement/(re)injury and muscular reactivity in chronic low back pain patients: An experimental investigation. *Pain, 82*, 297–304.

Vliagoftis, H., Dimitriadou, V., Boucher, W., Rozniecki, J. J., Correia, I., Raam, S., & Theoharides, T. C. (1992). Estradiol augments while tamoxifen inhibits rat mast cell secretion. *International Archives of Allergy and Immunology, 98*, 398–409.

Voller, B., Sycha, T., Gustorff, B., Schmetterer, L., Lehr, S., Eichler, H. G., Auff, E., & Schnider, P. (2003). A randomized, double-blind, placebo controlled study on analgesic effects of botulinum toxin A. *Neurology, 61*, 940–944.

Von Frey, M. (1896). Untersuchungen über die Sinnesfunktionen der menschlichen Haut: I. Druckempfindung und Schmerz. *Abhandlungen der Königlichen Sächsischen Gesellschaft der Wissenschaft zu Leipzig, Mathematische-Physiche Classe, 23*, 169–266.

Von Knorring, L., & Perris, C. (1981). Biochemistry of the augmenting-reducing response in visual evoked potentials. *Neuropsychobiology, 7*, 1–8.

Von Korff, M., Galer, B. S., & Stang, P. (1995). Chronic use of symptomatic headache medications. *Pain, 62*, 179–186.

Von Korff, M., Le Resche, L., & Dworkin, S. F. (1993). First onset of common pain symptoms: A prospective study of depression as a risk factor. *Pain, 55*, 251–258.

Von Korff, M., Ormel, J., Keefe, F. J., & Dworkin, S. F. (1992). Grading the severity of chronic pain. *Pain, 50*, 133–149.

Von Korff, M., Stewart, W. F., Simon, D. J., & Lipton, R. B. (1998). Migraine and reduced work performance. A population-based diary study. *Neurology, 50*, 1741–1745.

Von Korff, M., Wagner, E. H., Dworkin, S. F., & Saunders, K. W. (1991). Chronic pain and use of ambulatory health care. *Psychosomatic Medicine, 53*, 61–79.

Vosburgh, C. H., & Richards, A. N. (1903). An experimental study of the sugar content and extravascular coagulation of the blood after administration of adrenalin. *American Journal of Physiology, 9*, 35–51.

Vu, T. N. (2004). Current pharmacologic approaches to treating neuropathic pain. *Current Pain and Headache Reports, 8*, 15–18.

Vuilleumier, P., Chicherio, C., Assal, F., Schwartz, S., Slosman, D., & Landis, T. (2001). Functional neuroanatomical correlates of hysterical sensorimotor loss. *Brain, 124*, 1077–1090.

Wade, J. B., Dougherty, L. M., Hart, R. P., Rafii, A., & Price, D. D. (1992). A canonical correlation analysis of the influence of neuroticism and extraversion on chronic pain, suffering, and pain behavior. *Pain, 51*, 67–73.

Waersted, M., Bjørklund, R. A., & Westgaard, R. H. (1994). The effect of motivation on shoulder-muscle tension in attention-demanding tasks. *Ergonomics, 37*, 363–376.

Waersted, M., Eken, T., & Westgaard, R. H. (1996). Activity of single motor units in attention-demanding tasks: Firing pattern in the human trapezius muscle. *European Journal of Applied Physiology and Occupational Physiology, 72*, 323–329.

Waersted, M., & Westgaard, R. H. (1996). Attention-related muscle activity in different body regions during VDU work with minimal physical activity. *Ergonomics, 39*, 661–676.

Wagner, W., & Nootbaar-Wagner, U. (1997). Prophylactic treatment of migraine with gamma-linolenic and alpha-linolenic acids. *Cephalalgia, 17*, 127–130.

Wahren, L., Torebjörk, E., & New Yorkström, B. (1991). Quantitative sensory testing before and after regional guanethidine block in patients with neuralgia in the hand. *Pain, 46*, 23–30.

Wainer, H. (Ed.) (2000). *Computerized adaptive testing: A primer* (2nd ed.). Mahwah, NJ: Lawrence Erlbaum Associates.

Waldie, K. E., & Poulton, R. (2002). Physical and psychological correlates of primary headache in young adulthood: A 26 year longitudinal study. *Journal of Neurology, Neurosurgery, and Psychiatry, 72*, 86–92.

Waldstein, S. R., Bachen, E. A., & Manuck, S. B. (1997). Active coping and cardiovascular reactivity: A multiplicity of influences. *Psychosomatic Medicine, 59*, 620–625.

Walker, E. A., Katon, W. J., Harrop-Griffiths, J., Holm, L., Russo, J., & Hickock, L. R. (1988). Relationship of chronic pelvic pain to psychiatric diagnoses and childhood sexual abuse. *American Journal of Psychiatry, 145*, 75–80.

Wall, P. D. (1999). The placebo and the placebo response. In P. D. Wall & R. Melzack (Eds.), *Textbook of pain* (4th ed., pp. 1419–1430).

Wall, P. D. (2000). *Pain: The science of suffering.* New York: Columbia University Press.

Wallace, D. C. (1999). Mitochondrial diseases in man and mouse. *Science, 283*, 1482–1488.

Wallasch, T. M., Reinecke, M., & Langohr, H. D. (1991). EMG analysis of the late exteroceptive suppression period of temporalis muscle activity in episodic and chronic tension-type headaches. *Cephalalgia, 11*, 109–112.

Wallston, K. A., Wallston, B. S., & DeVellis, R. (1978). Development of the Multidimensional Health Locus of Control (MHLC) Scales. *Health Education Monographs, 6*, 160–170.

Walsh, D. M., & McAdams, E. T. (1997). *TENS: Clinical applications and related theory.* New York: Churchill Livingstone.

Walsh, N. E., Schoenfeld, L., Ramamurthy, S., & Hoffman, J. (1989). Normative model for cold pressor test. *American Journal of Physical Medicine and Rehabilitation, 68*, 6–11.

Walton, R. G., Hudak, R., & Green-Waite, R. J. (1993). Adverse reactions to aspartame: Double-blind challenge in patients from a vulnerable population. *Biological Psychiatry, 34*, 13–17.

Wang, G. K., Russell, C., & Wang, S.-Y. (2004). State-dependent block of voltage-gated Na$^+$ channels by amitriptyline via the local anesthetic receptor and its implication for neuropathic pain. *Pain, 110*, 166–174.

Wang, S.-J., Fuh, J.-L., Lu, S.-R., & Juang, K.-D. (2001). Quality of life differs among headache diagnoses: Analysis of SF-36 survey in 901 headache patients. *Pain, 89*, 285–292.

Wang, S-J., Fuh, J.-L., Lu, S.-R., & Juang, K.-D. (2006). Chronic daily headache in adolescents: Prevalence, impact, and medication overuse. *Neurology, 66*, 193–197.

Wang, S.-J., Fuh, J.-L., Lu, S.-R., Liu, C.-Y., Hsu, L.-C., Wang, P.-N., & Liu, H.-C. (2000). Chronic daily headache in Chinese elderly. *Neurology, 54*, 314–319.

Wang, S.-J., Silberstein, S. D., Patterson, S., & Young, W. B. (1998). Idiopathic intracranial hypertension without papilledema: A case-control study in a headache center. *Neurology, 51*, 245–249.

Wang, W., Timsit-Berthier, M., & Schoenen, J. (1996). Intensity dependence of auditory evoked potentials is pronounced in migraine: An indication of cortical potentiation and low serotonergic neurotransmission? *Neurology, 46,* 1404–1409.

Wang, W., Wang, Y.-H., Fu, X.-M., Sun, Z.-M., & Schoenen, J. (1999). Auditory evoked potentials and multiple personality measures in migraine and post-traumatic headaches. *Pain, 79,* 235–242.

Wantke, F., Gotz, M., & Jarisch, R. (1994). The red wine provocation test: Intolerance to histamine as a model for food intolerance. *Allergy Proceedings, 15,* 27–32.

Ward, N., Whitney, C., Avery, D., et al. (1991). The analgesic effects of caffeine in headache. *Pain, 44,* 151–155.

Wardlaw, S. L., Wehrenberg, W. B., Ferin, M., Antunes, J. L., & Frantz, A. G. (1982). Effects of sex steroids on β-endorphin in hypophyseal portal blood. *Journal of Clinical Endocrinology and Metabolism, 55,* 877–881.

Ware, J. E., Jr., Bjorner, J. B., & Kosinski, M. (2000). Practical implications of item response theory and computerized adaptive testing. *Medical Care, 38*(Suppl. II), II-73–II-82.

Ware, J. E., & Sherbourne, C. D. (1992). The MOS 36-item short-form health survey (SF-36): I. Conceptual framework and item selection. *Medical Care, 30,* 473–483.

Ware, J. E., Sherbourne, C. D., & Davies, A. R. (1992). Developing and testing the MOS 20-item short-form health survey: A general population application. In: A. L. Stewart & J. E. Ware (Eds.), *Measuring functioning and well-being: The Medical Outcomes Study approach* (pp. 277–290). Durham, NC: Duke University Press.

Warner, J. S., & Fenichel, G. M. (1996). Chronic post-traumatic headache often a myth? *Neurology, 46,* 915–916.

Watanabe, H., Kuwabara, T., Ohkubo, M., Tsuji, S., & Yuasa, T. (1996). Elevation of cerebral lactate detected by localized ¹H-magnetic resonance spectroscopy in migraine during the interictal period. *Neurology, 47,* 1093–1095.

Watanabe, Y., Saito, H., & Abe, K. (1993). Tricyclic antidepressants block NMDA receptor-mediated synaptic responses and induction of long-term potentiation in rat hippocampal slices. *Neuropharmacology, 32,* 479–486.

Waterink, W., & Van Boxtel, A. (1994). Facial and jaw-elevator EMG activity in relation to changes in performance level during a sustained information processing task. *Biological Psychology, 37,* 183–198.

Watkins, L. R., & Maier, S. F. (2000). The pain of being sick: Implications of immune-to-brain communication for understanding pain. *Annual Review of Psychology, 51,* 29–57.

Watson, D., & Clark, L. A. (1984). Negative affectivity: The disposition to experience aversive emotional states. *Psychological Bulletin, 96,* 465–490.

Watson, D., & Pennebaker, J. W. (1989). Health complaints, stress, and distress: Exploring the role of negative affectivity. *Psychological Review, 96,* 234–254.

Watson, J. F. (1887). *Annals of Philadelphia and Pennsylvania in the olden time.* Philadelphia: Edwin S. Stuart.

Wauquier, A., McGrady, A., Aloe, L, Klausner, T., & Collins, B. (1995). Changes in cerebral blood flow velocity associated with biofeedback-assisted relaxation treatment of migraine headaches are specific for the middle cerebral artery. *Headache, 35,* 358–362.

Waxman, S. G. (1999). The molecular basis for electrogenic computation in the brain: You can't step in the same river twice. *Molecular Psychiatry, 4,* 222–228.

Waxman, S. G., Kocsis, J. D., & Black, J. A. (1994). Type III sodium channel mRNA is expressed in embryonic but not adult spinal sensory neurons, and is re-expressed following axotomy. *Journal of Neurophysiology, 72,* 466–471.

Waxman, S. G., Cummins, T. R., Dib-Hajj, S. D., & Black, J. A. (2000). Voltage-gated sodium channels and the molecular pathogenesis of pain: A review. *Journal of Rehabilitation Research and Development, 37,* 517–528.

Weaver, M. T., & McGrady, A. (1995). A provisional model to predict blood pressure response to biofeedback-assisted relaxation. *Biofeedback and Self-Regulation, 20,* 229–240.

Weber, E. H. (1996). De tactu. In H. E. Ross & D. J. Murray (Ed. & Trans.), *E. H. Weber on the tactile senses* (2nd ed.). East Sussex, U.K: Erlbaum (UK) Taylor & Francis. (Original work published 1834).

Wehrenberg, W. B., Wardlaw, S. L., Frantz, A. G., & Ferin, M. (1982). Beta-endorphin in hypophyseal portal blood: Variations throughout the menstrual cycle. *Endocrinology, 111,* 879–881.

Weiller, C., May, A., Limmroth, V., Jüptner, M., Kaube, H., v. Schayck, R., Coenen, H. H., & Diener, H. C. (1995). Brain stem activation in spontaneous human migraine attacks. *Nature Medicine, 1,* 658–660.

Weinberger, D. A., & Davidson, M. N. (1994). Styles of inhibiting emotional expression: Distinguishing repressive coping from impression management. *Journal of Personality, 62,* 587–613.

Weisenberg, M., Aviram, O., Wolf, Y., & Raphaeli, N. (1984). Relevant and irrelevant anxiety in the reaction to pain. *Pain, 20,* 371–383.

Weiss, T., Miltner, W. H., & Dillmann, J. (2003). The influence of semantic priming on event-related potentials to painful laser-heat stimuli in migraine patients. *Neuroscience Letters, 340,* 135–138.

Weiss, T., Miltner, W. H., Liepert, J., Meissner, W., & Taub, E. (2004). Rapid functional plasticity in the primary somatomotor cortex and perceptual changes after nerve block. *European Journal of Neuroscience, 20,* 3413–3423.

Welch, K. M. A. (1993). Drug therapy of migraine. *New England Journal of Medicine, 329,* 1476–1483.

Welch, K. M. A. (1997). Pathogenesis of migraine. *Seminars in Neurology, 17,* 335–341.

Welch, K. M. A., Nagesh, V., Aurora, S. K., & Gelman, N. (2001). Periaqueductal gray matter dysfunction in migraine: Cause or the burden of illness? *Headache, 41,* 629–637.

Welch, K. M. A., & Ramadan, N. M. (1995). Mitochondria, magnesium and migraine. *Journal of the Neurological Sciences, 134,* 9–14.

Wernicke, J. F., Lu, Y., D'Souza, N., Waninger, A., & Tran, P. V. (2004). Duloxetine at doses of 60 mg QD and 60 mg BID is effective in treatment of diabetic neuropathic pain (DNP). *Neurology, 62*(Suppl. 5). Abstract P03.001.

Westgaard, R. H. (1996). Effects of psychological demand and stress on neuromuscular function. In S. D. Moon & S. L. Sauter (Eds.), *Psychosocial aspects of musculoskeletal disorders in office work* (pp. 75–89). London: Taylor and Francis.

Westgaard, R. H. (1999a). Effects of physical and mental stressors on muscle pain. *Scandinavian Journal of Work, Environment, and Health, 25*(Suppl. 4), 19–24.

Westgaard, R. H. (1999b). Muscle activity as a releasing factor for pain in the shoulder and neck. *Cephalalgia, 19*(Suppl. 25), 1–8.

Westgaard, R. H., & De Luca, C. J. (1997). Motor unit substitution during sustained contractions: Implications for ergonomics. In P. Seppälä, T. Luopajärvi, C.-H. Nygård, & M. Mattila (Eds.), *Proceedings of the 13th IEA congress* (Vol. 4, *Musculoskeletal disorders, rehabilitation*, pp. 237–239). Helsinki: Finnish Institute of Occupational Health.

Wheless, J. W., Castillo, E., Maggio, V., Kim, H. L., Breier, J. I., Simos, P. G., & Papanicolaou, A. C. (2004). Magnetoencephalography (MEG) and magnetic source imaging (MSI). *The Neurologist, 10,* 138–153.

White, A., Handler, P., & Smith, E. L. (1973). *Principles of biochemistry* (5th ed.). New York: McGraw-Hill.

White, W. B., Kent, J., Taylor, A., Verburg, K. M., Lefkowith, J. B., & Whelton, A. (2002). Effects of celecoxib on ambulatory blood pressure in hypertensive patients on ACE inhibitors. *Hypertension, 39,* 929–934.

Whiteside, G. T., & Munglani, R. (2001). Cell death in the superficial dorsal horn in a model of neuropathic pain. *Journal of Neuroscience Research, 64,* 168–173.

Whiteside, M. (1990). With tender loving care. *Cephalalgia, 10,* 107–110.

Widmer, C. G. (1991). Introduction III. Chronic muscle pain syndromes: An overview. *Canadian Journal of Physiology and Pharmacology, 69,* 659–661.

Wiertelak, E. P., Smith, K. P., Furness, L., Mooney-Heiberger, K., Mayr, T., Maier, S. F., & Watkins, L. R. (1994). Acute and conditioned hyperalgesic responses to illness. *Pain, 56,* 227–234.

Wilcox, G. L. (1991). Excitatory neurotransmitters and pain. In M. R. Bond, J. E. Charlton & C. J. Woolf (Eds.), *Pain research and clinical management* (Vol. 4, *Proceedings of the VIth World Congress on Pain*, pp. 97–117). New York: Elsevier.

Wilder-Smith, O. H. (2000). Changes in sensory processing after surgical nociception. *Current Review of Pain, 4*(3), 234–241.

Wilentz, J. (1996, March/April). The birth of the pain archive [Science writer's corner]. *APS Bulletin, 6*(2).

Wilkins, A. J. (1991). A tint to reduce eye-strain from fluorescent lighting? Preliminary observations. *Ophthalmology and Physiological Optics, 11,* 172–175.

Wilkins, A. J., Patel, R., Adjamian, P., & Evans, B. J. W. (2002). Tinted spectacles and visually sensitive migraine. *Cephalalgia, 22,* 711–719.

Wilkinson, F., & Crotogino, J. (2000). Orientation discrimination thresholds in migraine: A measure of visual cortical inhibition. *Cephalalgia, 20,* 57–66.

Wilkinson, S. M., Becker, W. J., & Heine, J. A. (2001). Opiate use to control bowel motility may induce chronic daily headache in patients with migraine. *Headache, 41,* 303–309.

Willems, E. W., Valdivia, L. F., Saxena, P. R., & Villalón, C. M. (2001). Pharmacological profile of the mechanisms involved in the external carotid vascular effects of the antimigraine agent isometheptene in anaesthetised dogs. *Naunyn Schmiedeberg's Archives of Pharmacology, 364,* 27–32.

Willer, J. C. (1985). Studies on pain. Effects of morphine on a spinal nociceptive flexion reflex and related pain sensation in man. *Brain Research, 331,* 105–114.

Willer, J. C., Boureau, F., & Albe-Fessard, D. (1979). Supraspinal influences on nociceptive flexion reflex and pain sensation in man. *Brain Research, 179,* 61–68.

Willer, J. C., Dehen, H., & Cambier, J. (1981). Stress-induced analgesia in humans: Endogenous opioids and naloxone-reversible depression of pain reflexes. *Science, 212,* 689–691.

Willer, J. C., & Ernst, M. (1986). Somatovegetative changes in stress-induced analgesia in man: An electrophysiological and pharmacological study. *Annals of the New York Academy of Sciences, 467,* 256–272.

Williams, D. E., Raczynski, J. M., Domino, J., & Davis, J. P. (1993). Psychophysiological and MMPI personality assessment of headaches: An integrative approach. *Headache, 33,* 149–154.

Williams, P., Dowson, A. J., Rapoport, A. M., & Sawyer, J. (2001). The cost effectiveness of stratified care in the management of migraine. *Pharmacoeconomics, 19,* 819–829.

Williamson, D. A., Epstein, L. H., & Lombardo, T. W. (1980). EMG measurement as a function of electrode placement and level of EMG. *Psychophysiology, 17,* 279–282.

Williamson, D. E., Birmaher, B., Ryan, N. D., Shiffrin, T. P., Lusky, J. A., Protopapa, J., et al. (2003). The Stressful Life Events Schedule for children and adolescents: Development and validation. *Psychiatry Research, 119,* 225–241.

Wilmshurst, P. T., Nightingale, S., Walsh, K. P., & Morrison, W. L. (2000). Effect on migraine of closure of cardiac right-to-left shunts to prevent recurrence of decompression illness or stroke or for haemodynamic reasons. *Lancet, 356,* 1648–1651.

Wiltse, L. L., & Rocchio, P. D. (1975). Preoperative psychological tests as predictors of success of chemonucleolysis in the treatment of the low-back syndrome. *Journal of Bone and Joint Surgery (American Volume), 57A,* 478–483.

Wind, J., & Punt, J. (1989). Migraine prophylaxis with low-dose aspirin: A promising new approach. In F. C. Rose (Ed.), *New advances in headache research* (pp. 265–267). London: Smith-Gordon.

Winter, J. E. (1912). The sensation of movement. *Psychological Review, 19,* 374–385.

Wittrock, D. A. (1997). The comparison of individuals with tension-type headache and headache-free controls on frontal EMG levels: A meta-analysis. *Headache, 37,* 424–432.

Woakes, E. (1868). On ergot of rye in the treatment of neuralgia. *British Medical Journal,* II, 360–361.

Wöber-Bingöl, C., Wöber, C., Karwautz, A., Schnider, P., Vesely, C., Wagner-Ennsgraber, C., Zebenholzer, K., & Wessely, P. (1996). Tension-type headache in different age groups at two headache centers. *Pain, 67,* 53–58.

Wolfe, F., Smythe, H. A., Yunus, M. B., Bennett, R. M., Bombardier, C., Goldenberg, D. L., et al. (1990). The American College of Rheumatology 1990 criteria for the classification of fibromyalgia. Report of the Multicenter Criteria Committee. *Arthritis and Rheumatism, 33,* 160–172.

Wolff, H. G. (1963). *Headache and other head pain.* New York: Oxford University Press.

Wolpe, J., & Lazarus, A. A. (1966). *Behavior therapy techniques.* New York: Pergamon Press.

Wood, J. N., Boorman, J. P., Okuse, K., & Baker, M. D. (2004). Voltage-gated sodium channels and pain pathways. *Journal of Neurobiology, 61,* 55–71.

Woodruff, P. G., & Fahy, J. V. (2001). Asthma: Prevalence, pathogenesis, and prospects for novel therapies. *JAMA, 286,* 395–398.

Woolf, C. J. (1991). Central mechanisms of acute pain. In M. R. Bond, J. E. Charlton & C. J. Woolf (Eds.), *Pain research and clinical management* (Vol. 4, *Proceedings of the VIth World Congress on Pain,* pp. 25–34). New York: Elsevier.

Woolf, C. J. (1996). Windup and central sensitization are not equivalent [editorial]. *Pain, 66,* 105–108.

Woolf, C. J., & Salter, M. W. (2000). Neuronal plasticity: Increasing the gain in pain. *Science, 288,* 1765–1768.

Workman, E. A., Tellian, F., & Short, D. (1992). Trazodone induction of migraine headache through mCPP. *American Journal of Psychiatry, 149,* 712–713.

Wray, S. H., Mijovic-Prelec, D., & Kosslyn, S. M. (1995). Visual processing in migraineurs. *Brain, 118* (Pt. 1), 25–35.

Wright, A. J. (1996, Feb.). From the history of anesthesia: Early electroanalgesia. *Educational Synopses in Anesthesiology and Critical Care, 3* (2).

Wu, G., & Morris, S. M. (1998). Arginine metabolism: Nitric oxide and beyond. *Biochemistry Journal, 336,* 1–17.

Wyllie, W. G., & Schlesinger, B. (1933). The periodic group of disorders in childhood. *British Journal of Childhood Diseases, 30*, 1–24.

Xing, J.-L., Hu, S.-J., Jian, Z., & Duan, J.-H. (2003). Subthreshold membrane potential oscillation mediates the excitatory effect of norepinephrine in chronically compressed dorsal root ganglion neurons in the rat. *Pain, 105*, 177–183.

Yale, S. H., & Glurich, I. (2005). Analysis of the inhibitory potential of *Ginkgo biloba, Echinacea purpurea*, and *Serenoa repens* on the metabolic activity of cytochrome P450 3A4, 2D6, and 2C9. *Journal of Alternative and Complementary Medicine*, 11, 433–439.

Yamaguchi, M. (1992). Incidence of headache and severity of head injury. *Headache, 32*, 427–431.

Yamamoto, M., & Meyer, J. S. (1980). Hemicranial disorder of vasomotor adrenoceptors in migraine and cluster headache. *Headache, 20*, 321–335.

Yanamoto, H., Hashimoto, N., Nagata, I., & Kikuchi, H. (1998). Infarct tolerance against temporary focal ischemia following spreading depression in rat brain. *Brain Research, 784*, 239–249.

Yang, T. T., Gallen, C., Schwartz, B., Bloom, F. E., Ramachandran, V. S., & Cobb, S. (1994). Sensory maps in the human brain. *Nature, 368*, 592–593.

Yang, W. H., Drouin, M. A., Herbert, M., Mao, Y., & Karsh, J. (1997). The monosodium glutamate symptom complex: Assessment in a double-blind, placebo-controlled, randomized study. *Journal of Allergy and Clinical Immunology, 99*, 757–762.

Yarnitsky, D., Goor-Aryeh, I., Bajwa, Z. H., Ransil, B. I., Cutrer, F. M., Sottile, A., & Burstein, R. (2003). 2003 Wolff Award: Possible parasympathetic contributions to peripheral and central sensitization during migraine. *Headache, 43*, 704–714.

Yarnitsky, D., Kunin, M., Brik, R., & Sprecher, E. (1997). Vibration reduces thermal pain in adjacent dermatomes. *Pain, 69*, 75–77.

Young, W. B., Hopkins, M. M., Shechter, A. L., & Silberstein, S. D. (2002). Topiramate: A case series study in migraine prophylaxis. *Cephalalgia, 22*, 659–663.

Young, W. B., Oshinsky, M. L., Shechter, A. L., Gebeline-Myers, C., Bradley, K. C., & Wassermann, E. M. (2004). Consecutive transcranial magnetic stimulation: Phosphene thresholds in migraineurs and controls. *Headache, 44*, 131–135.

Yu, X. M., & Mense, S. (1990). Response properties and descending control of rat dorsal horn neurons with deep receptive fields. *Neuroscience, 39*, 823–831.

Zachariae, R., & Bjerring, P. (1994). Laser-induced pain-related brain potentials and sensory pain ratings in high and low hypnotizable subjects during hypnotic suggestions of relaxation, dissociated imagery, focused analgesia, and placebo. *International Journal of Clinical and Experimental Hypnosis, 42*, 56–80.

Zakrzewska, J. M. (1999). Trigeminal, eye and ear pain. In P. D. Wall & R. Melzack (Eds.), *Textbook of pain* (4th ed., pp. 739–759). New York: Churchill Livingstone.

Zakrzewska, J. M. (2001). Cluster headache: Review of the literature. *British Journal of Oral and Maxillofacial Surgery, 39*, 103–113.

Zakrzewska, J. M. (2002). Diagnosis and differential diagnosis of trigeminal neuralgia. *Clinical Journal of Pain, 18*, 14–21.

Zambreanu, L., Wise, R. G., Brooks, J. C. W., Iannetti, G. D., & Tracey, I. (2005). A role for the brainstem in central sensitisation in humans. Evidence from functional magnetic resonance imaging. *Pain, 114*, 397–407.

Zecca, L., Youdim, M. B. H., Riederer, P., Connor, J. R., & Crichton, R. R. (2004). Iron, brain ageing and neurodegenerative disorders. *Nature Reviews. Neuroscience, 5*, 863–873.

Zeeberg, I., Orholm, M., Nielsen, J. D., Honore, P. F., & Larsen, J. J. V. (1981). Femoxetine in the prophylaxis of migraine—a randomized comparison with placebo. *Acta Neurologica Scandinavica, 64*, 452–459.

Zelman, D. C., Howland, E. W., Nichols, S. N., & Cleeland, C. S. (1991). The effects of induced mood on laboratory pain. *Pain, 46*, 105–111.

Zhuo, M., & Gebhart, G. F. (1997). Biphasic modulation of spinal nociceptive transmission from the medullary raphe nuclei in the rat. *Journal of Neurophysiology, 78*, 746–758.

Ziad, E. K., Rahi, A. C., Hamdan, S. A., & Mikati, M. A. (2005). Age, dose, and environmental temperature are risk factors for topiramate-related hyperthermia. *Neurology, 65*, 1139–1140.

Ziegler, D. K., Hurwitz, A., Hassanein, R. S., Kodanaz, H. A., Preskorn, S. H., & Mason, J. (1987). Migraine prophylaxis: A comparison of propranolol and amitriptyline. *Archives of Neurology, 44*, 486–489.

Ziegler, M. G. (1989). Catecholamine measurement in behavioral research. In N. Schneiderman, S. M. Weiss, & P. Kaufmann (Eds.), *Handbook of research methods in cardiovascular behavioral medicine* (pp. 167–183). New York: Plenum Press.

Zigelman, M., Kuritzky, A., Appel, S., Davidovitch, S., Zahavi, I., Hering, R., & Akselrod, S. (1992). Propranolol in the prophylaxis of migraine—evaluation by spectral analysis of beat-to-beat heart rate fluctuations. *Headache, 32*, 169–174.

Zornberg, A. G. (1995). *The beginning of desire: Reflections on Genesis.* New York: Doubleday.

Zwart, J.-A., Dyb, G., Hagen, K., Svebak, S., & Holmen, J. (2003). Analgesic use: A predictor of chronic pain and medication overuse headache. The Head-HUNT study. *Neurology, 61*, 160–164.

Zwart, J.-A., Dyb, G., Hagen, K., Svebak, S., Stovner, L. J., & Holmen, J. (2004). Analgesic overuse among subjects with headache, neck and low-back pain. The Head-HUNT Study. *Neurology, 62*, 1540–1544.

Zwarts, M. J., Drost, G., & Stegeman, D. F. (2000). Recent progress in the diagnostic use of surface EMG for neurological diseases. *Journal of Electromyography and Kinesiology, 10*, 287–291.

Credits

I would like to gratefully acknowledge the following sources:

Book epigraph is reprinted from *Garrison's history of neurology* by I. C. McHenry, 1969, Springfield, IL: Charles C. Thomas. Copyright 1969 Charles C. Thomas. Reprinted with permission.

Epigraph to Chapter 1 is reprinted from *Dr. Faustus* by Thomas Mann (Translated by H. T. Lowe-Porter), 1948, p. 342, NY: A.A. Knopf. Copyright by Random House. Reprinted with permission.

Epigraph to Chapter 2 is reprinted from "De la notion de temps dan l'évolution des processes pathologiques" by R. Leriche, *Press Médicale*, 1951, vol. 59, p. 1281. Copyright Masson, Paris. Reprinted with permission.

Epigraph to Chapter 3 is reprinted from *Studies on hysteria* by J. Breuer and S. Freud (J. Strachey, Trans.), 1893–1895/1957, p. 190, NY: Basic Books. Copyright Basic Books/Perseus Group. Reprinted with permission.

Epigraph to Chapter 6 is reprinted from *The challenge of pain* (updated, 2nd ed.) by R. Melzack and P. D. Wall, 1996, p. 189, NY: Penguin Books. Copyright R. Melzack and P. D. Wall. Reprinted with permission.

Epigraph to Chapter 7 is reprinted from *A treatise on the Canon of Medicine of Avicenna, incorporating a translation of the first book*, by O. C. Gruner, 1930, London: Luzac & Co. Copyright AMS Press. Reprinted with permission.

Epigraph to Chapter 10 is excerpted from "In Bed" by Joan Didion, *The White Album*, 1979, p. 172. Copyright 1979 by Joan Didion. Reprinted by permission of the author.

Epigraph to Chapter 15 is reprinted from *A treatise on the Canon of Medicine of Avicenna, incorporating a translation of the first book*, by O. C. Gruner, 1930, London: Luzac & Co. Copyright AMS Press. Reprinted with permission.

List of parafunctional oral behaviors (p. 297) is adapted from "Oral behavioral patterns in facial pain, headache and non-headache populations" by R. A. Moss, M. H. Ruff, and E. T. Sturgis, *Behaviour Research and Therapy*, 1984, vol. 22, p. 684. Copyright 1984 by Elsevier. Used with permission.

Author Index

Subject Index